Analysis of Human Genomics

Edited by Bryan Evans

hayle medical
New York

Hayle Medical,
750 Third Avenue, 9th Floor,
New York, NY 10017, USA

Visit us on the World Wide Web at:
www.haylemedical.com

ISBN: 978-1-63241-798-5

Printed in China.

Cataloging-in-Publication Data

Analysis of human genomics / edited by Bryan Evans.
p. cm.
Includes bibliographical references and index.
ISBN 978-1-63241-798-5
1. Human genome. 2. Genomics. 3. Human genetics. I. Evans, Bryan.

QH431 .A53 2019
611.018 166--dc23

Table of Contents

Preface

Genes are the determiners of human-inherited traits. The study of the human genome provides a way to understand diseases. Genetic tests can be performed to evaluate genetic conditions, such as Down syndrome, muscular dystrophy, Tay-Sachs disease, phenylketonuria, etc. The field of clinicogenomics is widely being used for personalized medicine such as oncogenomics and pharmacogenomics. It studies the entire human genome, thus allowing the detection of a wide number of mutations and structural anomalies. The future of human genomics holds immense potential as individuals may be sequenced at birth and also periodically throughout their lives to detect potential health risks. Thus, individuals will be able to change their lifestyles and behavior to minimize their predisposition to diseases. This book provides comprehensive insights into the field of human genomics. It elucidates new techniques and the applications of human genomics in a multidisciplinary manner. It aims to equip students and experts with the advanced topics and upcoming concepts in this area.

The researches compiled throughout the book are authentic and of high quality, combining several disciplines and from very diverse regions from around the world. Drawing on the contributions of many researchers from diverse countries, the book's objective is to provide the readers with the latest achievements in the area of research. This book will surely be a source of knowledge to all interested and researching the field.

In the end, I would like to express my deep sense of gratitude to all the authors for meeting the set deadlines in completing and submitting their research chapters. I would also like to thank the publisher for the support offered to us throughout the course of the book. Finally, I extend my sincere thanks to my family for being a constant source of inspiration and encouragement.

Editor

1

Nonparametric approaches for population structure analysis

Luluah Alhusain* and Alaaeldin M. Hafez

Abstract

The analysis of population structure has many applications in medical and population genetic research. Such analysis is used to provide clear insight into the underlying genetic population substructure and is a crucial prerequisite for any analysis of genetic data. The analysis involves grouping individuals into subpopulations based on shared genetic variations. The most widely used markers to study the variation of DNA sequences between populations are single nucleotide polymorphisms. Data preprocessing is a necessary step to assess the quality of the data and to determine which markers or individuals can reasonably be included in the analysis. After preprocessing, several methods can be utilized to uncover population substructure, which can be categorized into two broad approaches: parametric and nonparametric. Parametric approaches use statistical models to infer population structure and assign individuals into subpopulations. However, these approaches suffer from many drawbacks that make them impractical for large datasets. In contrast, nonparametric approaches do not suffer from these drawbacks, making them more viable than parametric approaches for analyzing large datasets. Consequently, nonparametric approaches are increasingly used to reveal population substructure. Thus, this paper reviews and discusses the nonparametric approaches that are available for population structure analysis along with some implications to resolve challenges.

Keywords: Population structure analysis, Clustering, Dimension reduction, Principal component analysis, Allele-sharing distance, Genetic data, Single nucleotide polymorphism, Population genetics

Background

Population structure analysis is a major area of interest within the field of genetics and bioinformatics. Population structure is the grouping of individuals into subpopulations based on observable characteristics, such as culture, language, geographical region, and physical appearance [1]. Since patterns of genetic variation exist among people, genetic research is concerned with characterizing the genetic variations of populations and summarizing the relationships between individuals from genetic data. Thus, the analysis of population structure involves the identification of shared genetic variations among individuals and, accordingly, the grouping of similar individuals into subpopulations.

The inference of population structure from genetic markers is very helpful in different applications, such as genome-wide association studies (GWAS) [2–8] and forensics [9]. In GWAS, case-control studies aim to scan a large portion of the genome to identify the responsible genes for different diseases via associations between a genetic marker and a disease. The presence of population structure might result in spurious associations between a marker and a disease, which occur when most of the samples in the case group are from a specific population. Subsequently, a marker appears significantly more frequently in the case than in the control group, so this marker is incorrectly considered to be associated with the disease. Consequently, inferring population structure is a prerequisite for association mapping studies to avoid making spurious correlations or missing genuine correlations, which would eventually reduce false positive rates. In forensics, identifying population substructure is a prerequisite for developing reference panels. Reference panels are composed of a set of genetic markers that can provide information on an individual's ancestry [10].

Populations are genetically structured into distinct subpopulations [11]. Thus, the main research question is how to assign n individuals using m genetic markers to K subpopulations. Therefore, research in population

* Correspondence: lalhusain@ksu.edu.sa
College of Computer and Information Sciences, King Saud University, Riyadh, Saudi Arabia

structure addresses the following problems: how to detect population structure, how to assign individuals to their corresponding subpopulation, how to determine the optimal number of subpopulations, how to reduce the number of genetic markers needed for inference of population structure, how to infer population structure at a fine scale, and finally, how to handle large genetic datasets [11–16].

Several methods can be utilized to uncover population substructure. In general, these methods can be categorized into two broad approaches: parametric and nonparametric. Parametric approaches use statistical models to infer population structure and assign individuals into subpopulations. However, these approaches suffer from many drawbacks that make them impractical for large datasets. Such drawbacks include an intensive computational cost, genetic assumptions that must be held, and sensitivity to sample size. In contrast, nonparametric approaches have the advantage of efficient computational cost and no modeling assumption requirements, making them more viable than parametric approaches for analyzing large datasets.

Advances in DNA sequencing technology have provided genome-wide single nucleotide polymorphisms (SNPs) that have enabled the study of genetic variation at an unprecedented resolution. Detailed characterization of genetic variations across all chromosomes is possible using thousands of markers spanning the entire genome. Consequently, nonparametric approaches are increasingly being used to reveal population structure because of their great advantage of efficiency in handling high-dimensional genetic datasets. Therefore, this paper reviews the literature on the topic of population structure analysis with an emphasis on nonparametric approaches. The purpose of this paper is to review the nonparametric methods available to infer population structure from genetic data. The paper comprises seven sections, including this background section. It begins by outlining the background information required to understand the genetic data used for the analysis, along with the data preprocessing. Then, an overview of the parametric and nonparametric approaches of population structure analysis is presented. Since nonparametric approaches are more viable than parametric approaches for analyzing large datasets, this paper is concentrated on the nonparametric approaches proposed to address the inference of population structure from genetic data. These approaches are categorized into dimension reduction-based methods and distance-based methods. Afterward, the paper discusses the literature on the selection of informative markers. Finally, the paper concludes with a comprehensive discussion of the literature. Figure 1 provides a general workflow for population structure analysis, where the input is the genetic dataset and the output is the population substructure as a set of subpopulations (i.e., clusters).

Genetic data

Data description

The most widely used markers to study the variation of DNA sequences are SNPs [17]. SNPs take the form of substitutions at a single base pair. An SNP occurs when a single nucleotide from a DNA sequence differs at the same position between individuals. Since SNPs arise in certain populations only, they are very useful to differentiate and analyze different populations. In practice, genotyping is an inexpensive process used to examine DNA samples to determine which alleles appear in particular loci. Therefore, genotyping produces a genotypic profile of an individual as an unordered set of alleles that appears at each locus. In this profile, the nucleotides are encoded as two alleles, allele (A) and allele (B). Therefore, three distinct genotypes can appear at a locus: wild-type homozygous (AA), homozygous (BB), and heterozygous (AB). Nevertheless, an SNP marker can be encoded as 0, 1, or 2 according to the number of reference alleles. Thus, it has the advantage of being handled as a numerical variable that represents the number of reference alleles.

Many datasets are available online to study population structure. These datasets consist of genotyped markers along with information about individuals, where the population label is the most required information for population structure analysis. The most well-known datasets are HapMap [18–20], 1000 Genomes Project [21], and Pan-Asian [22].

Data preprocessing

The preprocessing of genetic data is a necessary step to examine the quality of data and determine which markers or individuals can reasonably be included in the analysis [23]. First, the quality of the SNP markers is assessed, including the following:

- SNP call rate: SNP call rate is assessed to verify the amount of missing data for each marker. SNP call rate is the proportion of genotypes per marker with non-missing data. Usually, a threshold of 95% is used to remove these poorly genotyped SNPs. However, the threshold should be set carefully to avoid removing important markers.
- Hardy-Weinberg equilibrium (HWE): HWE [12] verifies the assumptions of Hardy-Weinberg. So, a statistical test is applied to determine whether a marker follows the Hardy-Weinberg equilibrium or not. If a marker deviates from the equilibrium, then

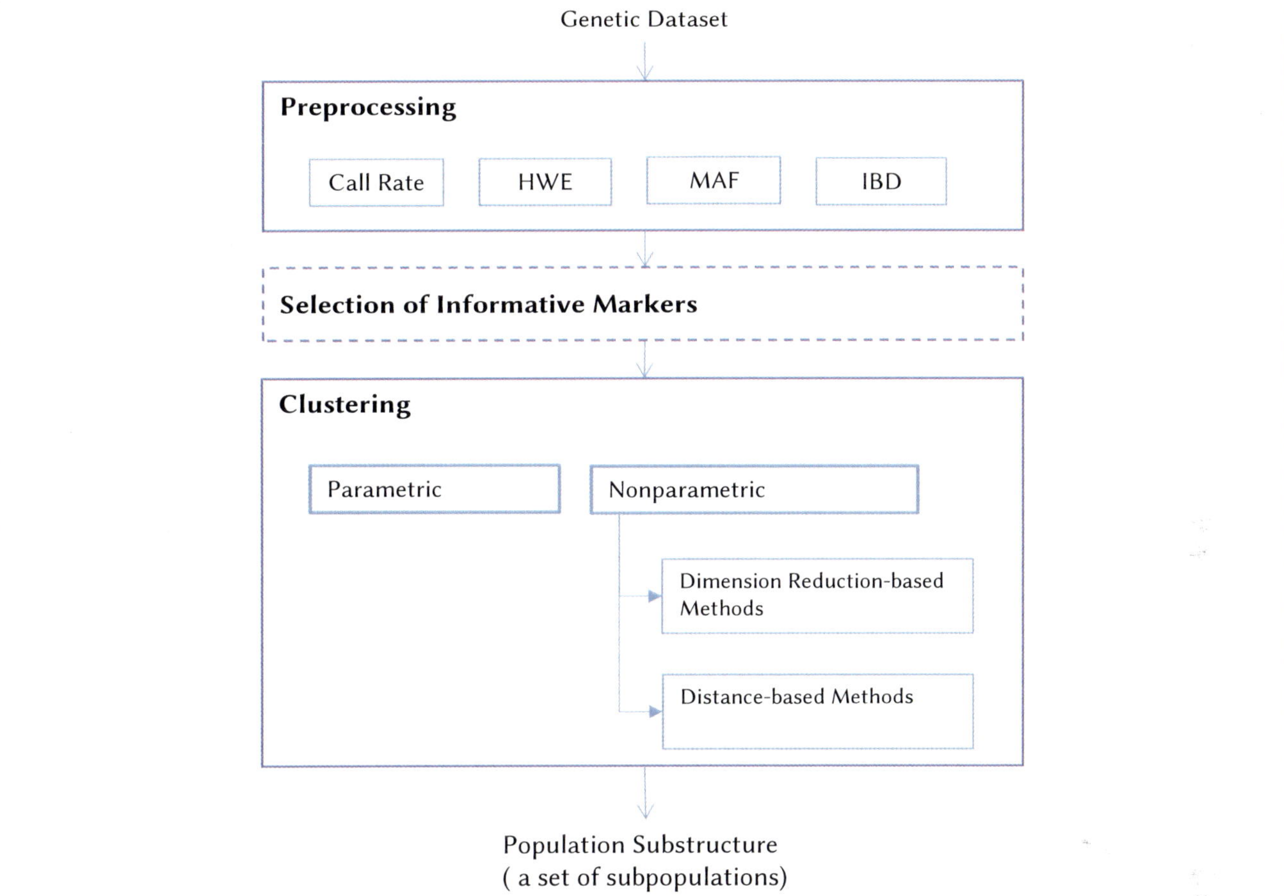

Fig. 1 A general workflow for population structure analysis

it may be because of genotyping errors; therefore, it should be excluded.

– Minor allele frequency (MAF): MAF denotes the frequency of a marker's less frequent allele in a given population. SNPs with low MAF should be excluded, and a threshold of 1–2% is typically applied.

For this assessment, PLINK [24] is typically used to prune SNPs with a minor allele frequency greater than 5%, a missing rate less than 5%, and a Hardy-Weinberg equilibrium (HWE) deviation p value of no less than 0.05.

Then, an assessment is performed to check the quality of the individuals, which includes the following:

- Individual call rate: Individual call rate refers to the proportion of genotypes per individual with non-missing data. The missingness rate should not exceed a certain threshold.
- Identity by descent (IBD): IBD [25] is calculated to assess which individuals are related. It indicates whether a pair of individuals has identical copies of the same ancestral allele. The proportion of shared alleles between a pair of individuals determines the relation between them, such as identical twins, first-degree relatives (i.e., full siblings, parent–offspring), second-degree relatives (i.e., half-siblings, uncle/aunt, nephew/niece), and third-degree relatives (i.e., cousins). Related individuals are excluded. In practice, relatedness can be assessed using kinship coefficients estimated by KING [26]. The KING command can be used to filter out related individuals, where a threshold of a degree relationship can be specified.

Parametric approaches

Parametric approaches use statistical models to infer population structure and assign individuals into subpopulations. These models are used to estimate population parameters, such as allele frequency, for the population and to calculate the likelihood that an individual belongs to a specific subpopulation [12, 27]. Parametric approaches are based on several genetic assumptions about the data, including the Hardy-Weinberg equilibrium

(HWE) [12] for populations and the linkage equilibrium (LE) [28] between loci within each population.

Essentially, a parametric approach infers ancestral proportions for each individual and then groups individuals who have similar patterns of inferred ancestry [16]. The majority of parametric methods for population structure analysis apply Bayesian inference. Bayesian inference is applied to model the probability of observed genotypes given the individual ancestry proportions and population allele frequencies. These methods simultaneously assign individuals to populations and identify populations from genotype data based on the estimation of the allele frequencies for each population [13, 29, 30].

STRUCTURE is a widely used parametric method that relies on Bayesian MCMC [12, 29]. In particular, Markov chain Monte Carlo (MCMC) based on Gibbs sampling is implemented to estimate the posterior distribution of allele frequency given the probability of ancestral populations of individuals and allele frequencies for all populations. Similar to STRUCTURE, PARTITION [31], BAPS/BAPS2 [32, 33], and GENELAND [34] take the same modeling approach, which is based on an MCMC algorithm, to sample the posterior distribution. Moreover, FRAPPE [35] and ADMIXTURE [30, 36] adopt the same modeling approach but rely on maximizing the likelihood using an expectation-maximization (EM) algorithm instead of sampling the posterior distribution. In contrast, L-POP [27] implements a maximum likelihood approach based on latent class analysis (LSA), whereas PSMIX [37] uses the same approach via the implementation of a mixture model. Recently, fast STRUCTURE [38] was developed to improve the inference model underlying STRUCTURE using a variational Bayesian method. Variational methods optimize the computation of posterior distributions and accelerate the inference process.

Parametric approaches estimate the observed allele frequency for each population using statistical inference models that include some parameters and are based on probability distribution. Before running these methods, parameters must be set, such as the number of populations *K*, the most critical parameter. Accordingly, a parametric approach suffers from many drawbacks: First and most importantly, the intensive computational cost makes it impractical for large-scale datasets containing thousands of individuals and thousands of markers [39–41]. Second, parametric approaches are developed on the basis of the genetic assumptions of the Hardy-Weinberg equilibrium (HWE) and the linkage equilibrium (LE) between loci within each population. As a result, they can be very misleading when data assumptions cannot be verified or are invalidated [35, 40]. In specific, LE does not hold when a vast amount of genetic data are used [42]. Third, parametric methods depend on an estimation of allele frequency that is sensitive to sample size. Consequently, allele frequency is subject to high variations when using small samples representing each subpopulation [29, 42]. Lastly, parametric methods are not applicable to analyzing large and highly structured population datasets because of the limited number of *K* clusters that can be inferred [16].

Nonparametric approaches

Nonparametric approaches have been proposed to address the problem of analyzing population structure from genetic data in order to overcome the drawbacks of parametric approaches. Nonparametric approaches group individuals with similar genetic profiles together [16]. In 2006, Liu and Zhao [40] proposed a two-stage nonparametric strategy for analyzing population structure from genetic data with the goal of facilitating the clustering process of the high-dimensional space of genotype data. The first stage involves reducing the dimensionality of the genotypic dataset using multivariate analysis methods, such as singular value decomposition (SVD) and principal component analysis (PCA). The second stage involves applying clustering algorithms to identify population substructure from the reduced data. Another nonparametric strategy is to calculate the pairwise distances between individuals and then perform clustering. Both strategies have the advantage of identifying a population structure and assigning individuals to their corresponding subpopulation. Indeed, both strategies provide a framework for population structure analysis from genetic data where different methods can fit into that framework.

Nonparametric approaches have many advantages, including an efficient computational cost and no modeling assumption requirements. Nonparametric approaches have a more efficient computational cost compared to parametric approaches, making the former more viable for analyzing large datasets [15]. Also, nonparametric approaches do not make any assumption on genetic data, which is a great advantage over parametric approaches [43]. Therefore, when a large amount of genotype data is available, nonparametric approaches are preferred, as there is no need to verify the assumptions of Hardy-Weinberg and the linkage equilibrium [44]. Moreover, since these approaches are not dependent on estimating allele frequencies, they are unaffected when the number of individuals representing a subpopulation is small [42].

There are many nonparametric methods. Some methods use a dimension reduction technique to reduce the dimensions of genetic markers before conducting a clustering. Other methods consider computing dis/similarity matrices of the data where a clustering technique is applied. Thus, nonparametric methods can be categorized into dimension reduction-based methods and distance-based methods.

Dimension reduction-based methods

Dimension reduction-based methods are based on mapping high-dimensional genetic data to low-dimensional space and then applying clustering on the reduced dimensions. Principal component analysis (PCA) is the most cited dimension reduction method used to detect population structure based on genetic data [45, 46]. Typically, PCA's scatterplots are used to visualize population structure, where the most genetically isolated subpopulations appear as distinct clusters of individuals. Most importantly, PCA can be used to infer spatial population genetic variations [47].

EIGENSTRAT\smartpca [39, 41] is the most used PCA-based tool for detecting population structure. In EIGENSTRAT\smartpca, eigenanalysis is used to detect population substructure, such that eigenvalues and eigenvectors capture the amount and axes of variation among individuals, respectively. Thus, the principal components (PCs), or eigenvectors, serve as the new reduced dimensions. Similar to EIGENSTRAT\smartpca, PLINK [24] and SNPRelate [48] can be used to apply PCA on genetic datasets.

Principal components analysis

Given $x = (x_{i,l})_{\substack{1 \le i \le n \\ 1 \le l \le p}}$ is an $n \times p$ matrix, where n is the number of individuals and p is the number of SNPs. Each entry $x_{i,\,l}$ corresponds to the genotype of individual i for the marker l, coded as 0, 1, or 2 according to the number of reference alleles present at the locus l.

To perform a principal components analysis (PCA) on the matrix x, the data are first centered and normalized. The column means μ_l and the observed allele frequency of each marker p_l are computed as follows:

$$\mu_l = \frac{\sum_{i=1}^{n} x_{il}}{n}$$

$$p_l = \frac{1 + \sum_{i=1}^{n} x_{il}}{2 + 2\,n}$$

The new genotype matrix $\tilde{x}$ is defined, such that each entry is:

$$\tilde{x}_{il} = \frac{x_{il} - \mu_l}{\sqrt{p_l(1-p_l)}}$$

Based on the $n \times n$ covariance matrix, a singular vector decomposition is computed as:

$$\frac{1}{p}\,\tilde{x}\,(\tilde{x}\,)^T$$

Then, a set of principal components $(PC_1, PC_2, \ldots, PC_{n-1})$ are generated [41, 49].

A major issue with PCA applied to genetic data is how to determine the number of significant principal components, which is the number of principal components needed to sufficiently describe a structure of the population [13]. The EIGENSTRAT algorithm applies a variant of eigenanalysis to determine the significant principal components based on Tracy-Widom (TW) theory [50]. TW theory states that the distribution of the largest eigenvalue approximately follows the TW distribution when the dimension of a matrix is suitably large [51]. Hence, the TW distribution is used to determine the probability of population substructure.

Principal components can be used as the axes of variations to provide a graphical overview of the population structure. This graphical representation of the individuals can highlight outlier individuals, or those which seem to lie farther out than the others. Also, the set of significant principal components can be used to cluster individuals into genetically homogeneous subpopulations. For instance, the Gaussian mixture model or *K*-means algorithm can be applied to these principal components [52].

Clustering based on principal components

Different clustering algorithms can be applied to the principal components. Since the principal components are normally distributed, they fit well with the Gaussian mixture model (GMM) clustering. Therefore, the PCAclust algorithm [52] was proposed as three steps. The first step involves applying PCA to the genetic data to compute the principal components (PCs). Then, a set of significant PCs is selected using the TW statistic at a 5% level. Finally, the selected PCs are clustered using the GMM algorithm to group the individuals into populations.

Moreover, Lee et al. [52] have proposed using PCA for dimension reduction with three clustering algorithms: *K*-means [53], the mixture model [54], and spectral clustering [55]. They used Gap statistics [56] and the Bayesian information criterion (BIC) [57] to predict the optimal number of clusters. In their experiment, they showed that all three algorithms have comparable results. However, the different clustering algorithms showed different degrees of sensitivity to noisy and non-informative markers, which demonstrated the importance of selecting a proper set of informative markers.

Furthermore, iterative pruning PCA (ipPCA) was proposed to resolve the highly structured population that appears as a conglomerate in PCA space. ipPCA does this by iteratively applying PCA to decompose the structure of the population. The ipPCA method has two versions, TW-ipPCA [11] and EigenDev-ipPCA, [16], which differ in their termination tests. Recently, HiClust-ipPCA [58] was proposed as a variation of EigenDev-ipPCA wherein hierarchical clustering is used.

The PCA-based ipPCA method [11] has been proposed to address the overlapping problem that appears in PCA space when analyzing closely related subpopulations. The ipPCA method can detect population structure at a fine scale by iteratively bisecting individuals based on a termination test that checks whether a significant structure is present. In ipPCA, PCA is applied, and then a termination test is verified to decide whether to advance to clustering or to stop. Clustering is performed based on significant PCs. The number of significant PCs depends on the number of individuals in the dataset, such that later iterations require fewer PCs for clustering than earlier iterations. Therefore, the new bisected datasets will have fewer individuals. ipPCA iterates until all individuals have been assigned to homogeneous subpopulations. At the end, the number of subpopulations K is determined by counting all the terminal nodes or subpopulations. ipPCA uses a fuzzy C-mean algorithm to split the dataset into two parts. Indeed, the iterative pruning nature of ipPCA offers a logical way to present the degree of relatedness between subpopulations.

ipPCA has two different versions: TW-ipPCA [11] and EigenDev-ipPCA [16]. TW-ipPCA applies the TW test as a termination criterion [41]. TW, as previously mentioned, is implemented in the EIGENSTRAT/smartpca algorithm for detecting whether a significant structure is present in the dataset. TW-ipPCA suffers from type 1 error when the sample size is large, and subsequently, a group of individuals belonging to a single subpopulation would be assigned into separate subpopulations.

EigenDev-ipPCA was proposed to address the spurious cluster problem using a heuristic called EigenDev as a termination criterion [16]. EigenDev is inspired by the Eigenvalue Grads heuristic [59], which is applied in the signal processing domain. The EigenDev statistic is based on the eigenvalues of the data matrix; it has no hidden parameters and is more robust to type 1 error. The application of EigenDev to ipPCA improves the accuracy of individuals' assignments and the estimation of the number of subpopulations, especially when using huge and complex datasets. EigenDev-ipPCA reveals subpopulations that are subclusters of subpopulations generated by TW-ipPCA.

HiClust-ipPCA [58] is another variation of ipPCA that employs hierarchical clustering instead of fuzzy C-mean within the ipPCA framework. In addition, a PCA-based feature selection is applied as a data preprocessing step. In each iteration, PCA is applied to select the most informative markers. Then, PCA is applied to the selected markers to map them to a reduced space. Next, a hierarchical clustering with Ward's minimum variance is applied to cluster data into two groups. This process is iterated until satisfying a termination condition. The experiments illustrate that hierarchical clustering provides better clustering results than fuzzy C-mean and that the use of the feature selection technique is effective for reducing data dimensions and increasing computational efficiency.

Other dimension reduction methods

There are many alternatives to PCA, such as singular value decomposition (SVD) [60]. Liu and Zhao [40] used SVD for dimension reduction and density-based mean clustering (DBMC) for clustering. SVD is used because it is efficient for a large matrix of markers and individuals. DBMC was proposed as a variant of K-means that can determine the number of clusters automatically, because K-means requires the number of clusters to be given. The similarity between individuals is measured using Cosine similarity. The performance of DBMC was compared with K-means and the mixture model [40], and it was found that the mixture model and DBMC performed better than K-means. Another alternative of PCA is multi-dimensional scaling (MDS), which uses a similarity matrix between the individuals instead of the data matrix to create axes of variation [61].

Table 1 describes the nonparametric dimension reduction-based methods in terms of dimension reduction and/or proximity measure, clustering technique, and the package/tool if it is available.

Distance-based methods

Distance-based methods are based on computing the pairwise similarities/distances between individuals. The allele-sharing distance (ASD) [44, 62] is a measure proposed for determining the genetic proximity between each pair of individuals. Distance-based methods usually apply a clustering on the ASD matrix to infer population structure. For instance, allele-sharing distance and Ward's minimum variance hierarchical clustering (AWclust) [42, 44] applies an agglomerative hierarchical clustering to ASD, while Spectral Hierarchical clustering for the Inference of Population Structure (SHIPS) [43] uses divisive clustering. Furthermore, NETVIEW [63] reveals the hierarchy of population substructures based on a representation of the genetic data as a network of individuals connected by edges representing the ASD between each pair. Iterative neighbor-joining tree clustering (iNJclust) [64] performs a graph-based clustering on a neighbor-joining (NJ) tree. Table 2 describes the distance-based methods in terms of the proximity measure, clustering technique, and available package/tool.

Allele-sharing distance

For clustering genetic data, allele-sharing distance (ASD) is used to identify closely related and distantly related

Table 1 Dimension reduction-based methods of population structure analysis

Reference	Dimension reduction	Distance matrix	Clustering	Tool/package
Patterson at el. (2006) [41]	PCA (TW)	–	–	EIGENSTRAT/smartpca [82]: Perl
Liu at el. (2006) [40]	SVD	Cosine similarity	Density-based mean clustering (DBMC)	–
Lee at el.(2009) [52]	PCA (TW)	–	Spectral clustering (*K*-means, mixture model)	–
Intarapanich at el. (2009) [11]	PCA (TW)	Euclidean distance	Fuzzy C-means	TW-ipPCA [83]: MATLAB
Limpiti at el.(2011) [16]	PCA (EigenDev)	Euclidean distance	Fuzzy C-means	EigenDev-ipPCA [83]: MATLAB
Amornbunchornvej at el. (2012) [58]	PCA	ASD	Ward's clustering	–

pairs of individuals. ASD is similar to identity by state (IBS) metric [25].

Given $x = (x_{i,l})_{\substack{1\le i\le n\\ 1\le l\le p}}$ is a $n \times p$ matrix where n is the number of individuals and p the number of SNPs. Each entry $x_{i,\ l}$ corresponds to the genotype of individual i for the marker l. Then, the ASD between individuals i and j at locus l, denoted as $D_l(i,j)$, is defined as follows:

$$D_l(i,j) = \begin{cases} 0 & \text{if same genotype} \\ 1 & \text{if one common allele} \\ 2 & \text{if no common allele} \end{cases}$$

Therefore, the total distance between individuals i and j can be calculated as:

$$D(i,j) = \frac{1}{p}\sum_{l=1}^{p}(D_l(i,j)) \qquad \text{for each } i \text{ and } j \in [1,n]$$

or as

$$D(i,j) = \frac{1}{p}\sum_{l=1}^{p}(|x_{i,l} - x_{j,l}|) \qquad \text{for each } i \text{ and } j \in [1,n]$$

where $x_{i,\ l}$, $x_{j,\ l}$ are the individuals' genotypes, coded as 0, 1, or 2 according to the number of reference alleles present at the locus l. The closer the pair of individuals are, genetically, the smaller the value of $D(i,j)$.

Using the function $D(i,j)$ to quantify the distance between each pair of individuals i and j, a distance matrix can be formed by combining the information for all pairs of individuals. The distance matrix, $= (D_{i,j})_{\substack{1\le i\le n\\ 1\le j\le n}}$, is a squared matrix of $n \times n$, where n is the number of individuals.

Based on ASD, a similarity measure can be inferred to measure the similarity between individuals i and j at locus l, denoted as $S_l(i,j)$, where:

$$S(i,j) = \frac{1}{p}\sum_{l=1}^{p}(2 - |x_{il} - x_{jl}|) \qquad \text{for each } i \text{ and } j \in [1,n]$$

Clustering based on ASD

Distance-based clustering methods use the ASD matrix as an input to group individuals into populations. AWclust, SHIPS, NETVIEW, and iNJclust all distance-based clustering methods, are summarized in Table 2.

AWclust [42, 44] is a distance-based population structure exploration method. The first step of AWclust is to construct the ASD matrix between all pairs of individuals in the sample. The second step is to apply hierarchical clustering to infer clusters of individuals from the ASD matrix using Ward's minimum variance algorithm [65, 66]. AWclust uses gap statistics [56] to select the optimal number of subpopulations K. The employment of gap statistics is computationally intensive as it involves an iterative statistical inference process [67]. To deal with the slow speed of calculating gap statistics, AWclust limits the number of inferred K to be 16 at maximum [67]. The execution of AWclust slows down dramatically when using a larger number of SNPs due to the increase in the size of the ASD matrix [67]. Deejai et al. [67] found that AWclust performs well only with a small number of SNP markers and in individuals with low diversity (i.e., the number of inferred subpopulations K is small), and thus, it is not suitable for

Table 2 Distance-based methods of population structure analysis

Reference	Clustering	Tool/package
Gao at el.(2007) [44]	Ward's minimum variance algorithm	AWclust [84]: R package
Bouaziz at el. (2012) [43]	Spectral clustering (GMM)	SHIPS [85]: R package
Neuditschko at el.(2012) [63]	Super paramagnetic clustering (SPC)	NETVIEW [86]: MATLAB
Limpiti at el. (2014) [64]	Neighbor-joining (NJ) tree-based clustering	iNJclust [87]: C++

performing large-scale population genetic analysis. The application of AWclust on HapMap project phase 1 [18] provided good results. It successfully differentiated the four ethnic populations in the dataset: African, European, Han Chinese, and Japanese individuals [44].

SHIPS [43, 68], or Spectral Hierarchical clustering for the Inference of Population Structure, is a distance-based method for inferring the structure of populations from genetic data. SHIPS applies a divisive strategy of hierarchical clustering followed by a pruning procedure to investigate population structure progressively. SHIPS constructs a binary tree to represent the substructure of a population using spectral clustering. Spectral clustering is applied to a pairwise distance matrix to divide a population into two subpopulations, and this is iterated for each of the two subpopulations. ASD is used within SHIPS; however, SHIPS can be used with any similarity matrix. SHIPS applies a pruning procedure along with gap statistics to determine the optimal number of subpopulations. A pruning procedure provides all possible clustering results. Thus, it allows a fast calculation of the gap statistics that requires all the clustering results of specified numbers of clusters. Moreover, because calculating gap statistics is time consuming, SHIPS applies a version of gap statistics that is less precise but has better experimental performance in estimating the optimal *K*. Experiments have involved applying SHIPS on two datasets: HapMap project phase 3 [19] and Pan-Asian [22]. These experiments have shown that SHIPS can accurately assign individuals to clusters with relatively low computational cost and estimate the number of clusters as well [43, 68]. In addition, SHIPS is quite robust such that several applications of SHIPS algorithm on the same dataset produce the same clustering result.

NETVIEW [63] is an analysis pipeline that combines a network-based clustering method with a visualization tool to infer fine-scale population structure. NETVIEW is composed of three key steps: distance matrix calculation, network construction and clustering, and network-based visualization. NETVIEW first calculates the ASD matrix that represents the relationships between all individuals in the dataset. Then, the ASD matrix is used to construct a population network using super paramagnetic clustering (SPC) [69]. In this network, nodes represent individuals, edges represent the relationship between a pair of individuals, and the thickness of edges represents the genetic distance. SPC is based on computing the *K*-nearest neighborhood to produce a cluster relationship matrix and a hierarchical tree of clusters. Specifically, SPC is implemented as Sorting Points Into Neighborhood (SPIN) [69, 70], which employs the Potts Hamiltonian model [71] to identify the number and size of clusters, known as cluster stability. The problem with SPC is how to specify the number of the nearest neighborhood an individual can have. Based on this number, NETVIEW produces clusters at optimal thresholds of genetic distance. The result of this algorithm provides a hierarchical clustering of individuals. However, NETVIEW uses a network-based visualization to present the population structure at a very fine scale, where highly interconnected individuals identify subpopulations. The empirical study in [63] involved applying NETVIEW on Human and Bovine HapMap datasets. The study demonstrated that NETVIEW could assign individuals to their corresponding subpopulations effectively and showed the genetic relatedness of individuals within their populations at a very fine scale.

iNJclust [64], or iterative Neighbor-Joining tree clustering, is an iterative application of graph-based clustering on a neighbor-joining (NJ) tree. The algorithm starts by computing the ASD matrix from the data. Then, an NJ tree is constructed based on the ASD matrix. Next, the algorithm performs a graph-based clustering to bisect the NJ tree into two subtrees. For each subtree, a new NJ tree is constructed based on the ASD matrix that contains only individuals within that subtree. The process of bisecting the NJ trees to create new subtrees is iterated until all subtrees become homogenous. The algorithm determines whether the cluster is homogeneous based on the fixation index. The fixation index (F_{ST}) is a measure of genetic population substructure used to examine the overall genetic divergence among subpopulations [72]. The construction of the NJ tree starts with all individuals as the leaf nodes. Then, the pair of nodes that are nearest to each other are merged. The merging process is repeated until all nodes are merged into the tree. The distance between nodes is measured using the minimum evolution criteria [73] based on the ASD. For NJ tree clustering, the NJ tree is split into two subtrees by cutting the edge between the two nodes with the longest length. iNJclust assigns the individuals into populations and estimates the optimal number of populations. The clustering result of iNJclust is a binary tree, where each leaf node represents a population of a set of individuals, and the tree structure represents the relationships between populations. The experimental results of applying iNJclust on real and simulated data have indicated that iNJclust yields a reasonable estimation of the number of populations, a robust assignment of individuals, and a meaningful representation of relationships among populations with the binary tree [64].

Selection of informative markers

Given that a large number of genetic markers can be used to infer population structure, reducing the number of markers is often desirable for efficient structure identification. In such settings, selecting ancestry informative markers (AIMs) aims to identify the minimum set of markers required to derive population structure and to reduce the genotyping cost. Selecting informative markers can be accomplished by using supervised or unsupervised methods. Supervised methods rely on prior knowledge of the ancestry of the individuals.

Informativeness for assignment (I_n) [74] is a supervised measure that computes mutual information based on allele frequencies and relies on self-reported ancestry information from individuals. In contrast, PCAIM [15] is an unsupervised algorithm proposed to identify a set of informative markers that captures the structure of a population. It does not demand prior information about the ancestry/origin of individuals. The PCAIM algorithm applies PCA to determine markers that are correlated with the significant principal components and then assigns a score to each marker. Then, the algorithm returns the top scoring markers that correlate well with the top few eigenvectors. The algorithm is efficient in selecting the informative markers. It is computationally fast and suitable for large datasets.

The performance of I_n and PCAIM in selecting informative markers has been evaluated in [15] and was found to attain comparable results; in addition, a considerable overlap was found between the selected markers. The overlapping was expected since PCAIM ranks markers based on how well they can reproduce the structure of the dataset, whereas I_n determines which markers are most likely to be associated with major clusters in the dataset. Therefore, PCAIM selects either the same markers or markers that are in high linkage disequilibrium (LD) with markers selected using the I_n measure.

The selection of informative markers could potentially suffer from redundant markers. Typically, redundancy exists due to the correlation among markers that are in the LD region. To select a minimal set of informative markers, a redundancy removal step should be applied after the initial markers selection step to avoid redundancy and determine the final set of AIMs.

In the literature, two different methods have been proposed to filter out redundant markers. The first method deals with the problem as a Column Subset Selection Problem, which is a well-known problem in linear algebra [75]. In [75], the algorithm Greedy QR [76, 77] is employed to select the minimally correlated subset of markers. The algorithm essentially works as an iterative process to pick up the uncorrelated markers. This algorithm has an implementation in MATLAB, and it can run efficiently in a shorter amount of time using thousands of markers. On the other hand, the redundancy removal problem can be resolved via the clustering technique. In particular, a clustering-based strategy was employed in [14] to minimize the number of markers to the most informative and uncorrelated ones, which was inspired by [78] in data analysis. In simpler terms, the strategy applies a clustering technique to cluster markers into K clusters and then returns one representative marker for each cluster. In [14], the Cluto toolkit [79] was used with default parameters for clustering using a cosine similarity matrix. The advantage of applying clustering to identify redundant markers is that it returns K lists of markers. Within each list, the markers are interchangeable, thus providing some flexibility in choosing any informative marker that falls into the same cluster. In contrast, the first method just returns one set of non-redundant markers. Although the two approaches of redundancy removal had comparable performance, clustering was slightly more accurate but was five times slower than the first method [14].

Discussion

Nonparametric approaches are increasingly being used to reveal population structure because of their great advantages of efficiency in handling high-dimensional genetic datasets [74]. Due to the high dimensionality of genetic data, it is imperative to reduce the dimensions of the data before clustering. In the literature of population structure analysis, PCA is employed as a dimension reduction technique for two purposes. The first purpose is feature extraction, where PCA is applied to transform the data to low-dimensional space where clustering will be performed. The second purpose is feature selection, where PCA is applied to select the informative genetic markers. To accomplish this, PCA is applied to a covariance matrix of genetic markers, and then the genetic markers that are well correlated with significant principal components are selected.

PCA is considered computationally efficient and performs well in detecting the genetic structure of populations. However, it is also argued that PCA not be efficient when used with correlated markers that naturally arise in any genetic data, especially in densely genotyped data. The problem is that a large number of redundant and correlated markers may mask the real structure of data. In practice, with large genotype data, there are linked markers due to linkage disequilibrium (LD) [28], which is considered dependent and redundant, and this may seriously distort the results of PCA. Moreover, dimension reduction methods, like PCA, consider the complete markers of the dataset to produce only one subspace, in which the clustering can then be performed. However, an issue would arise when the correlation between markers or the relevance of markers are significant for some clusters (i.e., populations) but not for complete datasets. Consequently, this issue can be resolved by subspace clustering. Subspace clustering computes multiple subspaces, where a different set of features is selected for each subspace. Then, individuals are clustered differently in each subspace according to the relevance of markers to describe those individuals. Subspace clustering may be a significant solution, inferring the population structure at a very fine scale.

Many distance-based methods have been developed to resolve the problem of clustering individuals into subpopulations. These methods have utilized different clustering techniques that required a matrix of pairwise distance/similarity between individuals. Allele-sharing distance (ASD) is widely used for this purpose. In [80], it is shown that the ASD between individuals from different subpopulations is always larger than that of individuals from the same subpopulations. Moreover, calculating the ASD for many SNP markers allows differentiation of the populations through the accumulated effect of SNP loci. However, distance assessment using ASD between individuals becomes increasingly meaningless as dimensionality increases. As with increasing the number of SNPs, the distances of the individual to its similar individuals and dissimilar individuals tend to be almost the same. Individuals appear almost alike because of correlated SNPs, which are considered "redundant," while ASD treats each marker independently. Therefore, the identification of correlated markers might improve the inference of population structure from high-dimensional genetic data. Filtering those markers before calculating ASD could contribute to more accurate clustering results, as achieved within HiClust-ipPCA [58].

The clustering techniques used to identify the population genetic substructure can be categorized into partitional clustering and hierarchical clustering. Partitional clustering produces a flat clustering which divides the data into a prespecified number of clusters *K* (e.g., K-means [81], DBMS [40], Lee's [52]). In contrast, hierarchical clustering produces a hierarchy of clusters (e.g., AWclust [44], SHIPS [43], NETVIEW [63], ipPCA [11, 16, 58], iNJclust [64]). Hierarchical clustering is preferable over partitional clustering in the context of population structure analysis. This is because it produces multiple nested partitions instead of one partition, which allows the choice of different partitions according to the desired level of similarity. Most importantly, a fine-scale population substructure can be obtained using hierarchical clustering because of the clustering's ability to capture data at different levels of granularity.

A major challenge in population structure analysis is the estimation of the optimal number of subpopulations (i.e., clusters). Gap statistics [56] have often been applied to determine the optimal number of clusters. However, gap statistics is computationally intensive and impractical for highly structured genetic datasets that comprise a large number of clusters. Some clustering methods can implicitly determine the optimal number of clusters—for instance, ipPCA [11, 16, 58], where the number of clusters is represented by the number of leaf nodes of the binary tree constructed by iterative applications of PCA. However, determining the number of populations as a single number is not practical and may have no biological meaning when there are hierarchical levels of population structure (i.e., subpopulations within populations). Furthermore, the researcher must be able to control the level of granularity to uncover the substructure of the population. Overall, these provide insights into the importance of presenting the clustering result as a hierarchy whereby the researcher can visually determine the optimal level of separation from the number of major clusters in the dendrogram. The dendrogram serves as a visual means for both understanding the structure of the data and selecting a reasonable number of clusters.

Conclusion

The analysis of population structure is used to obtain a clear insight into the underlying genetic population substructure and is a crucial prerequisite for any analysis of genetic data, such as genome-wide association studies, to eventually reduce false positive rates, and for forensics to develop reference panels that provide information on an individual's ancestry. Single nucleotide polymorphisms (SNPs) are the most widely used markers to study the variation of DNA sequences between populations. Data preprocessing is a necessary step to assess the quality of the data before analysis, including the assessment of the call rates of both SNPs and individuals, minor allele frequency, and relatedness between individuals, where a threshold is set to eliminate SNPs/individuals that do not meet that threshold. Additionally, the selection of ancestry informative markers (AIMs), which are the minimal set of markers required to derive population structure, is considered important in preprocessing to improve the accuracy of clustering results.

After preprocessing, several analysis methods, including parametric and nonparametric, are used. Parametric approaches are impractical for large datasets because of their intensive computational cost, genetic assumptions that must be held, and sensitivity to sample size. In contrast, nonparametric approaches have the advantage of efficient computational cost with no modeling assumption requirements, making them more viable than parametric approaches for analyzing large datasets. Nonparametric approaches can be categorized into dimension reduction-based and distance-based methods. On the one hand, dimension reduction techniques are used to reduce the dimensions of genetic markers before conducting a clustering. The most used dimension reduction technique is principal components analysis (PCA), as it is implemented in EIGENSTRAT\smartpca. On the other hand, distance-based methods include computing dis/similarity matrices of the data where the clustering method is applied, such as AWclust, SHIPS, NETVIEW, and iNJclust. In these methods, similarity is measured using allele-sharing distance (ASD). ASD is a measure to determine how genetically close each pair of individuals is.

All in all, as evident in the challenges introduced by the ever-growing sizes and complexity of genetic datasets, accurate and efficient analysis methods are increasingly desirable to take full advantage of these available genetic datasets.

Abbreviations

AIMs: Ancestry informative markers; ASD: Allele-sharing distance; AWclust: Allele-sharing distance and Ward's minimum variance hierarchical clustering; DBMC: Density-based mean clustering; GWAS: Genome-wide association studies; HWE: Hardy-Weinberg equilibrium; iNJclust: Iterative neighbor-joining tree clustering; ipPCA: Iterative pruning PCA; LD: Linkage disequilibrium; MDS: Multi-dimensional scaling; NJ: Neighbor-joining; PCA: Principal component analysis; SHIPS: Spectral Hierarchical clustering for the Inference of Population Structure; SVD: Singular value decomposition; TW: Tracy-Widom

Acknowledgements

This research project was supported by a grant from the "Research Center of the Female Scientific and Medical Colleges," Deanship of Scientific Research, King Saud University.

Authors' contributions

LA performed the literature review, analyzed the findings, and wrote the manuscript. AH assisted with the analysis and reviewed the manuscript. Both authors read and approved the final manuscript.

Competing interests

The authors declare that they have no competing interests.

References

1. Lawson DJ, Falush D. Population identification using genetic data. Annu Rev Genomics Hum Genet. 2012;13:337–61.
2. Pritchard JK, Donnelly P. Case-control studies of association in structured or admixed populations. Theor Popul Biol. 2001;60:227–37.
3. Hoggart CJ, Parra EJ, Shriver MD, Bonilla C, Kittles RA, Clayton DG, McKeigue PM. Control of confounding of genetic associations in stratified populations. Am J Hum Genet. 2003;72:1492–504.
4. Marchini J, Cardon LR, Phillips MS, Donnelly P. The effects of human population structure on large genetic association studies. Nat Genet. 2004; 36:512–7.
5. Helgason A, Yngvadóttir B, Hrafnkelsson B, Gulcher J, Stefánsson K. An Icelandic example of the impact of population structure on association studies. Nat Genet. 2005;37:90–5.
6. Ziv E, Burchard EG. Human population structure and genetic association studies. Pharmacogenomics. 2003;4:431–41.
7. Freedman ML, Reich D, Penney KL, McDonald GJ, Mignault AA, Patterson N, Gabriel SB, Topol EJ, Smoller JW, Pato CN. Assessing the impact of population stratification on genetic association studies. Nat Genet. 2004;36:388–93.
8. Price AL, Zaitlen NA, Reich D, Patterson N. New approaches to population stratification in genome-wide association studies. Nat Rev Genet. 2010;11:459.
9. Kidd KK, Pakstis AJ, Speed WC, Grigorenko EL, Kajuna SL, Karoma NJ, Kungulilo S, Kim J-J, Lu R-B, Odunsi A. Developing a SNP panel for forensic identification of individuals. Forensic Sci Int. 2006;164:20–32.
10. Kidd KK, Speed WC, Pakstis AJ, Furtado MR, Fang R, Madbouly A, Maiers M, Middha M, Friedlaender FR, Kidd JR. Progress toward an efficient panel of SNPs for ancestry inference. Forensic Sci Int Genet. 2014;10:23–32.
11. Intarapanich A, Shaw PJ, Assawamakin A, Wangkumhang P, Ngamphiw C, Chaichoompu K, Piriyapongsa J, Tongsima S. Iterative pruning PCA improves resolution of highly structured populations. BMC bioinformatics. 2009;10:382.
12. Pritchard JK, Stephens M, Donnelly P. Inference of population structure using multilocus genotype data. Genetics. 2000;155:945–59.
13. Liu Y, Nyunoya T, Leng S, Belinsky SA, Tesfaigzi Y, Bruse S. Softwares and methods for estimating genetic ancestry in human populations. Hum Genomics. 2013;7(1):1.
14. Paschou P, Lewis J, Javed A, Drineas P. Ancestry informative markers for fine-scale individual assignment to worldwide populations. J Med Genet. 2010;47:835–47.
15. Paschou P, Ziv E, Burchard EG, Choudhry S, Rodriguez-Cintron W, Mahoney MW, Drineas P. PCA-correlated SNPs for structure identification in worldwide human populations. PLoS Genet. 2007;3:e160.
16. Limpiti T, Intarapanich A, Assawamakin A, Shaw PJ, Wangkumhang P, Piriyapongsa J, Ngamphiw C, Tongsima S. Study of large and highly stratified population datasets by combining iterative pruning principal component analysis and structure. BMC bioinformatics. 2011;12:255.
17. Brookes AJ. The essence of SNPs. Gene. 1999;234:177–86.
18. The International HapMap C. A haplotype map of the human genome. Nature. 2005;437:1299–320.
19. Pemberton TJ, Wang C, Li JZ, Rosenberg NA. Inference of unexpected genetic relatedness among individuals in HapMap phase III. Am J Hum Genet. 2010;87:457–64.
20. Consortium IH. A second generation human haplotype map of over 3.1 million SNPs. Nature. 2007;449:851.
21. Consortium GP. An integrated map of genetic variation from 1,092 human genomes. Nature. 2012;491:56.
22. Ngamphiw C, Assawamakin A, Xu S, Shaw PJ, Yang JO, Ghang H, Bhak J, Liu E, Tongsima S, Consortium HP-AS. PanSNPdb: the Pan-Asian SNP genotyping database. PLoS One. 2011;6:e21451.
23. Laurie CC, Doheny KF, Mirel DB, Pugh EW, Bierut LJ, Bhangale T, Boehm F, Caporaso NE, Cornelis MC, Edenberg HJ. Quality control and quality assurance in genotypic data for genome-wide association studies. Genet Epidemiol. 2010;34:591–602.
24. Purcell S, Neale B, Todd-Brown K, Thomas L, Ferreira Manuel AR, Bender D, Maller J, Sklar P, de Bakker Paul IW, Daly Mark J, Sham Pak C. PLINK: a tool set for whole-genome association and population-based linkage analyses. Am J Hum Genet. 2007;81:559–75.
25. Stevens EL, Heckenberg G, Roberson ED, Baugher JD, Downey TJ, Pevsner J. Inference of relationships in population data using identity-by-descent and identity-by-state. PLoS Genet. 2011;7:e1002287.
26. Manichaikul A, Mychaleckyj JC, Rich SS, Daly K, Sale M, Chen W-M. Robust relationship inference in genome-wide association studies. Bioinformatics. 2010;26:2867–73.
27. Purcell S, Sham P. Properties of structured association approaches to detecting population stratification. Hum Hered. 2005;58:93–107.
28. Reich DE, Cargill M, Bolk S, Ireland J, Sabeti PC, Richter DJ, Lavery T, Kouyoumjian R, Farhadian SF, Ward R, Lander ES. Linkage disequilibrium in the human genome. Nature. 2001;411:199–204.
29. Porras-Hurtado L, Ruiz Y, Santos C, Phillips C, Carracedo Á, Lareu MV. An overview of STRUCTURE: applications, parameter settings, and supporting software. Front Genet. 2013;4:98.
30. Alexander DH, Lange K. Enhancements to the ADMIXTURE algorithm for individual ancestry estimation. BMC bioinformatics. 2011;12:246.
31. Dawson KJ, Belkhir K. A Bayesian approach to the identification of panmictic populations and the assignment of individuals. Genet Res. 2001;78:59–77.
32. Corander J, Waldmann P, Sillanpää MJ. Bayesian analysis of genetic differentiation between populations. Genetics. 2003;163:367–74.
33. Corander J, Waldmann P, Marttinen P, Sillanpää MJ. BAPS 2: enhanced possibilities for the analysis of genetic population structure. Bioinformatics. 2004;20:2363–9.
34. Guillot G, Mortier F, Estoup A. GENELAND: a computer package for landscape genetics. Mol Ecol Notes. 2005;5:712–5.

35. Tang H, Peng J, Wang P, Risch NJ. Estimation of individual admixture: analytical and study design considerations. Genet Epidemiol. 2005;28:289–301.
36. Alexander DH, Novembre J, Lange K. Fast model-based estimation of ancestry in unrelated individuals. Genome Res. 2009;19:1655–64.
37. Wu B, Liu N, Zhao H. PSMIX: an R package for population structure inference via maximum likelihood method. BMC bioinformatics. 2006;7:317.
38. Raj A, Stephens M, Pritchard JK. fastSTRUCTURE: variational inference of population structure in large SNP datasets. Genetics. 2014;197(2):573–89.
39. Price AL, Patterson NJ, Plenge RM, Weinblatt ME, Shadick NA, Reich D. Principal components analysis corrects for stratification in genome-wide association studies. Nat Genet. 2006;38:904–9.
40. Liu N, Zhao H. A non-parametric approach to population structure inference using multilocus genotypes. Human genomics. 2006;2:353.
41. Patterson N, Price AL, Reich D. Population structure and eigenanalysis. PLoS Genet. 2006;2:e190.
42. Gao X, Starmer JD. AWclust: point-and-click software for non-parametric population structure analysis. BMC bioinformatics. 2008;9:77.
43. Bouaziz M, Paccard C, Guedj M, Ambroise C. SHIPS: spectral hierarchical clustering for the inference of population structure in genetic studies. PLoS One. 2012;7:e45685.
44. Gao X, Starmer J. Human population structure detection via multilocus genotype clustering. BMC Genet. 2007;8:34.
45. Bryc K, Auton A, Nelson MR, Oksenberg JR, Hauser SL, Williams S, Froment A, Bodo J-M, Wambebe C, Tishkoff SA. Genome-wide patterns of population structure and admixture in West Africans and African Americans. Proc Natl Acad Sci. 2010;107:786–91.
46. Bryc K, Velez C, Karafet T, Moreno-Estrada A, Reynolds A, Auton A, Hammer M, Bustamante CD, Ostrer H. Genome-wide patterns of population structure and admixture among Hispanic/Latino populations. Proc Natl Acad Sci. 2010;107:8954–61.
47. Novembre J, Stephens M. Interpreting principal component analyses of spatial population genetic variation. Nat Genet. 2008;40:646–9.
48. Zheng X, Levine D, Shen J, Gogarten SM, Laurie C, Weir BS. A high-performance computing toolset for relatedness and principal component analysis of SNP data. Bioinformatics. 2012;28:3326–8.
49. McVean G. A genealogical interpretation of principal components analysis. PLoS Genet. 2009;5:e1000686.
50. Tracy CA, Widom H. Level-spacing distributions and the airy kernel. Commun Math Phys. 1994;159:151–74.
51. Johnstone IM. On the distribution of the largest eigenvalue in principal components analysis. Ann Stat. 2001;29(2):295–327.
52. Lee C, Abdool A, Huang C-H: PCA-based population structure inference with generic clustering algorithms. BMC bioinformatics 2009, 10:S73.
53. Hartigan JA, Wong MA. Algorithm AS 136: a k-means clustering algorithm. Appl Stat. 1979:100–8.
54. Fraley C, Raftery AE. Enhanced model-based clustering, density estimation, and discriminant analysis software: MCLUST. J Classif. 2003;20:263–86.
55. Ng AY, Jordan MI, Weiss Y. On spectral clustering: analysis and an algorithm. In: Proceedings of advances in neural information processing systems. Cambridge: MIT Press; 2001. p. 849–56.
56. Tibshirani R, Walther G, Hastie T. Estimating the number of clusters in a data set via the gap statistic. J Royal Stat Soc Series B (Statistical Methodology). 2001;63:411–23.
57. Schwarz G. Estimating the dimension of a model. Ann Stat. 1978;6:461–4.
58. Amornbunchornvej C, Limpiti T, Assawamakin A, Intarapanich A, Tongsima S: Improved iterative pruning principal component analysis with graph-theoretic hierarchical clustering. In 9th international conference on electrical engineering/electronics, computer, telecommunications and information technology; 16–18 2012. 2012: 1–4.
59. Luo J, Zhang Z: Using eigenvalue grads method to estimate the number of signal source. In 2000 5th International Conference on Signal Processing Proceedings; Beijing. IEEE; 2000: 223–225.
60. Wall ME, Rechtsteiner A, Rocha LM. Singular value decomposition and principal component analysis, A practical approach to microarray data analysis; 2003. p. 91.
61. Li M, Reilly C, Hanson T. A semiparametric test to detect associations between quantitative traits and candidate genes in structured populations. Bioinformatics. 2008;24:2356–62.
62. Mountain JL, Cavalli-Sforza LL. Inference of human evolution through cladistic analysis of nuclear DNA restriction polymorphisms. Proc Natl Acad Sci. 1994;91(14):6515–19.
63. Neuditschko M, Khatkar MS, Raadsma HW. NetView: a high-definition network-visualization approach to detect fine-scale population structures from genome-wide patterns of variation. PLoS One. 2012;7:e48375.
64. Limpiti T, Amornbunchornvej C, Intarapanich A, Assawamakin A, Tongsima S. iNJclust: iterative neighbor-joining tree clustering framework for inferring population structure. IEEE/ACM Trans Comput Biol Bioinformatics. 2014;11:903–14.
65. Ward Jr JH. Hierarchical grouping to optimize an objective function. J Am Stat Assoc. 1963;58:236–44.
66. Ward Jr JH, Hook ME. Application of an hierarchial grouping procedure to a problem of grouping profiles. Educ Psychol Meas. 1963;23(1):69–81.
67. Deejai P, Assawamakin A, Wangkumhang P, Poomputsa K, Tongsima S: On assigning individuals from cryptic population structures to optimal predicted subpopulations: an empirical evaluation of non-parametric population structure analysis techniques. In Computational Systems-Biology and Bioinformatics. Berlin: Springer; 2010. p. 58–70.
68. Bouaziz M: SHIPS: spectral hierarchical clustering for the inference of population structure. In Annals of Human Genetics; NJ,USA. WILEY-BLACKWELL; 2012: 413–413.
69. Blatt M, Wiseman S, Domany E. Superparamagnetic clustering of data. Phys Rev Lett. 1996;76:3251.
70. Tsafrir D, Tsafrir I, Ein-Dor L, Zuk O, Notterman DA, Domany E. Sorting points into neighborhoods (SPIN): data analysis and visualization by ordering distance matrices. Bioinformatics. 2005;21:2301–8.
71. Tetko IV, Facius A, Ruepp A, Mewes H-W. Super paramagnetic clustering of protein sequences. BMC Bioinformatics. 2005;6:82.
72. Holsinger KE, Weir BS. Genetics in geographically structured populations: defining, estimating and interpreting F ST. Nat Rev Genet. 2009;10:639.
73. Gascuel O, Steel M. Neighbor-joining revealed. Mol Biol Evol. 2006;23:1997–2000.
74. Rosenberg NA, Li LM, Ward R, Pritchard JK. Informativeness of genetic markers for inference of ancestry. Am J Hum Genet. 2003;73:1402–22.
75. Paschou P, Drineas P, Lewis J, Nievergelt CM, Nickerson DA, Smith JD, Ridker PM, Chasman DI, Krauss RM, Ziv E. Tracing sub-structure in the European American population with PCA-informative markers. PLoS Genet. 2008;4(7): e1000114.
76. Golub G. Numerical methods for solving linear least squares problems. Numer Math. 1965;7:206–16.
77. Gu M, Eisenstat SC. Efficient algorithms for computing a strong rank-revealing QR factorization. SIAM J Sci Comput. 1996;17:848–69.
78. Boutsidis C, Sun J, Anerousis N: Clustered subset selection and its applications on it service metrics. In Proceedings of the 17th ACM conference on Information and knowledge management. ACM; 2008: 599–608.
79. Zhao Y, Karypis G: Evaluation of hierarchical clustering algorithms for document datasets. In Proceedings of the eleventh international conference on Information and knowledge management. ACM; 2002: 515–524.
80. Gao X, Martin ER. Using allele sharing distance for detecting human population stratification. Hum Hered. 2009;68:182–91.
81. Jombart T, Devillard S, Balloux F. Discriminant analysis of principal components: a new method for the analysis of genetically structured populations. BMC Genet. 2010;11:94.
82. EIGENSTRAT/smartpca [http://www.hsph.harvard.edu/alkes-price/software/]. Accessed 20 Jan 2018.
83. ipPCA [http://www4a.biotec.or.th/GI/tools/ippca]. Accessed 20 Jan 2018.
84. AWclust [http://awclust.sourceforge.net/]. Accessed 20 Jan 2018.
85. SHIPS [http://www.math-evry.cnrs.fr/logiciels/ships]. Accessed 20 Apr 2018.
86. NETVIEW [http://sydney.edu.au/vetscience/reprogen/netview/]. Accessed 20 Jan 2018.
87. iNJclust [http://www4a.biotec.or.th/GI/tools/injclust]. Accessed 20 Jan 2018.

2

Recessive *VARS2* mutation underlies a novel syndrome with epilepsy, mental retardation, short stature, growth hormone deficiency, and hypogonadism

Abdulaziz Alsemari[1,3], Banan Al-Younes[2,3], Ewa Goljan[2,3], Dyala Jaroudi[2,3], Faisal BinHumaid[2,3], Brian F. Meyer[2,3], Stefan T. Arold[4] and Dorota Monies[2,3*]

Abstract

Background: Most mitochondrial and cytoplasmic aminoacyl-tRNA synthetases (aaRSs) are encoded by nuclear genes. Syndromic disorders resulting from mutation of aaRSs genes display significant phenotypic heterogeneity. We expand aaRSs-related phenotypes through characterization of the clinical and molecular basis of a novel autosomal-recessive syndrome manifesting severe mental retardation, ataxia, speech impairment, epilepsy, short stature, microcephaly, hypogonadism, and growth hormone deficiency.

Results: A G>A variant in exon 29 of *VARS2* (c.3650G>A) (NM_006295) was identified in the index case. This homozygous variant was confirmed by Sanger sequencing and segregated with disease in the family studied. The c.3650G>A change results in alteration of arginine to histidine at residue 1217 (R1217H) of the mature protein and is predicted to be pathogenic.

Conclusions: These findings contribute to a growing list of aaRSs disorders, broadens the spectrum of phenotypes attributable to *VARS2* mutations, and provides new insight into genotype-phenotype correlations among the mitochondrial synthetase genes.

Keywords: Syndromic, Angelman, Mitochondrial, Dysmorphism, Hypogonadism, Vitamin D deficiency

Background

Mental retardation (MR) affects approximately 1–3% of the human population. Both genetic and environmental factors are responsible for causing MR, but in almost 60% of the cases, the actual cause cannot be identified precisely [1, 2]. In developed countries, most severe forms of intellectual disability are thought to have a genetic cause [3]. Mutations in more than 400 genes have been linked to intellectual disability, but most of these mutations have a very low prevalence and their phenotypes are often indistinguishable [4].

* Correspondence: moniesdm@gmail.com
[2]Department of Genetics, King Faisal Specialist Hospital and Research Centre, MBC 03, PO Box 3354, Riyadh 11211, Saudi Arabia
[3]Saudi Human Genome Project, King Abdulaziz City for Science and Technology, Riyadh, Saudi Arabia
Full list of author information is available at the end of the article

A number of single-gene disorders result in mental retardation. Many of these are associated with atypical or dysmorphic physical characteristics. Such conditions include fragile X syndrome, neurofibromatosis, tuberous sclerosis, Noonan's syndrome, Cornelia de Lange's syndrome, and Angelman syndrome(AS) [5]. AS is usually considered as a diagnosis in individuals with severe developmental delay, in combination with seizures, ataxia, hypermotoric behaviors, and absence of speech. Ninety percent of these individuals have an identifiable molecular defect that results in the loss of expression of maternally inherited *UBE3A* (encoding E6AP) in the brain [6]. Over the last few years, many novel syndromes that mimic AS have been delineated and it is now recognized that some individuals who were clinically diagnosed with "test-negative AS" have one of these AS-like syndromes instead. Their phenotypes include severe intellectual disability, motor delay, variable degrees of speech delay ranging from being completely non-verbal to being able to speak in short sentences, autistic and maladaptive behaviors, short attention span, and seizures [7].

We report a novel autosomal recessive syndromic disorder with clinical resemblance to AS. The clinical spectrum includes severe mental retardation, ataxia, speech impairment, epilepsy, short stature, microcephaly, flap occiput, protruding tongue, prognathia, tremulous movement of limbs, apparent happy demeanor, easily excitable personality, and excessive chewing mouth behaviors. In addition, there were severe growth hormone deficiency, hypogonadism, and severe osteomalacia. Whole exome sequencing of the affected patients identified a homozygous mutation in *VARS2*.

Methods

Subjects and nucleic acid extraction

Four patients from a consanguineous extended family from the same region of Saudi Arabia were examined by a neurologist (AAS), in the department of Neurosciences, King Faisal Specialist Hospital and Research Center (KFSHRC). They were diagnosed with an Angelman-like syndrome. All subjects were enrolled under a KFSHRC IRB-approved (RAC# 13-MED2056-20) protocol with full-written informed consent. Genomic DNA was extracted from peripheral blood samples using standard procedures (Flexi Gene DNA Handbook, Qiagen). Samples were quantitated spectrophotometrically and stored at − 20 °C.

Linkage and homozygosity mapping

All participating individuals (affected and unaffected) were genotyped using an Affymetrix Axiom array (Affymetrix, Santa Clara, CA, USA) following the manufacturer's protocol (http://www.affymetrix.com/support/technical/manuals.affx). Resulting genotypes were analyzed for shared runs of homozygosity (ROH) using autoSNPa (http://dna.leeds.ac.uk/autosnpa/). Linkage analysis was performed using the Allegro module of Easy Linkage assuming autosomal recessive inheritance and 100% penetrance (http://genetik.charite.de/hoffmann/easyLINKAGE/index.html).

Whole exome sequencing and analysis

DNA was amplified to obtain a whole exome Ion Proton AmpliSeq library which was further used for emulsion PCR on an Ion OneTouch System followed by an enrichment process using an Ion OneTouch ES, both procedures following the manufacturer's instructions (Life Technologies, Carlsbad, CA, USA). The template-positive Ion PI Ion Sphere particles were processed for sequencing on the Ion Proton sequencer (Life Technologies, Carlsbad, CA, USA). Approximately 15–17 Gb of sequence was generated per sequencing run. Reads were mapped to UCSC hg19 (http://genome.ucsc.edu/) and variants identified using the Ion Torrent pipeline (Life Technologies, Carlsbad, CA, USA). The resultant variant caller file (vcf) was filtered to include only homozygous variants within the pre-determined ROH (shared by affecteds only) that were absent from dbSNP, 1000 genomes, approximately 2000 Saudi exomes. Included variants were further selected based upon pathogenicity predicted by Polyphen2 (http://genetics.bwh.harvard.edu/pph2/) and SIFT (http://sift.jcvi.org/). Potential causative variants were confirmed by Sanger sequencing and screened further for familial segregation based upon autosomal recessive inheritance. For confirmation, an amplicon incorporating the candidate variant was amplified and sequenced using a BigDye Terminator kit (Applied Biosystems, Foster City, CA) and run on an ABI 3730xl automated sequencer (Applied Biosystems, Foster City, CA). SeqScape v.2.6 software (Applied Biosystems, Foster City, CA) was used to align sequence data and identify variants.

Computational structural analysis of mutants

Sequences were retrieved from the Uniprot database. BLAST and SwissModel [8] were used to search for suitable structural templates in the Protein Data Bank (PDB). SwissModel, RaptorX [9], and I-Tasser [10] were used to produce homology models. Models were manually inspected, and mutations evaluated, using the Pymol program (pymol.org). Disorder and secondary structure elements were predicted using RaptorX. Transmembrane helices were predicted using Phobius [11]. Functional information was compiled from various resources, including Uniprot [12], InterPro [13], and publications associated with the model templates used.

Results

Clinical profile

The index case (V:3) (Fig. 1a), a 23-year-old male was a product of full-term pregnancy and normal delivery. He was well until the age of 4 months when he started to have generalized tonic clonic seizures. At the age of 1 year, the family noticed that the patient had delayed development. He had delayed sitting, delayed standing, and only started to crawl at the age of 2 years. The patient eventually exhibited severe developmental delay and severe speech impairment. The speech impairment was more receptive than expressive. Upon reviewing his family history, there were three other similarly affected siblings (one brother and two sisters). He also has four similarly affected cousins (two males and two females) (Fig. 1a).

Affected individuals usually have incoordination of movement until adolescence at which point they stop walking,

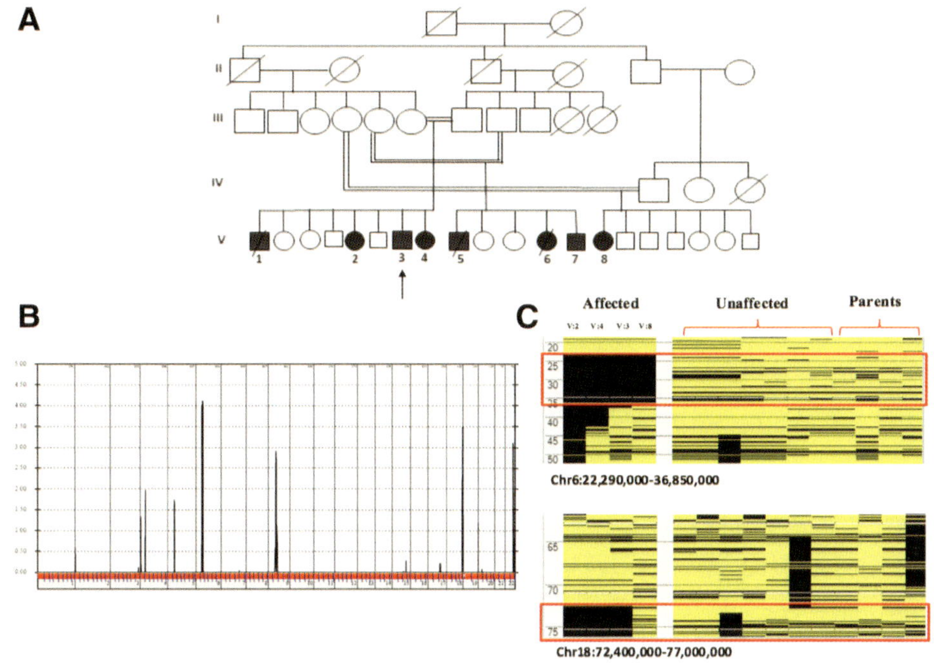

Fig. 1 Identification of disease locus on chromosome 6: **a** Pedigree of extended family with a novel syndromic disorder. **b** Genome-wide linkage analysis revealed a peak with a maximum LOD score of 4.11 on chromosome 6. **c** AutoSNPa output for chromosome 6 reveals an ROH (boxed in red) shared among affected members (V:2, V:3, V:4, and V:8) and not present in unaffected individuals or parents. Output for chromosome 18 excludes this locus because the ROH is not shared with affected individual V:10

consequent to flexed joint deformities of the lower limbs. Their behavioral pattern is best described as frequent episodic smiling and an apparent happy demeanor (Fig. 2a), with an easily excitable personality and habitual hand flapping movement. They also have a history of hyperphagia and usually eat a lot more than their normal siblings. Their examination showed severe mental retardation with expressive and receptive aphasia. Their speech and cognition deteriorates to a degree at which they became unable to produce words or to understand commands. There is no facial, axillae, or pubic hair. The affected male had small testicles. They have flat occiput and constant protruding tongue with tongue thrusting. They have microcephaly, prognathia, and wide-spaced teeth (Fig. 2b). During movement of the upper limbs, there are usually flexed arm positions (Fig. 2c). They are of short stature and increasingly become chair bound (Fig. 2d). They typically show an excessive chewing mouth behavior. Their examination showed brisk reflex of the upper and lower limbs. The older affected son (V:1) expired at the age of 23 because of a chest infection.

Laboratory investigations of the index case showed that he had a normal blood count, normal liver function test, and normal electrolytes and renal function test. His peripheral smear morphology was normal. His calcium was low at 2.3 mmol/l, while his phosphate amylase was normal. He had high alkaline phosphatase at 288 U/L (normal range is 40–135). The patient had normal synacthen test and a low IGF level (26 μg/l) (normal range between 116 and 358). IGF binding protein-3 was 1.8 mg/l, which is extremely low (normal range is 3.4–7.8 mg/l). His FSH was 1.8 IU/L and LH was 0.5 IU/L, both in the lower range. The prolactin level and TSH was normal. Testosterone was extremely low < 0.1 nmol/l (normal range is 9.9–27.8). Free androgen index is low < 0.1% (normal range is 14.8–94.8). The 25-hydroxy vitamin D level is undetectable in blood.

Twenty-four-hour urine collection for oligosaccharides was normal, and mucopolysaccharide was negative in the urine. Chromosomal analysis was 46,XY and attributed as no apparent chromosomal abnormalities. FISH analysis to test *SNRPN* deletion within the 15q11.2 locus for AS was negative. The patient also had a growth hormone stimulation test, and the result showed a flat response with a fasting growth hormone of 0.6 m U/L. After 10 min, it was 0.6 m U/L and after 1 h was 1.3 m U/L. This indicated severe growth hormone failure.

A skeletal survey was also done for the patient, and the result was in keeping with metabolic bone disease with evidence of severe osteomalacia and multiple looser zones and fractures, microcephaly, scoliosis, and kyphosis. Serum homocysteine was normal. MRI of the brain was performed and concluded that there were relative atrophic changes seen involving the cerebellum; otherwise, there was no evidence of white matter disease, cortical matter disease, or cortex abnormality.

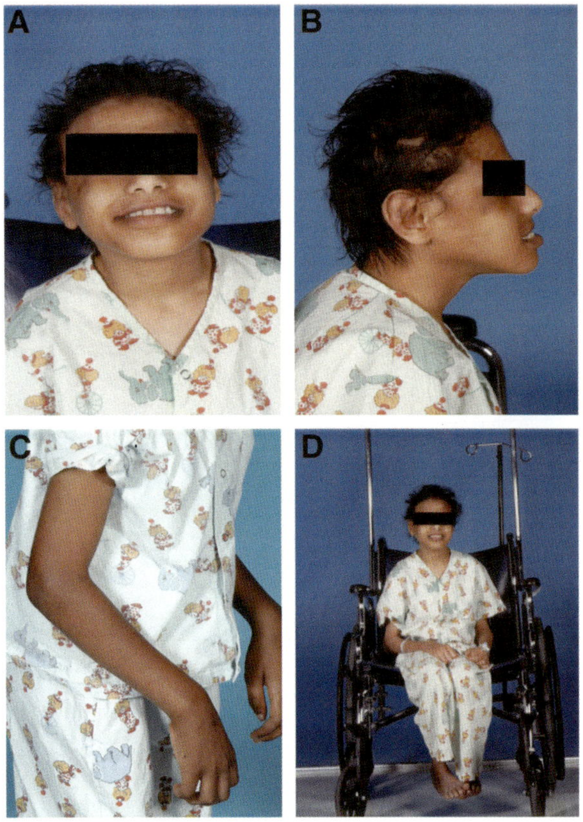

Fig. 2 Clinical features: **a** Apparent happy demeanor with easily excitable personality. **b** Microcephaly, prognathia, and wide spaced teeth. **c** There are usually flexed arm positions particularly during movement. **d** Short stature and increasingly chair bound

A muscle biopsy was studied for the index patient. It was interpreted as having type II fiber atrophy with glycogen excess associated with a mild increase in mitochondria. Similar findings were observed in his brother and sister. There were no deficiencies in mitochondrial electron transport chain enzymes. Citrate synthase activity was increased, suggesting increased mitochondrial proliferation.

Linkage and homozygosity mapping

Linkage analysis (Fig. 1b) localized the disease to a region on chromosome 6 defined proximally by rs743646 and distally by rs34811366 (chr6:4,536,241-6,670,705) with a maximum LOD score of 4.20. Based upon runs of homozygosity shared by all affecteds and absent in all unaffected individuals (Fig. 1c; red rectangle), we refined the critical interval to a 2.1 Mb region (chr6:4,231,133-6,018,243) containing approximately 60 RefSeq genes (hg19).

Whole exome sequencing and analysis

Whole exome sequencing of the index case (V:3) identified 25,168 variants relative to hg19, with 1342 variants on chr 6. These were further filtered to exclude all variants present outside our defined ROH (chr 6: 4,231,133-6,018,243) within which we identified 461 variants. By excluding previously reported variants (present in dbSNP, 1000 genomes and 2000 Arab exomes), the list was narrowed to 8. By only focusing on homozygous changes that were non-synonymous, splicing variants, frameshift insertions or deletions, and nonsense variants, we decreased the number of candidate variants to 1. It was a G>A change in exon 29 of *VARS2* (NM_006295:c.3650G>A:R1217H) (Fig. 3a). This homozygous variant was confirmed by Sanger sequencing, and the mutation segregated recessively with disease in the families studied (Fig. 3b).

Structure and function

VARS2 belongs to the class-I aminoacyl-tRNA synthetase family. The aminoacyl-tRNA synthetase (also known as aminoacyl-tRNA ligase) catalyzes the attachment of an amino acid to its cognate transfer RNA molecule in a highly specific two-step reaction. Class I aminoacyl-tRNA synthetases contain a characteristic Rossman fold catalytic domain and are mostly monomeric. tRNA binding involves an alpha-helical structure that is conserved between class I and class II synthetases. R1217 is located in the C-terminal coiled-coil domain of the tRNA synthetase domain of VARS2 (Fig. 4a). R1217 directly binds to the phosphate backbone of the tRNA D- loop. R1217 also forms a hydrogen bond with the ribose moiety of an adenosine that is flipped out and points toward the coiled-coil domain (Fig. 4b). R1217 has therefore an important function in the specific recognition of tRNA. The mutation of R1217 into a histidine abolishes this function. Hence, the R1217H mutant is expected to have compromised abilities to recognize the correct tRNA. This is consistent with the prediction of pathogenicity of this variant by models including Polyphen, SIFT, and CADD.

Discussion

Aminoacyl-tRNA synthetase enzymes (aaRSs) are involved in translation at the second step in creating a protein from a gene's instructions. The mRNA interacts with the ribosomal complex which reads the sequence of mRNA bases. Each sequence codes for one particular amino acid, and tRNA assembles the protein, one amino acid at a time. Subsequently, aaRSs help attach the amino acid to the tRNA [14].

A typical animal cell contains 37 cytoplasmic and mitochondrial synthetase genes, all of which are encoded on nuclear chromosomes. Mitochondrial synthetases are given the same name as cytosolic synthetases, appended with the numeral 2 (e.g., HARS and HARS2) [15]. Mitochondrial and cytoplasmic aaRSs are encoded by distinct nuclear genes, with the exception of GARS and KARS, which are present in both cellular compartments [16]. Mt-tRNA genes are located in three transcription units: the short H-strand unit (with the rRNA region and two

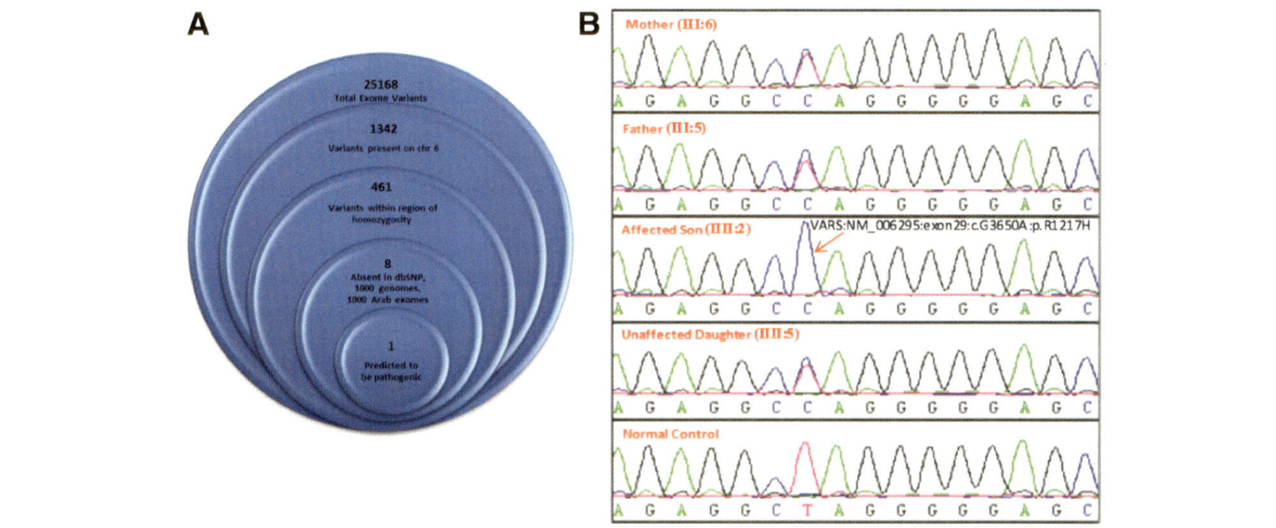

Fig. 3 *VARS2* mutation: **a** Filtering strategy used for identification of a causative mutation. **b** DNA electrophoregram with the G>A change in *VARS2* (NM_006295:exon29:c.G3650A:p.R1217H)

tRNA genes) is transcribed twice as fast as the L-strand that contains eight tRNA genes and more frequently the entire H-strand unit that produces 14 tRNAs [17]. Currently, pathological mutations that cause human diseases have been identified in many genes that encode cytoplasmic and mitochondrial tRNA-synthetases. The first cytoplasmic aaRSs mutation associated with a human disease, Charcot-Marie-Tooth, was discovered in glycyl-tRNA synthetase (GARS) [18]. Typically, defects in each mtARS have been identified in one tissue-specific disease (most commonly affecting the brain) or in one syndrome [19].

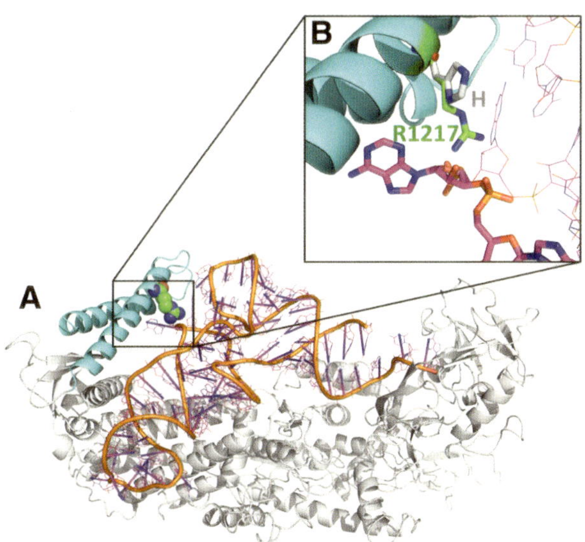

Fig. 4 Computational structural analysis of mutant: Homology model of the VARS2 tRNA synthetase domain, based on the PDB id 1gax (36% sequence id, RaptorX *p* value 1.12e-19). **a** The C-terminal coiled-coild domain is shown in cyan. R1217 is highlighted with carbon atoms shown in green. tRNA is shown with orange backbone. **b** Inlay: Zoom of the indicated region. H1217 is shown with gray carbon atoms. The tRNA D loop is shown with carbon atoms in magenta

VARS2 encodes mitochondrial valyl-tRNA (Val-tRNA) synthetase, which is involved in mitochondrial translation [16]. The deduced 993-amino acid protein has an N-terminal mitochondrial targeting signal with a predicted cleavage site after residue 29. VARS2 has characteristics of a class I mitochondrial aminoacyl-tRNA synthetase, including a classical Rossmann fold [20].

A homozygous mutation of *VARS2* was reported in a sporadic case with microcephaly and epilepsy [16]. It was associated with isolated deficiency of the mitochondrial respiratory chain (MRC) complex I. The disorder was secondary to a homozygous c.1100C>T transition in *VARS2*, resulting in a threonine 367 to isoleucine (T367I) substitution at a highly conserved residue. The affected patient was an 8-year-old with psychomotor delay, facial dysmorphisms, and microcephaly. At 4 years of age, there was onset of partial seizures. His brain MRI displayed hyperintense lesions in the periventricular regions, the insula, and the right fronto-temporal cortex. Brain proton magnetic resonance spectroscopy revealed a lactate peak in the frontal white matter. Muscle computerized tomography showed bilateral quadriceps hypotrophy, but no evident histological alteration was observed in a muscle biopsy [16].

In a British boy with combined oxidative phosphorylation deficiency-20, a compound heterozygous mutation of *VARS2*: a c.1135G>A transition, resulting in an alanine 379 to threonine (A379T) substitution, and a c.1877C-A transversion, resulting in an alanine 626 to

Table 1 Genetic and phenotypic heterogeneity

Clinical features	Diodato et al.	Taylor et al.	This study
	NM_001167734.1: c.1100C>T, p.Thr367Ile (Hom)	NM_001167734.1: c.1135G>A,p.Ala379Thr (Het) c.1877C>A, p.Ala626Asp (Het)	NM_006295: c.A3253G; p.S1085G
Mental retardation	X		X
Facial dysmorphisms	X		X
Ataxia		X	X
Combined oxidative phosphorylation deficiencies		X	
Microcephaly	X		X
Progressive external ophthalmoplegia		X	
Epilepsy	X		X
Short stature			X
Hyperintense lesions in the periventricular regions, the insula, and the right frontotemporal cortex	X		
Evidence of severe growth hormone deficiency			X
Hypogonadism			X
Severe osteomalacia			X

X : affected

aspartic acid substitution (A626D). He presented with progressive external ophthalmoplegia, ataxia, and combined oxidative phosphorylation deficiencies [21].

Our family share with the reported cases, the findings of microcephaly, epilepsy, and the progressive cerebral encephalopathy; however, several dysmorphic features were noticeable in clinical assessment of the affected members from our family. The hypogonadism, vitamin D resistant osteomalacia, and the growth hormone deficiency were significant and novel associations with the *VARS2* mutation in the family from this study (Table 1).

In our *VARS2* family, there were no apparent deficiencies in mitochondrial electron transport chain enzymes. However, citrate synthase activity was increased, suggesting increased mitochondrial proliferation. We identified a homozygous change *VARS2:*NM_006295:c.3650G>A:R1217H, segregating with disease in our family. This mutation is in the anticodon-binding domain of tRNA synthetase, while the reported isolated *VARS2* homozygous mutation [16] is located in the catalytic core domain of valyl-tRNA synthetase.

The lack of clear biochemical phenotypes of OXPHOS or mitochondrial protein synthesis defects in skin fibroblasts and myoblasts from most of mutant aaRSs patients prevented the use of cultured cells for functional studies. In a few RARS2 patients, fibroblasts showed OXPHOS defects, with RC enzymes variably affected; YARS2 patients presented deficient mitochondrial protein synthesis in myotubes but not in cultured fibroblasts [22].

Conclusions

In summary, we describe a novel autosomal recessive syndromic disorder associated with a mutation in *VARS2* (mitochondrial valyl tRNA synthetase). Clinical features included severe mental retardation, ataxia, speech impairment, epilepsy, short stature, microcephaly, dysmorphia, an easily excitable personality, and excessive chewing mouth behaviors. In addition, there was clinical and chemical evidence of severe growth hormone deficiency, hypogonadism, and severe osteomalacia. Our findings further expand the phenotypic spectrum of Aminoacyl-tRNA synthetase enzymes.

Acknowledgements

The authors would like to thank the family members for their participation in this study. We thank the Genotyping and Sequencing Core Facilities of King Faisal Specialist Hospital and Research Centre for their contributions. We would also like to acknowledge the support of King Abdulaziz City for Science and Technology (KACST) through the Saudi Human Genome Project (SHGP).

Funding

This work was funded through grants from King Faisal Specialist Hospital and Research Centre (RAC 2140029) and King Abdulaziz City for Science and Technology (KACST#13-MED2056-20).

Author's contributions

AA contributed to the conception and design, acquisition and analysis of data, and drafting of the manuscript. BA contributed to the acquisition and analysis of data and preparation of figures. EG contributed to the acquisition and analysis of data and preparation of figures. DJ contributed to the acquisition and analysis of data and preparation of figures. FB contributed to the acquisition and analysis of data. BFM contributed to the conception and design, acquisition and analysis of data, and drafting of the manuscript and figures. STA contributed to the acquisition and analysis of data. DM contributed to the conception and design, acquisition and analysis of data, and drafting of the manuscript and figures. All authors read and approved the final manuscript.

Competing interests
The authors declare that they have no competing interests.

Author details
[1]Department of Neurosciences, King Faisal Specialist Hospital and Research Centre, Riyadh, Saudi Arabia. [2]Department of Genetics, King Faisal Specialist Hospital and Research Centre, MBC 03, PO Box 3354, Riyadh 11211, Saudi Arabia. [3]Saudi Human Genome Project, King Abdulaziz City for Science and Technology, Riyadh, Saudi Arabia. [4]King Abdullah University of Science and Technology (KAUST), Computational Bioscience Research Center (CBRC), Division of Biological and Environmental Sciences and Engineering (BESE), Thuwal 23955-6900, Saudi Arabia.

References
1. Al-Mujadi H, AR AR, Katzarov MG, Dehrab NA, Batra YK, Al-Qattan AR. Preemptive gabapentin reduces postoperative pain and opioid demand following thyroid surgery. Can J Anaesth. 2006;53:268–73.
2. Fernell E. Aetiological factors and prevalence of severe mental retardation in children in a Swedish municipality: the possible role of consanguinity. Dev Med Child Neurol. 1998;40:608–11.
3. Ropers HH. Genetics of early onset cognitive impairment. Annu Rev Genomics Hum Genet. 2010;11:161–87.
4. de Ligt J, Willemsen MH, van Bon BW, Kleefstra T, Yntema HG, Kroes T, Vulto-van Silfhout AT, Koolen DA, de Vries P, Gilissen C, et al. Diagnostic exome sequencing in persons with severe intellectual disability. N Engl J Med. 2012;367:1921–9.
5. Fryns JP, de Ravel TJ. London Dysmorphology Database, London Neurogenetics Database and Dysmorphology Photo Library on CD-ROM [Version 3] 2001R. M. Winter, M. Baraitser, Oxford University Press, ISBN 019851-780, pound sterling 1595. Hum Genet. 2002;111:113.
6. Ramsden SC, Clayton-Smith J, Birch R, Buiting K. Practice guidelines for the molecular analysis of Prader-Willi and Angelman syndromes. BMC Med Genet. 2010;11:70.
7. Tan WH, Bird LM, Thibert RL, Williams CA. If not Angelman, what is it? A review of Angelman-like syndromes. Am J Med Genet A. 2014;164A:975–92.
8. Arnold K, Bordoli L, Kopp J, Schwede T. The SWISS-MODEL workspace: a web-based environment for protein structure homology modelling. Bioinformatics. 2006;22:195–201.
9. Kallberg M, Margaryan G, Wang S, Ma J, Xu J. RaptorX server: a resource for template-based protein structure modeling. Methods Mol Biol. 2014;1137:17–27.
10. Yang J, Yan R, Roy A, Xu D, Poisson J, Zhang Y. The I-TASSER Suite: protein structure and function prediction. Nat Methods. 2015;12:7–8.
11. Kall L, Krogh A, Sonnhammer EL. A combined transmembrane topology and signal peptide prediction method. J Mol Biol. 2004;338:1027–36.
12. UniProt C. UniProt: a hub for protein information. Nucleic Acids Res. 2015; 43:D204–12.
13. Hunter S, Jones P, Mitchell A, Apweiler R, Attwood TK, Bateman A, Bernard T, Binns D, Bork P, Burge S, et al. InterPro in 2011: new developments in the family and domain prediction database. Nucleic Acids Res. 2012;40:D306–12.
14. Francklyn C, Musier-Forsyth K, Martinis SA. Aminoacyl-tRNA synthetases in biology and disease: new evidence for structural and functional diversity in an ancient family of enzymes. RNA. 1997;3:954–60.
15. Abbott JA, Francklyn CS, Robey-Bond SM. Transfer RNA and human disease. Front Genet. 2014;5:158.
16. Diodato D, Melchionda L, Haack TB, Dallabona C, Baruffini E, Donnini C, Granata T, Ragona F, Balestri P, Margollicci M, et al. VARS2 and TARS2 mutations in patients with mitochondrial encephalomyopathies. Hum Mutat. 2014;35:983–9.
17. King MP, Attardi G. Post-transcriptional regulation of the steady-state levels of mitochondrial tRNAs in HeLa cells. J Biol Chem. 1993;268:10228–37.
18. Antonellis A, Ellsworth RE, Sambuughin N, Puls I, Abel A, Lee-Lin SQ, Jordanova A, Kremensky I, Christodoulou K, Middleton LT, et al. Glycyl tRNA synthetase mutations in Charcot-Marie-Tooth disease type 2D and distal spinal muscular atrophy type V. Am J Hum Genet. 2003;72:1293–9.
19. Euro L, Konovalova S, Asin-Cayuela J, Tulinius M, Griffin H, Horvath R, Taylor RW, Chinnery PF, Schara U, Thorburn DR, et al. Structural modeling of tissue-specific mitochondrial alanyl-tRNA synthetase (AARS2) defects predicts differential effects on aminoacylation. Front Genet. 2015;6:21.
20. Bonnefond L, Fender A, Rudinger-Thirion J, Giege R, Florentz C, Sissler M. Toward the full set of human mitochondrial aminoacyl-tRNA synthetases: characterization of AspRS and TyrRS. Biochemistry. 2005;44:4805–16.
21. Taylor RW, Pyle A, Griffin H, Blakely EL, Duff J, He L, Smertenko T, Alston CL, Neeve VC, Best A, et al. Use of whole-exome sequencing to determine the genetic basis of multiple mitochondrial respiratory chain complex deficiencies. JAMA. 2014;312:68–77.
22. Diodato D, Ghezzi D, Tiranti V. The mitochondrial aminoacyl tRNA synthetases: genes and syndromes. Int J Cell Biol. 2014;2014:787956.

3

Transcriptome analysis reveals manifold mechanisms of cyst development in ADPKD

Rita M. C. de Almeida[1,2], Sherry G. Clendenon[3], William G. Richards[4], Michael Boedigheimer[4], Michael Damore[4], Sandro Rossetti[5], Peter C. Harris[5], Britney-Shea Herbert[6], Wei Min Xu[7], Angela Wandinger-Ness[8], Heather H. Ward[9], James A. Glazier[3] and Robert L. Bacallao[7*]

Abstract

Background: Autosomal dominant polycystic kidney disease (ADPKD) causes progressive loss of renal function in adults as a consequence of the accumulation of cysts. ADPKD is the most common genetic cause of end-stage renal disease. Mutations in polycystin-1 occur in 87% of cases of ADPKD and mutations in polycystin-2 are found in 12% of ADPKD patients. The complexity of ADPKD has hampered efforts to identify the mechanisms underlying its pathogenesis. No current FDA (Federal Drug Administration)-approved therapies ameliorate ADPKD progression.

Results: We used the de Almeida laboratory's sensitive new transcriptogram method for whole-genome gene expression data analysis to analyze microarray data from cell lines developed from cell isolates of normal kidney and of both non-cystic nephrons and cysts from the kidney of a patient with ADPKD. We compared results obtained using standard Ingenuity Volcano plot analysis, Gene Set Enrichment Analysis (GSEA) and transcriptogram analysis. Transcriptogram analysis confirmed the findings of Ingenuity, GSEA, and published analysis of ADPKD kidney data and also identified multiple new expression changes in KEGG (Kyoto Encyclopedia of Genes and Genomes) pathways related to cell growth, cell death, genetic information processing, nucleotide metabolism, signal transduction, immune response, response to stimulus, cellular processes, ion homeostasis and transport and cofactors, vitamins, amino acids, energy, carbohydrates, drugs, lipids, and glycans. Transcriptogram analysis also provides significance metrics which allow us to prioritize further study of these pathways.

Conclusions: Transcriptogram analysis identifies novel pathways altered in ADPKD, providing new avenues to identify both ADPKD's mechanisms of pathogenesis and pharmaceutical targets to ameliorate the progression of the disease.

Keywords: Kidney, Transcriptogram, Cystic kidney disease, Autosomal dominant polycystic kidney disease, Bioinformatics, Pathway identification

Background

Autosomal dominant polycystic kidney disease (ADPKD) is a monogenic disorder associated with cystic renal disease, liver cysts, cardiac valve abnormalities, and berry aneurysms [1]. Progressive accumulation of renal cysts in ADPKD culminates in kidney failure, usually during the fifth or sixth decades of life. With a disease incidence of 1 in 800, ADPKD is one of the most common human genetic disorders. Despite extensive research, no Federal Drug Administration (FDA)-approved treatments prevent or delay disease progression, limiting patient treatment options to dialysis or kidney transplantation [2].

Two gene loci are responsible for ADPKD; HmPKD1 (human polycystic kidney disease gene 1) and HmPKD2 (human polycystic kidney disease gene 2) located on chromosomes 16 and 4, respectively. The gene products of these loci are polycystin-1 (PC-1) and polycystin-2 (PC-2), proteins that form a heteromeric complex in

* Correspondence: rbacalla@iupui.edu
[7]Division of Nephrology, Department of Medicine, Richard Roudebush VAMC and Indiana University School of Medicine, Indianapolis, IN 46202, USA
Full list of author information is available at the end of the article

primary cilium of renal cells [3–5]. Primary cilia are mechanically sensitive and serve as a flow sensor in renal tubular epithelia [6]. Due to the subcellular localization of polycystins, and the pleiotropic phenotypes associated with their mutations, Hildebrandt et al. called ADPKD the grandfather of ciliopathies [7].

Since ADPKD perturbs the Jnk/Stat (cJun N-terminal kinases/signal transducer and activator of transcription 1), MAPK (mitogen-activated protein kinase), mTOR (mammalian target of rapamycin), Wnt/Wgless (Wingless-related integration site/Wingless)and Erk (extracellular signal regulated kinase) kinase pathways [8], somatostatin analogues, vasopressin receptor antagonists, mTOR inhibitors, and statins have been tested for their ability to ameliorate the course of ADPKD. While mTOR inhibitors reduced cyst growth in murine polycystic kidney disease (PKD) models, they did not slow progression of renal impairment in human trials [9–11]. The FDA did not approve a recent vasopressin receptor antagonist, which inhibited cyst growth in several animal models of polycystic kidney disease, and slowed increases in total kidney volume and decreased estimated creatinine clearance in humans [12–14]. Because cyst formation in ADPKD begins in utero, drugs that can prevent initial cyst formation are not likely to be acceptable in a clinical setting [15, 16]. However, it is possible that the signaling pathways that initially drive cyst emergence are the unique entry points for treatment. We therefore concentrate on identifying the properties of ADPKD cells derived from normal nephrons and cysts from the same kidney to compare to kidney cells derived from an end-stage cystic kidney and normal human renal cortex. Our eventual goal would be to identify signaling pathways that provide a unique opening for targeted therapy in ADPKD.

The paucity of ADPKD drug candidates partially results from the difficulty in identifying pathways that promote cyst growth in renal cells but are not essential in other adult cell types. Standard gene-chip analysis of expressed mRNA shows that ADPKD perturbs Wnt/Wgless and Notch signaling [17, 18]. Decreased Notch signaling and mutated components in the Wnt pathway can cause renal cystic disease [18–20]. However, the Wnt/Wgless and Notch signaling pathways are essential to cell fate transitions and assignments in most cell types [21], so targeting these pathways would likely result in widespread and damaging bystander effects. Similarly, renal epithelial cells with an HmPKD1 mutation express many markers of immature cell differentiation, including increased proliferation rates, altered cell-ECM (extracellular matrix) adhesion, and increased apoptosis. However, most of these pathways are ubiquitous and thus not promising drug targets. To identify promising therapeutic targets, we need to compare expression patterns in cells from normal human renal cortex, normal nephrons in ADPKD patents, and in cysts from the same patients to identify pathways uniquely active in cystogenesis and not essential in other adult tissues. Identifying optimal drug targets also requires a coherent biological context that connects clusters of gene perturbations to the mechanisms of cyst formation, not just identification of individual perturbed genes in cystic ADPKD cells.

The de Almeida laboratory developed transcriptogram whole-genome gene expression data analysis to identify perturbed molecular networks and pathways more sensitively than conventional gene-chip analysis methods [22–24]. Transcriptogram analysis orders genes into a list using a Monte Carlo simulation that minimizes the distance within the list between associated gene products, so proximity in the list correlates with the degree of co-participation in biological processes. Calculating the average transcription level for genes within a moving window produces a transcriptogram profile which reveals any differentially expressed pathways. This robust statistical approach couples enhanced significance assessment with assessment of false discovery rates (FDRs). Transcriptogram analysis identifies rich sets of biological signaling interactions for later integrated hypothesis testing.

Results and discussion

We generated three different telomerase-immortalized cell lines, derived from isolates of (i) a normal kidney of a 57-year-old male (designated as normal cells, NK), (ii) non-cystic tissue from the kidney of a 36-year-old male (designated as non-cystic ADPKD cells, NC-ADPKD), and (iii) cystic tissue from the same donor (designated as cystic ADPKD cells, C-ADPKD). The additional ADPKD cell line in this paper is a previously characterized telomerase immortalized cell line isolated from an end-stage polycystic kidney [25]. We refer to the expression patterns of the NK cells as normal. We refer to expression of a gene or pathway in ADPKD, NC-ADPKD, or C-ADPKD cells as higher-than-normal if the expression level in those cells is significantly greater than in NK cells. Conversely, we refer to expression of a gene or pathway in ADPKD, NC-ADPKD, or C-ADPKD cells as lower-than-normal if the expression level in those cells is significantly lower than in NK cells. Differences between the NC-ADPKD and NK cells are particularly significant because they may identify early changes permissive for cyst formation in morphologically normal kidney tissue. We obtained microarray data for genome-wide gene expression for all cell lines in triplicate. We then analyzed the resulting data using three different, complementary methods: single gene expression analysis using QIAGEN's Ingenuity Pathway Analysis (IPA QIAGEN Redwood City), Gene Set Enrichment Analysis (GSEA) [26], and the transcriptogram method [22, 23, 27].

Mouse and human renal cells with aberrant polycystin-1 have impaired ciliary mechanosensation, and this impairment has been proposed as a cellular mechanism that promotes cystogenesis [28]. However, most cyst epithelia of human ADPKD kidneys express full-length polycystin-1 (PC-1) and polycystin-2 (PC-2) at normal or increased abundance [29–31]. Our PC-1 microarray data agrees with these observations (Fig. 1). Our microarray data show equal expression of PC-2 in NC-ADPKD and NK cells and reduced expression in C-ADPKD cells, a finding of uncertain significance.

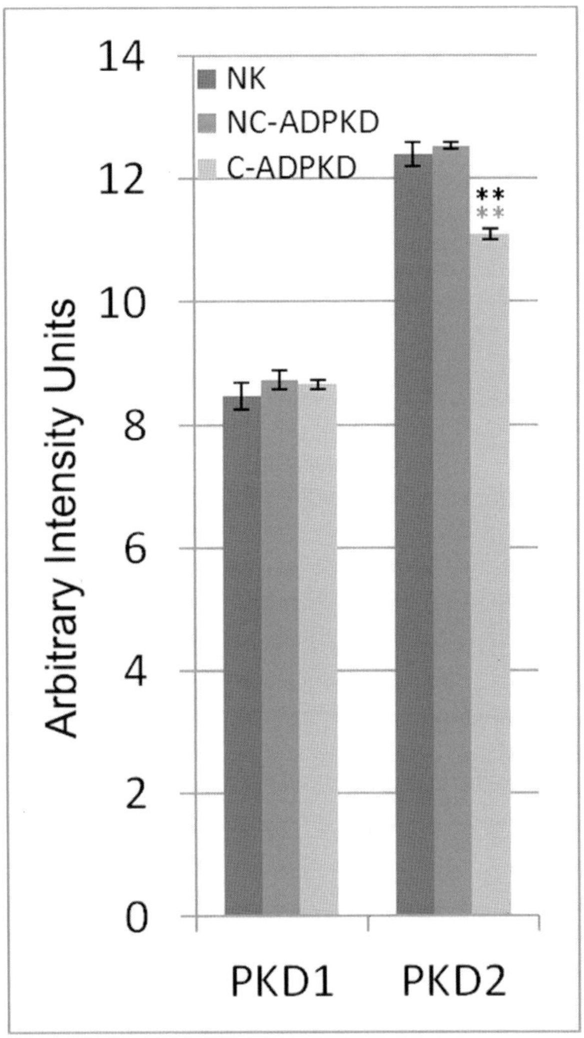

Fig. 1 PKD1 and PKD2 gene expression in the NK, NC-ADPKD, and C-ADPKD cells. PKD1 expression is not different from normal in the NC-ADPKD and C-ADPKD cells. PKD2 expression is normal in the NC-ADPKD cells but significantly lower than normal in C-ADPKD cells. Bars show mean ± s.e., $**p < 0.01$, $*p < 0.05$ (*black asterisk* is in comparison to NK, *gray asterisk* is in comparison to NC-ADPKD)

Volcano plots: single-gene analyses

Ingenuity pathway analysis scores each gene independently to create a list of all genes which change significantly in expression between two states. We averaged gene expression levels over the replicates for each cell line after normalization and compared cell lines by calculating the fold change (FC) as the ratio between the averages. We also obtained P values for each gene expressed. We present the results as Volcano plots (Fig. 2). Setting a significance threshold of FC > 2 and $P < 0.01$, we found 80 genes with significantly altered expression levels between the NK and NC-ADPKD cells, 968 genes with significantly altered expression levels between the NK and C-ADPKD cells, and 1182 genes with significantly altered expression levels between the C-ADPKD and NC-ADPKD cells (Additional file 1). These long lists of differentially expressed genes, by themselves, do not provide immediate insights into the biological mechanisms of ADPKD.

GSEA: Gene Set Enrichment Analyses

GSEA determines whether an a priori defined set of genes shows statistically significant, concordant differences between two biological states [26, 32, 33]. GSEA evaluates genome-wide expression profiles from cells belonging to two classes. We performed GSEA on the three pairs: NK versus NC-ADPKD cells, NK versus C-ADPKD cells, and NC-ADPKD versus C-ADPKD cells to identify differential expression in Kyoto Encyclopedia of Genes and Genomes (KEGG) pathways and in Gene Ontology: Biological Process (GO) terms. We set a significance threshold for the gene set permutation FDR <0.05. Table 1 summarizes the GSEA results and Table 2 lists all significantly altered KEGG pathway and GO term gene sets.

All GSEA-detected pathway differences between NK and NC-ADPKD cells related to 'metabolism' (We will use single '' to identify terms from GO and KEGG). GSEA-detected pathway differences between NK and C-ADPKD cells relate to 'chemokine signaling,' 'cell migration,' and 'cell-cell adhesion,' but not 'metabolism'. GSEA-detected pathway differences between NC-ADPKD and C-ADPKD cells relate to 'chemokine signaling,' 'cell migration,' and 'cell-cell adhesion' but not 'metabolism'. However, transcriptogram analyses (see below) show that expression of metabolome genes differs between these pairs as well, but too weakly for GSEA to detect, likely due to the competitive character of GSEA analysis [33].

Transcriptograms: genome-wide landscapes of gene expression

Transcriptograms project expression profiles onto a gene list that is ordered with genes belonging to the same KEGG pathway or GO term clustered in the list. We built an ordered list of 9684 genes (Additional file 2)

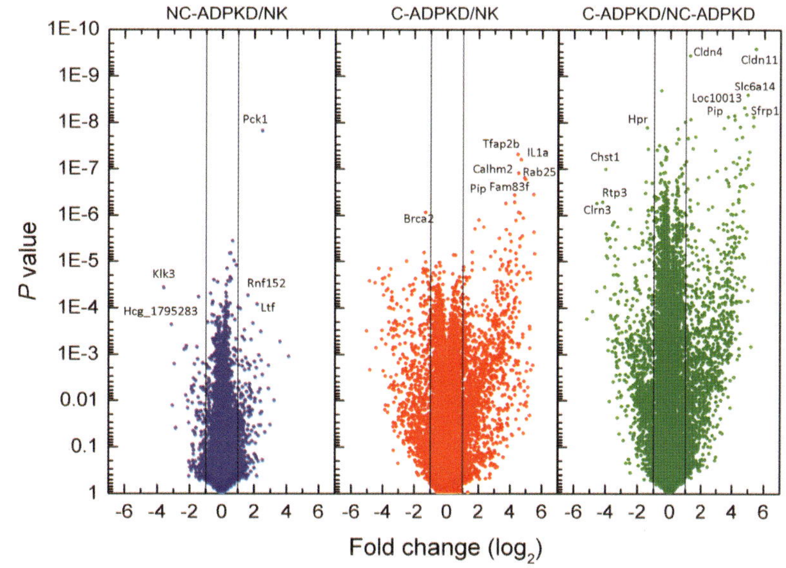

Fig. 2 Volcano plot of single gene analysis. Plots of log *P* value versus log$_2$ fold change for NC-ADPKD/NK, C-ADPKD/NK, and NC-ADPKD/C-ADPKD cells. The two *vertical lines* in each panel mark twofold change. *Labels* indicate representative genes with highly significant fold changes. See Additional file 1 for full lists of significantly changed genes

using a Monte Carlo Simulation that minimizes distances between associated gene products. Specifically, proximity in the list correlates with co-participation in biological processes, based on protein-protein association information available from the STRING database [34, 35]. Transcriptogram values then correspond to the average expression level of the genes located in a window of radius $r = 30$ (window size $2r + 1 = 61$) along the ordered list. Overlay of selected GO terms and KEGG pathways onto the ordered list then serves as a key to the biological correlates of expression differences and thus aids interpretation of transcriptograms of experimental

Table 1 GSEA analysis summary

GSEA summary for NC-ADPKD/NK						
Upregulated in		# gene sets	FDR < 0.25	FDR < 0.05	$P < 0.05$	$P < 0.01$
NK	KEGG	162	15	**5**	11	7
	GOBP	467	0	0	6	1
NC-ADPKD	KEGG	162	0	0	20	3
	GOBP	467	10	0	41	18
GSEA summary for C-ADPKD/NK						
Upregulated in		# gene sets	FDR < 0.25	FDR < 0.05	$P < 0.05$	$P < 0.01$
NK	KEGG	162	2	0	8	0
	GOBP	467	0	0	11	2
C-ADPKD	KEGG	162	15	**3**	17	12
	GOBP	467	1	**1**	46	13
GSEA summary for NC-ADPKD/C-ADPKD						
Upregulated in		# gene sets	FDR < 0.25	FDR < 0.05	$P < 0.05$	$P < 0.01$
NC-ADPKD	KEGG	162	11	0	10	4
	GOBP	467	17	0	24	13
C-ADPKD	KEGG	162	11	**4**	18	10
	GOBP	467	3	**1**	42	15

Numbers of gene sets that reach significance in comparisons of two GSEA classes, FDR < 0.05, are bold. *FDR* false discovery rate, *P* nominal *P* value, as described by Subramanian et al. 2005 [26]. GSEA expresses all differences as upregulation to minimize class bias due to the intrinsic asymmetry of the method

Table 2 KEGG pathways and GO terms identified as differentially expressed by GSEA analysis

	Size	ES	NES	Normal *P* value	FDR	FWER *P* value
NC-ADPKD/NK, upregulated in NK						
KEGG_drug_metabolism_cytochrome_p450	42	0.8	2.17	0	0	0
KEGG_metabolism_of xenobiotics_by_cytochrome p450	42	0.7	2.06	0	0	0.001
KEGG_histidine_metabolism	22	0.8	1.94	0	0.006	0.019
KEGG_glutathione_metabolism	38	0.7	1.86	0	0.013	0.049
KEGG_fatty_acid_metabolism	32	0.6	1.73	0.004	0.048	0.209
C-ADPKD/NK, upregulated in C-ADPKD						
KEGG_chemokine_signaling_pathway	144	−1	−1.73	0	0.01	0.011
KEGG_axon_guidance	99	−1	−1.68	0	0.03	0.066
KEGG_leukocyte_transendothelial_migration	86	−1	−1.66	0.001	0.028	0.092
GOBP_cell_cell_adhesion	48	0.8	1.8	0	0.001	0.001
NC-ADPKD/C-ADPKD, upregulated in C-ADPKD						
KEGG_leukocyte_transendothelial_migration	86	−1	−1.82	0	0	0
KEGG_chemokine_signaling_pathway	144	−1	−1.74	0	0.024	0.05
KEGG_tight_junction	101	−1	−1.73	0	0.02	0.063
KEGG_axon_guidance	99	−1	−1.73	0	0.016	0.066
GOBP_cell_cell_adhesion	48	0.8	1.8	0	0.007	0.008

Listing of KEGG pathways and GO terms with FDR < 5 %. GSEA expresses all differences as upregulation to minimize class bias due to the intrinsic asymmetry of the method

gene expression data (Fig. 3). The *x*-axis corresponds to the ordered gene list. Peaks represent regions of the list enriched with genes belonging to specific pathways or terms. We normalize the density profiles of term enrichment so that when all genes within a window participate in that pathway or term, the center point of that interval has a value of one. This paper presents transcriptograms as three-part panels, with the transcriptogram itself in the upper third of the panel, the *P* values for the transcriptogram in the middle third of the panel (with horizontal

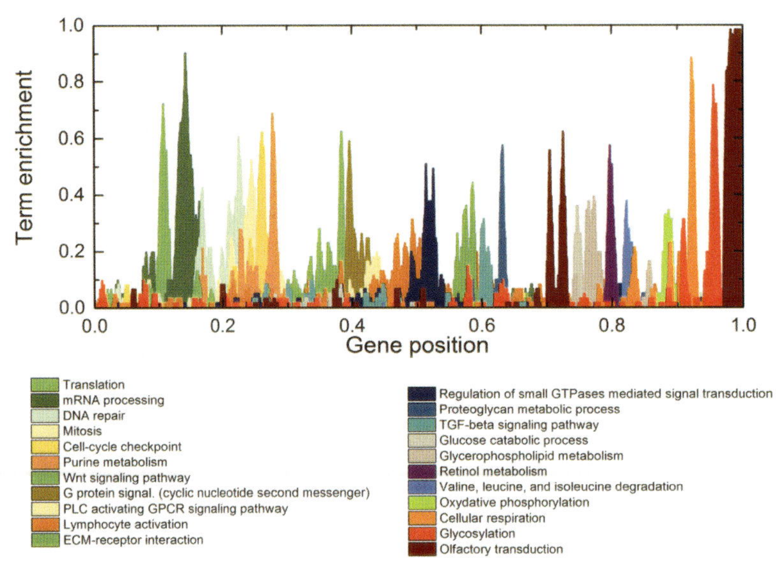

Fig. 3 Term enrichment map showing the correspondence between the ordered gene list and major biological terms and pathways. The *x*-axis indicates the relative position in the ordered list of 9684 genes. The colored profiles give the density distributions within the list of specific GO terms or KEGG pathways. A term enrichment value of 1 on the *y*-axis indicates that all genes in an interval of radius $r = 30$ participate in a given GO term or KEGG pathway. *Peaks* mark regions enriched with genes related to the term or pathway indicated in the legend. The legend orders the terms/pathways from left to right

lines indicating $p = 0.05$ and 0.01), and plots of peaks from the term enrichment density profile that correspond to significant peaks in the transcriptogram in the lower third of the panel. We calculated FDR values for all comparisons (Table 3).

Using transcriptogram analysis, we first compared the expression profiles of NK and NC-ADPKD samples (Fig. 4). Across most of the ordered list, the standard errors of the expression levels of genes for the NK and NC-ADPKD cells overlap, showing that gene expression levels of these genes in NC-ADPKD cells do not differ significantly from normal. However, gene positions between 0.22 and 0.26 and the intervals centered at positions 0.46 and 0.88 show significant differences ($P < 0.01$ and FDR < 0.12). The term enrichment profile shows that these significant peaks correspond to 'cell cycle,' 'locomotory behavior,' 'NOD (nucleotide-binding oligomerization domain)-like receptor signaling,' and 'Potassium ion transport' (Fig. 4). When we analyzed the gene lists from each interval of differential expression to identify additional pathways and terms, we found additional differentially expressed gene sets related to 'cell cycle,' 'nucleotide metabolism,' 'genetic information processing,' 'immune response,' and 'ion transport' (Figs. 7, 8, 9, 11, 13). We examined individual gene expression profiles from two of these pathways, 'NOD-like receptors' and 'potassium ion transport'. Genes differentially expressed at significant levels (Figs. 12a, 11b) may be potential targets for drug interventions to prevent or ameliorate very early stages of cyst growth.

Transcriptogram analysis comparing the NK and C-ADPKD samples (Fig. 5) detected additional regions of significant difference (where $P < 0.01$ and FDR < 0.12). The term enrichment profile shows that these significant peaks correspond to alterations in 'RNA processing,' 'cell cycle,' 'nucleic acid processing and metabolism,' 'G-protein signaling,' 'immune response,' and 'cell fate' related pathways including 'Calcium signaling' and 'JAK-STAT' pathways, 'wound healing,' 'extracellular matrix,' 'cell adhesion and tight junctions,' as well as energy-related gene sets for 'oxidative phosphorylation' and the 'TCA (tricarboxylic acid cycle) cycle,' and the 'drug-metabolism related cytochrome P450'. Analysis of the gene lists from each interval of differential expression identified additional related pathways and terms (Figs. 7, 8, 9, 10, 11, 12, 13, and 14). Overall, C-ADPKD cells have lower-than-normal metabolic rates and lower-than-normal expression levels of genes associated with 'cell proliferation,' 'RNA (ribonucleic acid) metabolism,' and 'sugar, lipid and energy metabolism'. Additionally, their interaction with the extracellular environment is strongly altered as indicated by enhanced expression of 'cell adhesion,' 'tight junction,' and 'cell surface signaling' pathways. Thus, C-ADPKD cells have abnormal interactions with their extracellular environment.

Table 3 False discovery rates

False discovery rates			
P value	NC-ADPKD/NK	C-ADPKD/NK	C-ADPKD/NC-ADPKD
0.1	0.131545	0.140392	0.0970966
0.05	0.137393	0.120033	0.0869387
0.01	0.100738	0.112763	0.0809876
0.005	0.100182	0.1156	0.0804989
0.001	0	0.106	0.0800862
0.0005	0	0	0.0800589
0.0001	0	0	0.08
5.00E−05	0	0	0.08

False discovery rates (FDR) for relative transcriptograms obtained using 500 sample-label permutations

Although cell cycle regulation is abnormal in both NC-ADPKD and C-ADPKD cells, expression of cell-cycle-related genes is higher-than-normal in NC-ADPKD samples and lower-than-normal in C-ADPKD samples. Additional pathways and terms identified from gene lists of the cell cycle or RNA metabolism-associated intervals (Figs. 7, 8, and 9) present a consistent pattern: expression in the NC-ADPKD sample is higher than normal and expression in C-ADPKD sample is lower than normal. This pattern of cell-cycle regulation disruption deserves future investigation since the genes included in this gene set initiate and regulate cell cycle progression making it difficult to predict the net effect on cell proliferation.

We then used transcriptogram analysis to compare NC-ADPKD and C-ADPKD samples (Fig. 6). Because NC-ADPKD and NK samples have very similar expression profiles (Fig. 4), the transcriptogram comparison of NC-ADPKD to C-ADPKD samples is similar to the transcriptogram comparison of NK to C-ADPKD samples. However, because NC-ADPKD and C-ADPKD samples derive from cystic and non-cystic tissues from the same kidney, standard errors and consequently, *P* values for this comparison are very small. However, the location of the most significant peaks and valleys are nearly identical in both comparisons. Many of the pathways and terms differentially expressed between NC-ADPKD and C-ADPKD samples (Figs. 6, 7, 8, 9, and 10) are also differentially expressed between NK and C-ADPKD samples.

Gene sets associated with significantly altered transcriptogram intervals

Transcriptogram values indicating significant differential expression do not directly refer to pathways or terms, but rather to intervals of the ordered list enriched with genes for specific pathways and terms. Therefore, subsequent to transcriptogram analysis (Figs. 3, 4, and 5), we fed the gene lists from each identified interval of differential expression into the publicly available David functional

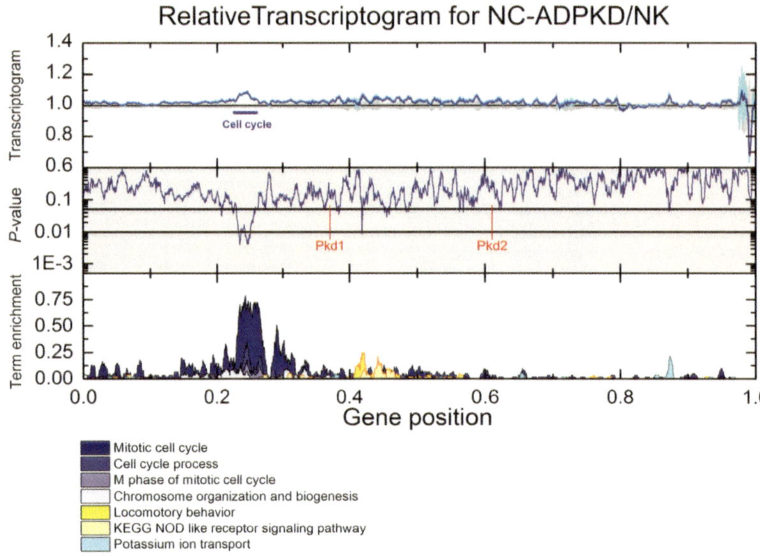

Fig. 4 Relative transcriptogram for NC-ADPKD/NK. The *x*-axis indicates the relative positon in the ordered list of 9684 genes. *Upper panel* the relative transcriptograms are presented as means ± s.e.m. with NC-ADPKD (*blue line ± cyan region*) and NK (*black line ± gray region*) given relative to NK. *Center panel* (*shaded gray*): *P* value from a two-tailed Weyl's *t* test is plotted for each point of the transcriptograms. *Horizontal lines* mark $P = 0.05$ and $P = 0.01$. Location in the ordered list of Pkd1 and Pkd2, the causative genes for ADPKD, is shown. *Lower panel* Term enrichment for transcriptogram regions with significantly changed expression. A term enrichment value of 1 on the *y*-axis indicates that all genes in an interval of radius $r = 30$ participate in a given GO term or KEGG pathway. As an example of how to read the relative transcriptogram figures, NC-ADPKD cells have higher-than-normal gene expression in the region of the peak labeled 'cell cycle' in the *upper panel* with a significance of $P < 0.01$ (*middle panel*). This region is enriched with genes associated with 'cell cycle' KEGG terms and GO pathways (marked with a *bar* and identified by referring to the *lower panel*, which shows term enrichment)

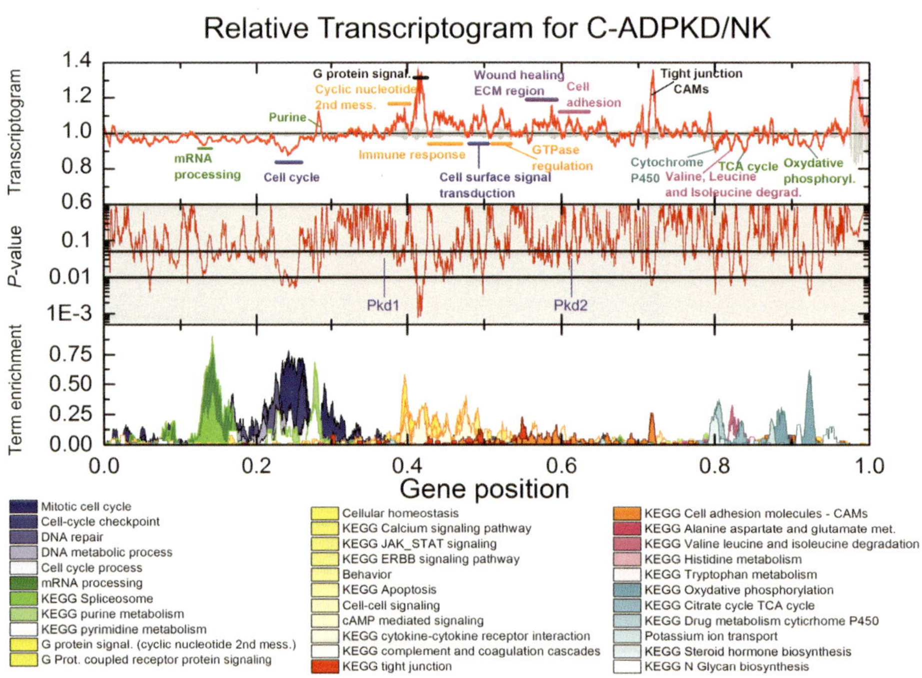

Fig. 5 Relative transcriptogram for C-ADPKD/NK. The *x*-axis indicates the relative position in the ordered list of 9684 genes. *Upper panel* We present the relative transcriptograms as means ± s.e.m. with C-ADPKD (*red line ± pink region*) and NK (*black line ± gray region*) given relative to NK. *Center panel* (*shaded gray*): *P* value from a two-tailed Weyl's *t* test for each point of the transcriptogram. *Horizontal lines* mark $P = 0.05$ and $P = 0.01$. We label the location in the ordered list of Pkd1 and Pkd2, the causative genes for ADPKD. *Lower panel* Term enrichment for transcriptogram regions with gene expression significantly different from normal. A term enrichment value of 1 on the y-axis indicates that all genes in an interval of radius $r = 30$ participate in a given GO term or KEGG pathway

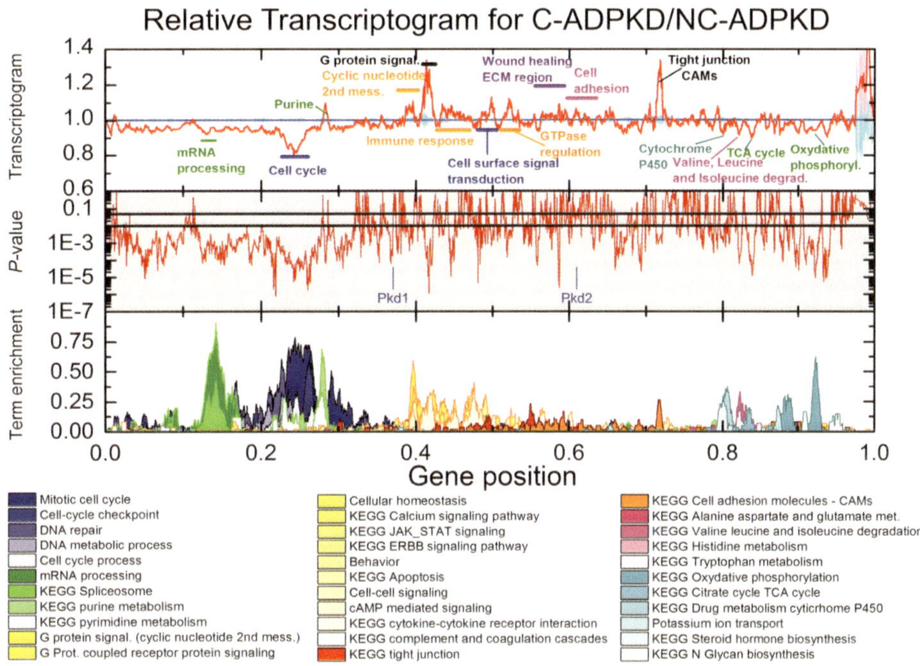

Fig. 6 Relative transcriptogram for C-ADPKD/NC-ADPKD. The *x*-axis indicates the relative positon in the ordered list of 9684 genes. *Upper panel* The relative transcriptograms are presented as means ± s.e.m. with C-ADPKD (red line ± pink region) and NC-ADPKD (blue line ± cyan region) relative to NC-ADPKD. Center panel (shaded gray): *P* value from a two tailed Weyl's *t* test for each point of the transcriptogram. Horizontal lines mark $P = 0.05$ and $P = 0.01$. We label the location in the ordered list of Pkd1 and Pkd2, the causative genes for ADPKD. Lower panel: Term enrichment for transcriptogram regions with gene expression significantly different from normal. A term enrichment value of 1 on the *y*-axis indicates that all genes in an interval of radius $r = 30$ participate in a given GO term or KEGG pathway. *P* values between C-ADPKD and NC-ADPKD cells are smaller than between either C-ADPKD or NC-ADPKD and NK cells (see Figs. 4 and 5) because C-ADPKD and NC-ADPKD cells were derived from the same individual, allowing us to discriminate additional differentially expressed regions

tools [36, 37] to identify additional KEGG pathways (pathways) and GO terms (terms) associated with those intervals. We then had to consider the differential expression of particular pathways and terms independently. For each of these pathways and terms, we calculated average expression levels and determined significance using Welch's two tail *t* test (Figs. 7, 8, 9, 10, 11, 12, 13, and 14). Finally, we categorized these pathways and terms according to the KEGG pathway map and GO term hierarchies, grouping together functionally overlapping pathways and terms from KEGG and GO.

Differentially regulated KEGG pathways and GO terms identified from gene set analyses

NC-ADPKD samples had higher-than-normal and C-ADPKD samples lower-than-normal expression of pathways and terms associated with 'cell proliferation' (Fig. 7). Both NC-ADPKD and C-ADPKD samples had higher-than-normal expression of 'cell-death-related' terms. These expanded results agree with the terms identified using the transcriptogram ordered gene list (Figs. 3, 4, and 5). Consistent with the changes seen in 'cell growth,' 'genetic information processing,' (Fig. 8) and 'amino acid metabolism' (Fig. 9), pathways and terms are higher than normal in NC-ADPKD samples and lower than normal in C-ADPKD samples. The one exception to this pattern, the KEGG 'ribosome pathway,' is higher than normal in both NC-ADPKD and C-ADPKD samples. These results suggest that treatments that target cell proliferation are likely to be effective in patients in which cysts have not yet begun to form and ineffective in patients with significant cyst formation. Pathways and terms with abnormal expression in NC-ADPKD samples pique our interest because changes that occur before cysts form have the greatest potential as targets for amelioration of cyst formation.

Conventional gene chip analysis has not identified pathways that explained the cell de-differentiation observed in cystic cells [38, 39]. Our analysis has revealed a group of signal transduction pathways and terms that are abnormal in ADPKD (Fig. 10). Both NC-ADPKD and C-ADPKD samples have higher-than-normal expression of most signal-transduction pathways. Elevated 'cyclic nucleotide related' pathways are not surprising, given cyclic AMP's role in promoting cyst expansion [40, 41]. Both NC-ADPKD and C-ADPKD samples have higher-than-normal expression of Wnt and Notch pathways, which enhance proliferation, increase resistance to apoptosis

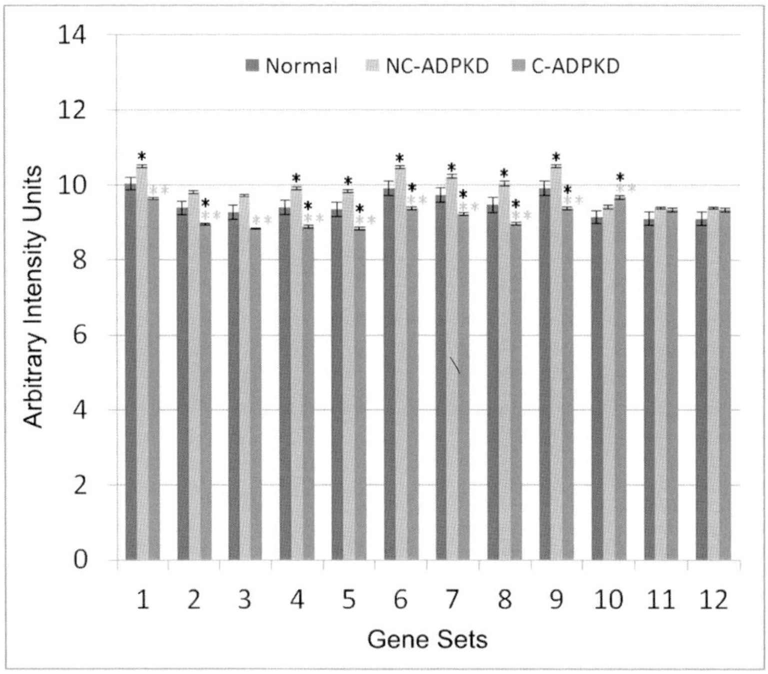

Fig. 7 Both cell growth and cell death are altered in ADPKD. NC-ADPKD cells have higher-than-normal expression and C-ADPKD cells have lower-than-normal expression of genes from 'cell growth' gene sets. Both NC-ADPKD and C-ADPKD cells have higher-than-normal expression of genes from 'cell death' gene sets. We present data as mean ± s.e.m., $^{**}P < 0.01$, $^{*}P < 0.05$ (*black asterisk* is in comparison to NK, *gray asterisk* is in comparison to NC-ADPKD). *Cell Growth Gene Sets:* (1) KEGG_CELL_CYCLE, (2) CELL_CYCLE, (3) CELL_CYCLE_CHECKPOINT, (4) CELL_CYCLE_PROCESS, (5) CELL_CYCLE_PHASE, (6) MITOTIC_M_PHASE, (7) MITOTIC_CELL_CYCLE, (8) M_PHASE, (9) MITOSIS. *Cell Death Gene Sets:* (10) KEGG_APOPTOSIS, (11) APOPTOTIC_PROCESS, (12) PROGRAMMED_CELL_DEATH

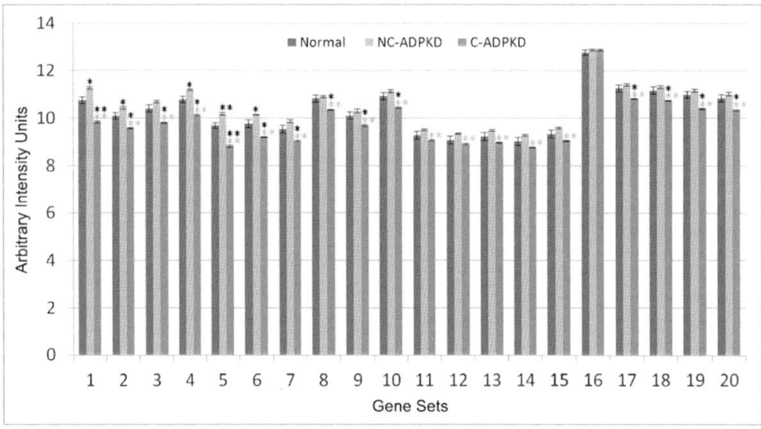

Fig. 8 Genetic information processing is altered in ADPKD. NC-ADPKD cells have higher-than-normal expression and C-ADPKD cells have lower-than-normal expression of genes from all 'Genetic information processing' gene sets except the KEGG ribosome gene set. We present data as mean ± s.e.m., $^{**}P < 0.01$, $^{*}P < 0.05$ (*black asterisk* is in comparison to NK, *gray asterisk* is in comparison to NC-ADPKD). *Genetic Information Processing Gene Sets:* (1) KEGG_DNA_REPLICATION, (2) KEGG_BASE_EXCISION_REPAIR, (3) KEGG_NUCLEOTIDE_EXCISION_REPAIR, (4) KEGG_MISMATCH_REPAIR, (5) KEGG_HOMOLOGOUS_RECOMBINATION, (6) DNA_REPLICATION, (7) DNA_REPAIR, (8) KEGG_RNA_POLYMERASE, (9) KEGG_BASAL_TRANSCRIPTION_FACTORS, (10) KEGG_SPLICEOSOME, (11) TRANSCRIPTION, (12) REGULATION_OF_TRANSCRIPTION, (13) TRANSCRIPTION_DNA_DEPENDENT, (14) REGULATION_OF_TRANSCRIPTION_DNA_DEPENDENT, (15) TRANSCRIPTION_FROM_RNA_POLYMERASE_II_PROMOTER, (16) KEGG_RIBOSOME, (17) RIBONUCLEOPROTEIN_COMPLEX_BIOGENESIS_AND_ASSEMBLY, (18) PROTEIN_RNA_COMPLEX_ASSEMBLY, (19) MRNA_PROCESSING_GO_0006397, (20) RNA_SPLICING_VIA_TRANSESTERIFICATION_REACTIONS

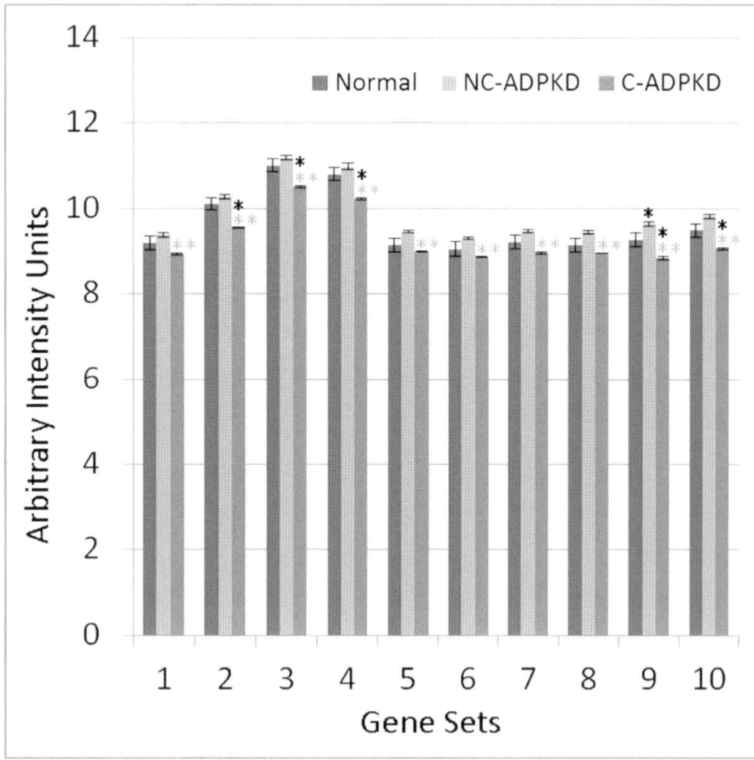

Fig. 9 Nucleotide metabolism is abnormal in ADPKD. NC-ADPKD cells have higher-than-normal expression and C-ADPKD cells have lower-than-normal expression of genes from all 'Nucleotide Metabolism' gene sets. We present data as mean ± s.e.m., $^{**}P < 0.01$, $^{*}P < 0.05$ (*black asterisk* is in comparison to NK, *gray asterisk* is in comparison to NC-ADPKD). *Nucleotide Metabolism Gene Sets:* (1) KEGG_PURINE_METABOLISM, (2) KEGG_PYRIMIDINE_METABOLISM, (3) RNA_SPLICING, (4) MRNA_METABOLIC_PROCESS, (5) NEGATIVE_REGULATION_OF_TRANSCRIPTION, (6) REGULATION OF NUCLEOBASE_NUCLEOSIDE_NUCLEOTIDE_AND_NUCLEIC_ACID_METABOLIC_PROCESS, (7) RNA_BIOSYNTHETIC_PROCESS, (8) NEGATIVE_REGULATION_OF NUCLEOBASE_NUCLEOSIDE_NUCLEOTIDE_AND_NUCLEIC_ACID_METABOLIC_PROCESS, (9) CHROMOSOME_ORGANIZATION_AND_BIOGENESIS, (10) DNA_METABOLIC_PROCESS

and inhibit differentiation of epithelial cells [42]. The excess expression is greater in NC-ADPKD than in C-ADPKD samples, again suggesting possible targets for prevention of cyst initiation.

Chronic non-resolving inflammation accompanies cyst accumulation in ADPKD [43]. Our analysis identified multiple 'immune response' pathways with abnormal expression (Fig. 11). All but one of the identified 'immune response' pathways had higher-than-normal expression in NC-ADPKD samples and further increased expression in C-ADPKD samples, consistent with increased inflammatory response as cysts accumulate. Notably, the morphologically normal NC-ADPKD-derived cells already showed higher-than-normal expression of 'immune response' pathways, suggesting that components of the immune response could provide targets to ameliorate the progression of ADPKD. An exception to this pattern was the lower-than-normal expression of the KEGG 'complement and coagulation' pathway in C-ADPKD samples.

'Response-to-stimulus' gene groups are overexpressed in kidney carcinoma [44]. Our analysis identifies multiple 'response-to-stimulus' terms with increased expression in ADPKD (Fig. 12), suggesting mechanistic similarities between PKD and kidney carcinoma [45]. All but one of the identified 'response-to-stimulus' terms had higher-than-normal expression in NC-ADPKD samples and further increased expression in C-ADPKD samples. In C-ADPKD samples, expression of 'response-to-endogenous-stimulus' genes was lower than normal and also lower than in NC-ADPKD samples.

Establishment and maintenance of epithelial cell polarity are prerequisites for normal function of all epithelial organs. Epithelia depend on cell adhesion molecules to adapt and respond to mechanical forces and cell density, while tight junctions control diffusion across the epithelial layer. Transcriptogram analysis shows that both NC-ADPKD and C-ADPKD cells have higher-than-normal expression of genes in the 'cell-adhesion-molecule' and 'tight-junction' KEGG pathways (Fig. 12). Nephron segments differentially express multiple tight-junction proteins which may determine segment specific paracellular permeability [46]. ADPKD cyst epithelia express claudin-7 in an abnormal distribution on the apical and basolateral membrane [47]. Decreased presence of strong E-cadherin

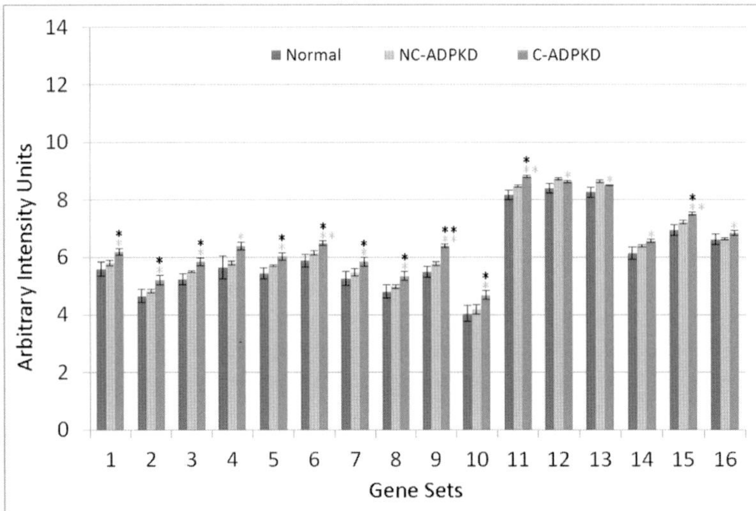

Fig. 10 ADPKD upregulates signal transduction. NC-ADPKD and C-ADPKD cells have higher-than-normal expression of genes from all signal transduction gene sets. Expression levels in NC-ADPKD cells are intermediate between those of NK and C-ADPKD cells, exception that expression levels of Wnt and Notch signaling pathways are higher in NC-ADPKD cells. These pathways are normally active primarily during embryonic development. We present data as mean ± s.e.m., $^{**}P < 0.01$, $^{*}P < 0.05$ (*black asterisk* is in comparison to NK, *gray asterisk* is in comparison to NC-ADPKD). *Signal Transduction Gene Sets:* (1) G_PROT._COUPLED_RECEPTOR_PROTEIN_SIGNALING, (2) G_PROT._SIGNALING_COUPLED_TO_CYCLIC_NUCLEOTIDE_2ND_MESS, (3) G_PROT._SIGNALING_COUPLED_TO_CAMP_NUCLEOTIDE_2ND_MESS, (4) G_PROT._SIGNALING_ADENYLATE_CYCLASE_ACTIVATING, (5) CAMP_MEDIATED_SIGNALING, (6) CELL_CELL_SIGNALING, (7) SYNAPTIC_TRANSMISSION, (8) CYCLIC_NUCLEOTIDE_MEDIATED_SIGNALING, (9) KEGG_CYTOKINE_CYTOKINE_RECEPTOR_INTERACTION, (10) KEGG_NEUROACTIVE_LIGAND_RECEPTOR_INTERACTION, (11) KEGG_ERBB_SIGNALING_PATHWAY, (12) KEGG_WNT_SIGNALING_PATHWAY, (13) KEGG_NOTCH_SIGNALING_PATHWAY, (14) KEGG_CALCIUM_SIGNALING_PATHWAY, (15) KEGG_JAK_STAT_SIGNALING_PATHWAY, (16) KEGG_ABC_TRANSPORTERS

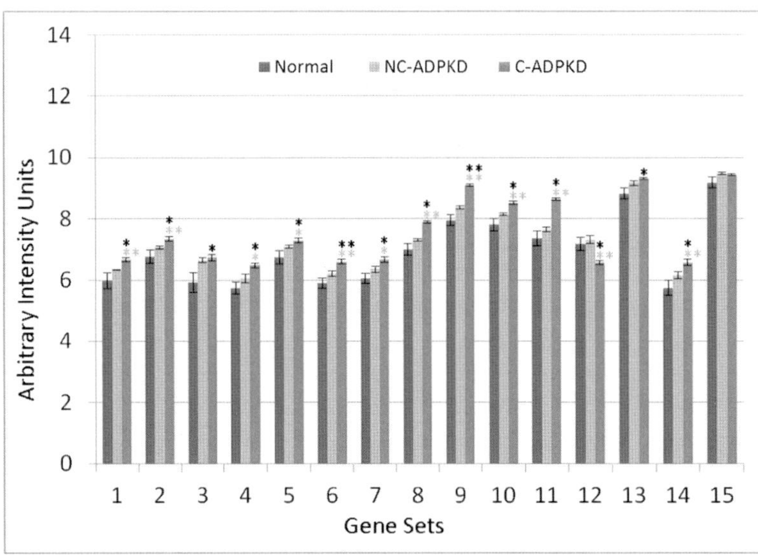

Fig. 11 Immune response is abnormal in ADPKD. NC-ADPKD and C-ADPKD cells both express higher-than-normal levels of genes from 'immune response' gene sets, exception that C-ADPKD cells have lower-than-normal expression of the KEGG 'Complement and Coagulation cascade' gene set (12). We present data as mean ± s.e.m., $^{**}P < 0.01$, $^{*}P < 0.05$ (*black asterisk* is in comparison to NK, *gray asterisk* is in comparison to NC-ADPKD). *Immune Response Gene Sets:* (1) INFLAMMATORY_RESPONSE, (2) IMMUNE_RESPONSE, (3) HUMORAL_IMMUNE_RESPONSE, (4) CELL_ACTIVATION, (5) IMMUNE_SYSTEM_PROCESS, (6) LEUKOCYTE_ACTIVATION, (7) LYMPHOCYTE_ACTIVATION, (8) KEGG_CHEMOKINE_SIGNALING_PATHWAY, (9) KEGG_NOD_LIKE_RECEPTOR_SIGNALING_PATHWAY, (10) KEGG_T_CELL_RECEPTOR_SIGNALING_PATHWAY, (11) KEGG_LEUKOCYTE_TRANSENDOTHELIAL_MIGRATION, (12) KEGG_COMPLEMENT_AND_COAGULATION_CASCADES, (13) KEGG_CYTOSOLIC_DNA_SENSING_PATHWAY, (14) KEGG_HEMATOPOIETIC_CELL_LINEAGE, (15) KEGG_FC_GAMMA_R_MEDIATED_PHAGOCYTOSIS

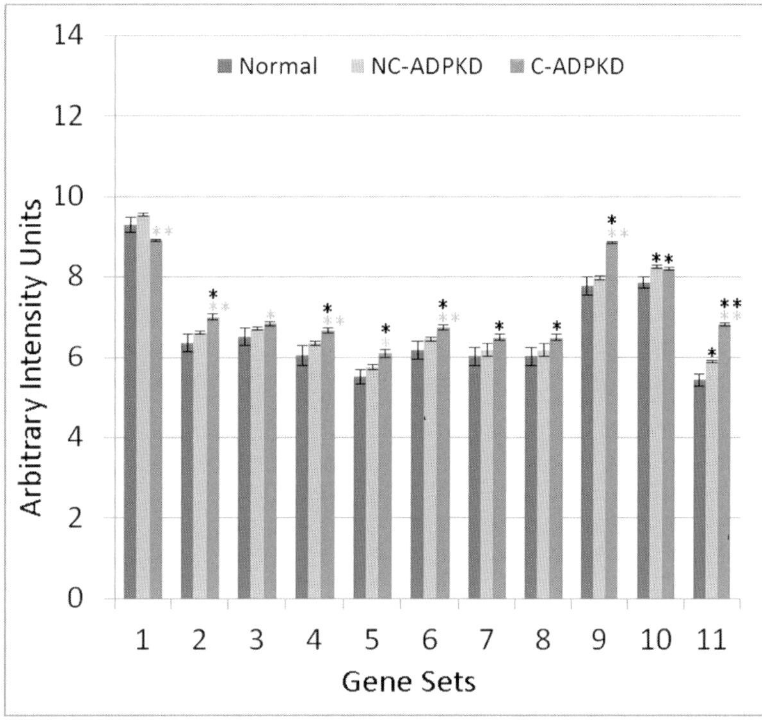

Fig. 12 Response to stimulus and cellular processes are abnormal in ADPKD. Both NC-ADPKD and C-ADPKD cells have higher-than-normal expression of genes in the 'response to stimulus' gene sets (1–8), except that C-ADPKD cells have lower-than-normal expression of genes in the 'response to endogenous stimulus' gene set. C-ADPKD cells have higher-than-normal expression of genes in the 'cellular processes' gene sets (9–11). Data are represented as mean ± s.e.m., $^{**}P < 0.01$, $^{*}P < 0.05$ (*black asterisk* is in comparison to NK, *gray asterisk* is in comparison to NC-ADPKD). *Response to Stimulus Gene Sets:* (1) RESPONSE_TO_ENDOGENOUS_STIMULUS, (2) RESPONSE_TO_EXTERNAL_STIMULUS, (3) REGULATION_OF_RESPONSE_TO_STIMULUS, (4) DEFENSE_RESPONSE, (5) CELLULAR_DEFENSE_RESPONSE, (6) RESPONSE_TO_WOUNDING, (7) COAGULATION, (8) BLOOD_COAGULATION. *Cellular Processes Gene Sets:* (9) KEGG_TIGHT_JUNCTION, (10) KEGG_GAP_JUNCTION, (11) LOCOMOTORY_BEHAVIOR

adhesion molecules on the tubule cell surface, accompanied by upregulation of weaker cell-cell adhesion by N-cadherin and cadherin-8 are also known components of ADPKD [48, 49]. This lower-than-normal cell-cell adhesion accompanies higher-than-normal expression of cell motility terms, both hallmarks of epithelial to mesenchymal transition and cellular de-differentiation.

Defects in urine concentration are a well-established component of ADPKD [50]. NC-ADPKD samples had slightly higher-than-normal and C-ADPKD samples had significantly lower-than-normal expression of 'vasopressin-regulated water reabsorption' [51] and 'proximal tubule bicarbonate reclamation' [52] pathways (Fig. 13).

ADPKD causes widespread disruptions of metabolism (Fig. 14). Of the metabolic pathways and terms identified, 'cofactor and vitamin metabolism' and 'amino acid and energy metabolism' were all decreased in C-ADPKD samples. 'Carbohydrate, drug, lipid and glycan metabolism' pathways were lower than normal in C-ADPKD samples with the exception of 'fructose and mannose,' 'galactose,' and 'amino sugar and nucleotide sugar metabolism'. 'Drug metabolism cytochrome P450' pathway expression levels were lower than normal in both NC-ADPKD and C-ADPKD samples. 'Lipid metabolism' pathway expression was significantly abnormal, but with mixed expression effects. 'Glycan metabolism' pathway expression was slightly higher than normal in NC-ADPKD samples and lower than normal in C-ADPKD samples.

The differential expression of pathways and terms (Figs. 7, 8, 9, 10, 11, 12, 13, and 14) in the gene sets associated with significantly altered transcriptogram intervals (Figs. 4, 5, and 6) provides strong evidence that:

1) 'Proliferation,' 'genetic information processing,' and 'nucleotide metabolism' pathways and terms are higher-than-normal in NC-ADPKD and lower-than-normal in C-ADPKD, while 'apoptosis' is higher-than-normal in both NC-ADPKD and C-ADPKD.
2) 'Immune response' pathways and terms overall are upregulated in both NC-ADPKD and C-ADPKD.
3) Changes in 'signal transduction' and 'cellular process' pathways are consistent with de-differentiation of epithelial cells in ADPKD.
4) 'Metabolism' pathways and terms overall are downregulated in ADPKD.

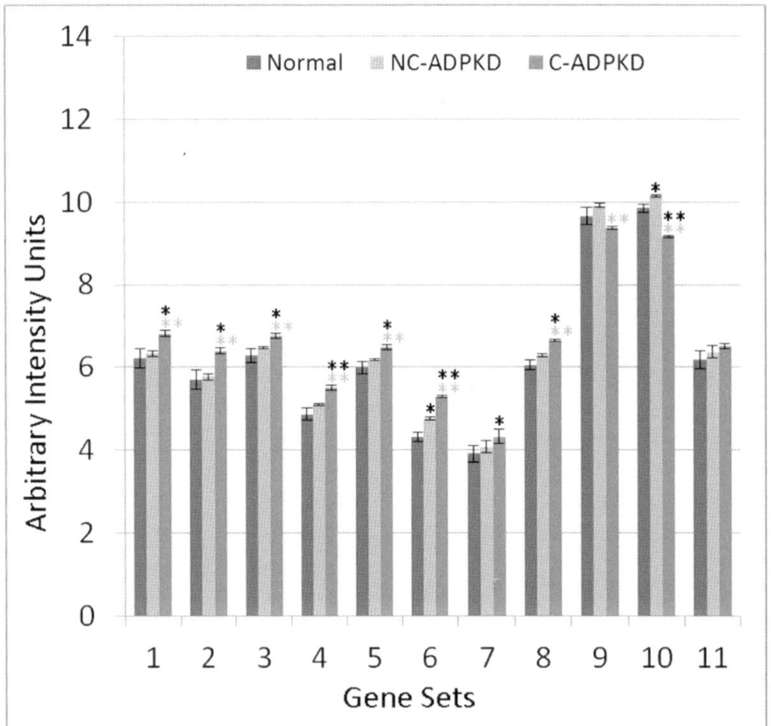

Fig. 13 Ion homeostasis and transport are abnormal in ADPKD. NC-ADPKD cells have higher-than-normal and C-ADPKD cells have much higher-than-normal expression of genes in 'ion homeostasis' gene sets (1–8). NC-ADPKD cells have higher-than-normal expression of genes in 'transport' gene sets (9–11). We represent data as mean ± s.e.m, $^{**}P < 0.01$, $^{*}P < 0.05$ (*black asterisk* is in comparison to NK, *gray asterisk* is in comparison to NC-ADPKD). *Ion Homeostasis Gene Sets:* (1) ION_HOMEOSTASIS, (2) CELLULAR_CATION_HOMEOSTASIS, (3) ION_TRANSPORT, (4) METAL_ION_TRANSPORT, (5) CATION_TRANSPORT, (6) POTASSIUM_ION_TRANSPORT, (7) CALCIUM_ION_TRANSPORT, (8) MONOVALENT_INORGANIC_CATION_TRANSPORT. *Transport Gene Sets:* (9) KEGG_VASOPRESSIN_REGULATED_WATER_REABSORPTION, (10) KEGG_PROXIMAL_TUBULE_BICARBONATE_RECLAMATION, (11) REGULATION_OF_BODY_FLUID_LEVELS

We therefore posit that genes from the pathways and terms that are uniquely altered in NC-ADPKD samples (e.g., before cysts have formed) have the greatest potential as drug targets for ameliorating cyst formation.

Finding individual candidate genes

We next examine the expression levels of the individual genes (Fig. 15) in selected pathways and terms which transcriptogram analysis identifies as differentially expressed at a significant level (Figs. 7, 8, 9, 10, 11, 12, 13 and 14). Selection of pathways and terms for further examination was based on significance level and relevance to the existing literature. These genes likely play key roles in development of ADPKD and are thus potential targets for drug therapies to prevent or delay ADPKD. Figure 15 shows the levels of expression of individual genes from three pathways and terms, 'Nod-like receptor signaling' a term from 'immune response,' 'potassium ion transport' a term from 'ion homeostasis,' and 'oxidative phosphorylation' a term from 'energy metabolism'. We then confirmed expression levels of individual genes in these pathways and terms using qRT-PCR (Additional file 3).

The intracellular NOD-like receptor (NLR) family plays a central role in regulation of the innate immune response. The NLRs NOD1 and NOD2 sense bacterial peptidoglycan fragments and respond by stimulating the activation of NF-κB (nuclear factor kappa beta) and MAPK, cytokine production, and apoptosis. The NLRs NALP1 (NLR-pyrin containing), NALP3 and Ipaf activate caspase-1 through inflammasomes, which generate pro-inflammatory cytokines. NOD-like receptor signaling contributes to multiple renal diseases with inflammatory components, including ureteric obstruction, ischemia reperfusion injury, glomerulonephritis, sepsis, hypoxia, glycerol-induced renal failure, and crystal nephropathy [53–55]. However, neither the Volcano plots nor GSEA analysis found abnormal activity of NOD-like receptor signaling in ADPKD cells. We examined expression of the 20 individual genes involved in the KEGG 'NOD-like receptor signaling' pathway (Fig. 15a) that were present in our microarrays. In NC-ADPKD cells, all but one of the 20 NOD-like receptor signaling genes had higher-than-normal expression (Fig. 15a), suggesting that that reducing NOD-like receptor signaling early in ADPKD might ameliorate the progression of the disease. C-ADPKD cells

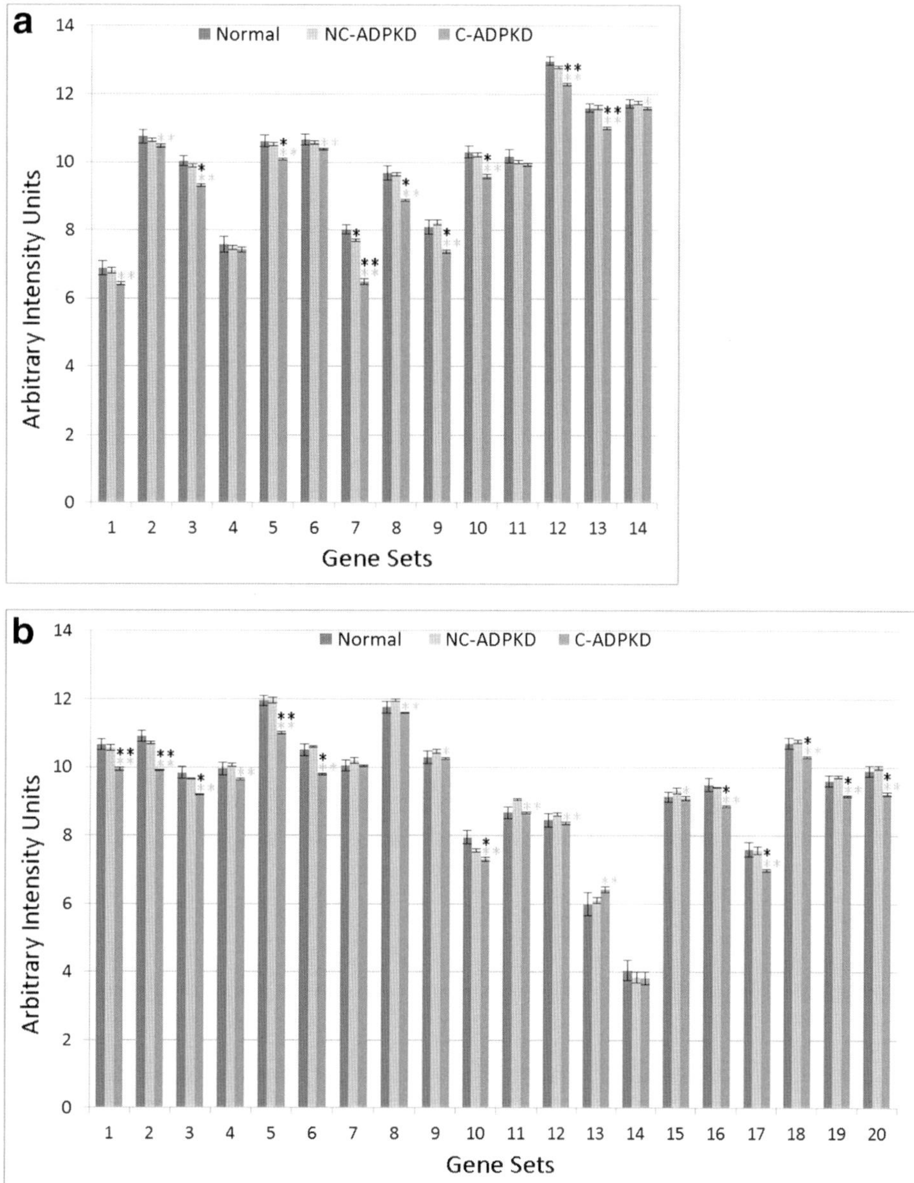

Fig. 14 (See legend on next page.)

(See figure on previous page.)

Fig. 14 ADPKD broadly perturbs metabolism. **a** Cofactor and vitamin, amino acid, and energy metabolism and **b** carbohydrate, drug, lipid, and glycan metabolism. C-ADPKD cells have lower-than-normal expression of genes in 'cofactor and vitamin' gene sets (A1-2) compared to both NK and NC-ADPKD cells. Both NC-ADPKD and C-ADPKD cells have lower-than-normal expression of genes in 'amino acid' gene sets (A3-11). C-ADPKD cells have lower-than-normal expression of genes in 'energy metabolism' gene sets (A12-14). C-ADPKD cells have lower-than-normal expression of genes in all 'carbohydrate metabolism' gene sets (B1-9) except for the KEGG 'histidine metabolism' gene set. C-ADPKD cells have lower-than-normal expression of genes in the 'drug metabolism' gene set (B10). C-ADPKD cells have lower-than-normal expression of genes in all 'lipid metabolism' (B11-18) gene sets except for the KEGG 'arachidonic acid metabolism' gene set (B13). C-ADPKD cells have lower-than-normal expression of genes in 'glycan metabolism' gene sets (B19-20). We present data as mean ± s.e.m., $^{**}P < 0.01$, $^{*}P < 0.05$ (*black asterisk* is in comparison to NK, *gray asterisk* is in comparison to NC-ADPKD). **a** Cofactor and vitamin, amino acid, and energy metabolism gene sets. *Cofactor and Vitamin Gene Sets:* (1) KEGG_RETINOL_METABOLISM, (2) KEGG_PORPHYRIN_AND_CHLOROPHYLL_METABOLISM. *Amino Acid Metabolism Gene Sets:* (3) KEGG_ALANINE_ASPARTATE_AND_GLUTAMATE_METABOLISM, (4) KEGG_GLYCINE_SERINE_AND_THREONINE_METABOLISM, (5) KEGG_VALINE_LEUCINE_AND_ISOLEUCINE_DEGRADATION, (6) KEGG_ARGININE_AND_PROLINE_METABOLISM, (7) KEGG_HISTIDINE_METABOLISM, (8) KEGG_TRYPTOPHAN_METABOLISM, (9) KEGG_BETA_ALANINE_METABOLISM, (10) KEGG_SELENOAMINO_ACID_METABOLISM, (11) KEGG_GLUTATHIONE_METABOLISM. *Energy Metabolism Gene Sets:* (12) KEGG_OXIDATIVE_PHOSPHORYLATION, (13) MITOCHONDRIAL_TRANSPORT, (14) MITOCHONDRION_ORGANIZATION_AND_BIOGENESIS. **b** Carbohydrate, drug, lipid and glycan metabolism gene sets. *Carbohydrate Metabolism Gene Sets:* (1) KEGG_GLYOXYLATE_AND_DICARBOXYLATE_METABOLISM, (2) KEGG_PROPANOATE_METABOLISM, (3) KEGG_BUTANOATE_METABOLISM (4) KEGG_GLYCOLYSIS_GLUCONEOGENESIS, (5) KEGG_CITRATE_CYCLE_TCA_CYCLE, (6) KEGG_PYRUVATE_METABOLISM, (7) KEGG_FRUCTOSE_AND_MANNOSE_METABOLISM, (8) KEGG_GALACTOSE_METABOLISM, (9) KEGG_AMINO_SUGAR_AND_NUCLEOTIDE_SUGAR_METABOLISM. *Drug Metabolism Gene Sets;* (10) KEGG_DRUG_METABOLISM_CYTOCHROME_P450. *Lipid Metabolism Gene Sets:* (11) KEGG_GLYCEROLIPID_METABOLISM, (12) KEGG_GLYCEROPHOSPHOLIPID_METABOLISM, (13) KEGG_ARACHIDONIC_ACID_METABOLISM, (14) KEGG_LINOLEIC_ACID_METABOLISM, (15) KEGG_SPHINGOLIPID_METABOLISM, (16) KEGG_FATTY_ACID_METABOLISM, (17) KEGG_STEROID_HORMONE_BIOSYNTHESIS, (18) PHOSPHOLIPID_BIOSYNTHETIC_PROCESS. *Glycan Metabolism Gene Sets:* (19) KEGG_N_GLYCAN_BIOSYNTHESIS, (20) KEGG_GLYCOSYLPHOSPHATIDYLINOSITOL_GPI_ANCHOR_BIOSYNTHESIS

also had higher-than-normal expression levels of several of these genes, including tumor necrosis factor (TNF). TNF blockers are an approved treatment for debilitating chronic inflammatory diseases, in particular rheumatoid arthritis (RA) so tumor necrosis factor (TNF) blockers specifically and NOD-like receptor signaling blockers in general may be worth testing for treatment of ADPKD. Even if they do not slow cyst progression, they may reduce the chronic pain associated with inflammatory diseases like ADPKD.

The kidney is the primary regulator of total body potassium content. Maintenance of proper levels and distribution of potassium across the cell membrane is critical for normal cell function [56]. Further, potassium channels are critical for cAMP-dependent chloride secretion and cyst growth in ADPKD [57]. We examined expression of the 11 individual genes in our microarrays with the GO 'potassium ion transport' label (Fig. 15c). Our analysis revealed changes of expression of 'potassium ion transport' as a category and of individual genes within that category, which neither Volcano plotting or GSEA analysis was able to identify.

$Pkd1^{-/-}$ cells and kidneys from cystic mice preferentially rely on aerobic glycolysis for their energy demands, a metabolic switch similar to the Warburg effect in cancer cells [58]. Our analysis revealed changes in pathways and terms related to 'energy metabolism' that conventional volcano and GSEA analysis missed. We examined expression of the 20 individual genes in the KEGG 'oxidative phosphorylation' pathway (Fig. 15b) that were present in our microarrays. Expression of all oxidative phosphorylation related genes was significantly lower than normal in both C-ADPKD and NC-ADPKD samples, with greater reduction in C-ADPKD samples. Volcano plotting also identified phosphoenolpyruvate carboxy-kinase 1 (Pck1) as significantly differentially expressed (Fig. 1); the Pck1 enzyme is a main control point for the regulation of gluconeogenesis. Pck1 expression in NC-ADPKD samples is 5.58 times higher than normal ($p = 1.54 \times 10^{-8}$) and is 0.58 times lower than normal (not significant) in C-ADPKD samples.

Discussion

In this communication, we compare gene expression profiles between a paired age and sex-matched pair of telomerase immortalized human cell lines (NK and PKD). A second grouped pair of immortalized human cell lines (NC-ADPKD and C-ADPKD) was derived from renal cysts and normal appearing nephrons from the same human male polycystic kidney. The choice to use immortalized cell lines as the source material to isolate RNA was based on our prior unsuccessful attempts to obtain good-quality RNA from polycystic kidneys. Due to their large size and the need to cross clamp the kidneys at the renal pedicle, we obtained poor-quality RNA isolated from the nephrectomy specimen likely because of prolonged warm ischemia time. While the use of cell lines allowed us to eliminate the issue of RNA degradation, it also brings forward the question as to how generalizable is the data presented in this communication. In our review, the group that solved the problem of obtaining high-quality RNA from polycystic kidney surgical specimens was Song et al. [17]. Our preliminary analysis of that data set using the transcriptogram approach shows a close concordance between our data and Song's data. This comparison will be the subject of a future communication.

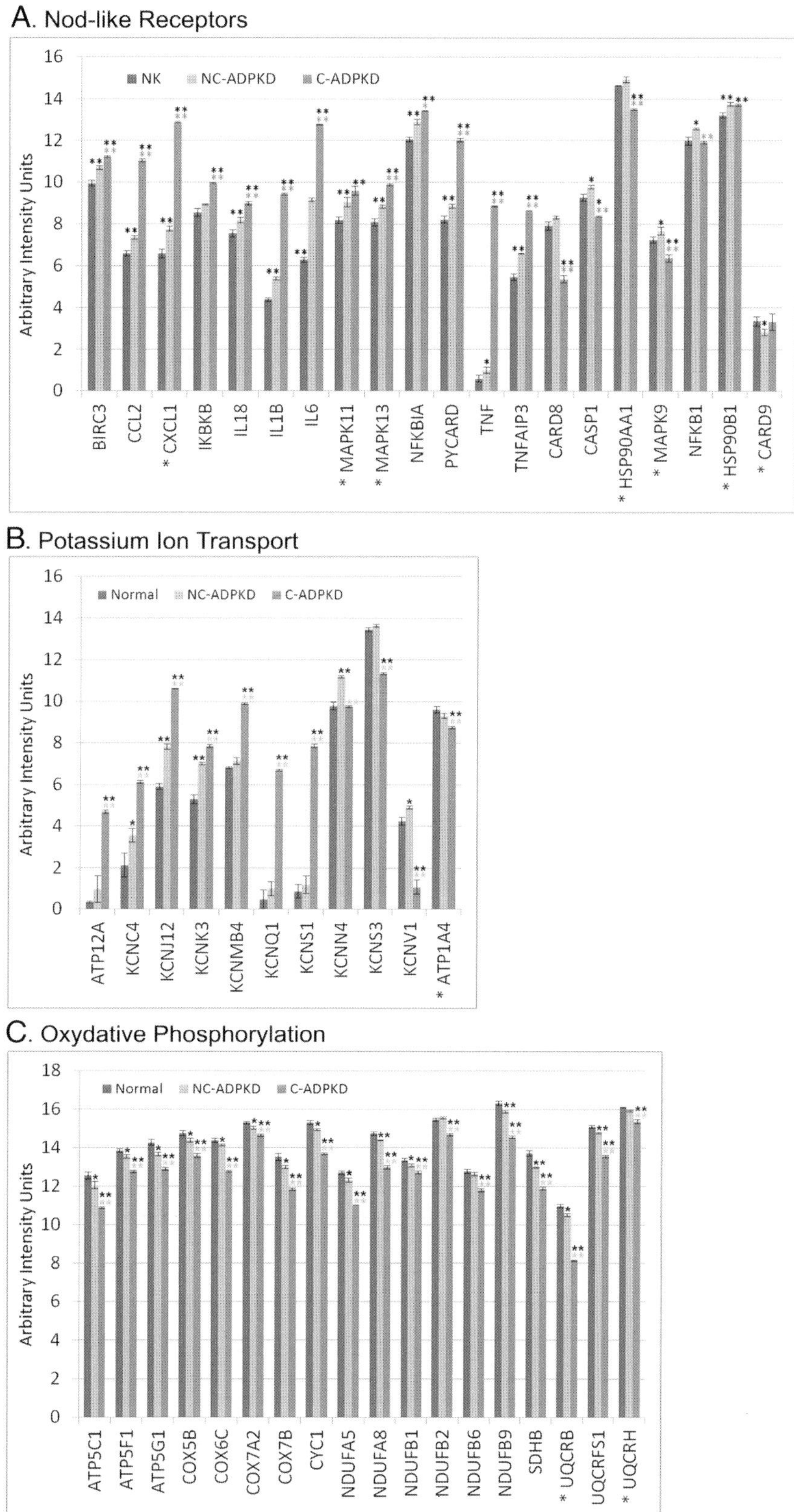

Fig. 15 (See legend on next page.)

(See figure on previous page.)
Fig. 15 Comparisons of individual gene expression levels for genes selected from differentially expressed gene sets. **a** NOD-like receptor signaling, **b** potassium ion transport, and **c** oxidative phosphorylation. To simplify presentation of these gene sets, where we used two or more probes in the microarray for a single gene, we give mean values and mark the gene names with an "asterisk". Within gene sets, we can discern changes in individual genes responsible for differential expression of the pathways. We present data as mean ± s.e.m., $^{**}P < 0.01$, $^{*}P < 0.05$ (*black asterisk* is in comparison to NK, *gray asterisk* is in comparison to NC-ADPKD). Additional file 4 provides additional information on each gene

Other evaluations of gene expression data have relied on murine cell lines or RNA isolated from newly formed cysts from conditional knockout models, and results from these studies identify similar themes for aberrant signaling such as immune defense, cell structure and motility, cellular proliferation, apoptosis, and metabolic control [59–62]. These are GSEA findings that are also observed in our study suggesting that a subset of findings observed in our cell lines are generalizable.

Current analyses of genome-wide gene expression measurements (microarrays or RNASeq, for example) such as single gene Volcano plots (Fig. 1) and GSEA gene set analysis (Tables 1 and 2) have failed to identify patterns of gene expression that define specific diseases or reveal the entirety of their molecular mechanisms of pathogenesis. Our ADPKD transcriptogram analysis (Figs. 4, 5, and 6) identified more significantly altered KEGG pathways and GO terms than either Volcano plots (Fig. 2) or GSEA analysis (Tables 1 and 2). Importantly, transcriptogram analysis identifies additional pathways and terms which are consistent with what we know about signaling, functional, and morphological changes that occur in ADPKD, clarifying the mechanisms by which PKD mutations drive cyst formation.

Comparing global gene expression profiles between NK, ADPKD, NC-ADPKD, and C-ADPKD shows that the NC-ADPKD gene profile is most similar to the NK line expression profile. The NK cell line profile is markedly different from both the C-ADPKD and end-stage ADPKD cell line gene expression profiles (Additional file 5: Figure S5). NC-ADPKD, C-ADPKD, and ADPKD cell lines all have truncation mutations in one allele of the PC-1 gene. However, when we sequenced the PC-1 genomic clones, we found no evidence for second somatic mutations in the PC-1 gene [25]. Additionally, there were no differences in total polycystin-1 and 2 protein expression in the ADPKD cell line [25]. The sole distinguishing feature between the NK and ADPKD cell lines was the absence of polycystin-1 in the cilia of the ADPKD cells [63]. Our transcriptogram analysis suggests that some other genetic event, i.e., a second hit, causes the dramatic shift in gene expression which transforms non-cystic ADPDK cells into cystic ADPKD cells [64]. The transition in expression profiles may have been determined during the early steps of cyst emergence that set the subsequent gene expression profile to reflect a fundamentally altered differentiation profile [17] [65]. Alternatively, a second somatic mutation that launched cyst emergence occurred in some other cystogenic gene site where we have incomplete information at present [66, 67]. Notably, in a murine conditional PKD1 knockout, cyst formation is most robust with PKD1 inactivation up to post-natal day 14 [68]. In other knock out models, cyst formation also requires a kidney injury and repair cycle to yield robust cystogenesis suggesting that there is a developmental window, recapitulated during cell repair that leads to a risk of cyst formation when polycystin-1 levels are abnormal [69].

Several of the many signaling pathways altered in cystic epithelia deserve special consideration [70]. Several potassium channel genes are overexpressed in our cystic cell lines. These potassium channel genes are KCNC4 (potassium voltage-gated channel subfamily C member 4), KCNJ12 (potassium voltage-gated channel subfamily J member 12), KCNK3 (potassium two pore domain channel subfamily K member 3), KCNMB4 (potassium calcium-activated channel subfamily M regulatory beta subunit 4), KCNQ1 (potassium voltage-gated family Q member 1), and KCNS1 (potassium voltage-gated channel modifier subfamily S member 1). NC-ADPKD cells have higher-than-normal and C-ADPKD cells have lower-than-normal expression of KCNN4 (potassium calcium-activated channel subfamily N member 4), KCNV1 (potassium voltage gated channel modifier subfamily V member 1), and KCNS3 (potassium voltage-gated channel subfamily A member 3). Notably, KCNN4 is responsible for calcium-dependent cyst fluid secretion and is thus a potential therapeutic target to inhibit cyst growth [57]. Many of these channels act to hyperpolarize the cell membrane, and voltage-sensitive K channel membrane depolarization induces nano-scale assembly of phosphatidyl serine, which in turn results in nano-scale clustering sites for K-ras, thereby promoting cell cycle progression via MAPK downstream signaling [71, 72]. Experimental studies have demonstrated that cyst expansion results in cell stretching [73]. Since some K channels are stretch activated, K channel activation of proliferation could lead to feedback, where cyst expansion driven by fluid secretion directly accelerates cell-cycle progression [73–76].

Our transcriptogram analysis found significantly higher-than-normal expression of downstream mediators of the 'inflammasome signaling' pathway in NC-ADPKD and C-ADPKD samples, which may accelerate disease pathogenesis [53, 77–80]. This signaling cascade includes nucleotide-binding oligomerization domain receptors or

NOD-like receptors, which have been implicated in renal diseases including ureteric obstruction, ischemia reperfusion injury, glomerulonephritis, sepsis, hypoxia, glycerol-induced renal failure, and crystal nephropathy [53–55, 81]. Our data show that NOD-like receptor signaling may also play an important role in ADPKD. NC-ADPKD and C-ADPKD samples had higher-than-normal ($p < 0.01$) expression of a number of other inflammasome signaling genes, including: interleukin (IL) 6, IL1β, NFκB1A, CCL2 (chemokine (C-C motif) ligand), BIRC3, TNFAIP3, IL18, PYCARD (also called ASC), and MAPK13.

Inflammasome signaling, a part of the innate immune system, includes membrane receptors that recognize conserved pathogen-associated molecular patterns (PAMPs) on invading pathogens or host-derived danger-associated molecular patterns (DAMPs) released in response to stress, reactive oxygen species generation, or cell death [78]. Both Toll-like receptors and C-type lectin pattern recognition receptors (PRRs) can initiate inflammasome signaling at the cell membrane [55]. Additional PRRs include the retinoic acid-inducible gene (RIG-1)-like receptors which recognize double-stranded RNAs (dsRNA) and NOD-like receptors which recognize microbe-associated molecular pattern signatures (MAMPS) and DAMPs. Other intracellular monitors of the system include HIN-200 receptors and RIG-1-like receptors [82–84]. Inflammasome signaling begins with a priming phase, initiated by receptors that signal through myeloid differentiation primary response (MyD88) pathways and other NFκB activating pathways such as IL-1R and the tumor necrosis factor receptor (TNFR) [55, 85]. Priming promotes IL1β, NRLP3, and IL18 transcription and protein synthesis and requires interleukin 1 receptor-associated kinase (IRAK1) activation [86]. K^{-+}efflux, adenosine tri-phosphate (ATP), reactive oxygen species (ROS), pore-forming toxins, or crystals [87–91] all lead to inflammasome activation. The purinergic receptor P2X7 [78, 89, 92, 93] is another inflammasome activator, which is more active under conditions of low fluid shear stress. ADPKD cells, lining cyst walls, are sheltered from fluid shear normally found in tubule lumens; hence, it is likely that in vivo P2X7 is more active [29]. Following inflammasome activation, NOD-like receptors such as NLRP3 form macromolecular complexes with ASC (apoptosis-associated speck-like protein, PYCARD), an adaptor with a caspase recruitment domain (CARD) that bridges NLRs and caspase-1 [94]. This macromolecular complex activates caspace-1, which enzymatically cleaves the pro-inflammatory cytokines IL-1β and IL-18 [95]. Inflammasome signaling has transcriptional effects mediated via MAPK to induce NFκB and the pro-inflammatory cytokines IL-1β and IL-18 [86].

The cystic epithelial cells in our study have higher-than-normal expression of the inflammasome adaptor PYCARD/ASC and the signal modulators BIRC3, preparing them to over-respond to inflammasome signals [80, 95]. The cystic epithelial cells also have higher-than-normal levels of the mRNAs encoding downstream effectors of inflammasome signaling, which likely increase expression of IL1β, IL-18, TNFα, monocyte chemotactic protein-1 (MCP-1), and IL-6 [96–98]. While many of these protein biomarkers correlate with disease severity in either animal models of renal cyst disease or urine from patients with ADPKD [99, 100], our analysis indicates that they may also drive cyst genesis and expansion.

Intense fibrosis and loss of functional parenchyma accompany kidney enlargement during ADPKD disease progression [101, 102]. Our transcriptome analysis suggest that cystic epithelial cells can excessively augment innate inflammatory responses that may accelerate fibrosis and stimulate a chronic inflammatory state by driving macrophage polarization and activation [103]. Since intracellular levels of calcium are low in ADPKD cells [70, 104, 105] and levels of P2X7 gene expression are lower than normal [25], reactive oxygen species are the most likely trigger of inflammasome assembly [88]. Even though P2X7 message levels are lower than normal in ADPKD cells, primary cultured cyst epithelial cells secrete high levels of ATP [29, 106], leading to maximal stimulation of any P2X7 receptors that are present. Since P2X7 activation co-stimulates formation of the NALP inflammasome, cystic epithelial cells may be the primary sources of the IL18 and IL1β identified in cyst fluid [100, 107].

Recent evidence suggests that other K channels can activate transport vesicle release in response to inflammasome activation, and the resultant vesicle cargo protein composition depends on the K channel responsible for membrane depolarization [92]. Thus, aberrant endogenous K-channel expression in cystic epithelia may impair auto regulatory responses to interleukin secretion.

We propose a scenario for the persistent inflammation seen in ADPKD kidneys based on our transcriptogram analysis. Our findings show higher-than-normal mRNA expression of MCP-1 in C-ADPKD cells, which would promote mononuclear cell infiltration into cystic kidney parenchyma. Within the parenchyma, IL1β, IL-18, and IL-6 can all activate infiltrated mononuclear cells. High levels of DAMPs released by apoptotic cells, and DAMPs such as hyaluronic acid and protein fragments resulting from proteolytic extracellular matrix fragments in ADPKD cystic kidneys would then further push mononuclear cells towards an M2 phenotype [99, 107–111]. These M2-like monocytes would continuously secrete transforming growth factor (TGF-β) and connective tissue growth factor (CTGF), which would convert cells in the interstitium to myofibroblasts [78, 102]. Other M2-like monocytes would stimulate epithelial cell proliferation thereby driving cyst expansion [103]. The same signals would stimulate Th1 cells to secrete IFN-γ, IL-13, and Th2 cells to secrete IL-4 and IL-5 and Treg cells to secrete IL-10 and TGF-β, exacerbating the dysregulated inflammatory cascade [86]. This pathogenic picture suggests that pharmacologic interventions which attenuate the inflammatory cascade should delay cyst expansion and fibrosis in ADPKD.

Conclusions

Our analysis of ADPKD provides a workflow which applies to the hierarchical analysis of any large-scale microarray study. We begin with transcriptogram analysis as a method of global triage to identify intervals of altered expression in the ordered gene list, then determine which genes in those intervals of KEGG pathways or GO terms that are differentially expressed (e.g.,'potassium ion transport' in Fig. 14), and finally explore the significance of altered expression profiles of single genes within those altered pathways and terms (Fig. 15). The transcriptograms provide crucial mechanistic context for understanding the significance of altered gene expression.

Methods

Cell lines and culture conditions

All cell lines derived from human kidneys under a protocol were approved by the Indiana University Institutional Review Board. We immortalized all cell lines with human telomerase as previously described and maintained them in continuous culture [25]. We grew cells with renal epithelial growth media supplemented with 5% fetal bovine serum (Lonza, Bazel, Switzerland and GE Healthcare HyClone, Little Chalfont, Buckinghamshire, UK) and maintained them at 37 °C, 5% CO_2 atmosphere. We passaged cells twice-weekly using trypsin-EDTA (Sigma-Aldrich, St. Louis, MO). We micro-dissected the source tissue for the NC-ADPKD and C-ADPKD cell lines from an early stage polycystic kidney from a 36-year-old male. We isolated NC-ADPKD cells from intact renal tubules and C-ADPKD cells from surface cysts. All cell lines expressed the proximal tubule markers ANPEP (alanyl aminopeptidase, membrane), FAH (fumarylacetoacetate hydrolase), SLC5A2 (sodium glucose transporter 5A2), LRP2 (LDL receptor related protein), and HNF1A (hepatocyte nuclear factor 1 homeobox A). They did not express proximal marker CUBN (cubulin). All lines expressed the cortical thick ascending limb marker UMOD (uromodulin). No lines expressed SLC12A1 (solute carrier family 12 member 1) or KCNJ1 (potassium voltage-gated channel subfamily J) . All cell lines expressed the distal convoluted tubule markers KLK1 (kallikrein-1) and KL (klotho). Only the NC-ADPKD cells expressed SLC12A3 (solute carrier family 12 member 3). The NK cell line expressed PVALB (parvalbumin). All cell lines expressed the collecting duct markers, AQP2 (aquaporin 2), and SCNN1G (sodium channel epithelial 1 subunit gamma), while no cell lines expressed FXYD2 (sodium/potassium-transporting ATPase gamma). The gene-expression profiles suggest that the cultured cells likely originate from proximal tubule segments. In contrast, the NK kidney cell line is a mixed cell population made from whole kidney collagenase digest. Herbert et al. have described the NK and ADPKD Q4004X cells [25]. We sequenced the HmPKD1 gene using a protocol of Herbert et al., revealing a heterozygous truncation mutation at amino acid 2556 (Q2556X) [25].

Chemicals and reagents

We purchased all buffers and inorganic chemicals from Sigma-Aldrich (Sigma-Aldrich, St. Louis, MO). We isolated total RNA from cells using TRIzol Reagent (Thermo Fischer Scientific, Waltham, MA) according to manufacturer's directions. We plated cells onto Costar membrane filter supports at a density of 50,000 cells/cm^2 and grew them for 5 days to ensure confluence [25].

We labeled 200 ng of purified total RNA using the Agilent QuickAmp labeling kit, 1-color (Agilent Technologies, Palo Alto, CA) and hybridized purified cRNA to a custom Agilent Human Whole Genome 4x180K array, which replicates the content of the v2 4x44k array at least four times (AMIDID 026822). After hybridization at 65 °C, 20 rpm for 17 h, we washed arrays in wash buffer 1 (6XSSC (saline sodium citrate), 0.005 % TritonX-102) for 5 min at room temperature and wash buffer 2 (0.06X SSC, 0.005 % Triton X-102) for 5 min at 37 °C. We scanned arrays on the Agilent High-Resolution Microarray B-series Scanner (G2505B) and quantified the images using Agilent Feature Extraction software (version 10.7).

Microarray data preprocessing and normalization

We processed extracted feature (reporter) intensities from each array separately by subtracting a constant to bring the minimum intensity to 1 and then taking the log, base 2. We mapped the transformed intensities using a non-linear function to ensure that the cumulative distribution profiles of the intensities were comparable between all arrays. We present the resulting comparable feature intensities in arbitrary units. We removed features with low intensity from the analysis if the 90th percentile was below the limit of detection (LoD), which we estimated as the mean of a set of negative controls plus 1.96 times the standard deviation of the negative controls. We also removed features with low range across all samples, which we defined as having a difference between the 95th percentile and 5th percentile of less than log 2 (1.5-fold). We summarized the replicate probes by averaging and constructed a mixed-effects linear model of expression using factors for tissue type (cysts or kidney), status (ADPKD or NK), and cell line (NK, C-ADPKD, NC-ADPKD, ADPKD), treating cell line as a random effect.

Volcano plotting

We averaged gene expression levels over the replicates for each cell line after normalization and compared the cell lines by calculating the FC. We defined FC as the ratio between the averages and we determined P values for each gene expressed. Volcano plots use FC as the x-axis and the P value as the y-axis (Fig. 2). We defined significantly changed genes as those with thresholds of $FC > 2$ and $P < 0.01$.

Gene Set Enrichment Analysis (GSEA)

We performed gene set enrichment analysis using the application available at the Broad Institute Gene Set Enrichment Analysis website [26, 33]. We estimated the signal-to-noise ratio and false discovery rates (FDR), from 1000 gene-set permutations, due to the low number of samples in each class ($n = 3$). We tested the Gene Ontology: Biological Process terms and KEGG pathways gene sets. Since we used gene permutations, we considered gene sets to be differentially expressed if FDR < 0.05. We calculated GSEA for NC-ADPKD versus NK, C-ADPKD versus NK, and C-ADPKD versus C-ADPKD.

Transcriptogram analysis

Ordering the gene list

Transcriptograms give an integrated visualization of genome-wide gene expression data by projecting expression levels onto a functionally ordered gene list to produce a genome-wide expression profile [23, 27, 34]. The gene list ordering is based on STRING database protein-protein interactions [34] with confidence scores over 0.800 drawn from all methods to infer associations, with the exception of text mining. The ordering process is performed using a Monte Carlo algorithm that minimizes a cost function:

$$F = \sum_{i=1}^{N-1} \sum_{j=i+1}^{N} d_{i\,j}^{\alpha} \left(|A_{i\,j}-A_{i+1\,j}| + |A_{i\,j}-A_{i-1\,j}| + |A_{i\,j}-A_{i\,j+1}| + |A_{i\,j}-A_{i\,j-1}| \right), \tag{1}$$

where N is the number of genes in the list and A is the association matrix. $A_{i\,j} = 1$ when the products of the genes at positions i and j in the list associate and $A_{i\,j} = 0$ otherwise. $d_{i\,j} = |i - j|$ measures the distance between the locations of genes i and j in the list. Minimizing F causes associated genes to cluster in the list. Minimization starts with a randomly ordered list of all genes whose products have at least one association. Each step chooses a pair of genes randomly, tentatively swaps their positions, and calculates the change in the cost function ΔF. The algorithm accepts the position swap whenever $\Delta F \le 0$. If $\Delta F > 0$, the algorithm accepts the swap with probability $\exp - \frac{\Delta F}{T}$. T is a fluctuation amplitude that allows the configuration to escape from local minima of ΔF. One Monte-Carlo step (MCS) equals N attempted gene-pair exchanges. The simulated annealing algorithm starts with T large and decreases T by a small amount once every 100 MCS. The ordering algorithm produces a gene list (Additional file 2) where the probability that any two genes associate decays exponentially with their distance in the list.

Visualizing KEGG pathway and GO term profiles in the ordered list

Because STRING database interactions use KEGG pathway maps for benchmarking and calibration [112], genes in close proximity in the list are probably in the same KEGG pathway. Consequently, the ordered list groups genes by biological function. We used David's Annotational Tools [113] to obtain a list of the GO terms and KEGG pathways that associate to intervals of the ordered list. For each of these GO terms and KEGG pathways, we obtain a profile by creating an N-element vector, $\vec{h}$, and setting $h_i = 1$, if the gene at position i in the list participates in the specified GO term or KEGG pathway and $h_i = 0$, if the gene at position i in the list does not participate in the specified GO term or KEGG pathway [113, 114]. For each pathway or term, we obtained a profile for $r = 30$. A value of 1 indicates that all genes in an interval participate in a given GO term or KEGG pathway. We read the resulting profiles along the ordered list as indicative of the level of enrichment with genes of a given GO term or KEGG pathway. Interpretation of transcriptograms is then facilitated by comparing the enrichment profiles from regions with significant difference in their transcriptograms.

Transcriptogram calculation

We next map the microarray data onto the ordered list. We then smooth the raw profile to obtain a final *transcriptogram profile*, a new $N - 2r - 1$ element vector, $\vec{k}$ using a running average with a window of size $2r + 1$ ($r = 30$):

$$k_i = \frac{1}{2r+1} \sum_{j=-r}^{r} h_{i+j}, \tag{2}$$

where $i \in \{r + 1, N - r - 1\}$. The resulting profile is the transcriptogram for the expression data. Profile peaks in $\vec{k}$ can be interpreted by comparison with the KEGG pathways and GO terms enriched in that region of the ordered list.

Class comparison

We next compare transcriptograms between sample classes. First, we produce the transcriptograms. We next average the transcriptograms for all the samples of each class, producing a class-average transcriptogram profile, $\left\langle \vec{k} \right\rangle$ and corresponding standard error profile $\vec{\sigma}_k$. To compare a reference (R) and perturbed (P) expression pattern, we divide the perturbed by the normal value for each averaged transcriptogram profile element to obtain the relative transcriptogram $\vec{\Delta}_{P/R}$:

$$\Delta_i = \frac{k_i^P}{k_i^R}. \tag{3}$$

Regions in $\vec{\Delta}_{P,R}$ with $\Delta_i \gg 1$ or $\ll 1$ indicate specific perturbed gene expression. The upper panels in Figs. 4, 5, and 6 show the relative transcriptograms.

Significance evaluation

We estimate the significance of differences between two transcriptogram classes using a two-tailed Welch's t test on the class averages to obtain a P value for each list position and by creating 500 random permutations of the sample labels (phenotypes) to estimate the FDR. The middle panels in Figs. 4, 5, and 6 show the P value for each list position.

Abbreviations

ADPKD: Autosomal dominant polycystic kidney disease; ANPEP: Alanyl aminopeptidase, membrane; ASC: Apoptosis-associated speck-like protein; ATP: Adenosine tri-phosphate; C-ADPKD: Cystic autosomal dominant polycystic kidney disease; CARD: Caspase recruitment domain; CCL2: Chemokine (C-C motif) ligand 2; CTGF: Connective tissue growth factor; CUBN: Cubulin; DAMPs: Damage-associated molecular patterns; DNA: Deoxyribonucleic acid; ECM: Extracellular matrix; Erk: Extracellular signal regulated kinase; FAH: Fumarylacetoacetate hydrolase; FC: Fold change; FDA: Federal Drug Administration; FDR: False discovery rate; FXYD: Sodium/potassium-transporting ATPase gamma; G PROT: G protein; GO: Gene ontology; GSEA: Gene Set Enrichment Analysis; HmPKD1: Human polycystic kidney disease gene 1; HmPKD2: Human polycystic kidney disease gene 2; HNF1A: Hepatocyte nuclear factor 1 homeobox A; IL: Interleukin; IRAK1: Interleukin 1 receptor associated kinase 1; Jnk: cJun N-Terminal kinase; KCNC4: Potassium voltage-gated channel subfamily C member 4; KCNJ1: Potassium voltage-gated channel subfamily J; KCNJ12: Potassium voltage-gated channel subfamily J member 12; KCNK3: Potassium two pore domain channel subfamily k member 3; KCNMB4: Potassium calcium-activated channel subfamily M regulatory beta subunit 4; KCNN4: Potassium calcium-activated channel subfamily N member 4; KCNQ1: Potassium voltage gated family Q member 1; KCNS1: Potassium voltage gated channel modifier subfamily S member 1; KCNS3: Potassium voltage gated channel subfamily A member 3; KCNV1: Potassium voltage gated channel modifier subfamily V member 1; KEGG: Kyoto Encyclopedia of Genes and Genomes; KL: Klotho; KLK1: Kallikrein-1; LRP: LDL receptor-related protein; MAPK: Mitogen-activated protein kinase; MCP: Monocyte chemotactic protein; mTOR: Mammalian target of rapamycin; MyD88: Myeloid differentiation primary response 88; NALP1: NLR pyrin containing; NC ADPKD: Non-cystic autosomal dominant polycystic kidney disease; NF-kB: Nuclear factor kappa beta; NK: Normal kidney; NLR: NOD-like receptor; NLRP3: NOD-like receptor protein; NOD: Nucleotide-binding oligomerization domain; P2X: Purinergic receptor; PAMPs: Pathogen associated molecular patterns; PC-1: Polycystin 1; PC-2: Polycystin 2; Pck1: Phosphoenolpyruvate carboxy-kinase 1; PKD: Polycystic kidney disease; PRRs: Pattern recognition receptors; PVALB: Parvalbumin; qRT-PCR: Quantitative reverse transcriptase polymerase chain reaction; RA: Rheumatoid arthritis; RIG-1: Retinoic acid inducible protein; RNA: Ribonucleic acid; ROS: Reactive oxygen species; SCNN1G: Sodium channel epithelial 1 subunit gamma; SLC12A1: Solute carrier family 12 member 1; SLC12A3: Solute carrier family 12 member 3; SLC5A2: Sodium glucose transporter 5A2; Stat: Signal transducer and activator of transcription 1; TCA: Tricarboxylic acid; TGF: Transforming growth factor; TNF: Tumor necrosis factor; Treg: Regulatory T cell; UMOD: Uromodulin; Wgless: Wingless; Wnt: Wingless-related integration site

Acknowledgements

The authors thank Dr. Swenson-Fields from Kansas University Medical Center, Dr. Seth Alper from Harvard University, and Dr. Purvi Mehrotra from Indiana University School of Medicine for helpful discussions.

Funding

Brazilian agencies CNPq, CAPES, and FAPERGS provided partial support for this project. RMCA acknowledges the kind hospitality of the Biocomplexity Institute, Indiana University, Bloomington. RLB acknowledges support from a Merit Review, BX001736, NIH NIDDK grant R01 DK079312, and a Dr. Ralph and Marian Falk Medical Research Trust Award. An Indiana University Collaborative Research Grant supported the initial collaboration between the RLB and JAG groups. We acknowledge additional generous support from Amgen and Indiana University. RLB thanks the Bloch family for continued support. JAG acknowledges support from NIH NIGMS/NIEHS/NIBIB grants R01 GM11243, R01 GM076692, R01 GM077138, and a Dr. Ralph and Marian Falk Medical Research Trust Award. AWN acknowledges support from NIH NIDDK grant R01 DK050141 and NIH NCI grant P30 CA118100. HHW acknowledges support from NIH NIDDK grant K01 DK097206 and Paul Teschan Research Fund project #3RX05.

Authors' contributions

RMCA performed all calculations for GSEA and transcriptogram analyses and all statistical analyses. RMCA, SGC, JAG, and RLB participated in the design and coordination of the study and writing of the manuscript. BSH, HHW, AWN, and RLB developed the cell lines. WX assisted in the development and maintenance of the cell lines and isolated all RNA samples for these studies. BR, MB, and MD performed the microarray experiments and performed Volcano plots analyses. HHW participated in the initial analyses of the microarray data and made critical suggestions concerning the direction of further analyses. BSH, AWN, and HHW provided critical input for interpretation of the transcriptogram analysis results. RLB oversaw the project. WGR analyzed Agilent human gene array data. SR and PCH analyzed the genetic changes in the HmPKD1 loci in the human cystic epithelial cell lines. All authors read and approved the final manuscript.

Competing interests

The authors declare that they have no competing interests.

Review Board (IRB) deemed this research as exempt from IRB review. Therefore, IRB approval was waived.

Author details

[1]Biocomplexity Institute and Department of Physics, Indiana University, Bloomington, IN 47405, USA. [2]Instituto de Física and Instituto Nacional de Ciência e Tecnologia, Universidade Federal do Rio Grande do Sul, 91501-970 Porto Alegre, RS, Brazil. [3]Biocomplexity Institute and Department of Intelligent Systems Engineering, Indiana University, Bloomington, IN 47405, USA. [4]AMGEN Inc., One Amgen Center Drive, Thousand Oaks, CA 91320-1799, USA. [5]Division of Nephrology, Mayo Clinic, 200 First Street SW, Rochester, MN 55905, USA. [6]Department of Medical and Molecular Genetics, Indiana University School of Medicine, Indianapolis, IN 46202, USA. [7]Division

of Nephrology, Department of Medicine, Richard Roudebush VAMC and Indiana University School of Medicine, Indianapolis, IN 46202, USA. [8]Department of Pathology MSC08-4640 and Cancer Research and Treatment Center, University of New Mexico Health Sciences Center, Albuquerque, NM 87131, USA. [9]Division of Nephrology, Department of Medicine, University of New Mexico Health Sciences Center, Albuquerque, NM 87131, USA.

References

1. Torres VE, Harris PC, Pirson Y. Autosomal dominant polycystic kidney disease. Lancet. 2007;369(9569):1287–301.
2. Santoro D, Pellicanò V, Visconti L, Trifirò G, Buemi M, Cernaro V. An overview of experimental and early investigational therapies for the treatment of polycystic kidney disease. Expert Opin Investig Drugs. 2015;24(9):1199–218.
3. Qian F, Germino FJ, Cai Y, Zhang X, Somlo S, Germino GG. PKD1 interacts with PKD2 through a probable coiled-coil domain. Nat Genetics. 1997;16(2):179–83.
4. Yoder BK, Hou X, Guay-Woodford LM. The polycystic kidney disease proteins, polycystin-1, polycystin-2, polaris, and cystin, are co-localized in renal cilia.[see comment]. J Am Soc Nephrol. 2002;13(10):2508–16.
5. Gainullin VG, Hopp K, Ward CJ, Hommerding CJ, Harris PC. Polycystin-1 maturation requires polycystin-2 in a dose-dependent manner. J Clin Invest. 2015;125(2):607–20.
6. Praetorius HA, Spring KR. A physiological view of the primary cilium. Annu Rev Physiol. 2005;67:515–29.
7. Hildebrandt F, Benzing T, Katsanis N. Ciliopathies. N Engl J Med. 2011; 364(16):1533–43.
8. Gallagher AR, Hidaka S, Gretz N, Witzgall R. Molecular basis of autosomal-dominant polycystic kidney disease. Cell Mol Life Sci. 2002;59(4):682–93.
9. Walz G, Budde K, Mannaa M, Nürnberger J, Wanner C, Sommerer C, et al. Everolimus in patients with autosomal dominant polycystic kidney disease. N Engl J Med. 2010;363(9):830–40.
10. He Q, Lin C, Ji S, Chen J. Efficacy and safety of mTOR inhibitor therapy in patients with early-stage autosomal dominant polycystic kidney disease: a meta-analysis of randomized controlled trials. Am J Med Sci. 2012;344(6):491–7.
11. Torres VE, Chapman AB, Devuyst O, Gansevoort RT, Grantham JJ, Higashihara E, et al. Tolvaptan in patients with autosomal dominant polycystic kidney disease. N Engl J Med. 2012;367(25):2407–18.
12. Gattone VH, Maser RL, Branden MG, Tiam C, Resenberg J. Collecting duct gene expression and effect of an AVP-V2 receptor antagonist on the progression of PKD in pcy mice. J Am Soc Nephrol. 1998;9:18A.
13. Wang X, Gattone 2nd V, Harris PC, Torres VE. Effectiveness of vasopressin V2 receptor antagonists OPC-31260 and OPC-41061 on polycystic kidney disease development in the PCK rat.[see comment]. J Am Soc Nephrol. 2005;16(4):846–51.
14. Torres VE, Higashihara E, Devuyst O, Chapman AB, Gansevoort RT, Grantham JJ, et al. Effect of tolvaptan in autosomal dominant polycystic kidney disease by CKD stage: results from the TEMPO 3:4 trial. Clin J Am Soc Nephrol. 2016;11(5):803–11.
15. Harris PC, Bae KT, Rossetti S, Torres VE, Grantham JJ, Chapman AB, et al. Cyst number but not the rate of cystic growth is associated with the mutated gene in autosomal dominant polycystic kidney disease. J Am Soc Nephrol. 2006;17(11):3013–9.
16. Waldherr R, Zerres K, Gall A, Enders H. Polycystic kidney disease in the fetus. Lancet. 1989;2(8657):274–5.
17. Song X, Di Giovanni V, He N, Wang K, Ingram A, Rosenblum ND, et al. Systems biology of autosomal dominant polycystic kidney disease (ADPKD): computational identification of gene expression pathways and integrated regulatory networks. Hum Mol Genet. 2009;18(13):2328–43.
18. Surendran K, Selassie M, Liapis H, Krigman H, Kopan R. Reduced Notch signaling leads to renal cysts and papillary microadenomas. J Am Soc Nephrol. 2010;21(5):819–32.
19. Romaker D, Puetz M, Teschner S, Donauer J, Geyer M, Gerke P, et al. Increased expression of secreted frizzled-related protein 4 in polycystic kidneys. J Am Soc Nephrol. 2009;20(1):48–56.
20. Liu M, Shi S, Senthilnathan S, Yu J, Wu E, Bergmann C, et al. Genetic variation of DKK3 may modify renal disease severity in ADPKD. J Am Soc Nephrol. 2010;21(9):1510–20.
21. Hayward P, Kalmar T, Arias AM. Wnt/Notch signalling and information processing during development. Development. 2008;135(3):411–24.
22. da Silva SR, Perrone GC, Dinis JM, de Almeida RM. Reproducibility enhancement and differential expression of non predefined functional gene sets in human genome. BMC Genomics. 2014;15:1181.
23. Rybarczyk-Filho JL, Castro MA, Dalmolin RJ, Moreira JC, Brunnet LG, de Almeida RM. Towards a genome-wide transcriptogram: the Saccharomyces cerevisiae case. Nucleic Acids Res. 2011;39(8):3005–16.
24. de Almeida RMC. The Transcriptogramer: a software for genome wide expression analysis. http://lief.if.ufrgs.br/pub/biosoftwares/transcriptogramer [Available from: lief.if.ufrgs.br/pub/biosoftwares/transcriptogramer. Accessed 14 Nov 2016.
25. Herbert BS, Grimes BR, Xu WM, Werner M, Ward C, Rossetti S, et al. A telomerase immortalized human proximal tubule cell line with a truncation mutation (Q4004X) in polycystin-1. PLoS One. 2013;8(1):e55191.
26. Subramanian A, Tamayo P, Mootha VK, Mukherjee S, Ebert BL, Gillette MA, et al. Gene set enrichment analysis: a knowledge-based approach for interpreting genome-wide expression profiles. Proc Natl Acad Sci U S A. 2005;102(43):15545–50.
27. da Silva SRM, Perrone GC, Dinis JM, de Almeida RMC. Transcriptograms: signal to noise enhancement in transcriptome analysis. BMC Genomics. 2014;15:1181–99.
28. Nauli SM, Alenghat FJ, Luo Y, Williams E, Vassilev P, Li X, et al. Polycystins 1 and 2 mediate mechanosensation in the primary cilium of kidney cells. [comment]. Nat Genetics. 2003;33(2):129–37.
29. Xu C, Shmukler BE, Nishimura K, Kaczmarek E, Rossetti S, Harris PC, et al. Attenuated, flow-induced ATP release contributes to absence of flow-sensitive, purinergic Cai2+ signaling in human ADPKD cyst epithelial cells. Am J Physiol Renal Physiol. 2009;296(6):F1464–76.
30. Ong AC, Ward CJ, Butler RJ, Biddolph S, Bowker C, Torra R, et al. Coordinate expression of the autosomal dominant polycystic kidney disease proteins, polycystin-2 and polycystin-1, in normal and cystic tissue. Am J Pathol. 1999;154(6):1721–9.
31. Ong ACM, Wheatley DN. Polycystic kidney disease—the ciliary connection. Lancet. 2003;361(9359):774–6.
32. Irizarry RA, Wang C, Zhou Y, Speed TP. Gene set enrichment analysis made simple. Stat Methods Med Res. 2009;18(6):565–75.
33. Mootha VK, Lindgren CM, Eriksson KF, Subramanian A, Sihag S, Lehar J, et al. PGC-1alpha-responsive genes involved in oxidative phosphorylation are coordinately downregulated in human diabetes. Nat Genet. 2003; 34(3):267–73.
34. Szklarczyk D, Franceschini A, Wyder S, Forslund K, Heller D, Huerta-Cepas J, et al. STRING v10: protein-protein interaction networks, integrated over the tree of life. Nucleic Acids Res. 2015;43(Database issue):D447–52.
35. Jensen LJ, Kuhn M, Stark M, Chaffron S, Creevey C, Muller J, et al. STRING 8—a global view on proteins and their functional interactions in 630 organisms. Nucleic Acids Res. 2009;37(Database issue):D412–6.
36. Huang dW, Sherman BT, Zheng X, Yang J, Imamichi T, Stephens R, et al. Extracting biological meaning from large gene lists with DAVID. Curr Protoc Bioinformatics. 2009;Chapter 13:Unit 13.1.
37. Huang dW, Sherman BT, Lempicki RA. Bioinformatics enrichment tools: paths toward the comprehensive functional analysis of large gene lists. Nucleic Acids Res. 2009;37(1):1–13.
38. Thomson RB, Mentone S, Kim R, Earle K, Delpire E, Somlo S, et al. Histopathological analysis of renal cystic epithelia in the Pkd2WS25/-mouse model of ADPKD. Am J Physiol Renal Physiol. 2003;285(5):F870–80.
39. Carone FA, Nakamura S, Caputo M, Bacallao R, Nelson WJ, Kanwar YS. Cell polarity in human renal cystic disease. Lab Invest. 1994;70(5):648–55.
40. Yamaguchi T, Reif GA, Calvet JP, Wallace DP. Sorafenib inhibits cAMP-dependent ERK activation, cell proliferation, and in vitro cyst growth of human ADPKD cyst epithelial cells. Am J Physiol Renal Physiol. 2010;299(5):F944–51.
41. Belibi FA, Reif G, Wallace DP, Yamaguchi T, Olsen L, Li H, et al. Cyclic AMP promotes growth and secretion in human polycystic kidney epithelial cells. [see comment]. Kidney Int. 2004;66(3):964–73.
42. Chuang PY, Menon MC, He JC. Molecular targets for treatment of kidney fibrosis. J Mol Med (Berl). 2013;91(5):549–59.
43. Fearn A, Sheerin NS. Complement activation in progressive renal disease. World J Nephrol. 2015;4(1):31–40.
44. Yang W, Yoshigoe K, Qin X, Liu JS, Yang JY, Niemierko A, et al. Identification of genes and pathways involved in kidney renal clear cell carcinoma. BMC Bioinformatics. 2014;15 Suppl 17:S2.
45. Seeger-Nukpezah T, Geynisman DM, Nikonova AS, Benzing T, Golemis EA. The hallmarks of cancer: relevance to the pathogenesis of polycystic kidney disease. Nat Rev Nephrol. 2015;11(9):515–34.
46. Hou J, Rajagopal M, Yu AS. Claudins and the kidney. Annu Rev Physiol. 2013;75:479–501.
47. Yu AS, Kanzawa SA, Usorov A, Lantinga-van Leeuwen IS, Peters DJ. Tight junction composition is altered in the epithelium of polycystic kidneys. J Pathol. 2008;216(1):120–8.

48. Kher R, Sha EC, Escobar MR, Andreoli EM, Wang P, Xu WM, et al. Ectopic expression of cadherin 8 is sufficient to cause cyst formation in a novel 3D collagen matrix renal tubule culture. Am J Physiol Cell Physiol. 2011; 301(1):C99–C105.
49. Roitbak T, Ward CJ, Harris PC, Bacallao R, Ness SA, Wandinger-Ness A. A polycystin-1 multiprotein complex is disrupted in polycystic kidney disease cells. Mol Biol Cell. 2004;15(3):1334–46.
50. Martinez-Hernandez A, Amenta PS. The basement membrane in pathology. Lab Invest. 1983;48(6):656–77.
51. Boone M, Deen PM. Physiology and pathophysiology of the vasopressin-regulated renal water reabsorption. Pflugers Arch. 2008;456(6):1005–24.
52. Nakhoul N, Batuman V. Role of proximal tubules in the pathogenesis of kidney disease. Contrib Nephrol. 2011;169:37–50.
53. Turner CM, Arulkumaran N, Singer M, Unwin RJ, Tam FW. Is the inflammasome a potential therapeutic target in renal disease? BMC Nephrol. 2014;15:21.
54. Du P, Fan B, Han H, Zhen J, Shang J, Wang X, et al. NOD2 promotes renal injury by exacerbating inflammation and podocyte insulin resistance in diabetic nephropathy. Kidney Int. 2013;84(2):265–76.
55. Anders HJ, Lech M. NOD-like and Toll-like receptors or inflammasomes contribute to kidney disease in a canonical and a non-canonical manner. Kidney Int. 2013;84(2):225–8.
56. Palmer BF. Regulation of potassium homeostasis. Clin J Am Soc Nephrol. 2015;10(6):1050–60.
57. Albaqumi M, Srivastava S, Li Z, Zhdnova O, Wulff H, Itani O, et al. KCa3.1 potassium channels are critical for cAMP-dependent chloride secretion and cyst growth in autosomal-dominant polycystic kidney disease. Kidney Int. 2008;74(6):740–9.
58. Rowe I, Chiaravalli M, Mannella V, Ulisse V, Quilici G, Pema M, et al. Defective glucose metabolism in polycystic kidney disease identifies a new therapeutic strategy. Nat Med. 2013;19(4):488–93.
59. Menezes LF, Germino GG. Systems biology of polycystic kidney disease: a critical review. Wiley Interdiscip Rev Syst Biol Med. 2015;7(1):39–52.
60. Menezes LF, Zhou F, Patterson AD, Piontek KB, Krausz KW, Gonzalez FJ, et al. Network analysis of a Pkd1-mouse model of autosomal dominant polycystic kidney disease identifies HNF4α as a disease modifier. PLoS Genet. 2012;8(11):e1003053.
61. Chen WC, Tzeng YS, Li H. Gene expression in early and progression phases of autosomal dominant polycystic kidney disease. BMC Res Notes. 2008;1:131.
62. Gresh L, Fischer E, Reimann A, Tanguy M, Garbay S, Shao X, et al. A transcriptional network in polycystic kidney disease. EMBO J. 2004;23(7):1657–68.
63. Xu C, Rossetti S, Jiang L, Harris PC, Brown-Glaberman U, Wandinger-Ness A, et al. Human ADPKD primary cyst epithelial cells with a novel, single codon deletion in the PKD1 gene exhibit defective ciliary polycystin localization and loss of flow-induced Ca2+ signaling. Am J Physiol Renal Physiol. 2007;292(3):F930–45.
64. Germino GG. Autosomal dominant polycystic kidney disease: a two-hit model. Hosp Pract. 1997;32(3):81–2. 5-8, 91-2 passim.
65. Grantham JJ. Polycystic kidney disease (PKD): neoplasia in disguise. Am J Kidney Dis. 1990;15:110–6.
66. Woo DD, Nguyen DK, Khatibi N, Olsen P. Genetic identification of two major modifier loci of polycystic kidney disease progression in pcy mice. J Clin Invest. 1997;100(8):1934–40.
67. Iakoubova OA, Dushkin H, Beier DR. Genetic analysis of a quantitative trait in a mouse model of polycystic kidney disease. Am J Respir Crit Care Med. 1997;156(4 Pt 2):S72–7.
68. Piontek K, Menezes LF, Garcia-Gonzalez MA, Huso DL, Germino GG. A critical developmental switch defines the kinetics of kidney cyst formation after loss of Pkd1. Nat Med. 2007;13(12):1490–5.
69. Verdeguer F, Le Corre S, Fischer E, Callens C, Garbay S, Doyen A, et al. A mitotic transcriptional switch in polycystic kidney disease. Nat Med. 2010;16(1):106–10.
70. Harris PC, Torres VE. Genetic mechanisms and signaling pathways in autosomal dominant polycystic kidney disease. J Clin Invest. 2014;124(6):2315–24.
71. Zhou Y, Wong CO, Cho KJ, van der Hoeven D, Liang H, Thakur DP, et al. Membrane potential modulates plasma membrane phospholipid dynamics and K-Ras signaling. Science. 2015;349(6250):873–6.
72. Zhou Y, Hancock JF. Ras nanoclusters: versatile lipid-based signaling platforms. Biochim Biophys Acta. 2015;1853(4):841–9.
73. Tanner GA, McQuillan PF, Maxwell MR, Keck JK, McAteer JA. An in vitro test of the cell stretch-proliferation hypothesis of renal cyst enlargement. J Am Soc Nephrol. 1995;6(4):1230–41.
74. Gin E, Tanaka EM, Brusch L. A model for cyst lumen expansion and size regulation via fluid secretion. J Theor Biol. 2010;264(3):1077–88.
75. Sachs F. Stretch-activated ion channels: what are they? Physiology (Bethesda). 2010;25(1):50–6.
76. Sharif-Naeini R, Folgering JH, Bichet D, Duprat F, Lauritzen I, Arhatte M, et al. Polycystin-1 and -2 dosage regulates pressure sensing. Cell. 2009;139(3):587–96.
77. Anders HJ, Muruve DA. The inflammasomes in kidney disease. J Am Soc Nephrol. 2011;22(6):1007–18.
78. Anders HJ, Schaefer L. Beyond tissue injury-damage-associated molecular patterns, toll-like receptors, and inflammasomes also drive regeneration and fibrosis. J Am Soc Nephrol. 2014;25(7):1387–400.
79. Chang A, Ko K, Clark MR. The emerging role of the inflammasome in kidney diseases. Curr Opin Nephrol Hypertens. 2014;23(3):204–10.
80. Darisipudi MN, Knauf F. An update on the role of the inflammasomes in the pathogenesis of kidney diseases. Pediatr Nephrol. 2016;31(4):535–44.
81. Gasse P, Riteau N, Charron S, Girre S, Fick L, Pétrilli V, et al. Uric acid is a danger signal activating NALP3 inflammasome in lung injury inflammation and fibrosis. Am J Respir Crit Care Med. 2009;179(10):903–13.
82. Dawson MJ, Trapani JA. HIN-200: a novel family of IFN-inducible nuclear proteins expressed in leukocytes. J Leukoc Biol. 1996;60(3):310–6.
83. Pichlmair A, Schulz O, Tan CP, Näslund TI, Liljeström P, Weber F, et al. RIG-I-mediated antiviral responses to single-stranded RNA bearing 5'-phosphates. Science. 2006;314(5801):997–1001.
84. Yoneyama M, Kikuchi M, Natsukawa T, Shinobu N, Imaizumi T, Miyagishi M, et al. The RNA helicase RIG-I has an essential function in double-stranded RNA-induced innate antiviral responses. Nat Immunol. 2004;5(7):730–7.
85. Correa-Costa M, Braga TT, Semedo P, Hayashida CY, Bechara LR, Elias RM, et al. Pivotal role of Toll-like receptors 2 and 4, its adaptor molecule MyD88, and inflammasome complex in experimental tubule-interstitial nephritis. PLoS One. 2011;6(12):e29004.
86. Stutz A, Golenbock DT, Latz E. Inflammasomes: too big to miss. J Clin Invest. 2009;119(12):3502–11.
87. Rivers-Auty J, Brough D. Potassium efflux fires the canon: potassium efflux as a common trigger for canonical and noncanonical NLRP3 pathways. Eur J Immunol. 2015;45(10):2758–61.
88. Heid ME, Keyel PA, Kamga C, Shiva S, Watkins SC, Salter RD. Mitochondrial reactive oxygen species induces NLRP3-dependent lysosomal damage and inflammasome activation. J Immunol. 2013;191(10):5230–8.
89. Latz E, Xiao TS, Stutz A. Activation and regulation of the inflammasomes. Nat Rev Immunol. 2013;13(6):397–411.
90. Martinon F. Mechanisms of uric acid crystal-mediated autoinflammation. Immunol Rev. 2010;233(1):218–32.
91. Franchi L, Muñoz-Planillo R, Núñez G. Sensing and reacting to microbes through the inflammasomes. Nat Immunol. 2012;13(4):325–32.
92. de Torre-Minguela C, Barberà-Cremades M, Gómez AI, Martín-Sánchez F, Pelegrín P. Macrophage activation and polarization modify P2X7 receptor secretome influencing the inflammatory process. Sci Rep. 2016;6:22586.
93. Chen K, Zhang J, Zhang W, Yang J, Li K, He Y. ATP-P2X4 signaling mediates NLRP3 inflammasome activation: a novel pathway of diabetic nephropathy. Int J Biochem Cell Biol. 2013;45(5):932–43.
94. Stutz A, Horvath GL, Monks BG, Latz E. ASC speck formation as a readout for inflammasome activation. Methods Mol Biol. 2013;1040:91–101.
95. Schroder K, Tschopp J. The inflammasomes. Cell. 2010;140(6):821–32.
96. Tai YH, Flick J, Levine SA, Madara JL, Sharp GW, Donowitz M. Regulation of tight junction resistance in T84 monolayers by elevation in intracellular Ca2+: a protein kinase C effect. J Membr Biol. 1996;149(1):71–9.
97. Cowley Jr BD, Ricardo SD, Nagao S, Diamond JR. Increased renal expression of monocyte chemoattractant protein-1 and osteopontin in ADPKD in rats. Kidney Int. 2001;60(6):2087–96.
98. Yoo JK, Kwon H, Khil LY, Zhang L, Jun HS, Yoon JW. IL-18 induces monocyte chemotactic protein-1 production in macrophages through the phosphatidylinositol 3-kinase/Akt and MEK/ERK1/2 pathways. J Immunol. 2005;175(12):8280–6.
99. Zheng D, Wolfe M, Cowley BD, Wallace DP, Yamaguchi T, Grantham JJ. Urinary excretion of monocyte chemoattractant protein-1 in autosomal dominant polycystic kidney disease. J Am Soc Nephrol. 2003;14(10):2588–95.
100. Parikh CR, Dahl NK, Chapman AB, Bost JE, Edelstein CL, Comer DM, et al. Evaluation of urine biomarkers of kidney injury in polycystic kidney disease. Kidney Int. 2012;81(8):784–90.
101. Carone FA, Kanwar Y. Pathobiology of tubular basement membranes in renal cystic disease. In: Hatano M, editor. Nephrology. New York: Springer Verlag; 1991. p. 876–84.

102. Norman J. Fibrosis and progression of autosomal dominant polycystic kidney disease. Biochimica et Biophysica Acta (BBA) Mol Basis Dis. 2011;1812(10):1327–36.
103. Swenson-Fields KI, Vivian CJ, Salah SM, Peda JD, Davis BM, van Rooijen N, et al. Macrophages promote polycystic kidney disease progression. Kidney Int. 2013;83(5):855–64.
104. Mekahli D, Parys JB, Bultynck G, Missiaen L, De Smedt H. Polycystins and cellular Ca2+ signaling. Cell Mol Life Sci. 2013;70(15):2697–712.
105. Mekahli D, Sammels E, Luyten T, Welkenhuyzen K, van den Heuvel LP, Levtchenko EN, et al. Polycystin-1 and polycystin-2 are both required to amplify inositol-trisphosphate-induced Ca2+ release. Cell Calcium. 2012;51(6):452–8.
106. Wilson PD, Hovater JS, Casey CC, Fortenberry JA, Schwiebert EM. ATP release mechanisms in primary cultures of epithelia derived from the cysts of polycystic kidneys. J Am Soc Nephrol. 1999;10(2):218–29.
107. Gardner KJ, Burnside J, Elzinga L, Locksley R. Cytokines in fluids from polycystic kidneys. Kidney Int. 1991;39(4):718–24.
108. Carone FA, Kanwar Y. Tubular cell and matrix changes in renal cystic disease. Contrib Nephrol. 1993;101:1–6.
109. Jin H, Carone FA, Nakamura S, Liu ZZ, Kanwar YS. Altered synthesis and intracellular transport of proteoglycans by cyst-derived cells from human polycystic kidneys. J Am Soc Nephrol. 1992;2(12):1726–33.
110. Wilson PD, Norman JT, Kuo NT, Burrow CR. Abnormalities in extracellular matrix regulation in autosomal dominant polycystic kidney disease. Contrib Nephrol. 1996;118:126–34.
111. Woo D. Apoptosis and loss of renal tissue in polycystic kidney diseases. NE J Med. 1995;333:18–25.
112. Kanehisa M, Goto S, Sato Y, Kawashima M, Furumichi M, Tanabe M. Data, information, knowledge and principle: back to metabolism in KEGG. Nucleic Acids Res. 2014;42(Database issue):D199–205.
113. Huang DW, Sherman BT, Tan Q, Collins JR, Alvord WG, Roayaei J, et al. The DAVID Gene Functional Classification Tool: a novel biological module-centric algorithm to functionally analyze large gene lists. Genome Biol. 2007;8(9):R183.
114. Huang dW, Sherman BT, Stephens R, Baseler MW, Lane HC, Lempicki RA. DAVID gene ID conversion tool. Bioinformation. 2008;2(10):428–30.

4

Genetic variation in neurodegenerative diseases and its accessibility in the model organism *Caenorhabditis elegans*

Yiru Anning Wang[1,2], Jan Edward Kammenga[2] and Simon Crawford Harvey[1*]

Abstract

Background: Neurodegenerative diseases (NGDs) such as Alzheimer's and Parkinson's are debilitating and largely untreatable conditions strongly linked to age. The clinical, neuropathological, and genetic components of NGDs indicate that neurodegeneration is a complex trait determined by multiple genes and by the environment.

Main body: The symptoms of NGDs differ among individuals due to their genetic background, and this variation affects the onset and progression of NGD and NGD-like states. Such genetic variation affects the molecular and cellular processes underlying NGDs, leading to differential clinical phenotypes. So far, we have a limited understanding of the mechanisms of individual background variation. Here, we consider how variation between genetic backgrounds affects the mechanisms of aging and proteostasis in NGD phenotypes. We discuss how the nematode *Caenorhabditis elegans* can be used to identify the role of variation between genetic backgrounds. Additionally, we review advances in *C. elegans* methods that can facilitate the identification of NGD regulators and/or networks.

Conclusion: Genetic variation both in disease genes and in regulatory factors that modulate onset and progression of NGDs are incompletely understood. The nematode *C. elegans* represents a valuable system in which to address such questions.

Keywords: Neurodegenerative diseases, Natural variation, Quantitative genetics, *C. elegans*

Background

Neurodegenerative diseases (NGDs) cause disability and premature death, primarily among older people. These chronic and fatal illnesses include Alzheimer's disease (AD), Parkinson's disease (PD), Huntington's diseases (HD), spinocerebellar ataxia, prion diseases (PrD) (i.e., transmissible spongiform encephalopathies), frontotemporal dementia (FTD), and amyotrophic lateral sclerosis (ALS) [88]. Most NGDs are age dependent with their incidence increasing with advancing age. This makes understanding NGDs increasingly important given the recent increase in human lifespan seen in many countries. Many disease-causing mutations underlying different NGDs have phenotypic effects that result from the misfolding of proteins and/or mitochondrial dysfunctions leading to widespread damage in different parts of the nervous system (Fig. 1). This damage leads to a range of symptoms, and the overlap between symptoms in different NGDs can make it difficult to precisely diagnose patients. Diagnosis is further complicated by the individual variability apparent from the onset of disease [99]. For example, PD is characterized by motor issues, including tremor, slowing of movement, and an unstable gait, and by cognitive symptoms, but only some patients suffer from cognitive impairment and develop dementia [20].

The rate of disease progression (i.e., the duration of a given neuropathological stage) and clinical presentation also vary from one patient to another. Young onset PD patients, for example, often have a more frequent family history of PD and a more variable survival rate relative to those without the familial history [79]. Several studies of the amyloid-β protein aggregates, which cause AD, also indicate that the existence of distinct shapes in beta amyloid peptide (Aβ) aggregates, 40 residue Aβ (Aβ40)

* Correspondence: simon.harvey@canterbury.ac.uk
[1]Biomolecular Research Group, School of Human and Life Science, Canterbury Christ Church University, Canterbury CT1 1QU, UK
Full list of author information is available at the end of the article

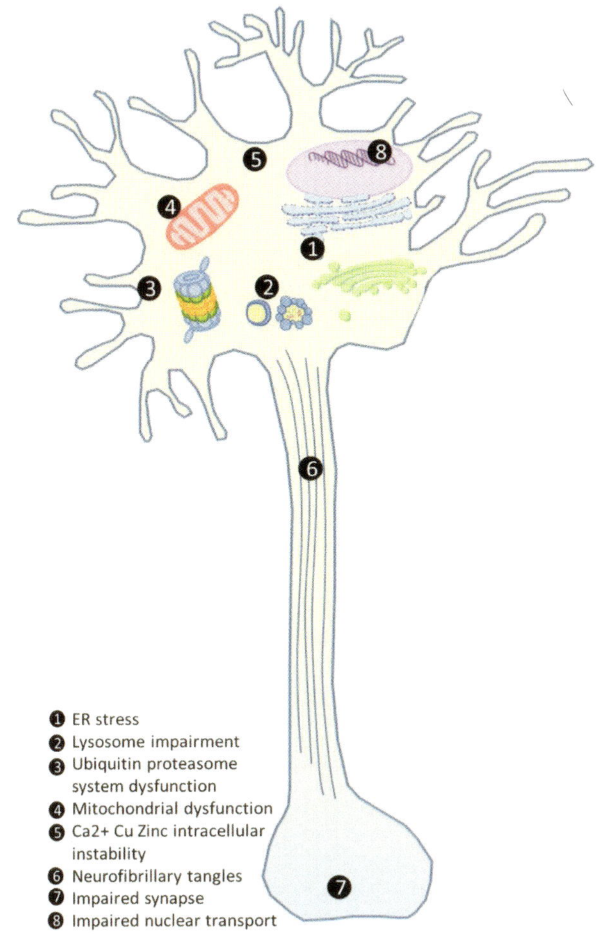

Fig. 1 Schematic diagram of the pathological mechanisms associated with neurodegeneration in neurons. Eight main events exist in the cellular biological processes related to neurodegeneration: *1* The protein-misfolding process inhibits ER to Golgi trafficking and alters ER-associated degradation, inducing the ER stress [55]; *2* Damaged lysosomes disrupt processes that maintains lysosomal homeostasis [78]; *3* Accumulation of misfolded proteins generates positive feedback exacerbating other effects [15]; *4* Dysfunctional mitochondrial maintenance directly affects mitochondrial biogenesis and induction of autophagy [75], e.g., the production of ROS and ATP in the cell; *5* Altered homeostasis generates excessive influx of calcium, copper, and zinc, due to ER and mitochondrial stresses [78]; *6* Plaques and neurofibrillary tangles, due to tau phosphorylation and aggregates, reduce neurotransmitter release, which also *7* weaken synaptic strength [15]; *8* Signaling pathways in the stressed organelle or the cytoplasm induce the transductions of the signals to the nucleus, which provoke DNA damage [10, 80]

and 42 residue Aβ fibril structures [51], and identify the distinct strain-specific traits (defined as "strainness") of the forms of AD by the different conformation of the aggregates [91, 104].

There is however limited knowledge about the mechanisms that determine individual variation. Individuals that carry the same mutation in the same disease-causing gene may display a range of different clinical symptoms. For example, assessing 6-year change in verbal memory, processing speed, and executive function in AD identified effects of MS4A4E, CLU, and NME8 in whites and of ZCWPW1 and CDS33 variants in African Americans. For MS4A4E and CLU, this association was only significant in individuals bearing at least one *APOE ϵ4* allele (AD risk gene) [9]. Apart from lifestyle and environment, these individual differences are caused by the unique genetic background of each person. The genetic background, thus, could be defined as the genetic makeup of all alleles that interact with the disease related to the "disease-causing" mutation.

Detailed mechanistic studies into background modifiers of NGDs are however difficult to conduct at the individual level in humans for ethical and technical reasons. Model organisms such as yeast, insects, worms, fish, and rodents are therefore critical to furthering our understanding of differences between individual in NGDs. This use is facilitated by the range of methods and approaches available to construct transgenic models of human diseases in model species with different genetic backgrounds [1, 19, 32, 53]. They are likewise an important resource for investigating the genetic underpinnings of quantitative traits, including complex disease phenotypes. Here, we review the onset and progression of NGDs in the context of genetic background and illustrate how work on the model species *Caenorhabditis elegans* can illuminate the underlying mechanisms of individual variation.

NGD phenotypes depend on the genetic background

Individual genetic backgrounds differ from thousands to millions of genetic variants that will range from single-nucleotide polymorphisms (SNPs) to, potentially very large, copy number variants (CNVs) [92, 109]. This genetic variation is a major determinate of differences in predisposition to disease [1, 41], where risk-increasing variants are numerous, display intricate patterns of interaction with each other as well as with non-genetic variables, and unlike classical Mendelian ("monogenic") disorders will often exhibit no simple mode of inheritance. Differential phenotypes for most NGDs arise from multiple genetic variants and their interaction with each other, as well as environmental factors. Hence, the genetics of these diseases is considered "complex" based on the heterogeneity in pathology and the disease polygenicity [8].

Genetic background can affect an important feature shared by different NGDs, specifically the formation of cerebral deposits of misfolded protein aggregates (also called prion-like proteins). For example, AD is characterized by the presence of neurofibrillary tangles and beta amyloid peptide (Aβ) in neural plaques, which are abnormal accumulations of microtubule-associated protein tau in a hyperphosphorylated state [82]. Similarly, the accumulation of proteins with polyglutamine-rich extensions is characteristic of HD and associated polyglutamine diseases [13], while PD involves the loss of dopaminergic neurons and the presence of Lewy bodies and Lewy neurites that are the aggregates of the synaptic protein alpha-synuclein. However, exactly how genetic variation modifies and affects specific parts of the NGD pathways is mostly unclear. We suggest that the genetic variation associated with NGDs can be grouped into two classes. Firstly, variation present directly in disease genes. Secondly, variation in regulatory factors that modulate onset and progression of the NGDs. Critically, this distinction separates those variations that are causative of disease from those that modify the disease but that on their own, cannot cause NGD.

In an example of the first such class of variants, multiple rare mutations in amyloid precursor protein (APP), or in the presenilin-1 and 2 genes (*PSEN1* and *PSEN2*), can cause early-onset AD (Fig. 3). Similarly, multiple mutations in leucine-rich repeat kinase 2 (*LRRK2*), a gene associated with PD, are known to be related to the sporadic late-onset form of the disease. Here, the G2385R and R1628P *LRRK2* variants are validated risk factors for PD in Asian populations, while the G2019S variant has been identified in different populations worldwide [57]. Examples of the second class of variants are those known to act in the IIS/mTOR pathway (Figs. 2 and 3). This pathway modulates response to a range of stresses and in the NGDs has been linked to a range of pathological processes (Fig. 1 and Table 1). For instance, Baleriola et al. [4] reported moderate eIF2α activation by Aβ and a greater frequency of ATF4 (the eIF2α effector) transcripts were identified in axons in the brain of AD patients. ATF4 is also known to activate the Parkin gene in PD and also to be related to stress pathways [55]. ATF4 therefore induces transcriptional expression of genes mediated by the UPR, including genes involved in amino acid metabolism, resistance to oxidative stress, and the proapoptotic transcription factor *CHOP*, which are related to disease processing [4, 24]. However, rare coding variation in ATF4 has been also found with pathway impairment in patients with sporadic cervical dystonia [69]. Additionally, Chaudhry et al. [11], using gene-based analyses for late-onset AD, revealed associations with the WT1, ZC3H12C, DLGAP2, and GPR1 genes, suggesting a possible role in AD pathogenesis.

Genetic variants therefore produce a broad spectrum of biological effects. This can be seen in analysis of natural variants affecting late-onset AD (LOAD), where more than 20 genes involved in a range of processes including metabolism, inflammation, synaptic activity, and intracellular trafficking have been identified [45]. CNVs are also associated with variation in NGD phenotypes, with, for example, a rare duplication of the amyloid-β protein precursor linked to early-onset AD [35]. Thus, the question of how genetic variants affect mechanisms in diseases such as AD and PD remains challenging. Here, model species like the nematode *C. elegans* might offer a solution and provide more insight into the mechanism(s) underlying individual variation in NGD disease phenotypes.

Natural variation associated with complex traits in *C. elegans* NGD models

C. elegans is a globally distributed nematode, and its level of natural genetic diversity is similar to human genetic variation [18]. Studying NGDs in a genetically tractable model species, such as *C. elegans*, allows detailed insight into the molecular pathogenesis. *C. elegans* models of AD, PD, HD, and other several NGDs have been established [22, 30, 31, 50, 84]. These models involve the transgenic expression of human genes under the control of a *C. elegans* promotor, with the resulting protein often linked to GFP or YFP. Applying fluorescent proteins (e.g., YFP) allows tracking of target proteins over time and the visualization of aggregation in vivo via the observation of the fluorescent foci (e.g., [101]). Such studies of AD using transgenic *C. elegans* have been carried out for many years. More recently, McColl et al. [53] have generated an improved model with human DA-Aβ 1–42 under the control of the muscle-specific promoter *unc-54* promotor. In this line, the full-length Aβ1-42 (the predominant Aβ species in human brain) is expressed in worm body wall muscle cells, and its oligomerizations and aggregations develop and result in severe. This fully penetrant, age progressive paralysis also shows more rapid than that caused from Aβ3-42 expression [53].

These transgenic models have all been generated in the N2 strain of *C. elegans* and have been widely used in screens for gene function analysis. However, such analyses in a single background have constrained the analysis and detection of natural allelic variants associated with complex traits. The most striking demonstration of this is a comparison of the RNAi phenotypes of ~1400 genes between N2 and CB4856 that showed that ~20% of genes differ in the severity of phenotypes between just these two genetic backgrounds [103]. Crucially, the natural variation found in *C. elegans* is also sufficient to cause significant changes in signaling pathways both at the gene expression (transcript and protein abundance) and phenotypic levels [87]. Accordingly, these could contribute to understanding how allelic variation affects gene expression, at the level of translation, in the multiple pathways and/or networks of complex traits involved in development and disease progression. For comparative investigations on mammalian genetics (including metabolism, aging, cancer, and neurodegeneration diseases), we therefore suggest that taking the different genetic backgrounds of the worm into consideration could be

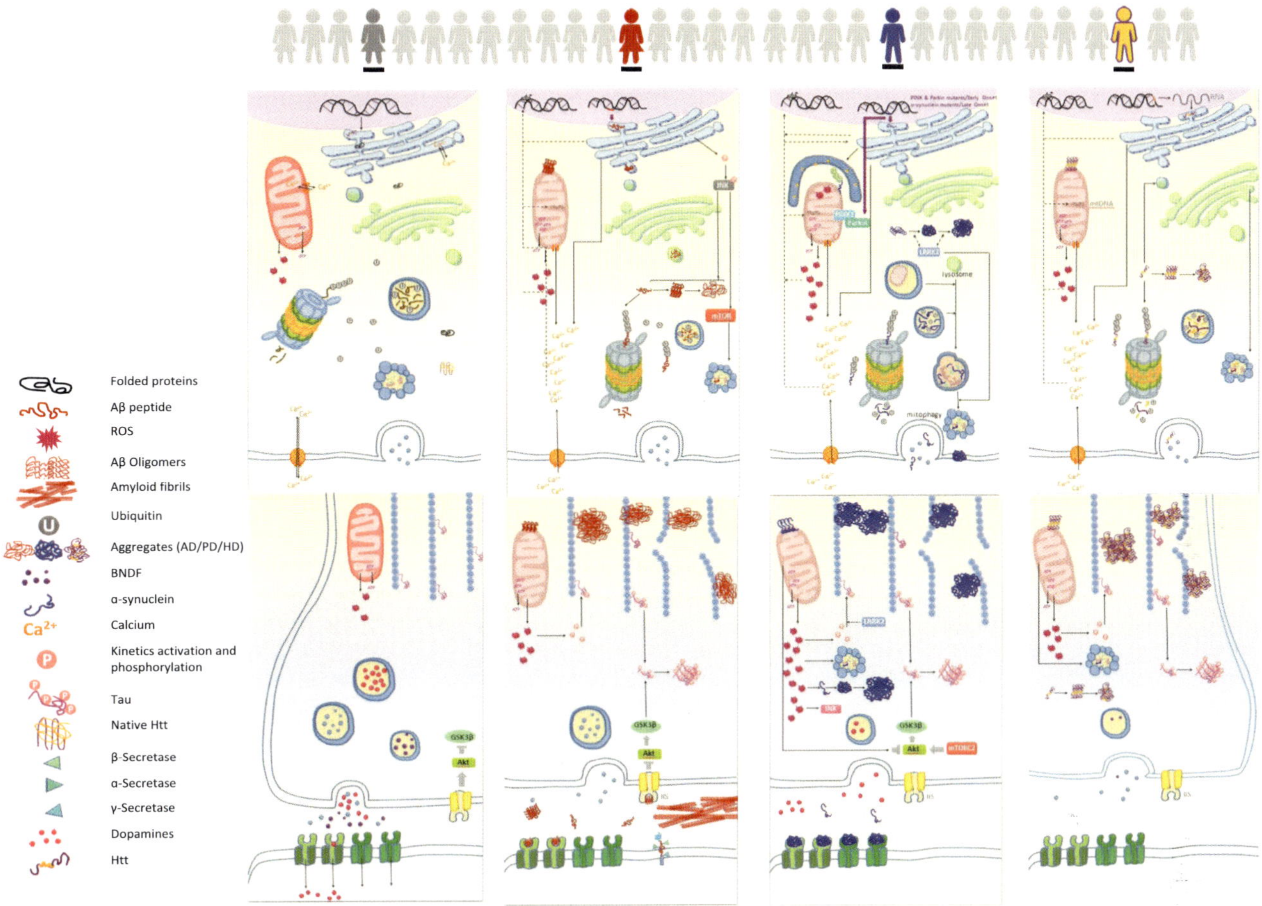

Fig. 2 The molecular processes implicated in neurodegeneration in the neurons of a normal healthy individual (*gray*) and in AD (*red*), PD (*blue*), and HD (*yellow*) patients. The schematic neuron is divided into the soma and axonal terminal bouton. For simplicity, postsynaptic/dendritic events are not included. Misfolded proteins aggregate first into oligomers and then into higher-molecular-weight insoluble protofibrils and further aggregates [17, 37, 104]. In AD patients with mutations in APP, PSEN1, PSEN2, or APOE, the JNK pathway is activated, increasing levels of phospho-JNK in neurons. This mediates the phosphorylation of APP and FoxO-dependent autophagy [52, 63]. Moreover, the soluble Aβ oligomers activate the mTOR pathways again promoting autophagy [52]. Further phosphorylation of tau and impaired Aβ activate the IIS/Akt pathways and affect cognitive function and synaptic plasticity [38]. In PD, mutations in PINK and Parkin (related to EOPD) or α-synuclein mutations (LOPD) lead to the inhibition of α-synuclein degradation as well as accumulation of autophagic vacuoles, which result in neuronal death [16, 96]. Misfolded α-synuclein also interacts with membranes and mitochondria, causing calcium dysregulation and a reduction of mitochondrial activity. This results in mtDNA damage as well as impairments to the ubiquitin-proteasome system (UPS) and mitophagy. The significant pathological etiology of HD is the enlargement of the polyglutamine (polyQ) domain within the HTT protein's N-terminus [110]. MLH1 (MutL homolog 1) and an SNP within a nuclear factor-κB binding site (Nf-KB) in the HTT promoter play a role in the altered onset of HD. In comparison with AD and PD, proteasome efficiency is strongly reduced in HD patients. Meanwhile, the polyQ domain of mutant HTT contributes increased toxicity by attracting and binding to other cytoplasmic and nuclear structures that contain polyglutamine (reviewed by [6]). Additionally, a major loss of brain-derived neurotrophic factor (BDNF) protein has been shown in HD and may due to the deficits in BDNF delivery and/or loss of BDNF gene transcription by mutant Htt [23, 39]

valuable. This approach would be likely to clarify proteostasis mechanisms and more fully reveal the relationships between genotype and phenotype. For example, in *Drosophila*, Chow et al. [14] showed 114 lines from the sequenced *Drosophila* Genetic Reference Panel of wild-derived inbred strains that exhibit the high heterogeneity in survival under endoplasmic reticulum (ER) stress conditions, and showed that 17 of 25 tested candidate genes were active in the putative response to ER stress [14].

Genetic and phenotypic differences between *C. elegans* populations have been identified with many traits shown to be variable between isolates (e.g., [2, 33, 40, 42, 90, 102]; for review, see [67]). Next to the canonical wild type Bristol N2, the most extensively characterized *C. elegans* isolate is the Hawaiian strain CB4856. This isolate is extensively diverged from N2, with a recent de novo assembly of the CB4856 genome suggesting that many variations have been maintained by balancing

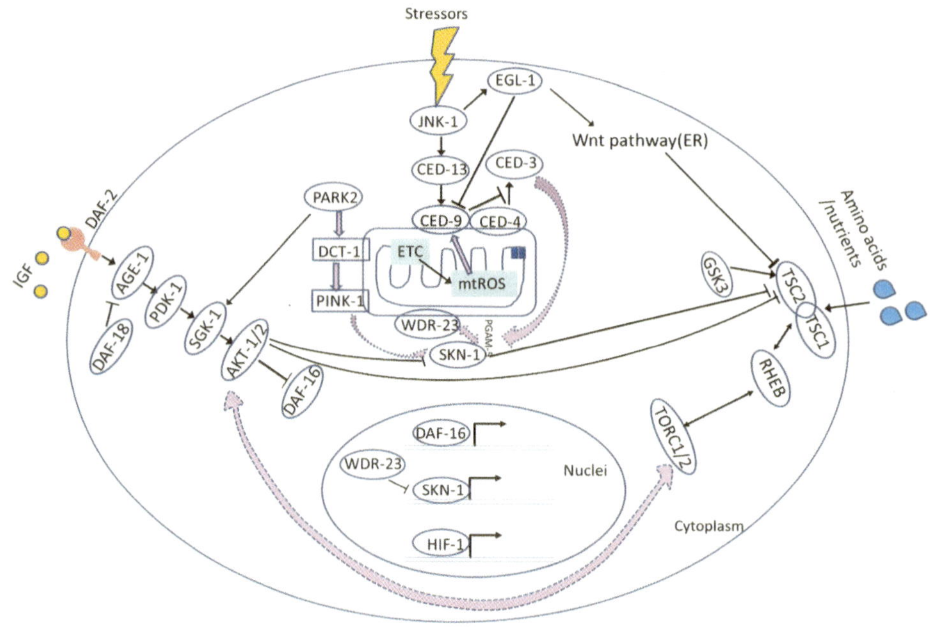

Fig. 3 *C. elegans* cellular pathways and their crosstalk, relating to aging and the stress response. Shown (from *left to right*) are the insulin/insulin-like growth factor (IIS) signaling pathway, the mitochondrial signaling pathways, and the mechanistic target of rapamycin (TOR) pathway. *Arrows* indicate positive regulatory events and *bars* indicate inhibitory interactions. *Purple block arrows* represent interactions between the different pathways, whereas *dashed purple block arrows* indicate possible indirect interactions. The oval molecules and their corresponding mammalian homologs involved in IIS [28, 56, 62, 72] are as below: AGE-1/PI3K, phospatidylinositol-3-kinase; PDK-1, 3-phosphoinositide-dependent kinase 1 ortholog; SGK-1, a serine/threonine protein kinase that is orthologous to the mammalian serum- and glucocorticoid-inducible kinases (SGKs); Akt/PKB, the serine/threonine kinase; DAF-16/FOXO, forkhead box O (FOXO) transcription factor. Mitochondrial dysfunctions [90–96] are associated with apoptotic/programmed cell death (PCD), aberrant autophagic regulation, endoplasmic reticulum dysfunction, and intracellular calcium, including c-Jun N-terminal kinase (JNK) subgroup of mitogen-activated protein (MAP) kinases; CED-4, CED-9, and EGL-1 belong to a conserved genetic pathway to regulate apoptosis during *C. elegans* development [63]; PINK-1, a predicted serine/threonine kinase which is similar with human *PINK1*, PTEN-induced kinase-1; *SKN-1/Nrf*, skin in excess transcription factor 1/NF-E2-related factor; *mtROS*, mitochondrial reactive oxygen species; *ATP*, adenosine-5′-triphosphate; *HIF-1*, hypoxia-inducible transcription factor 1. Major molecules in TOR pathways include *TSC1/2*, tuberous sclerosis complexes 1 and 2; *RHEB*, Ras homolog enriched in brain; *TOR*, target of rapamycin kinase; *GSK3*, glycogen synthase kinase ortholog. See text in Table 1 for further details

selection over long evolutionary timescales [94]. Wild *C. elegans* populations have also been shown to display significant local adaptation to their environment at multiple levels from the genotype and transcriptome [102]. Given this genetic and phenotypic variation, it is likely that variable natural genetic backgrounds of *C. elegans* will harbor abundant genetic variation that will modify the severity of NGD phenotypes. Wider analysis of more recently isolated wild isolates is also important as recent research has revealed specific adaptations to laboratory conditions that exist in the canonical wild-type Bristol N2 [5, 54, 66].

Studies into genetic background effects on NGDs in *C. elegans* have focused on a polyglutamine model. Here, Gidalevitz et al. [27] looked at the effects of natural genetic variation on susceptibility to aggregation and to toxicity [27]. This work introgressed a polyQ40 transgene from an N2 background into three wild genetic backgrounds, including the California-derived isolate DR1350, the Madeira isolate JU258, and the genetically distant Hawaiian isolate CB4856. A series of markers of pathology progression, such as onset of toxicity aggregation and the differential cell-specific susceptibility to aggregation, showed wide variation among the new introgression lines and between polyQ40 carrying recombinant inbred lines (RILs) derived from DR1350 and N2. This indicates that natural variation in genetic background can control resistance to misfolded protein aggregations and act to bind its associated cellular dysfunctions, which encourages further dissection on natural genetic variation susceptibility to age-related protein homeostasis in disease mechanisms.

Li et al. [49] mapped a large fraction of the *C. elegans* protein-protein interaction network. This was extended when the initial version of a human interactome map came out, adding more than 300 new connections to over 100 disease-associated proteins, including proteins related to NGD [73]. Lejeune et al. [48] accomplished a large-scale RNA interference screen in *C. elegans* strains that express N-terminal huntingtin in touch receptor neurons. Then, a subset of high-confidence modifier genes in pathways of interest in HD was identified by

Table 1 Pathways regulating longevity, stress, and disease responses

Insulin/Insulin-like growth factor (IIS) signaling pathway. The insulin-like receptor *DAF-2* is one of the main molecular components of IIS pathway in *C. elegans*, which is activated by binding insulin-like peptides (IPs) [44]. *DAF-2* activation by IPs results in recruitment and activation of AKT and SGK-1 (which are activated by phosphorylation of PDK-1 at the plasma membrane) to phosphorylate and sequester DAF-16 in the cytosol [95]. When activated by stresses, dephosphorylated DAF-16 enter the nucleus and regulates the transcription of a large number of genes involved in resistance to abiotic and biotic stresses, dauer larvae formation, metabolism, and longevity [63, 98]. DAF-16 can become dephosphorylated by the absence of the IP ligand(s), by inhibition from upstream pathway members—e.g., DAF-18 opposes the activity of PDK-1 and AKT-1 via inhibition of AGE-1—or by mutations in upstream genes, leading to lifespan extension [28, 56, 62, 72]. Strikingly, downregulation of IIS via *daf-2* or *age-1* mutations in *C. elegans* delays the formation of small aggregates in nematode models of NGDs and also slows the onset and decreases the severity of associated pathologies in a *daf-16*-dependent manner [17].

Mechanistic target of rapamycin (mTOR) pathway. The kinase mTOR integrates nutrient and anabolic signals to promote growth [52, 106, 112]. The TSC1/TSC2 complex acts as a negative regulator of mTORCs upstream, RHEB, but can be activated by AKT kinase (which belongs to IIS pathway) [36]. The mTORC signaling regulates a large number of developmental processes. TORC1 signaling transactivates/represses PH4-4 that induces pro-survival factors expression for life extension under nutrient restriction [85]. Moreover, TORC1 can increase protein synthesis and extends lifespan by both activating the ribosomal subunit S6 kinase (S6K) and inhibiting 4E-BP1 (a negative regulator of translation) [81, 97]. Meanwhile, investigations in *C. elegans* as well as other organisms have shown that autophagy is induced by inhibition of TORC1 [46]. An inadequate level of autophagy has been implicated in physiological responses to exercise and aging as well as in pathophysiological processes, such as cancer and metabolic and neurodegenerative disorders [47]. Although mammalian TORC2 (mTORC2) signaling shows insensitivity to nutrients in comparison to mTORC1, it does respond to growth factors like insulin through a poorly defined mechanism that requires PI3K (the *C. elegans* homolog is AGE-1) [111]. Moreover, mTORC2 directly activates AKT and SCK-1 which regulate cellular processes such as metabolism, survival, apoptosis, growth, and proliferation through the phosphorylation of several effectors [47]. In addition, TORC2 controls the cell cycle-dependent polarization of the actin cytoskeleton, which is involved in complex liposome mechanism, inducing several processes required for cancer cell growth, survival, and proliferation. Functioning as a nutrient sensor—detecting nutrients and amino acids—mTOR has a complex influence on several crucial cellular functions and shows clear effects on aging, protein synthesis and autophagy, and the homeostasis pathways that play a key role in the mechanisms that affect NGDs.

Mitochondrial signaling pathway. Mitochondria play important roles in aging and disease through apoptotic/programmed cell death (PCD), aberrant autophagic regulation, endoplasmic reticulum dysfunction, and intracellular calcium (see review [108]). The intrinsic apoptosis machinery of *C. elegans* comprises CED-9, CED-4, and CED-3, which is conserved from nematode to vertebrates and stimulates a protective response to mitochondrial dysfunction. JNK-1 promotes the expression of EGL-1 and CED-13. EGL-1 is required for all apoptosis, but CED-13 is required for pro-longevity signaling through the intrinsic pathway, i.e., mitochondrial reactive oxygen species (mROS) signaling pathway [80, 107]. Several stress factors, such as low IIS, heat stress, mitochondrial stress, and oxidative stress, among others, have been found to simulate the autophagic degradation of mitochondria (mitophagy). Besides sharing crucial regulatory factors with the general autophagy pathways, stressful conditions, specific components are also recruited for mitochondrial degradation. Outer mitochondrial membrane kinase PINK1 and its recruitment the cytosolic E3 ubiquitin ligase PARK2/parkin (also on the organelle) as well as their downstream signaling mediator, DCT-1, participate in mitophagy induction, mitochondrial homoeostasis protection, and survival promotion under stress conditions [65]. Mutations in PINK1 and PARK2 result in recessive familial forms of human Parkinson's disease and

Table 1 Pathways regulating longevity, stress, and disease responses *(Continued)*

correlate with mitochondrial dysfunction in mouse models [13, 58]. Similar to DAF-16, the transcription of SKN-1, which plays a key regulator in mitochondrial signaling pathway, has an influence on longevity and stress responses as well as NGDs [12, 107]. SKN-1 activation can be triggered by increased numbers of damaged mitochondria as well as increased cytoplasmic calcium levels upon mitophagy inhibition [65]. However, phosphorylation of SKN-1 by GSK-3 and kinases downstream from the *DAF-2* insulin-like pathway (AKT-1, AKT-2, and SGK-1) negatively regulate SKN-1 nuclear accumulation and activation [12, 98]. Prohibitin PHB complex, PHB1/PHB2, affect mitochondrial metabolism by sensing free radicals and/or mediating ROS production to influence longevity [3]. Interestingly, another negative regulator of SNK-1, WDR-23, has been found to interact with and regulate nuclear accumulation of SKN-1 but function independently of DAF-16 [12, 89].

Furthermore, Ca2+ released from the endoplasmic reticulum (ER) can also lead to ROS accumulation. The perturbation of ER Ca2+ homeostasis causes mitochondrial dysfunction, activating the mitochondrial-mediated apoptotic pathway, which has also been implicated in neuronal death in AD mouse model [59, 65]. Additionally, protein-folding stress at the ER stimulates the unfolded protein response (UPR), which is involved in the pathogenesis of many human diseases. For example, the basal activity of the UPR is beneficial under normal conditions but accelerates the pathology caused by toxic Ab protein in a *C. elegans* model of AD [74].

network-based analysis, including metabolic, neurodevelopmental, and pro-survival pathways. These results and those of similar large-scale analyses support the investigation of human disease pathways using *C. elegans* as a model (Table 1).

C. elegans offers the opportunity to investigate the genetic background modifiers affecting complex disease pathways (Table 2). For example, comparisons of RAS/MAPK signaling—a pathway critical in many complex human diseases, including AD [43]—across two different genetic backgrounds, N2 and CB4856, as well as their derived recombinant inbred lines identified the polymorphic monoamine oxidase *amx-2* (MAOA) as a negative regulator of RAS/MARK [77]. It was found that MAOA's effects on RAS/MAPK signaling are produced by its effects on the level of the serotoninmetabolite 5 hydroxyindoleacetic acid (5-HIAA), the first endogenous small molecule identified to act as a systemic inhibitor of RAS/MAPK signaling [77].

Genetic networks in stress and aging leverage the detection of NGD modifiers

NGDs are associated with other complex diseases (e.g., cancers). In part, this is a consequence of the involvement of the cellular systems that deal with various types of stress. For instance, variation in the genes that regulate the brain's molecular response to oxidative stress are associated with differential neural vulnerability to the damaging effects of amyloid-β [34]. Here, oxidative phosphorylation takes place within mitochondria, to meet the elevated energy demands of neurons (Figs. 1, 2, and 3). However, this can also accelerate the accumulated oxidative damage, which could trigger impaired

Table 2 Quantitative genetic studies of genomic and phenotypic variation

The majority of quantitative trait locus (QTL) mapping approaches require inbred strains that have different alleles at loci affecting variation in the trait of interest and a polymorphic molecular marker linkage map. A cross between two genetically distinct parental strains or a series of crosses among parental lines produces recombinant inbred lines (RILs) or other segregating populations, such as introgression lines (IL). In most cases, the final panel is repeatedly inbred to obtain isogenic, and thus genetically stable, lines. As a consequence of random recombination events, each RIL combines different parts of the two (or more) parental genomes. In most previous research on *C. elegans*, the Hawaiian CB4856 strain—a strain that is highly divergent from N2 at many loci—and N2 have been used to detect QTLs [7, 70]. Various N2xCB4856 RILs and ILs present variable transgressive traits, and large genetic and phenotypic differences for a wide range of traits including reproduction, growth, and gene expression.

QTL mapping has however a number of shortcomings. Since the location of identified QTLs is indicated only by looking at which markers give the greatest differences between genotype class averages, QTL effects are often poor estimates of the true allele(s) effect. Moreover, when QTLs are far from markers—as has often been the case in earlier work when the markers are widely spaced—the mapping resolution is low. Furthermore, the network of genes as well as by environmental factors can regulate the complex dynamic process, such as disease progressing. Therefore, the QTLs or nucleotides (QTNs) that underlie a complex dynamic trait are expected to be characterized. Despite functional mapping provides a useful quantitative and testable framework for assessing the interplay between gene actions or interactions and developmental changes [105], further investigations are still needed through its opportunity to study development in a comprehensive manner and to study the dynamic network of genes that determine the physiology of an individual organism over time.

For understanding genetic pathways and gene networks, mapping of gene expression levels as quantitative trait loci (called eQTLs) has also been increasingly used for determining how a given variant affects gene expression. Sequence variants in eQTLs affect the expression of a gene, while other QTLs impact on any given trait of interest except from the trait causing by gene expression [71]. Owing to available measurement of either traits or phenotypes, eQTLs have been identified by evaluating gene expression in panels of genetically distinct genotyped individuals [29, 71].

mitochondrial energy production and upregulate oxidative phosphorylation causing further DNA damage and significant levels of neuronal apoptosis [21].

A large number of genome-wide association studies (GWAS) in humans have identified pathways modulating the rate of aging and simultaneously influencing multiple age-related diseases such as NGDs [68, 76]. These GWAS studies have been invaluable in identifying and characterizing genetic variants associated with variation in disease phenotypes. For example, Seshadri et al. [83] identified 38 SNPs within 10 loci by integrating data from multiple studies and also identified CLU, PICALM, and CR1 as novel genes for late-onset AD (LOAD). A similar meta-analysis of GWAS studies of PD identified six more risk loci associated with the disease [60], while a combination of GWAS and whole-exome sequencing (WES) identified variants in the CEL gene/locus associated with PD [86]. Similarly, N'Songo et al. [61] identified ABCA7 missense variants that play a role in conferring AD risk in African Americans by performing WES with previously identified AD GWAS loci. According to their highlighted allelic heterogeneity at this locus, they also suggested the presence of additional AD risk variants in MS4A6A, PTK2B, and ZCWPW1.

NGDs are also strongly associated with aging, indicating that there is a link between protein misfolding and aging. This is very clear when the ILS (FOXO) pathway, a representative aging-related pathway, is considered. In *C. elegans*, this pathway ultimately controls the localization of DAF-16—a FOXO transcription factor that regulates a large number of genes involved in abiotic and biotic stress resistance, metabolism, and longevity—with dephosphorylation of DAF-16 allowing it to enter the nucleus [32]. The phosphorylation of DAF-16 is controlled by the insulin/IGF-1 transmembrane receptor ortholog *DAF-2*, with reductions in *daf-2* activity resulting in *daf-16*-dependent increases in lifespan. Loss of function *daf-2* mutations also increase lifespan in PD mutants of *C. elegans*, delaying the accumulation of small aggregates of alpha-synuclein in the body wall muscle and rescuing deficiencies in resistance to different stresses [17]. In humans, the age of onset of HD has a strong association with the length of polyQ expansion in the huntingtin protein but also varies between individuals with the same repeat length. In laboratory mouse strains, different genetic backgrounds can induce differential somatic expansion of CAG repeat.

Perspectives: what is the genetic architecture of variation in NGD responses in *C. elegans*?

C. elegans quantitative genetics (Table 2) has yielded considerable insights into understanding complex human disease pathways, but there has been limited work in extending this to the analysis of NGDs. To this end, powerful and serviceable datasets relating to causal genetic variant exploration based on genomic analysis have been collected and can be obtained from WormQTL^{HD} (human disease) www.WormQTL-HD.org [100]. WormQTL^{HD} allows for systematically investigating phenotypic expression of *C. elegans* at levels equivalent to those of human diseases, by catalyzing integration of reported disease candidate gene associations, gene orthologue data, molecular profiles, phenotypic variations, and QTL results [93, 100]. Thus, this will support relevant available meta-datasets for human-worm studies and database exploration.

Taken together, *C. elegans*, a powerful model organism, can be used to study how variation affects the onset and progression of protein-misfolding disease and how the susceptibility to proteotoxicity performs in genetically diverse but phenotypically general individuals. This may explain the higher propensity to aggregation of the mutant disease-related proteins, in order to uncovering onset and phenotypes of disease patterns [27]. Regardless of the toxicity and aggregation of misfolded proteins, other factors leading to the variable complex traits could possibly include multiple additive or allele interactions, with the consequence of underlying intervention strategies at onset and/or in progression of disease. In addition, Paaby et al. [64] revealed cryptic genetic variations (CGVs) in the gene networks of *C. elegans* embryogenesis. CGVs are silent alleles in general and can be only activated to influence phenotype, when other functional genes are perturbed. The seemingly omnipresent cryptic-effect loci segregate at intermediate frequencies in the wild. However, they reveal low developmental pleiotropy. In the specific perturbations, e.g., changes of the molecular, cellular, or developmental processes that govern its phenotypic expression in complex metabolic human diseases, CGVs are required to be revealed [42, 56]; for reviews, see [25, 26]. Above all, the natural variation play an important role in neurodegeneration, involving inherently plastic genetic and molecular pathways, and might allow for description of complex etiology and implementation in eluding the harmful influences.

Conclusions

Given the molecular conservation in neuronal signaling between *C. elegans* and vertebrates, including humans, this nematode is a valuable model species for studying NGD pathways and the alleles that affect them. Despite progress in identification of several AD- and PD-related genes, the effect of natural alleles underlying protein misfolding in these diseases remains mostly unclear. Here, we reviewed how natural variation could influence the severity of disease phenotypes. Experiments that rely solely on induced mutants in Bristol N2 limit the ability to explore how naturally varying alleles alter signaling pathways. Thus, further research should go beyond classic mutant screens on the genetic pathway analysis of complex traits, i.e., phenotypic differences among individuals, to also consider the allelic interactions in different genetic backgrounds. Consequently, the predictive nematode models of human genetic diseases could provide a more complete genetic and molecular understanding of how genetic variation shapes gene expression and cell biology for personalized genomic medicine.

Abbreviations

5-HIAA: Serotoninmetabolite 5 hydroxyindoleacetic acid; AD: Alzheimer's disease; ALS: Amyotrophic lateral sclerosis; APP: Amyloid precursor protein; Aβ: Beta amyloid peptide; BDNF: Brain-derived neurotrophic factor; CGVs: Cryptic genetic variations; CNV: Copy number variants; eQTLs: Expression quantitative trait loci; ER: Endoplasmic reticulum; FOXO: Forkhead box O protein; FTD: Frontotemporal dementia; GWAS: Genome wide association studies; HD: Huntington's disease; HTT: Huntingtin; IIS: Insulin/insulin-like growth factor; ILs: Introgression lines; JNK: c-Jun N-terminal kinase; LOAD: Late-onset Alzheimer s disease; LRRK2: Leucine-rich repeat kinase 2; MAOA: Monogeamine oxidase *amx-2*; MAPK: Mitogen-activated protein kinases; MLH1: MutL homolog 1; mROS: Mitochondrial reactive oxygen species; mTOR: Mechanistic target of rapamycin; mTORC2: Mammalian TORC2; NGDs: Neurodegenerative diseases; PCD: Programmed cell death; PD: Parkinson's disease; polyQ: Polyglutamine; PrD: Prion diseases; QTLs: Quantitative trait locus; QTNs: Quantitative trait nucleotides; RILs: Recombinant inbred lines; ROS: Reactive oxygen species; S6K: Subunit S6 kinase; SNP: Single nucleotide polymorphism; UPR: Unfolded protein response; UPS: Ubiquitin/proteasome system; WES: Whole-exome sequencing

Acknowledgements

We thank Mark Sterken, Basten Snoek, Jana Stastna, Katharina Jovic, Yu Nie, and the members of our laboratories for helpful advice and discussions. We also thank Bei Tian, Jun Qiu, Yongran Ji, Chunyue Wei, and Dianfan Zhou for assistance.

Funding

YW is supported by a PhD Scholarship from Canterbury Christ Church University. JK is supported by the Human Frontiers Science Program. SH is supported by the Leverhulme Trust.

Authors' contributions

YW, JK, and SH wrote the manuscript. All authors read and approved the final manuscript.

Competing interests

The authors declare that they have no competing interests.

Author details

[1]Biomolecular Research Group, School of Human and Life Science, Canterbury Christ Church University, Canterbury CT1 1QU, UK. [2]Laboratory of Nematology, Wageningen University, 6708 PB Wageningen, The Netherlands.

References

1. Albert FW, Kruglyak L. The role of regulatory variation in complex traits and disease. Nat Rev Genet. 2015;16:197–212.
2. Andersen EC, Shimko TC, Crissman JR, et al. A powerful new quantitative genetics platform, combining *Caenorhabditis elegans* high-throughput fitness assays with a large collection of recombinant strains. G3 (Bethesda). 2015;5:911–20.
3. Artal-Sanz M, Tavernarakis N. Prohibitin and mitochondrial biology. Trends Endocrinol Metab. 2009;20:394–401.
4. Baleriola J, Walker CA, Jean YY, et al. Axonally synthesized ATF4 transmits a neurodegenerative signal across brain regions. Cell. 2014;158:1159–72.
5. Balla KM, Andersen EC, Kruglyak L, Troemel ER. A wild *C. elegans* strain has enhanced epithelial immunity to a natural microsporidian parasite. PLoS Pathog. 2015;11:1–21.
6. Becanovic K, Norremolle A, Neal SJ, et al. A SNP in the HTT promoter alters NF-[kappa]B binding and is a bidirectional genetic modifier of Huntington disease. Nat Neurosci. 2015;18:807–16.
7. Bendesky A, Pitts J, Rockman M V, et al. Long-range regulatory polymorphisms affecting a GABA receptor constitute a quantitative trait locus (QTL) for social behavior in *Caenorhabditis elegans*. PLoS Genet. 2012; 8(12):e1003157.
8. Bertram L, Bertram L, Tanzi RE, Tanzi RE. The genetic epidemiology of neurodegenerative disease. J Clin Invest. 2005;115:1449–57.
9. Bressler J, Mosley TH, Penman A, et al. Genetic variants associated with risk of Alzheimer's disease contribute to cognitive change in midlife: the Atherosclerosis

Risk in Communities Study. Am J Med Genet Part B Neuropsychiatr Genet. 2017;174:269–82.
10. Chakraborty S, Bornhorst J, Nguyen TT, Aschner M. Oxidative stress mechanisms underlying Parkinson's disease-associated neurodegeneration in *C. elegans*. Int J Mol Sci. 2013;14:23103–28.
11. Chaudhry M, Wang X, Bamne MN, et al. Genetic variation in imprinted genes is associated with risk of late-onset Alzheimer's disease. J Alzheimers Dis. 2015;44:989–94.
12. Choe KP, Przybysz AJ, Strange K. The WD40 repeat protein WDR-23 functions with the CUL4/DDB1 ubiquitin ligase to regulate nuclear abundance and activity of SKN-1 in *Caenorhabditis elegans*. Mol Cell Biol. 2009;29:2704–15.
13. Choi AMK, Ryter SW, Levine B. Autophagy in human health and disease. N Engl J Med. 2013;368:651–62.
14. Chow CY, Wolfner MF, Clark AG. Using natural variation in Drosophila to discover previously unknown endoplasmic reticulum stress genes. Proc Natl Acad Sci. 2013;110:9013–8.
15. Ciechanover A, Kwon YT. Degradation of misfolded proteins in neurodegenerative diseases: therapeutic targets and strategies. Exp Mol Med. 2015;47:e147.
16. Collier TJ, Redmond DE, Steece-Collier K, et al. Is alpha-synuclein loss-of-function a contributor to parkinsonian pathology? Evidence from non-human primates. Front Neurosci. 2016;10:1–7.
17. Cooper JF, Dues DJ, Spielbauer KK, et al. Delaying aging is neuroprotective in Parkinson's disease: a genetic analysis in *C. elegans* models. npj Park Dis. 2015;1:15022.
18. Cutter AD. Nucleotide polymorphism and linkage disequilibrium in wild populations of the partial selfer *Caenorhabditis elegans*. Genetics. 2006;172:171.
19. Dawson TM, Ko HS, Dawson VL. Genetic animal models of Parkinson's disease. Neuron. 2010;66:646–61.
20. Del Tredici K, Braak H. Lewy pathology and neurodegeneration in premotor Parkinson's disease. Mov Disord. 2012;27:597–607.
21. Driver JA. Inverse association between cancer and neurodegenerative disease: review of the epidemiologic and biological evidence. Biogerontology. 2014;15:547–57.
22. Faber PW, Voisine C, King DC, et al. Glutamine/proline-rich PQE-1 proteins protect *Caenorhabditis elegans* neurons from huntingtin polyglutamine neurotoxicity. Proc Natl Acad Sci U S A. 2002;99:17131–6.
23. Ferrer I, Goutan E, Marín C, et al. Brain-derived neurotrophic factor in Huntington disease. Brain Res. 2000;866:257–61.
24. Fusakio ME, Willy JA, Wang Y, et al. Transcription factor ATF4 directs basal and stress-induced gene expression in the unfolded protein response and cholesterol metabolism in the liver. Mol Biol Cell. 2016;27:1536–51.
25. Gaertner BE, Parmenter MD, Rockman MV, et al. More than the sum of its parts: a complex epistatic network underlies natural variation in thermal preference behavior in *Caenorhabditis elegans*. Genetics. 2012;192:1533–42.
26. Gaertner BE, Phillips PC. *Caenorhabditis elegans* as a platform for molecular quantitative genetics and the systems biology of natural variation. Genet Res (Camb). 2010;92:331–48.
27. Gidalevitz T, Wang N, Deravaj T, et al. Natural genetic variation determines susceptibility to aggregation or toxicity in a *C. elegans* model for polyglutamine disease. BMC Biol. 2013;11:100.
28. Gil EB, Malone Link E, Liu LX, et al. Regulation of the insulin-like developmental pathway of *Caenorhabditis elegans* by a homolog of the PTEN tumor suppressor gene. Proc Natl Acad Sci. 1999;96:2925–30.
29. Gutteling EW, Riksen J a G, Bakker J, Kammenga JE. Mapping phenotypic plasticity and genotype-environment interactions affecting life-history traits in *Caenorhabditis elegans*. Heredity (Edinb). 2007;98:28–37.
30. Harrington AJ, Hamamichi S, Caldwell GA, Caldwell KA. *C. elegans* as a model organism to investigate molecular pathways involved with Parkinson's disease. Dev Dyn. 2010;239:1282–95.
31. Hassan WM, Dostal V, Huemann BN, et al. Identifying Aβ-specific pathogenic mechanisms using a nematode model of Alzheimer's disease. Neurobiol Aging. 2015;36:857–66.
32. Hesp K, Smant G, Kammenga JE. *Caenorhabditis elegans* DAF-16/FOXO transcription factor and its mammalian homologs associate with age-related disease. Exp Gerontol. 2015;72:1–7.
33. Hodgkin J, Doniach T. Natural variation and copulatory plug formation in *Caenorhabditis elegans*. Genetics. 1997;146:149–64.
34. Hohman TJ, Koran MEI, Thornton-Wells TA. Genetic variation modifies risk for neurodegeneration based on biomarker status. Front Aging Neurosci. 2014;6:1–11.
35. Hooli BV, Kovacs-Vajna ZM, Mullin K, et al. Rare autosomal copy number variations in early-onset familial Alzheimer's disease. Mol Psychiatry. 2013;19:676–81.
36. HUANG J, MANNING BD. The TSC1–TSC2 complex: a molecular switchboard controlling cell growth. Biochem J. 2008;412:179–90.
37. Imarisio S, Carmichael J, Korolchuk V, et al. Huntington's disease: from pathology and genetics to potential therapies. Biochem J. 2008;412:191–209.
38. Jack CR, Knopman DS, Jagust WJ, et al. Tracking pathophysiological processes in Alzheimer's disease: an updated hypothetical model of dynamic biomarkers. Lancet Neurol. 2013;12:207–16.
39. Jeon J, Kim W, Jang J, et al. Gene therapy by proteasome activator, PA28γ, improves motor coordination and proteasome function in Huntington's disease YAC128 mice. Neuroscience. 2016;324:20–8.
40. Kamkina P, Snoek LB, Grossmann J, et al. Natural genetic variation differentially affects the proteome and transcriptome in *C. elegans*. Mol Cell Proteomics. 2016;15(5):1670–80.
41. Kammenga JE. The background puzzle: how identical mutations in the same gene lead to different disease symptoms. The FEBS Journal. 2017. doi:10.1111/febs.14080.
42. Kammenga JE, Phillips PC, De Bono M, Doroszuk A. Beyond induced mutants: using worms to study natural variation in genetic pathways. Trends Genet. 2008;24:178–85.
43. Kim EK, Choi E-J. Pathological roles of MAPK signaling pathways in human diseases. Biochim Biophys Acta - Mol Basis Dis. 2010;1802:396–405.
44. Kimura KD, Tissenbaum HA, Liu Y, Ruvkun G. *daf-2*, an insulin receptor-like gene that regulates longevity and diapause in *Caenorhabditis elegans*. Science. 1997;277:942–6.
45. Lambert J-C, Ibrahim-Verbaas CA, Harold D, et al. Meta-analysis of 74,046 individuals identifies 11 new susceptibility loci for Alzheimer's disease. Nat Genet. 2013;45:1452–8.
46. Lapierre LR, Meléndez A, Hansen M. Autophagy links lipid metabolism to longevity in *C. elegans*. Autophagy. 2012;8:144–6.
47. Laplante M, Sabatini DM. Regulation of mTORC1 and its impact on gene expression at a glance. J Cell Sci. 2013;126:1713–9.
48. Lejeune FX, Mesrob L, Parmentier F, Bicep C, Vazquez-Manrique RP, Parker JA, Vert JP, Tourette C, Neri C. Large-scale functional RNAi screen in *C. elegans* identifies genes that regulate the dysfunction of mutant polyglutamine neurons. BMC genomics. 2012;13(1):91.
49. Li S, Armstrong CM, Bertin N, et al. A map of the interactome network of the metazoan *C. elegans*. Science. 2004;303:540–3.
50. Link CD. *C. elegans* models of age-associated neurodegenerative diseases: lessons from transgenic worm models of Alzheimer's disease. Exp Gerontol. 2006;41:1007–13.
51. Lu J-X, Qiang W, Yau W-M, et al. Molecular structure of β-amyloid fibrils in Alzheimer's disease brain tissue. Cell. 2013;154:1257–68.
52. Ma XM, Blenis J. Molecular mechanisms of mTOR-mediated translational control. Nat Rev Mol Cell Biol. 2009;10:307–18.
53. McColl G, Roberts BR, Pukala TL, et al. Utility of an improved model of amyloid-beta (Aβ1-42) toxicity in *Caenorhabditis elegans* for drug screening for Alzheimer's disease. Mol Neurodegener. 2012;7:57.
54. McGrath PT, Xu Y, Ailion M, et al. Parallel evolution of domesticated Caenorhabditis species targets pheromone receptor genes. Nature. 2011;477:321–5.
55. Mercado G, Valdés P, Hetz C. An ERcentric view of Parkinson's disease. Trends Mol Med. 2013;19:165–75.
56. Mihaylova VT, Borland CZ, Manjarrez L, et al. The PTEN tumor suppressor homolog in *Caenorhabditis elegans* regulates longevity and dauer formation in an insulin receptor-like signaling pathway. Proc Natl Acad Sci U S A. 1999;96:7427–32.
57. Monfrini E, Di Fonzo A. In: Rideout HJ, editor. Leucine-rich repeat kinase (LRRK2) genetics and Parkinson's disease BT—leucine-rich repeat kinase 2 (LRRK2). Cham: Springer International Publishing; 2017. p. 3–30.
58. Morris BJ, Willcox DC, Donlon TA, Willcox BJ. FOXO3: a major gene for human longevity—a mini-review. Gerontology. 2015;61:515–25.
59. Mota SI, Costa RO, Ferreira IL, et al. Oxidative stress involving changes in Nrf2 and ER stress in early stages of Alzheimer's disease. Biochim Biophys Acta - Mol Basis Dis. 2015;1852:1428–41.
60. Nalls MA, Pankratz N, Lill CM, et al. Large-scale meta-analysis of genome-wide association data identifies six new risk loci for Parkinson's disease. Nat Genet. 2014;46:989–93.

61. N'Songo A, et al. Comprehensive screening for disease risk variants in early-onset Alzheimer's disease genes in African Americans identifies novel PSEN variants. J Alzheimers Dis. 2017;56(4):1215–22.
62. Ogg S, Ruvkun G. The *C. elegans* PTEN Homolog, DAF-18, acts in the insulin receptor-like metabolic signaling pathway. Mol Cell. 2016;2:887–93.
63. Oh SW, Mukhopadhyay A, Svrzikapa N, et al. JNK regulates lifespan in *Caenorhabditis elegans* by modulating nuclear translocation of forkhead transcription factor/DAF-16. Proc Natl Acad Sci U S A. 2005;102:4494–9.
64. Paaby A, White A, Riccardi D. *C. elegans* harbors pervasive cryptic genetic variation for embryogenesis *C. elegans* harbors pervasive cryptic genetic variation for embryogenesis. 2014. p. 1–31.
65. Palikaras K, Lionaki E, Tavernarakis N. Coupling mitogenesis and mitophagy for longevity. Autophagy. 2015;11:1428–30.
66. Petersen C, Dirksen P, Schulenburg H. Why we need more ecology for genetic models such as *C. elegans*. Trends Genet. 2015;31:120–7.
67. Phillips PC. Epistasis—the essential role of gene interactions in the structure and evolution of genetic systems. Nat Rev Genet. 2008;9:855–67. doi:10.1038/nrg2452.
68. Ramanan VK, Saykin AJ. Pathways to neurodegeneration: mechanistic insights from GWAS in Alzheimer's disease, Parkinson's disease, and related disorders. Am J Neurodegener Dis. 2013;2:145–75.
69. Rittiner JE, Caffall ZF, Hernandez-Martinez R, et al. Functional genomic analyses of mendelian and sporadic disease identify impaired eIF2α signaling as a generalizable mechanism for dystonia. 2016.
70. Rockman MV. The QTN program and the alleles that matter for evolution: all that's gold does not glitter. Evolution (NY). 2012;66:1–17.
71. Rodriguez M, Snoek LB, Riksen JAG, et al. Genetic variation for stress-response hormesis in *C. elegans* lifespan. Exp Gerontol. 2012;47:581–7.
72. Rouault J-P, Kuwabara PE, Sinilnikova OM, et al. Regulation of dauer larva development in *Caenorhabditis elegans* by *daf-18*, a homologue of the tumour suppressor *PTEN*. Curr Biol. 2016;9:329–34.
73. Rual J-F, Venkatesan K, Hao T, et al. Towards a proteome-scale map of the human protein-protein interaction network. Nature. 2005;437:1173–8.
74. Safra M, Ben-Hamo S, Kenyon C, Henis-Korenblit S. The ire-1 ER stress-response pathway is required for normal secretory-protein metabolism in *C. elegans*. J Cell Sci. 2013;126:4136–46.
75. Saito T, Sadoshima J (2016) HHS Public Access. 116:1477–1490.
76. Sanchez-Mut JV, Heyn H, Vidal E, et al. Human DNA methylomes of neurodegenerative diseases show common epigenomic patterns. Transl Psychiatry. 2016;6:e718.
77. Schmid T, Snoek LB, Fröhli E, et al. Systemic regulation of RAS/MAPK signaling by the serotonin metabolite 5-HIAA. PLoS Genet. 2015;11:e1005236.
78. Schneider L, Zhang J. Lysosomal function in macromolecular homeostasis and bioenergetics in Parkinson's disease. Mol Neurodegener. 2010;5:14.
79. Schrag A, Schott JM. Epidemiological, clinical, and genetic characteristics of early-onset parkinsonism. Lancet Neurol. 2006;5:355–63.
80. Schumacher B, Hanazawa M, Lee MH, et al. Translational repression of *C. elegans* p53 by GLD-1 regulates DNA damage-induced apoptosis. Cell. 2005;120:357–68.
81. Selman C, Tullet JMA, Wieser D, et al. Ribosomal protein S6 Kinase 1 signaling regulates mammalian life span. Science. 2009;326:140–4.
82. Serrano-Pozo A, Frosch MP, Masliah E, Hyman BT. Neuropathological alterations in Alzheimer disease. Cold Spring Harb Perspect Med. 2011;1:a006189.
83. Seshadri S, Fitzpatrick AL, Arfan Ikram M, et al. Genome-wide analysis of genetic loci associated with Alzheimer's disease. JAMA. 2010;303:1832–40.
84. Settivari R, VanDuyn N, LeVora J, Nass R. The Nrf2/SKN-1-dependent glutathione S-transferase π homologue GST-1 inhibits dopamine neuron degeneration in a *Caenorhabditis elegans* model of manganism. Neurotoxicology. 2013;38:51–60.
85. Sheaffer KL, Updike DL, Mango SE. The target of rapamycin (TOR) pathway antagonizes pha-4/FoxA to control development and aging. Curr Biol. 2008;18:1355–64.
86. Siitonen A, Nalls MA, Hernández D, et al. Genetics of early-onset Parkinson's disease in Finland: exome sequencing and genome-wide association study. Neurobiol Aging. 2017;53:195.e7–195.e10.
87. Singh KD, Roschitzki B, Snoek LB, *et al.* Natural genetic variation influences protein abundances in *C. elegans* developmental signalling pathways. PLoS One. 2016;11(3):e0149418.
88. Soto C. Protein misfolding in neurodegenerative diseases : the key pending questions. 2013. p. 19–22.
89. Staab TA, Griffen TC, Corcoran C, et al. The conserved SKN-1/Nrf2 stress response pathway regulates synaptic function in *Caenorhabditis elegans*. PLoS Genet. 2013;9(3):e1003354.
90. Stastna JJ, Snoek LB, Kammenga JE, Harvey SC. Genotype-dependent lifespan effects in peptone deprived *Caenorhabditis elegans*. Sci Rep. 2015;5:16259.
91. Stöhr J, Condello C, Watts JC, et al. Distinct synthetic Aβ prion strains producing different amyloid deposits in bigenic mice. Proc Natl Acad Sci. 2014;111:10329–34.
92. Stranger BE, Forrest MS, Dunning M, et al. Relative impact of nucleotide and copy number variation on gene expression phenotypes. Science. 2007;315:848–53.
93. Swertz MA, van der Velde KJ, Tesson BM, et al. XGAP: a uniform and extensible data model and software platform for genotype and phenotype experiments. Genome Biol. 2010;11:R27.
94. Thompson D, Regev A, Roy S. Comparative analysis of gene regulatory networks: from network reconstruction to evolution. Annu Rev Cell Dev Biol. 2015;31:399–428.
95. Tissenbaum HA. Genetics, life span, health span, and the aging process in *Caenorhabditis elegans*. J Gerontol A Biol Sci Med Sci. 2012;67(A):503–10.
96. Triplett JC, Zhang Z, Sultana R, et al. Quantitative expression proteomics and phosphoproteomics profile of brain from PINK1 knockout mice: Insights into mechanisms of familial Parkinson's disease. J Neurochem. 2015;133:750–65.
97. Troulinaki K, Bano D. Mitochondrial deficiency: a double-edged sword for aging and neurodegeneration. Front Genet. 2012;3:1–10.
98. Tullet JMA. DAF-16 target identification in *C. elegans*: past, present and future. Biogerontology. 2015;16:221–34.
99. Ukraintseva SV, Arbeev KG, Akushevich I, et al. Trade-offs between cancer and other diseases: do they exist and influence longevity? Rejuvenation Res. 2010;13:387–96.
100. Van Der Velde KJ, De Haan M, Zych K, et al. WormQTLHD—a web database for linking human disease to natural variation data in *C. elegans*. Nucleic Acids Res. 2014;42:794–801.
101. Van Ham TJ, Thijssen KL, Breitling R, et al. *C. elegans* model identifies genetic modifiers of alpha-synuclein inclusion formation during aging. 2008.
102. Volkers RJM, Snoek LB, van H Hubar CJ, et al. Gene-environment and protein-degradation signatures characterize genomic and phenotypic diversity in wild *Caenorhabditis elegans* populations. BMC Biol. 2013;11:93.
103. Vu V, Verster AJ, Schertzberg M, et al. Natural variation in gene expression modulates the severity of mutant phenotypes. Cell. 2015;162:391–402.
104. Watts JC, Condello C, Stöhr J, et al. Serial propagation of distinct strains of Aβ prions from Alzheimer's disease patients. Proc Natl Acad Sci U S A. 2014; 111:10323–8.
105. Wu RL, Lin M. Opinion: functional mapping—how to map and study the genetic architecture of dynamic complex traits. Nat Rev Genet. 2006;7:229–37.
106. Wullschleger S, Loewith R, Hall MN. TOR signaling in growth and metabolism. Cell. 2006;124:471–84.
107. Yee C, Yang W, Hekimi S. The intrinsic apoptosis pathway mediates the pro-longevity response to mitochondrial ROS in C elegans. Cell. 2014;157:897–909.
108. Zaltieri M, Longhena F, Pizzi M, et al. Mitochondrial dysfunction and alpha-synuclein synaptic pathology in Parkinson's disease: who's on first? Parkinsons Dis. 2015;2015:1–10.
109. Zhang F, Gu W, Hurles ME, Lupski JR. Copy number variation in human health, disease, and evolution. Annu Rev Genomics Hum Genet. 2009;10:451–81.
110. Zhang X, Abels ER, Redzic JS, et al. Potential transfer of polyglutamine and CAG-repeat RNA in extracellular vesicles in Huntington's disease: background and evaluation in cell culture. Cell Mol Neurobiol. 2016;36:459–70.
111. Zinzalla V, Stracka D, Oppliger W, Hall MN. Activation of mTORC2 by association with the ribosome. Cell. 2011;144:757–68.
112. Zoncu R, Efeyan A, Sabatini DM. mTOR: from growth signal integration to cancer, diabetes and ageing. Nat Rev Mol Cell Biol. 2011;12:21–35.

5

Mutational analysis of COL1A1 and COL1A2 genes among Estonian osteogenesis imperfecta patients

Lidiia Zhytnik[1*], Katre Maasalu[1,2], Ene Reimann[3,4], Ele Prans[4], Sulev Kõks[3,4] and Aare Märtson[1,2]

Abstract

Background: Osteogenesis imperfecta (OI) is a rare bone disorder. In 90% of cases, OI is caused by mutations in the *COL1A1/2* genes, which code procollagen α1 and α2 chains. The main aim of the current research was to identify the mutational spectrum of *COL1A1/2* genes in Estonian patients. The small population size of Estonia provides a unique chance to explore the collagen I mutational profile of 100% of OI families in the country.

Methods: We performed mutational analysis of peripheral blood gDNA of 30 unrelated Estonian OI patients using Sanger sequencing of *COL1A1* and *COL1A2* genes, including all intron-exon junctions and 5′UTR and 3′UTR regions, to identify causative OI mutations.

Results: We identified *COL1A1/2* mutations in 86.67% of patients (26/30). 76.92% of discovered mutations were located in the *COL1A1* ($n = 20$) and 23.08% in the *COL1A2* ($n = 6$) gene. Half of the *COL1A1/2* mutations appeared to be novel. The percentage of quantitative *COL1A1/2* mutations was 69.23%. Glycine substitution with serine was the most prevalent among missense mutations. All qualitative mutations were situated in the chain domain of pro-α1/2 chains.

Conclusion: Our study shows that among the Estonian OI population, the range of collagen I mutations is quite high, which agrees with other described OI cohorts of Northern Europe. The Estonian OI cohort differs due to the high number of quantitative variants and simple missense variants, which are mostly Gly to Ser substitutions and do not extend the chain domain of *COL1A1/2* products.

Keywords: Osteogenesis Imperfecta, Collagen I, *COL1A1*, *COL1A2*, Sanger sequencing

Background

Despite being a rare genetic bone fragility disorder, osteogenesis imperfecta (OI) is among the most widely occurring of rare congenital skeletal dysplasias [1]. OI prevalence is estimated 1/10,000–20,000 at birth [2, 3]. OI is characterized by low bone mineral density, recurrent fractures, skeletal deformations, and blue eye sclera [2, 4–6]. Other remarkable features of OI include Dentinogenesis Imperfecta, triangular face, hearing loss, joint laxity, short stature, and easy bruising [2, 4–6].

OI has many manifestations and is considered a group of disorders. Phenotypes range from mild osteopenia to severe deformities or even mortality. In 1979, Sillence described four OI types (I–IV) according to phenotype severity [5]. Recent updated classification distinguishes three additional types with specific histologies (V–VII) [4, 7]. Genetic OI classification considers every OI gene as a separate OI type and so far includes OI types I–XVII [4, 8, 9].

The genetics of the disorder reflect the complexity of the OI phenotype range. Up to 21 different genes have been associated with occurrence of OI [10–19]. Previous studies have shown that the primary cause of OI are mutations in the *COL1A1/2* genes, which code procollagen type I α1 and α2 chains, respectively [20]. Despite the approximately 1500 mutations already described in collagen type I genes, investigators continue to report novel mutations [21]. Moreover, there is still some

* Correspondence: Lidiia.Zhytnik@ut.ee
[1]Department of Traumatology and Orthopedics, University of Tartu, Puusepa 8, 51014 Tartu, Estonia
Full list of author information is available at the end of the article

controversy regarding the proportion of collagen mutations reported in different populations, which have ranged from 60 to 95% [9, 10]. In this context, we believe that population-based studies of OI genetics might broaden current knowledge of collagen I mutations and OI.

Due to Estonia's small population (1.3 million) and centered treatment, follow-up, and research of all OI patients at the OI Center of the Traumatology and Orthopedics Clinic, Tartu University (TU) Hospital, it was possible to perform analysis of *COL1A1/2* mutations among the whole Estonian OI population [22]. Herein, we describe for the first time the mutational spectrum of *COL1A1/2* genes among 30 unrelated OI patients, from 30 Estonian OI families, which we estimate to constitute ~ 100% of OI cases in Estonia.

Methods

Subjects

The patients included in the study are treated and followed-up by the OI Center of the Traumatology and Orthopedics Clinic, TU Hospital.

A total of 30 OI patients from 30 unrelated families were included in the study. Data regarding the OI types of the subjects were obtained from the medical records of TU Hospital [23]. All new OI cases across Estonia are registered by and treated at TU Hospital's OI Center. Thus, it can be estimated that as of May 2017, the current patient cohort represented ~ 100% of the Estonian OI population.

No patient came from a consanguineous family. Mutational analysis of the *COL1A1/2* genes was performed on a younger affected member of every OI family included in the study.

In accordance with the Declaration of Helsinki, all patients or their legal representatives signed an informed consent form prior to participation. The study was approved by the University of Tartu's Ethical Review Committee on Human Research (permit no. 221/M-34).

Genealogical description

Genealogical data of OI history in the family, consanguinity, and miscarriages was obtained from each patient or their representative. We constructed pedigree trees per kindred using the "Kinship2" package in R v3.3.2 [24].

Mutational analysis of the *COL1A1/2* genes

Genomic DNA (gDNA) was purified from 3 ml of ethylenediaminetetraacetic acid (EDTA) preserved whole blood samples—stored at −80 °C—using a Gentra Puregene Blood Kit (Quiagen, Germany) following the manufacturer's protocol.

PCR amplification and Sanger sequencing were performed as described previously [25]. Sequence products were analyzed using Applied Biosystems' Sequence Scanner v1.0 and Mutation Surveyor DNA Variant analysis software v5.0.1. (Softgenetics, USA) and aligned to the GenBank human reference genome sequences of *COL1A1* (gDNA NG_007400.1, complementary (cDNA) NM_000088.3), and *COL1A2* (gDNA NG_007405.1, cDNA NM_000089.3). Raw sequencing data are available from the authors upon request. We focused on non-synonymous and splice-site variants absent from the publicly available normal datasets (including dbSNP135 and the 1000 Genomes Project) [26, 27]. We used the PolyPhen-2, SIFT, and MutationTaster software tools to predict the functional effects and pathogenicity of mutations [28–30]. Variants absent from the osteogenesis imperfecta mutation database were considered novel (http://www.le.ac.uk/ge/collagen/) [21, 31].

All statistical analyses were carried out with R v3.3.2. software (R Team, Austria) [32]. To assess the distribution of *COL1A1/2* mutations and compare them to other studied OI populations, percentage differences were used.

Results

Mutational analysis of the *COL1A1/2* genes of Estonian OI patients highlighted OI causative mutations in 26 of 30 patients (86.67%) (Fig. 1a). The number of patients harboring *COL1A1* mutations was 20 (76.92%); *COL1A2* mutations were found in 6 patients (23.08%) (Fig. 1b). A list of the mutations and their characteristics can be found in Table 1.

The number of novel mutations was 13/26 (50%) (Table 1). Half of the *COL1A1* and *COL1A2* mutations appeared to be undescribed in the collagen type I mutation database. Patient EE26 had a heterozygous non-synonymous rs1800215 SNP (p.Ala1075Thr) in the *COL1A1* gene, which was described before as a benign variant (data not shown). [33]

Twenty-five mutations had an autosomal dominant inheritance pattern (Table 1). Of these, eight patients had no previous history of OI in the family. Thus, we assumed that their parents and relatives, who did not have any clinical features of OI, are not carriers of these mutations.

Patient EE07 had a recessive missense mutation. Mutational analysis showed that their parents are not carriers of the mutation, which confirmed the de novo nature of the mutation.

We found 12/26 mutations (46.15%) had altering splice sites, 10 and 2 in the *COL1A1* and *COL1A2* genes, respectively. One of the patients harbored a deletion capturing both coding and intronic sequence, in exon-intron 34 (EE30). Nonsense mutations were present in 6

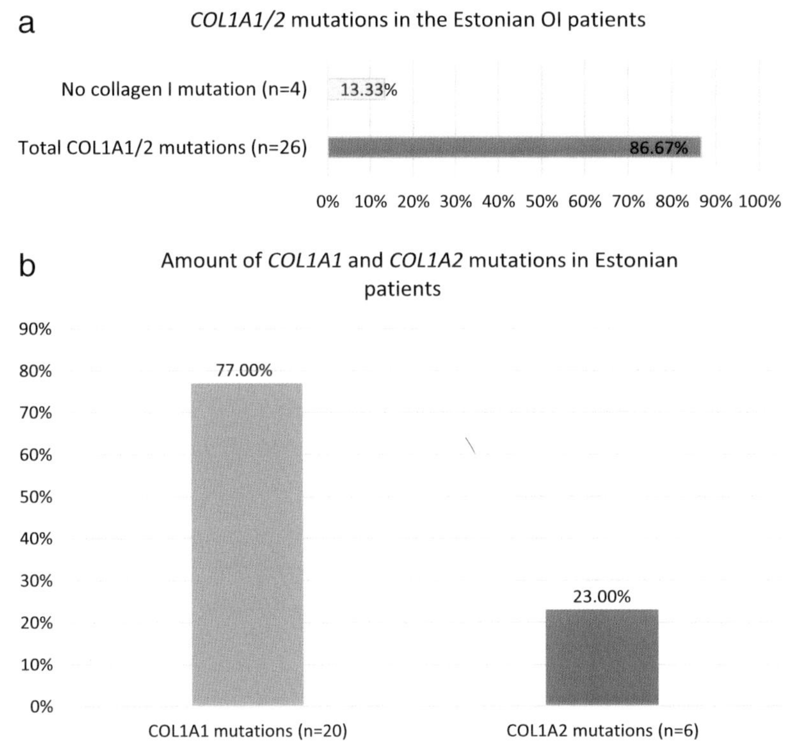

Fig. 1 Diagram of collagen type I mutation distribution Estonian OI patients. **a** Percentage of patients with *COL1A1/2* mutations vs patients negative for collagen I mutations. **b** Percentage of mutations in the *COL1A1* and *COL1A2* genes

patients (23.08%), all in the *COL1A1* gene. Overall, quantitative mutations were present in 18 patients (16 in *COL1A1* and 2 in *COL1A2* genes) (Fig. 2).

Missense mutations, associated with collagen I quality defects, were indicated in eight patients (30.77%), four in *COL1A1* and four in *COL1A2* genes. Of these, seven were Glycine substitutions (four of the *COL1A2* and three of the *COL1A1* missense mutations). In four cases, Glycine was substituted with Serine, two in the *COL1A1* and *COL1A2* genes, respectively (Fig. 2).

A c.3262G>T (*COL1A1*) mutation was detected in two patients (EE21 and EE22), who were thought to be unrelated (Table 1). Investigation of the pedigree trees revealed a distant relationship between the families four generations back, of which the patients were not aware. Two identical splice site mutations at c.1821 + 1G>A (*COL1A1*) in intron 26 were identified in patients EE02 (type III OI) and EE05 (type I OI) (Table 1). This mutation arose independently in the patients and caused phenotypes of different severity.

Discussion

Collagen I mutations were found in 26/30 (87%) studied OI patients. Previous findings have suggested collagen mutations ranging from 60 to 90% among different OI populations and study cohorts [25]. In a Finnish OI study, 90.7% of patients harbored collagen I mutations [34], which is higher than we found among Estonian OI patients. In Pollitt et al.'s study, collagen I mutations were revealed in 75% of OI patients [35], which is slightly lower than our Estonian cohort. Our data is in good agreement with research on the genetic epidemiology of the Swedish OI population, of which 87% had collagen I mutations [36]. The results of our study are also in concordance with Bardai et al.'s recent study of a large number (598) of OI individuals, where collagen type I mutations were found in 86% of OI patients of all types and different ethnic groups [19].

In some population studies, the amount of collagen I mutations were also lower. For example, in 51.4% of Taiwanese patients ($N = 72$), 52.2% of Korean patients ($N = 67$), and 59.4% of Vietnamese OI patients ($N = 91$) [25, 37, 38]. Due to the difficulties in arranging large cross-population studies of a rare disorder in populous countries, results can often be fragmented, which complicates population-wide estimates [39, 40]. However, questions about the lower collagen type I mutational pattern of OI patients from Asian populations remain.

The proportions of *COL1A1* and *COL1A2* in Estonian, Finnish, and Swedish OI populations were surprisingly similar, 77 and 23%, 78 and 22%, and 79 and 21%, respectively [34, 36]. Similar values were reported by Pollitt et al., where 77% of mutations occurred in the *COL1A1* and 23% in the *COL1A2* gene ($N = 83$) [35]. In

Table 1 Mutational spectrum of the *COL1A1* and the *COL1A2* genes among Estonian OI patients

No	Patient ID	Gene	Mutation	Exon	Mutation type	Protein alteration	Sillence OI type
1	EE01#	COL1A2	c.1630G>GT*	Exon 28	Missense	p.Gly544Cys	III
2	EE02	COL1A1	c.1821 + 1G>GA	Intron 26	Splice site	–	III
3	EE03	COL1A1	c.1897G>GT*	Exon 26	Nonsense	p.Glu633*	IV
4	EE04	COL1A1	c.750 + 2T>TA*	Intron 10	Splice site	–	IV
5	EE05	COL1A1	c.1821 + 1G>GA	Intron 26	Splice site	–	I
6	EE07#	COL1A1	c.2317G>T*	Exon 33_34	Missense	p.Gly773Cys	II
7	EE08	COL1A1	c.3217G>GA*	Exon 45	Missense	p.Gly1073Ser	III
8	EE09	COL1A1	c.1155 + 2T>TG*	Intron 17	Splice site	–	I
9	EE10	COL1A1	c.1128_hetdelT	Exon 17	Frameshift	p.Gly377Alafs*164	I
10	EE11#	COL1A1	c.3235G>GA	Exon 45	Missense	p.Gly1079Ser	I
11	EE13	COL1A1	c.2089C>CT	Exon 31	Nonsense	p.Arg697*	IV
12	EE14#	COL1A1	c.904-9G>GA	Intron 13	Splice site	–	I
13	EE15	COL1A2	c.1009G>GA	Exon 19	Missense	p.Gly337Ser	III
14	EE16#	COL1A2	c.2324G>GA	Exon 38	Missense	p.Gly775Glu	III
15	EE17#	COL1A1	c.3045 + 1G>GA	Intron 42	Splice site	–	IV
16	EE18	COL1A1	c.505G>GA*	Exon 6	Missense	p.Glu169Lys	I
17	EE19	COL1A1	c.299-1G>GC*	Intron 3	Splice site	–	IV
18	EE20	COL1A2	c.937-3C>CT	Intron 18	Splice site	–	I
19	EE21	COL1A1	c.3262G>GT*	Exon 46	Nonsense	p.Gly1088*	IV
20	EE22	COL1A1	c.3262G>GT*	Exon 46	Nonsense	p.Gly1088*	I
21	EE24	COL1A1	c.1767 + 5G>GA*	Intron 25	Splice site	–	IV
22	EE25	COL1A1	c.1354-2A>AG	Intron 20	Splice site	–	I
23	EE27#	COL1A1	c.3208-1G>GA*	Intron 44	Splice site	–	I
24	EE29#	COL1A2	c.865G>AG	Exon 17	Missense	p.Gly289Ser	III
25	EE30	COL1A2	c.2026-1_2031het dup*	Intron-Exon 34	Splice site, frameshift	–	III/IV
26	EE31#	COL1A1	c.1081C>CT	Exon 17	Nonsense	p.Arg361*	I

Patients with de novo mutations and without OI history in the family are marked with an octothorp (#). Novel mutations unreported in the collagen type I variant database (http://www.le.ac.uk/ge/collagen/) are marked with an asterisk (*). In cases of heterozygous mutation, both the wild type and the mutated allele are indicated after an arrow (>)

Bardai et al.'s 2016 study, 69% were *COL1A1* and 31% *COL1A2* mutations, which is similar to the beforementioned results [19].

The Estonian cohort also has a high proportion of quantitative mutations compared to qualitative collagen mutations, 69 and 31%, respectively. In the Finnish OI cohort, 67% of mutations were quantitative and 33% qualitative [34]. In the work of Pollitt et al., 35% of mutations were qualitative and 65% quantitative [35]. In the Swedish population, the proportions were almost equal (53 and 47%) [36]. Interestingly, we found only two quantitative mutations in the *COL1A2* gene, which matches previous reports about comparatively lower numbers of quantitative mutations of this gene [34–36]. Due to the higher number of mutations leading to haploinsufficiency in the *COL1A1* gene compared to the *COL1A2* gene, patients harboring mutations in the *COL1A1* gene had milder phenotypes (I, IV) compared to patients with *COL1A2* mutations (type III, except EE20 who had a splice site mutation and OI type I).

Glycine substitutions composed the vast majority of missense mutations (7 of 8 cases), with serine being the most substituted amino acid (4 of 7 cases), which supports previous findings. Curiously, all missense mutations were situated in triple helical chain domains (aa residues 162–1218 α1; aa residues 80–1102 α2) of *COL1A1/2* gene products. Only one mutation (patient EE07 with OI type II) altered the "lethal cluster" proposed by Marini et al. [41].

Half of the mutations (50%) we found appeared to be novel. Despite the numerous works on collagen I mutations and a growing list of identified mutations, the number of revealed novel variants was high, which underlines the individual nature of OI mutations [19, 35, 36]. Half of the glycine substitutions (4 of 7) were even absent from the collagen I mutational database.

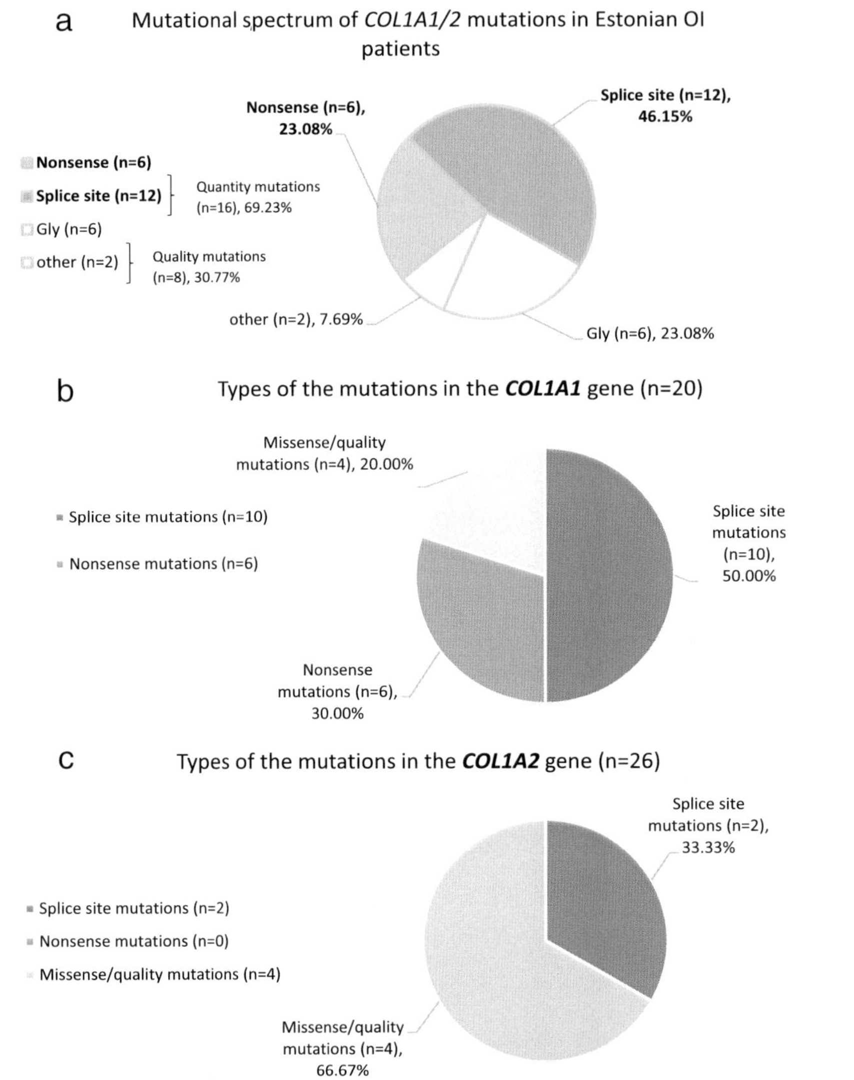

Fig. 2 a Mutational spectrum of *COL1A1/2* mutations in Estonian OI patients. Distribution of the *COL1A1* (**b**) and *COL1A2* (**c**) mutations according to mutation type

Despite sharing of the same mutation, patients may develop different phenotypes, as in the case of patients EE02 and EE05, who had type III and I OI, respectively. Genotype-phenotype correlations remain an unresolved issue in our understanding of OI. Cases of inter- and intra-familial OI diversity are not rare. Not only genetics, but additional factors, such as epigenetics and environment might contribute to the development of specific OI phenotypes. This leads to many questions and the need to further investigate potential OI factors.

Sanger sequencing is a powerful and accurate method of mutational analysis and allows the identification of frameshift, and missense and nonsense mutations in the coding regions of genes. Moreover, due to the special design of the primers distant from intron-exon junction regions, we could asses splice site mutations of the *COL1A1/2* genes, which are the cause of quantitative collagen defects. However, the current study had some limitations. We could not identify whole gene or exon deletions and duplications, which could have slightly reduced the number of discovered *COL1A1/2* mutations. In addition, due to the small population size of Estonia, our cohort was limited. We cannot exclude the possibility that the small sample size might be the cause of differences compared to the results of other studies.

Conclusion

This paper has described the mutational spectrum of *COL1A1/2* genes among 30 Estonian OI patients, which were estimated to represent ~ 100% of OI families in Estonia at the time. We identified collagen I mutations in 87% of Estonian OI families. The number of quantitative mutations (69%) was high compared to other European OI cohorts. All missense mutations of our Estonian patients altered the triple helical chain domain of α1 and α2 procollagen chains. One mutation was situated in the lethal cluster. A normal distribution of novel collagen mutations (50%) among the *COL1A1* (77%) and *COL1A2* (23%) genes, and mostly glycine substitutions were observed, compared to other OI cohorts of Northern Europe. Four patients that showed no collagen type I mutations will be further studied using whole exome sequencing analysis to identify disease causing variants.

Abbreviations
3'UTR: Three prime untranslated region; 5'UTR: Five prime untranslated region; cDNA: Complementary DNA; EDTA: Ethylenediaminetetraacetic acid; gDNA: Genomic DNA; OI: Osteogenesis Imperfecta; TU: University of Tartu

Acknowledgements
We would like to thank the following people and organizations for their help and support with data collection: workers of the Department of Traumatology and Orthopedics and Department of Pathophysiology, University of Tartu, and Ardo Birk and Madis Karu for the development of the online OI database of the Clinic of Traumatology and Orthopedics, TU Hospital.

Funding
This study was supported by the Estonian Science Agency project IUT20-46 (TARBS14046I), the European Regional Development Fund and the Archimedes Foundation to the Centre of Excellence on Translational Medicine, the University of Tartu's Development Fund, University of Tartu's Baseline Funding, and the HypOrth Project funded by the European Union's 7th Framework Programme grant agreement no. 602398.

Authors' contributions
LZ conceived the study, carried out the genetic studies, performed the data analysis, participated in the design of the study, and drafted the manuscript. EP, SK, and ER carried out the genetic studies, performed the data analysis, and helped to draft the manuscript. KM participated in the design of the study, interacted with the patients, coordinated the blood sample collection, and helped to draft the manuscript and perform analysis. SK and AM participated in the designing of the study, coordinated the data interpretation and statistical analysis, and helped to draft the manuscript. All authors read and approved the final manuscript.

Competing interests
The authors declare that they have no competing interests.

Author details
[1]Department of Traumatology and Orthopedics, University of Tartu, Puusepa 8, 51014 Tartu, Estonia. [2]Clinic of Traumatology and Orthopedics, Tartu University Hospital, Puusepa 8, 51014 Tartu, Estonia. [3]Centre of Translational Medicine, University of Tartu, Ravila 14a, 50411 Tartu, Estonia. [4]Department of Pathophysiology, University of Tartu, Ravila 19, 50411 Tartu, Estonia.

References
1. Martin E, Shapiro JR. Osteogenesis imperfecta: epidemiology and pathophysiology. Curr Osteoporos Rep. 2009;5(3):91–7. doi:10.1007/s11914-007-0023-z.
2. Byers PH, Steiner RD. Osteogenesis imperfecta. Annu Rev Med. 1992;43:269–82. doi:10.1146/annurev.me.43.020192.001413.
3. Martin E, Shapiro JR. Osteogenesis imperfecta: epidemiology and pathophysiology. Curr Osteoporos Rep. 2007;5(3):91–7. http://www.ncbi.nlm.nih.gov/pubmed/17925189. Accessed 5 Apr 2017
4. Van Dijk FS, Sillence DO. Osteogenesis imperfecta: clinical diagnosis, nomenclature and severity assessment. Am J Med Genet A. 2014;164A(6):1470–81. doi:10.1002/ajmg.a.36545.
5. Sillence DO, Senn A, Danks DM. Genetic heterogeneity in osteogenesis imperfecta. J Med Genet. 1979;16(2):101–16. http://www.pubmedcentral.nih.gov/articlerender.fcgi?artid=1012733&tool=pmcentrez&rendertype=abstract. Accessed 18 Sept 2014
6. Ben Amor M, Rauch F, Monti E, Antoniazzi F. Osteogenesis imperfecta. Pediatr Endocrinol Rev. 2013;10(Suppl 2):397-405. http://www.ncbi.nlm.nih.gov/pubmed/23858623. Accessed 11 Dec 2014.
7. Fratzl-Zelman N, Misof BM, Roschger P, Klaushofer K. Classification of osteogenesis imperfecta. Wien Med Wochenschr. 2015;165(13-14):264–70. doi:10.1007/s10354-015-0368-3.
8. Home - OMIM - NCBI. http://www.ncbi.nlm.nih.gov/omim. Accessed 18 Feb 2015.
9. Shapiro JR. Clinical and genetic classification of osteogenesis imperfecta and epidemiology. In: Osteogenesis Imperfecta. Elsevier; 2014:15-22. doi:10.1016/B978-0-12-397165-4.00002-2.
10. Cho T-J, Lee K-E, Lee S-K, et al. A single recurrent mutation in the 5'-UTR of IFITM5 causes osteogenesis imperfecta type V. Am J Hum Genet. 2012;91(2):343–8. doi:10.1016/j.ajhg.2012.06.005.
11. Semler O, Garbes L, Keupp K, et al. A mutation in the 5'-UTR of IFITM5 creates an in-frame start codon and causes autosomal-dominant osteogenesis imperfecta type V with hyperplastic callus. Am J Hum Genet. 2012;91(2):349–57. doi:10.1016/j.ajhg.2012.06.011.
12. Amor IM, Ben F, Rauch K, Gruenwald M, Weis DR, Eyre P. Roughley FH, Glorieux and RM. Severe osteogenesis imperfecta caused by a small in-frame deletion in CRTAP. Am J Med Genet A. 2011;42(11):157–62. doi:10.1002/ajmg.a.34269. Severe.
13. van Dijk FS, Zillikens MC, Micha D, et al. PLS3 mutations in X-linked osteoporosis with fractures. N Engl J Med. 2013;369(16):1529–36. doi:10.1056/NEJMoa1308223.
14. Becker J, Semler O, Gilissen C, et al. Exome sequencing identifies truncating mutations in human SERPINF1 in autosomal-recessive osteogenesis imperfecta. Am J Hum Genet. 2011;88(3):362–71. doi:10.1016/j.ajhg.2011.01.015.
15. Christiansen HE, Schwarze U, Pyott SM, et al. Homozygosity for a missense mutation in SERPINH1, which encodes the collagen chaperone protein HSP47, results in severe recessive osteogenesis imperfecta. Am J Hum Genet. 2010;86(3):389–98. doi:10.1016/j.ajhg.2010.01.034.
16. Willaert a, Malfait F, Symoens S, et al. Recessive osteogenesis imperfecta caused by LEPRE1 mutations: clinical documentation and identification of the splice form responsible for prolyl 3-hydroxylation. J Med Genet. 2009;46:233–41. doi:10.1136/jmg.2008.062729
17. Marini JC, Reich A, Smith SM. Osteogenesis imperfecta due to mutations in non-collagenous genes: lessons in the biology of bone formation. Curr Opin Pediatr. 2014;26(4):500–7. doi:10.1097/MOP.0000000000000117.
18. Alanay Y, Avaygan H, Camacho N, et al. Mutations in the gene encoding the RER protein FKBP65 cause autosomal-recessive osteogenesis imperfecta. Am J Hum Genet. 2010;86(4):551–9. doi:10.1016/j.ajhg.2010.02.022.
19. Bardai G, Moffatt P, Glorieux FH, Rauch F. DNA sequence analysis in 598 individuals with a clinical diagnosis of osteogenesis imperfecta: diagnostic yield and mutation spectrum. Osteoporos Int. 2016;27(12):3607–13. doi:10.1007/s00198-016-3709-1.
20. van Dijk FS, Cobben JM, Kariminejad A, et al. Osteogenesis imperfecta: a review with clinical examples. Mol Syndromol. 2011;2(1):1–20. doi:000332228.
21. Dalgleish R. The human collagen mutation database 1998. Nucleic Acids Res. 1998;26(1):253–5. http://www.ncbi.nlm.nih.gov/pubmed/9399846. Accessed 5 Apr 2017
22. Statistics Estonia. The population of Estonia increased last year—statistics Estonia. http://www.stat.ee/news-release-2017-008. Accessed 5 Apr 2017.
23. Maasalu K, Haviko T, Märtson A. Treatment of children with osteogenesis imperfecta in Estonia. Acta Paediatr. 2007;92(4):452–5. doi:10.1111/j.1651-2227.2003.tb00577.x.
24. Sinnwell JP, Therneau TM, Schaid DJ. The kinship2 R package for pedigree data. Hum Hered. 2014;78(2):91–3. doi:10.1159/000363105.
25. Ho Duy B, Zhytnik L, Maasalu K, et al. Mutation analysis of the COL1A1 and COL1A2 genes in Vietnamese patients with osteogenesis imperfecta. Hum Genomics. 2016;10(1):27. doi:10.1186/s40246-016-0083-1.
26. Home - SNP - NCBI. https://www.ncbi.nlm.nih.gov/snp. Accessed 11 Apr 2017.
27. Genomes | A deep catalog of human genetic variation. http://www.internationalgenome.org/. Accessed 11 Apr 2017.

28. Kumar P, Henikoff S, Ng PC. Predicting the effects of coding non-synonymous variants on protein function using the SIFT algorithm. Nat Protoc. 2009;4(7):1073–81. doi:10.1038/nprot.2009.86.
29. Adzhubei IA, Schmidt S, Peshkin L, et al. A method and server for predicting damaging missense mutations. Nat Methods. 2010;7(4):248–9. doi:10.1038/nmeth0410-248.
30. Schwarz JM, Rödelsperger C, Schuelke M, Seelow D. MutationTaster evaluates disease-causing potential of sequence alterations. Nat Methods. 2010;7(8):575–6. doi:10.1038/nmeth0810-575.
31. Dalgleish R. The human type I collagen mutation database. Nucleic Acids Res. 1997;25(1):181–7. http://www.ncbi.nlm.nih.gov/pubmed/9016532. Accessed 5 Apr 2017
32. Chen R, Mias GI, Li-Pook-Than J, et al. Personal omics profiling reveals dynamic molecular and medical phenotypes. Cell. 2012;148(6):1293–307. doi:10.1016/j.cell.2012.02.009.
33. Bodian DL, Chan T-F, Poon A, et al. Mutation and polymorphism spectrum in osteogenesis imperfecta type II: implications for genotype-phenotype relationships. Hum Mol Genet. 2009;18(3):463–71. doi:10.1093/hmg/ddn374.
34. Hartikka H, Kuurila K, Körkkö J, et al. Lack of correlation between the type of *COL1A1* or *COL1A2* mutation and hearing loss in osteogenesis imperfecta patients. Hum Mutat. 2004;24(2):147–54. doi:10.1002/humu.20071.
35. Pollitt R, McMahon R, Nunn J, et al. Mutation analysis of COL1A1 and COL1A2 in patients diagnosed with osteogenesis imperfecta type I–IV. Hum Mutat. 2006;27(7):716. doi:10.1002/humu.9430.
36. Lindahl K, Åström E, Rubin C-J, et al. Genetic epidemiology, prevalence, and genotype–phenotype correlations in the Swedish population with osteogenesis imperfecta. Eur J Hum Genet. 2015;23(8):1042–50. doi:10.1038/ejhg.2015.81.
37. Lin H-Y, Chuang C-K, Su Y-N, et al. Genotype and phenotype analysis of Taiwanese patients with osteogenesis imperfecta. Orphanet J Rare Dis. 2015;10:152. doi:10.1186/s13023-015-0370-2.
38. Lee K-S, Song H-R, Cho T-J, et al. Mutational spectrum of type I collagen genes in Korean patients with osteogenesis imperfecta. Hum Mutat. 2006;27(December 2005):599. doi:10.1002/humu.9423
39. Yang Z, Ke ZF, Zeng C, Wang Z, Shi HJ, Wang LT. Mutation characteristics in type I collagen genes in Chinese patients with osteogenesis imperfecta. Genet Mol Res. 2011;10(1):177–85. doi:10.4238/vol10-1gmr984.
40. Zhang Z-L, Zhang H, Ke Y, et al. The identification of novel mutations in COL1A1, COL1A2, and LEPRE1 genes in Chinese patients with osteogenesis imperfecta. J Bone Miner Metab. 2012;30(1):69–77. doi:10.1007/s00774-011-0284-6.
41. Marini JC, Forlino A, Cabral WA, et al. Consortium for osteogenesis imperfecta mutations in the helical domain of type I collagen: regions rich in lethal mutations align with collagen binding sites for integrins and proteoglycans. Hum Mutat. 2007;28(3):209–21. doi:10.1002/humu.20429.

6

Overexpressed HSF1 cancer signature genes cluster in human chromosome 8q

Christopher Q. Zhang[1,4], Heinric Williams[3,4], Thomas L. Prince[3,4†] and Eric S. Ho[1,2*†]

Abstract

Background: HSF1 (heat shock factor 1) is a transcription factor that is found to facilitate malignant cancer development and proliferation. In cancer cells, HSF1 mediates a set of genes distinct from heat shock that contributes to malignancy. This set of genes is known as the HSF1 Cancer Signature genes or simply HSF1-CanSig genes. HSF1-CanSig genes function and operate differently than typical cancer-causing genes, yet it is involved in fundamental oncogenic processes.

Results: By utilizing expression data from 9241 cancer patients, we identified that human chromosome 8q21-24 is a location hotspot for the most frequently overexpressed HSF1-CanSig genes. Intriguingly, the strength of the HSF1 cancer program correlates with the number of overexpressed HSF1-CanSig genes in 8q, illuminating the essential role of HSF1 in mediating gene expression in different cancers. Chromosome 8q21-24 is found under selective pressure in preserving gene order as it exhibits strong synteny among human, mouse, rat, and bovine, although the biological significance remains unknown. Statistical modeling, hierarchical clustering, and gene ontology-based pathway analyses indicate crosstalk between HSF1-mediated responses and pre-mRNA 3′ processing in cancers.

Conclusions: Our results confirm the unique role of chromosome 8q mediated by the master regulator HSF1 in cancer cases. Additionally, this study highlights the connection between cellular processes triggered by HSF1 and pre-mRNA 3′ processing in cancers.

Keywords: Heat shock factor 1 (HSF1), HSF1 cancer signature (CanSig), Malignancy, Pre-mRNA 3′ processing, Chromosome 8q, Synteny

Introduction

Heat-shock factor 1 (HSF1) is a master transcription factor that initiates the expression of heat shock proteins (HSPs) and other genes in response to cellular stress, thus allowing cells to adapt and prolong survival. Cancer cells, however, hijack this protective mechanism to allow them to continue proliferating in their toxic microenvironments. Several studies have linked increased HSF1 activity to malignant cell growth [1]. This pro-malignant activity is associated with HSF1 binding to the promoters and initiating the expression of certain genes independent of heat shock [1]. Identified by Mendillo, Santagata, and coworkers, the HSF1 Cancer Signature (HSF1-CanSig) is a set of 475 genes overexpressed in a number of highly malignant cancer cells and primary tumors [1].

HSF1 itself is observed to be overexpressed in across different tumor types and to promote proliferation, migration, and invasion [2–5]. Frequently, overexpressed genes across different tumors or cancer types are understood to be likely oncogenic and contribute to tumorigenesis [6]. Consequently, this drives the overexpression of the HSF1-CanSig in tumor cells and possibly the surrounding stroma leading to metastasis and poor clinical outcomes [1, 2]. The biological processes and features that link the HSF1-CanSig to malignant cell growth, however, are still unclear.

To elucidate the role of the HSF1-CanSig in cancer, we mined and analyzed the overexpression in 9241 cancer cases from 27 unique primary tumor sites from The Cancer Genome Atlas (TCGA) hosted in cBioPortal [7]. We found that 27 of the top 100 most frequently overexpressed HSF1-CanSig genes are clustered in a highly syntenic region of chromosome 8q. We observed that

* Correspondence: hoe@lafayette.edu
†Equal contributors
1 Department of Biology, Lafayette College, Easton, PA 18042, USA
2 Department of Computer Science, Lafayette College, Easton, PA 18042, USA
Full list of author information is available at the end of the article

this HSF1-driven chromosome 8q gene is set to be overexpressed in a majority of cancer types. Furthermore, our gene ontology analysis indicates a link between HSF1-driven transcription and mRNA processing located on chromosome 8q.

Results

Top 100 high-scoring HSF1-CanSig genes are disproportionately located in chromosome 8q

We devised an overexpression score to quantify the prevalence of HSF1-CanSig genes being overexpressed among cancer cases (see the "Materials and methods" section for details). The overexpression score reflects the prevalence of a gene being overexpressed ≥ 2 standard deviations above the control reference as calculated by cBioPortal for different primary tumor sites [8]. A gene associated with a high overexpression score indicates that the gene is often upregulated in cancer cases. Overexpression scores of all 475 HSF1-CanSig genes from different primary tumor sites were aggregated, ranked, and examined by their percentage distribution per chromosome arm in tiers: top 100, 200, 300, and all HSF1-CanSig genes. If ranking has no effect on distribution, the distribution of genes in each tier should resemble the distribution of all HSF1-CanSig genes, meaning that they distribute like the result of random sampling of HSF1-CanSig genes. Intriguingly, 27% of the top 100 groups comprises of genes encoded in chromosome 8q (Fig. 1a, leftmost light blue bar) given that 8q consists of only 6% (29 of 475) of all HSF1-CanSig (leftmost gray bar). Such percentage declines continuously with from the top 200 group to top 300 group.

To assess the statistical significance of the distribution exhibited in Fig. 1a, we tested the probability of observing certain number of genes per chromosome arm in different tiers by hypergeometric test and Fisher's exact test (Additional file 1: Table S1). The four chromosome arms that encode the highest number of HSF1-CanSig genes are 1p (30), 8q (29), 11q (29), and 17q (30). When genes were examined in tiers by ranking, HSF1-CanSig genes encoded in 8q are included most disproportionately in different tiers but not for genes in the other three chromosome arms, i.e., 1p, 11q, and 17q. The group that attained the smallest p value of Fisher's test was the top 100 group ($5.41e^{-20}$), whereas hypergeometric test found that the top 50 group achieved the lowest p value ($3.13e^{-18}$) followed by the top 100 group ($1.09e^{-17}$). But the former captures only 22 8q genes out of 29 versus 27 8q genes by the latter. To balance statistical rigor and coverage, we decided to focus on the top 100 frequently overexpressed HSF1-CanSig genes. Importantly, regardless of which tier we choose, the most striking finding is that a large proportion of top-ranking genes are encoding in chromosome 8q as supported by Additional file 1: Table S1.

Next, we examine whether the skew distribution of 8q genes in the top 100 group is influenced by the intrinsic distribution of cancer or protein-coding genes. To rule out this possibility, the aggregated overexpression scores of the top 100 high-scoring HSF1-CanSig genes were compared with two null models or references: census cancer gene and all protein-coding genes, which consist of only 2–3% of 8q genes (gray and black bars in Fig. 1b, respectively). A high correlation between the two references based on the percentage of genes per chromosome arm was shown ($R = 0.92$, $p < 5.98e^{-8}$), suggesting that cancer genes exhibit similar distribution as protein coding genes in the human genome. To ascertain the bias of HSF1-CanSig 8q genes quantitatively, a hypergeometric test was used. The probability of observing 27 or more HSF1-CanSig 8q genes (listed in Table 1) in a sample of 100 genes by chance is 1.02×10^{-22}.

Overexpression of HSF1-CanSig 8q genes is primary tumor site-specific

Furthermore, we examined the distribution of HSF1-CanSig 8q genes by individual primary tumor sites. Skewed distribution of HSF1-CanSig genes on chromosome 8q, similar to that in Fig. 1b, was observed in 22 out of 27 primary sites with a variable degree of 8q bias (plots for individual primary site can be found in Additional file 2). The five primary tumor sites that showed no bias are the adrenal gland, kidney, nervous system, thymus, and thyroid. An exponential distribution ($p_i = \lambda e^{-\lambda i}$ or in linear form: $\ln p_i = -\lambda i + \ln \lambda$) was used to quantify the extent of skewness: p_i is the probability or proportion of the ith-ranked chromosome, λ is a coefficient, and i is the rank in the range 1 to 10. A large magnitude of λ indicates a high degree of skewness and vice versa. The λ values of primary sites span a wide spectrum of chromosome 8q bias as shown in Fig. 2, where higher 8q bias are observed in breast and liver cancers than in lymph nodes and soft tissue, for instance. Primary sites lacking 8q bias primary tumor sites tend to be cornered at a region with small λ value (labeled in gray). This result reveals that the overexpression of these HSF1-CanSig 8q genes is primary tumor site-specific.

HSF1-CanSig genes clustered at a 44-Mbp region near the end of chromosome 8q

The 27 HSF1-CanSig 8q genes ranked in the top 100 high-scoring HSF1-CanSig genes are tabulated in Table 1. Remarkably, all HSF1-CanSig 8q genes including HSF1 itself occupy the last three cytogenetic bands of chromosome 8q, i.e., 8q21.3 to 8q.24.3 (~ 44 Mbps). The 3′-

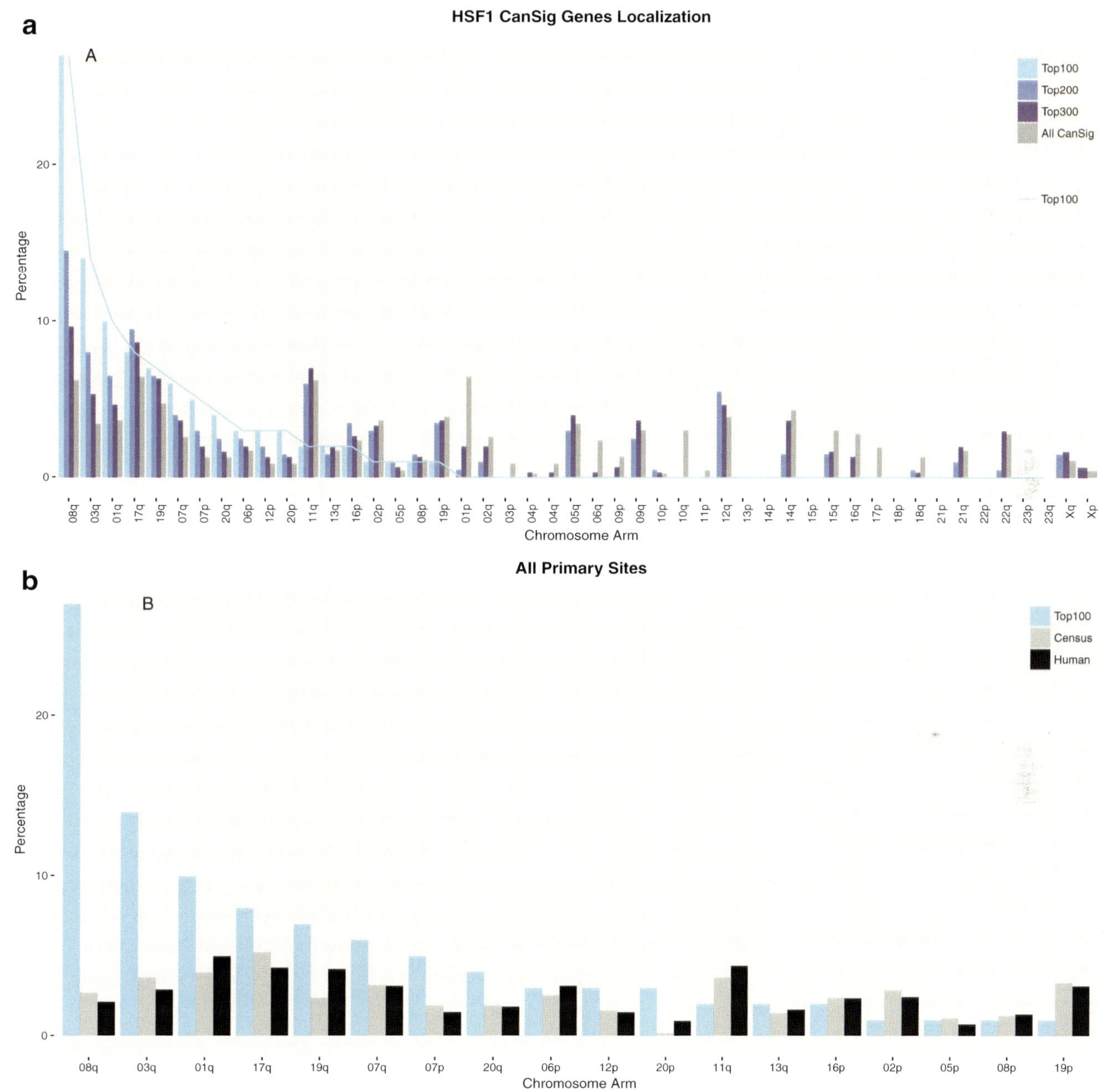

Fig. 1 **a** Percentage distribution of HSF1-CanSig genes by chromosome arms from different tiers: top 100, top 200, top 300, and all HSF1-CanSign genes. **b** Percentage distribution of the top 100 high-scoring HSF1-CanSig genes by chromosome arm. Two references were used for comparison: 633 cancer census genes (labeled census) from COSMIC [49] and 19,073 human protein-coding genes (labeled all) based on HuGO [48]

most gene ZNF250 is ~237 Kbps from the chromosome's 3′ end with only three genes encoded further downstream.

Frequently overexpressed HSF1 associates with the overexpression of HSF1-CanSig genes in 8q

Cancer is heterogeneous both within and between cancer types. Hence, we sought to rank individual HSF1-CanSig 8q genes in different primary tumor sites (Table 2). To cover the entire chromosomal segment encoding all 29 HSF1-CanSig 8q genes, two 8q genes, GPT and KLF10, were included even though they were not ranked in the top 100. The one-sample two-sided Student's t test was used to assess the ranking distribution of them (the second column from the right in Table 2) for each primary tumor site where the p values of the t test are shown in the last column of Table 2. At 95% confidence level, ranks of 8q genes in 20 primary tumor sites (from the ovary to pleura in Table 2) are detected with statistically significant deviation from the

Table 1 Twenty-seven out of the top 100 high-scoring HSF1-CanSig genes are clustered near the end of chromosome 8q

Gene symbol	Name	Location	Rank
PUF60	Poly(U) binding splicing factor 60	08q24.3	1
HSF1	Heat shock transcription factor 1	08q24.3	2
NUDCD1	Nudc domain containing 1	08q23.1	3
MRPL13	Mitochondrial ribosomal protein L13	08q24.12	4
ENY2	ENY2, transcription and export complex 2 subunit	08q23.1	5
CPSF1	Cleavage and polyadenylation specific factor 1	08q24.3	7
SHARPIN	SHANK associated RH domain interactor	08q24.3	8
AZIN1	Antizyme inhibitor 1	08q22.3	9
MAF1	MAF1 homolog, negative regulator of RNA polymerase III	08q24.3	10
PABPC1	Poly(A) binding protein cytoplasmic 1	08q22.3	11
TRAPPC9	Trafficking protein particle complex 9	08q24.3	12
ZNF250	Zinc finger protein 250	08q24.3	13
ZNF34	Zinc finger protein 34	08q24.3	15
NBN	Nibrin	08q21.3	16
JRK	Jrk helix-turn-helix protein	08q24.3	19
DPY19L4	Dpy-19 Like 4 (*C. elegans*)	08q22.1	22
CYHR1	Cysteine and histidine rich 1	08q24.3	23
TPD52	Tumor protein D52	08q21.13	28
PLEC	Plectin	08q24.3	32
MFSD3	Major facilitator superfamily domain containing 3	08q24.3	35
KIFC2	Kinesin family member C2	08q24.3	40
C8ORF37	Chromosome 8 open reading frame 37	08q22.1	49
NDRG1	N-Myc downstream regulated 1	08q24.22	54
SLC45A4	Solute carrier family 45 member 4	08q24.3	56
MROH6	Maestro heat like repeat family member 6	08q24.3	59
LY6K	Lymphocyte antigen 6 family member K	08q24.3	66
LRP12	LDL receptor related protein 12	08q22.3	69

Rank is based on the aggregated overexpression score of all primary tumor sites

mean rank of 233 (see the “Materials and methods” section for the determination of the mean rank). No single primary tumor site had all 29 HSF1-CanSig 8q genes overexpressed in the top 100 HSF1-CanSig genes. Surprisingly there were no primary tumor sites with significant low-average rank (the lowest two are the thymus, $p = 0.896$, and the thyroid, $p = 0.283$, in Table 2), suggesting the absence of a strong suppression among HSF1-CanSig 8q genes in those primary tumor sites.

While no single HSF1-CanSig 8q gene is ranked in the top 100 across all primary sites, HSF1 is frequently overexpressed in most primary tumor sites with kidney as the only exception (26 out of 27, shown at the bottom of HSF1 column in Table 2). HSF1 is also the gene with the highest average rank (33) followed by CPSF1 (52). Additionally, the rank of HSF1 correlates with the average rank of primary sites ($R = 0.71$), but the most correlated 8q gene is CYHR1, not HSF1. Importantly, HSF1 is the only gene in which its rank is always lower than the average rank (Additional file 3: Figure S1).

Lastly, primary tumor sites associated with a small number of high-scoring HSF1-CanSig 8q genes, such as the lymph nodes, soft tissue, thymus, and thyroid, tend to exhibit lower skewness (see Fig. 2). These results suggest a minor role of HSF1-mediated activities in those primary tumor sites.

Primary tumor sites are segregated by ranks

We next asked if the ranks of HSF1-CanSig 8q genes in different primary tumor sites share similar patterns. By using hierarchical clustering with two distinct distance methods, primary sites were clustered using the ranks of HSF1-CanSig 8q genes as shown in Fig. 3. Both panels in Fig. 3 show that primary tumor sites can be reliably split into two groups by the average rank, namely, the top-ranking and the low-ranking groups. The medians

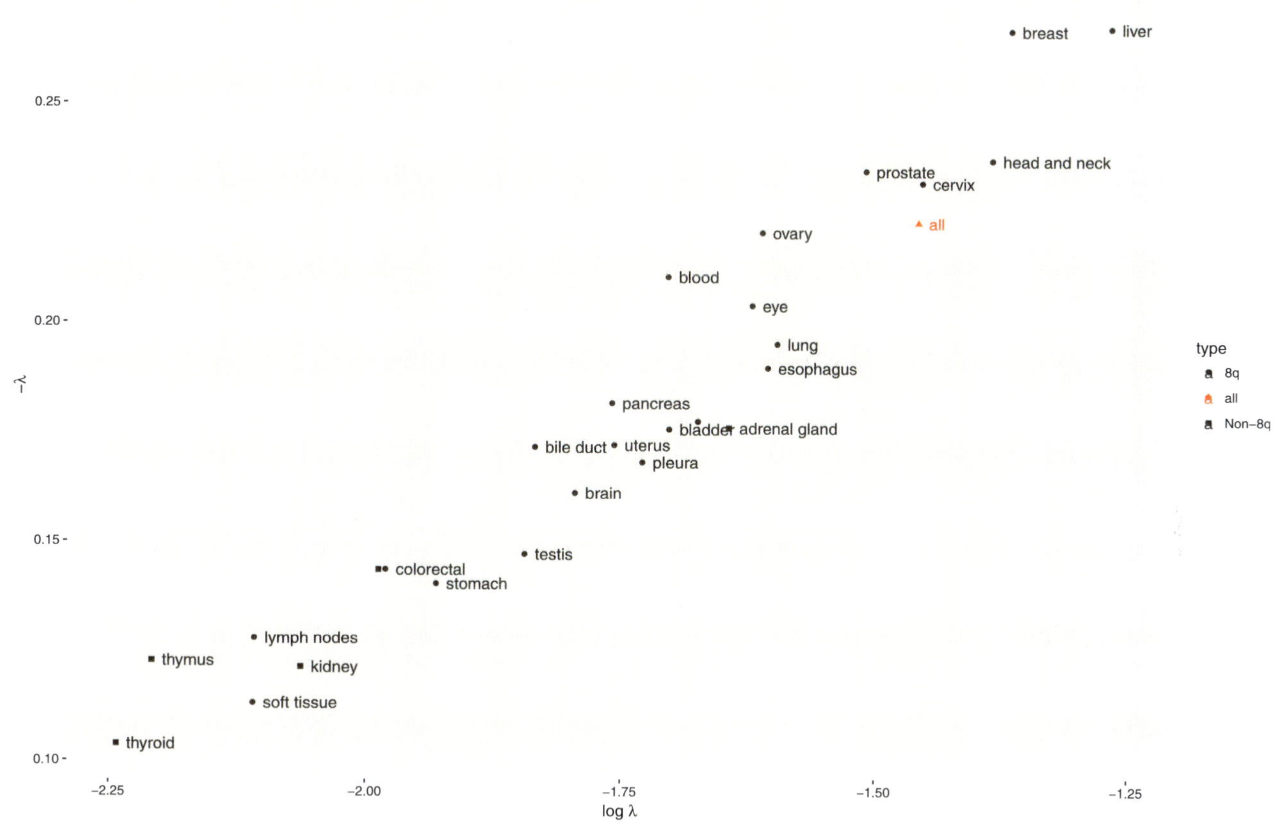

Fig. 2 Quantification of 8q skewness. The percentages of the top 10 chromosomes were fitted to an exponential model. The model outputs (λ = slope, ln(λ) = intercept) are plotted. Primary tumor sites with 8q and without 8q clustering are in blue and gray, respectively. The red triangle represents the fitting of data when 8q genes from all primary sites are ranked together

of the top-ranking groups produced by the two distance methods reflect higher consistency as they vary within a narrow range of 65–68. But the medians of the low-ranking groups show a larger difference from 148 to 198.

Regarding the range of average rank within each group, if the outlier, i.e., soft tissue with average rank 213, is taken out from the top-ranking correlation-distance group in Fig. 3b, the range of average ranks in both becomes identical, 34 to 102. A cutoff value of 102 seems to divide the two groups. Moreover, top-ranking groups created by the two distance methods share 13 out of 14 to 17 primary sites (marked by asterisks in Fig. 3). The low-ranking groups however display a larger variation in rank medians 146–198, but 9 out of 10 to 13 primary sites are clustered together by both methods (marked by plus signs in Fig. 3). This result suggests the feasibility of stratifying primary tumor sites by the over-expression of HSF1-CanSig 8q genes.

HSF1-CanSig 8q genes are highly syntenic in mammals

Since the proximity of HSF1-CanSig 8q genes seems to be a contributing factor for their cohesive expression pattern, we asked whether their proximity reveals biological significance. We sought answers in the light of evolution by examining the synteny of the genomic region spanning the 5′- and 3′-most HSF1-CanSig 8q genes, i.e., TPD53 and ZNF250, respectively. It means that other non-HSF1-CanSig genes were also included in the syntenic analysis. This region consists of 267 genes with known genomic coordinates in human where 29 of them are HSF1-CanSig genes. We aligned these human genes with homologs from bovine, mouse, and rat. Their pairwise percentage of synteny can be found in Table 3A, which varies from the lowest 50% (mouse and bovine) to the highest 84% (human and mouse). As our focus is on the HSF1-CanSig genes, we highlighted their genomic order in Table 3B. Syntenic information of all 267 genes can be found in Additional file 1: Table S5.

Twenty-three out of 29 human HSF1-CanSig 8q genes are syntenic to mouse and rat. Although three non-syntenic genes (Nbn, Dpy19l4, and 2610301B20Rik in mouse and Nbn, Dpy19l4, and MGC94199 in rat) reside in other chromosomes, the order of their locations still agrees with that in humans. If these three genes are included in calculating the percentage of synteny, human-

Table 2 Ranks of HSF1-CanSig 8q genes by primary tumor site. The bracketed number next to the name of a primary site denotes the number of cases recruited in the study. Genes displayed in the table heading are arranged in a syntenic order. The number inside a cell denotes the rank of the gene among HSF1-CanSig genes with the most frequently overexpressed genes ranked 1. Ranks ≤ 100 are highlighted in solid black. Some genes may share the same rank if they have the same overexpression score. Count includes only genes with rank ≤ 100. Average rank is the arithmetic mean of ranks. HSF1-CanSig genes GPT and LRP12 are not part of the top 100 high-scoring genes. *p* value is determined by one-sample two-sided Student's *t* test. The table is sorted by average rank and count in ascending and descending order, respectively

Primary Site	TPD52	NBN	DPY19L4	C8ORF37	PABPC1	KLF10	AZIN1	LRP12	NUDCD1	ENY2	MRPL13	NDRG1	TRAPPC9	SLC45A4	JRK	LY6K	MROH6	PUF60	PLEC	SHARPIN	MAF1	HSF1	CPSF1	CYHR1	KIFC2	GPT	MFSD3	ZNF34	ZNF250	Count	Average Rank	p-value
ovary (558)	30	18	49	85	35	60	11	40	23	25	28	40	6	32	33	136	70	2	9	1	5	3	29	16	50	120	15	4	7	27	34	1.47E-23
eye (80)	29	10	23	27	332	245	7	21	17	2	4	25	16	12	6	42	42	3	23	8	14	21	6	9	16	37	2	11	21	27	36	9.29E-15
prostate (498)	2	11	28	45	1	120	5	30	5	3	8	154	16	87	22	135	59	11	28	15	9	6	18	28	13	135	35	30	7	25	37	4.70E-20
breast (1100)	25	34	23	43	9	187	7	58	2	3	1	46	12	92	35	27	64	4	56	22	17	5	29	104	40	163	59	13	10	26	41	1.44E-19
colorectal (382)	55	35	8	62	13	34	7	60	12	17	30	104	22	113	41	177	60	9	132	18	12	20	23	24	120	342	42	19	22	23	56	7.09E-14
skin (472)	129	63	32	93	25	250	32	164	65	17	16	129	27	38	15	173	74	5	108	53	39	15	6	3	53	59	42	11	38	23	61	2.26E-15
bladder (408)	41	16	16	29	3	125	5	125	11	4	9	83	32	117	67	37	63	6	146	44	12	1	27	83	202	188	117	146	21	21	61	2.92E-15
liver (373)	29	19	25	113	2	376	14	113	3	6	1	74	13	72	20	415	21	4	30	5	7	11	9	17	33	356	23	15	10	24	63	1.08E-08
lung (517)	26	29	32	59	7	257	19	111	6	13	48	43	20	304	39	39	59	1	155	22	5	4	11	18	39	461	48	9	15	24	65	2.23E-09
head and neck (522)	209	45	70	70	21	26	31	75	16	21	51	16	84	280	112	23	152	3	23	14	19	2	10	33	28	447	84	29	53	24	71	7.05E-10
esophagus (185)	50	69	32	91	75	270	26	188	14	31	9	38	34	75	50	20	170	4	22	19	15	2	26	19	57	299	188	69	99	24	71	7.89E-12
pancreas (179)	39	97	31	153	21	383	4	97	2	3	1	465	50	12	12	60	39	21	9	18	50	24	9	78	60	153	18	153	19	24	72	9.73E-09
stomach (415)	13	25	22	97	12	450	4	161	9	10	7	31	33	180	92	128	55	3	142	45	59	8	14	17	59	148	31	274	110	21	77	2.62E-09
uterus (177)	83	223	16	104	12	386	27	262	4	23	56	27	71	18	35	188	43	56	35	27	7	7	10	47	65	310	65	23	16	23	77	3.21E-09
cervix (306)	167	53	67	167	16	149	34	118	34	41	19	96	149	135	96	41	268	18	268	36	21	20	28	46	53	393	82	62	72	20	95	5.10E-09
testis (156)	51	5	152	17	8	101	16	127	183	183	51	86	26	101	21	338	40	51	9	56	152	35	14	295	56	127	463	6	127	17	100	4.14E-07
brain (530)	241	22	114	262	15	319	319	202	28	13	23	163	68	114	18	35	449	22	42	42	10	8	13	35	96	37	163	28	30	19	101	1.46E-06
blood (179)	20	33	177	25	25	128	15	100	37	249	33	100	9	33	2	462	3	79	47	100	79	79	177	47	289	464	58	79	9	22	102	3.56E-06
bile duct (36)	9	14	41	74	414	144	414	414	74	144	41	414	6	74	9	22	74	74	269	74	144	41	41	41	144	269	269	41	22	18	131	4.44E-04
pleura (87)	230	230	230	300	58	386	91	230	58	18	91	230	58	58	143	300	386	143	143	91	58	5	91	143	18	29	91	91	230	15	146	1.71E-04
adrenal gland (79)	138	82	69	82	232	329	393	138	23	82	113	232	138	329	100	466	466	100	82	69	159	46	35	192	232	138	393	439	82	12	185	7.45E-02
nervous system (528)	245	145	272	272	145	190	272	26	166	99	190	409	125	215	112	442	332	99	215	59	59	22	59	442	426	190	190	39	22	9	189	7.60E-02
lymph nodes (48)	106	56	358	56	106	211	358	358	211	106	106	358	106	211	11	56	358	358	358	358	211	56	26	211	458	211	211	358	56	7	207	3.06E-01
soft tissue (263)	334	38	110	285	72	257	68	215	4	22	2	215	285	309	196	426	387	72	110	285	232	93	82	410	447	460	447	126	196	9	213	4.75E-01
kidney (534)	70	196	437	344	63	131	80	175	217	30	429	241	344	450	241	450	48	70	149	48	58	196	63	407	217	437	283	283	379	9	225	7.80E-01
thymus (120)	29	90	133	350	213	350	213	281	133	406	281	213	90	281	350	406	52	90	350	52	281	52	213	281	281	281	461	350	281	7	236	8.96E-01
thyroid (509)	443	452	421	207	352	278	421	124	400	57	180	352	96	452	400	421	57	278	96	36	43	96	324	443	207	207	180	352	236	7	262	2.83E-01
Count	17	22	17	16	20	3	20	9	21	22	21	13	21	12	20	11	18	24	14	25	21	26	24	17	16	4	15	18	20	17\19		
Average Rank	105	78	111	130	85	227	107	149	65	60	68	162	72	155	84	202	144	59	113	60	66	33	52	129	139	239	150	113	81		112	

rat and human-mouse share 72 and 84% of synteny, respectively. In comparison between bovine and human, all 8q homologs in bovine are found in a single chromosome, i.e., chromosome 14, but in the complementary strand of the bovine's reference genome. Twenty-five of the 29 8q genes are syntenic. If the entire 8q region is considered, bovine's genes share only 57% of synteny with human versus 61–71% in rat and mouse, indicating bovine genome has accumulated a larger scale of genome rearrangement than human, mouse, and rat since divergence. Regardless, the gene order is largely preserved between human and bovine. This finding is congruent with the estimated divergence time among these four mammals [9]. According to the report, bovine and human and mouse and human diverge in about 71–113 million years ago (MYA) and 62–101 MYA, respectively. Furthermore, our findings concur with the synteny analyses from the genome sequencing project of human (Figure 46 of [10]), Brown Norway rat (Figure 4 of [11]), and Taurine cattle (Figure S12 of [12]). To further investigate the synteny of human 8q in mouse, rat, and bovine, the tool Cinteny [13] was used to visualize the extent of synteny and they can be found in Additional file 3: Figure S2.

There are two possible explanations to account for the observed syntenic conservation among these genes: (i) the divergence time between taxa is insufficient to observe significant rearrangement or (ii) the proximity of genes is essential for biological functions. Classic examples are the Hox and globin gene clusters. As the estimation from [9] is adequate to disregard the former, we were intrigued to explore the latter, i.e., the biological function shared among these genes.

Synteny does not explain coexpression

To determine whether or not the overexpression of HSF1-CanSig 8q genes in cancers is related to synteny, we analyzed the expression pattern of genes flanking HSF1 (genomic coordinates of HSF1's neighboring genes can be found in Additional file 1: Table S7) in each cancer case to shed light on the clustering of HSF1-CanSig 8q genes. We reasoned that if the expression level of HSF1's neighboring genes correlates with their distance from HSF1, synteny may be a factor accounting for the clustering of CanSig 8q genes; otherwise reasons other than synteny may shape the clustering.

We selected 1682 cancer cases with HSF1 overexpressed two or more standard deviations above the reference. As shown in Fig. 4a, expression of HSF1 and its neighboring genes do not correlate with the distance between them. Genes close to HSF1 such as MROH1, BOP1, and DGAT1 do not show higher correlation (in terms of overexpression with HSF1) than HSF1-CanSig 8q genes that are farther from them. For example,

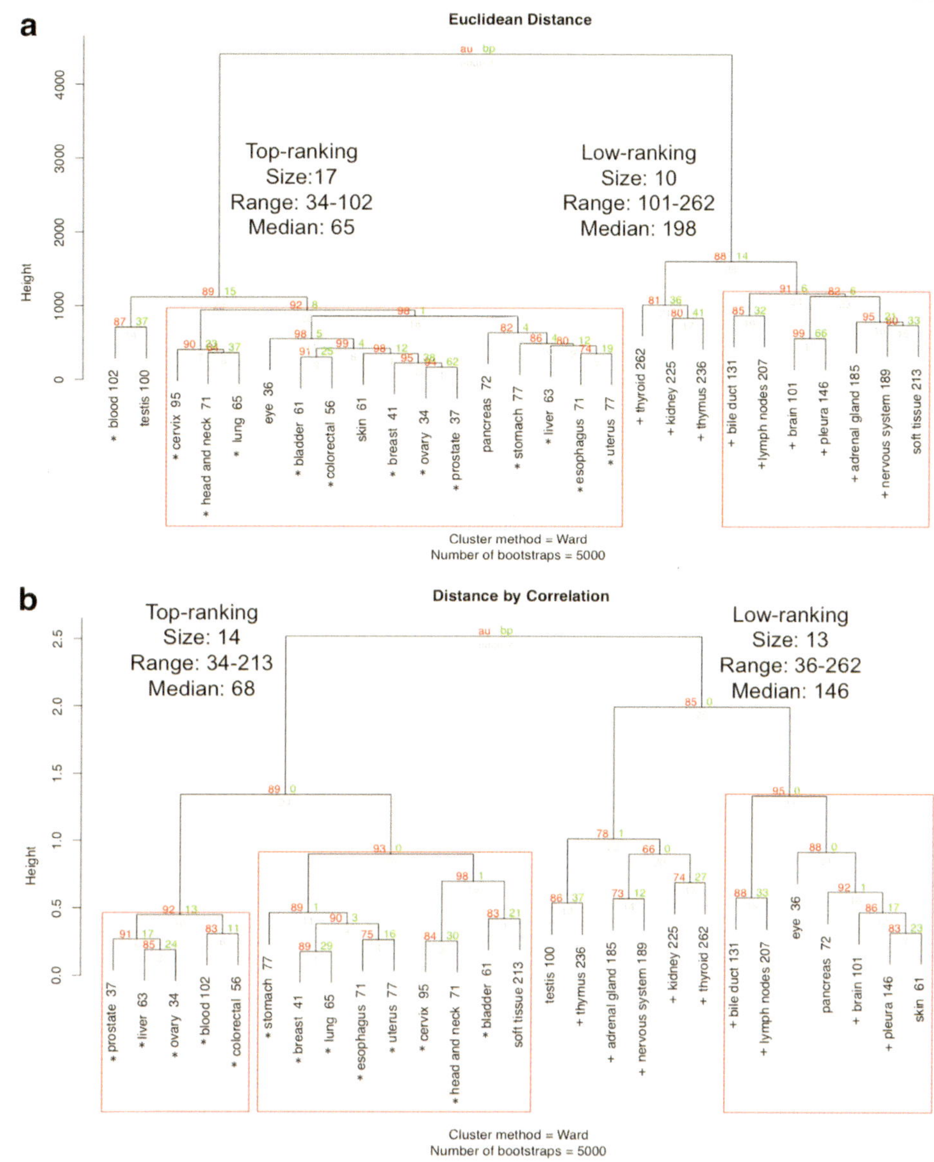

Fig. 3 Rank analysis by hierarchical clustering with bootstrapping. The number beside each primary tumor site is the average rank. Subtrees with high bootstrap value (≥ 90) are highlighted in red boxes. Each dendrogram was built after bootstrapping 5000 times. The red and green numbers at the branch point represent approximately unbias (AU) *p* value and bootstrap probability (BP), respectively. AU is recommended as a better parameter than BP to assess the clustering reliability at each branch point [54]. Cluster subtree highlighted by red box indicates AU ≥ 90. For the top-ranking groups, primary tumor sites shared between two distance methods are marked by asterisks. Similarly, for the low-ranking groups, primary sites are marked by plus signs. **a** Cluster dendrogram based on Euclidean distance. **b** Same input data as panel **a** but correlation was used as the distance calculation method

although 8q genes SHARPIN, MAF1, and CPSF1 are far apart from HSF1 than MROH1, BOP1, and DGAT1, they exhibit higher correlation with HSF1's expression. Similar variability is also observed when correlations are examined by individual primary tumor site (Additional file 4). Thus, our data suggests that synteny is not a contributing factor for the co-overexpression of HSF1-CanSig genes clustered in chromosome 8q21-24. It is however intriguing to see that several overexpressed non-HSF1-CanSig genes are correlated with HSF1 such as MAF1 ($R = 0.7$), CYC1 ($R = 0.6$), and SLC52A2 ($R = 0.6$) (see Fig. 4b).

Network analysis links HSF1-mediated responses to pre-mRNA 3′ processing

Next, we took a systems approach to determine if HSF1-CanSig 8q genes work cooperatively in biological networks. WebGestalt gene network (or pathway) analysis was performed to determine whether shared biological processes are common to these genes. The basic

Table 3 Synteny analysis of HSF1-CanSig 8q genes. A. Percentage of syntenic genes between species. Percentages are based on the number of genes in the column's species. The percentages in lower triangle excluded the separated chr4q in mouse and chr5q in rat. Whereas, the percentages in the upper triangle (shaded) include the separated chr4q in mouse and chr5q in rat. B. Order of human genes is used as the reference. Genes are ordered in 5'-to-3' direction according to respective reference genomes from top to bottom except for bovine, which is in reverse order. Non-syntenic genes are marked in boxes. Superscript + indicates the chromosomal location of the gene was determined by BLAT. Exact genomic coordinates of these genes can be found in Additional file 1: Table S6

A	Human	Mouse	Rat	Bovine
Human		84	72	57
Mouse	71		82	59
Rat	61	69		65
Bovine	57	50	55	

B			
Bovine (bosTau8)	Human (hg38)	Mouse (mm10)	Rat (rn6)
Chr14	Chr8q	Chr15q	Chr7q
MRPL13			
	TPD52	*Chr4q*$^{\#}$	*Chr5q*$^{\#}$
NBN	NBN	*Nbn*$^{\#}$	*Nbn*$^{\#}$
DPY19L4^{+}	DPY19L4	*Dpy19l4*$^{\#}$	*Dpy19l4*$^{\#}$
C14H8orf37^{+}	C8orf37	*2610301B20Rik*$^{\#}$	*MGC94199*$^{\#}$
PABPC1	PABPC1	Pabpc1	Pabpc1
KLF10	KLF10	Klf10	Klf10
AZIN1	AZIN1	Azin1	Azin1
LRP12	LRP12	Lrp12	Lrp12
NUDCD1	NUDCD1	Nudcd1	Nudcd1
ENY2	ENY2	Eny2	Eny2
	MRPL13	Mrpl13	Mrpl13
TPD52 SLC45A4^{+}			
NDRG1	NDRG1	Ndrg1	Ndrg1
TRAPPC9^{+}	TRAPPC9	Trappc9	Trappc9
	SLC45A4	Slc45a4	Slc45a4^{+}
JRK^{+}	JRK	Jrk	Jrk
N.A.	LY6K	N.A.	N.A.
MROH6^{+}	MROH6	Mroh6	Mroh6^{+}
PUF60	PUF60	Puf60	Puf60
PLEC^{+}	PLEC	Plec	Plec
SHARPIN	SHARPIN	Sharpin	Sharpin
MAF1	MAF1	Maf1	Maf1^{+}
HSF1	HSF1	Hsf1	Hsf1
CPSF1	CPSF1	Cpsf1	Cpsf1
CYHR1	CYHR1	Cyhr1	Cyhr1
KIFC2	KIFC2	Kifc2	Kifc2
GPT	GPT	Gpt	Gpt
MFSD3^{+}	MFSD3	Mfsd3	Mfsd3
ZNF34	ZNF34	N.A.	N.A.
ZNF250^{+}	ZNF250	Zfp647^{+}	Zfp647^{+}

mechanism of WebGestalt is to detect the enrichment of Gene Ontology (GO) terms associated with a set of genes with statistical support. We used 29 HSF1-CanSig 8q genes to query 33 TCGA RNA-Seq studies in various primary tumor sites (the list of studies queried can be found in Additional file 1: Table S8). A sample of result generated by WebGestalt can be found in Additional file 3.

Out of the 33 TCGA datasets, eight studies were found to be enriched by HSF1-CanSig 8q genes: adrenocortical carcinoma, colon adenocarcinoma, esophageal carcinoma, kidney chromophobe, hepatocellular carcinoma,

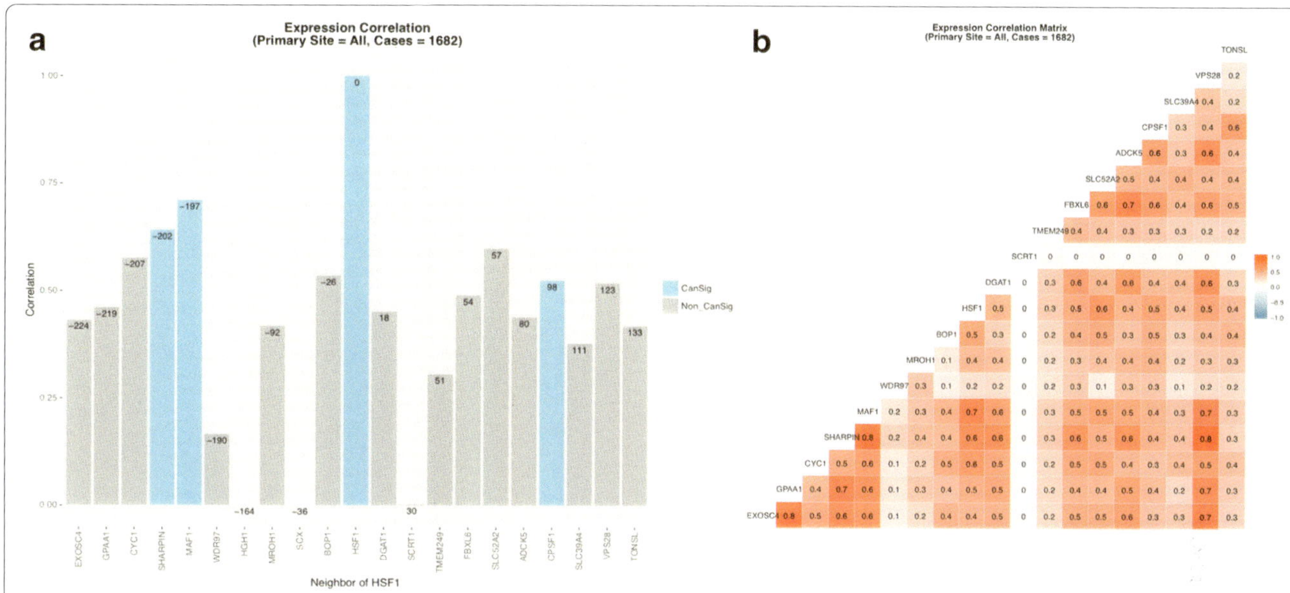

Fig. 4 Expression correlation between genes in the neighborhood of HSF1. **a** HSF1 is set as the focal gene. No expression data can be obtained for HGH1 and SCX in cBioPortal; therefore, their correlations were set to zero. The numbers on the top of the bars represent the distance of the gene from HSF1 in Kbps. Negative signs indicate genes are located upstream of HSF1. **b** Correlation matrix of all 21 genes. Blank boxes represent insufficient number of cases to determine the correlation

lung adenocarcinoma, ovarian serous cystadenocarcinoma, and stomach adenocarcinoma. Intriguingly, all results pointed to the enrichment of RNA polyadenylation (GO:0043631, p values 2.40e-3 to 4.34e-2), mRNA polyadenylation (GO:0006378, p values 2.40e-3 to 4.34e-2), and 3′ end processing (GO:0031124, p values 3.03–4.30e-2). With no exception, the CanSig 8q genes that contributed to these hits were HSF1, PABPC1, and CPSF1.

To corroborate WebGestalt's results, we repeated the hierarchical clustering analysis of rank data (Table 2) but using only HSF1 and three pre-mRNA 3′ processing genes: PABPC1, CPSF1, and PUF60. (Note that the clustering method requires a minimum of four genes; therefore, PUF60, a RNA processing factor, was included here even though WebGestalt did not highlight it.) If these four genes dominate the average rank of HSF1-CanSig 8q genes in different primary tumor sites, the clustering results produced by them should highly resemble to the results in Fig. 3. Figure 5a, b shows two cluster dendrograms produced by the two distance methods which share high similarity with Fig. 3a, b, respectively. When the two cluster dendrograms generated by the Euclidean distance (Figs. 3a and 5a) are compared, the top-ranking and low-ranking groups are found to share 15 and 9 common primary sites, respectively, which means 24 out of 27 primary sites. Similarly, the two dendrograms using correlation distance method (Figs. 3b and 5b) share 12 and 9 common primary sites, respectively. It means that these four genes are representative for all HSF1-CanSig 8q genes, indicating influential role played by them. It also suggests that HSF1 mediates pre-mRNA 3′ processing in cancer development.

Discussion

We have undertaken a cancer bioinformatics approach to study the clustering of HSF1-CanSig genes in chromosome 8q. Based on the TCGA expression data obtained from cancer cases, we found that HSF1-CanSig genes are clustered at chromosome 8q substantiated by compelling statistical evidence under two null models: all protein-coding genes and all HSF1-CanSig genes. λ value analysis further reveals variation of 8q prevalence in 27 primary tumor sites (Fig. 2). This result may support the use of λ to characterize the strength of HSF1 cancer program in various cancers: bone [14], breast [1], colon [1], esophagus [3], head and neck [15], liver [16], lung [1], ovarian [5], pancreas [17], prostate [18], uterine [4], and skin cancer [19]. Crucially, this perspective has been confirmed by the hierarchical clustering analysis as all of the above cancers, except bone, are members of the top-ranking group (Figs. 3 and 5).

The rank analysis discovers the association between HSF1 and HSF1-CanSig genes encoded in chromosome 8q in 27 primary tumor sites. HSF1's rank correlates with and always falls below the average rank across primary sites (Additional file 3: Figure S1). The ranks of 20 out of 27 primary tumor sites are asymmetrically skewed to high ranks with statistical significance, suggesting the overexpression of HSF1-CanSig 8q genes is coordinated

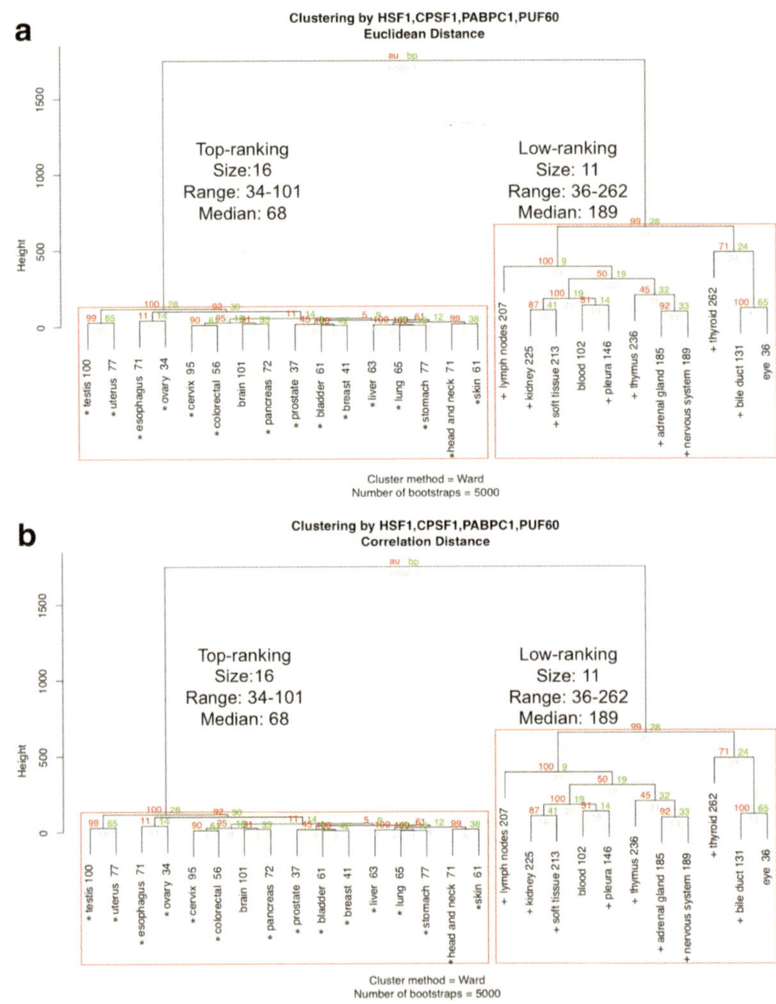

Fig. 5 a Hierarchical clustering of rank data (Table 2) by HSF1 and three pre-mRNA 3′ processing factors: PABPC1, CPSF1, and PUF60. Distance method is based on the Euclidean distance. In the top-ranking group, the asterisk denotes the primary tumor site shared with Fig. 3a. In the low-ranking group, the plus sign indicates the primary site shared with Fig. 3a. **b** Clustering by correlation distance

in those tumor sites. In contrast, when the rank of HSF1 is greater than the cutoff rank ~ 102, more diverse overexpression patterns are observed among HSF1-CanSig 8q genes, implying the diminishing control of HSF1 in those cancers. These observations engender HSF1 to be an important target for the development of cancer treatment.

Clustered HSF1-CanSig 8q genes co-express at a high level in several primary tumor sites. Is the clustering of HSF1-CanSig 8q genes a contributing factor for co-expression biologically? As "Nothing in biology makes sense except in the light of evolution" [20], we sought answers from synteny. Our results (Table 3B) indicate the majority (22–23) of HSF1-CanSig 8q genes are syntenic among human, mouse, rat, and bovine. Despite the neighboring gene model suggesting an evolutionary explanation of this co-expression [21, 22], our results do not align with such a model. When the expressions of genes flanking HSF1 were examined, our results demonstrate incoherent overexpression levels attributed to distance. Thus, other forces such as the transcriptional activation by HSF1 or its downstream products may be the cause of the co-expression of HSF1-CanSig 8q genes in tumors. It still remains as a question whether this is common for other cancer-related transcription factors. Related to this analysis is the finding that a few non-HSF1-CanSig genes encoded in chromosome 8q whose expressions correlate with HSF1: GPAA1 ($R \sim 0.8$) and EXOSC4 ($R \sim 0.75$) in the ovary and FBXL6 ($R \sim 0.8$) in the prostate (Additional file 4). These findings concur with previous studies that genes in regions 8q21, 8q22, and 8q24 are notable for cancers [23–25].

Hierarchical clustering and network analysis have fostered the connection between HSF1 and pre-mRNA 3′ processing. Three essential pre-mRNA processing factors are discovered in relation to the overexpression of

HSF1-CanSig genes through network analysis: PABPC1, CPSF1, and PUF60. CPSF1 is an essential polyadenylation factor. To date, no biochemical evidence supports any association between HSF1 and CPSF1. However, the interaction between the two processes, heat shock and polyadenylation, has been confirmed by two previous studies [26, 27], suggesting intermediaries may be involved in the crosstalk between these two processes. The poly(A) tail of a mRNA serves as a checkpoint for mRNA nuclear export. Intriguingly, HSF1-TRP interaction had been reported to facilitate the export of HSP70 mRNA under stress [28]. HSF1 had also been shown to form complexes with two core polyadenylation factors: symplekin and CstF64 [29, 30]. Alternative polyadenylation (APA) is ubiquitous and tissue-specific in mammals [31–33]. Importantly, it has been confirmed to play an essential role in many tumor types [34–43]. In rare cases, APA interferes with the protein encoded by the gene. Two classic, non-cancer examples are calcitonin-related polypeptide-alpha gene (CALCA) [44] and immunoglobulin M (IgM) [45]. But more often, APA alters the 3′ untranslated regions (UTRs) by either shortening or lengthening the constitutive 3′ UTRs. 3′ UTR is known to harbor binding sites of regulatory proteins, and miRNAs, in addition to secondary structures [46]. Their binding can either attenuate or bolster mRNA stability, affecting downstream protein synthesis and subsequently the proteome of cells.

It is noteworthy that two other HSF1-CanSig 8q genes are associated with pre-mRNA 3′-end processing: PUF60 and PABPC1. PUF60 is a member of the highly conserved nucleic acid-binding protein family: pumilio and FBF homology protein (PUF). PUF60 involves in pre-mRNA splicing and transcriptional regulation. Notably, PABPC1 binds to poly(A) tail of eukaryotic mRNA, promoting mRNA translatability. A proteomic study had identified the presence of PUF60 and PABPC1 in the polyadenylation complex [47], ascertaining the linkage between heat shock and polyadenylation.

Conclusion

The role of HSF1 played in cancer proliferation and malignancy is critical and well established. The cancer bioinformatics approach taken by us provides new information about the overexpression of HSF1-CanSig 8q genes mediated by HSF1 in different tumor types, illuminating the connection between malignancy progression driven by HSF1 and pre-mRNA 3′ processing. However, the true underlying biological mechanisms that drives HSF1 relationship with chromosome 8q is multifaceted and largely unknown but may hold the key to understanding tumor development in certain tissues and organs. As the activation of the master regulator HSF1 varies among different primary tumor sites, HSF1-CanSig 8q genes may be developed as prognosis biomarkers for improving clinical outcomes.

Materials and methods

HSF1-CanSig genes and cancer expression data

The list of 456 HSF1 CanSig genes was downloaded from Table S5 of [1]. To facilitate searching by gene symbols, they were adhered to the standard HUGO Gene Nomenclature [48]. As a result, 87 non-HuGO gene symbols from [1] were replaced by the official HuGO gene symbols. Six of them were converted to multiple gene symbols, expanding the original list to 475 HSF1-CanSig genes. The complete list of HSF1-CanSig genes and their full names and chromosome locations can be found in Additional file 1: Table S2.

mRNA expression (in fold change) of the HSF1-CanSig genes in different cancer primary sites were retrieved from cBioPortal via its Web API [7]. At the time of writing, cBioPortal contains 159 cancer studies conducted in 29 primary tumor sites (Additional file 1: Table S3). Our goal is to include one RNA-Seq study per primary site. The following criteria were used to select expression data for our analysis:

1. The study is focused on a specific primary tumor.
2. Transcriptome data is generated by the study.
3. Only one study is selected per primary tumor site. If multiple transcriptome datasets are found for a primary site, the study recruited the largest number of cancer cases is chosen.
4. Only expressions of HSF1-CanSig genes are considered.

Transcriptome data were found in the majority, but not all, of cancer studies. In this report, 27 studies were selected according to the above criteria and they are tabulated in Additional file 1: Table S9.

Overexpression score of HSF1-CanSig genes

A cancer study consists of a group of cancer cases or patients, and each cancer case is associated with a set of mRNA expression *z*-scores of genes. But in this report, our focus is solely on the 475 HSF1-CanSig genes mentioned above. cBioPortal pre-computes a *z*-score for each gene, representing the number of standard deviations of its expression deviates from the reference gene population [8]. For example, a *z*-score value 2.8318 for gene ANAT in the case TCGA-OR-A5J1-01 from the Adrenocortical Carcinoma study indicates that the gene ANAT is overexpressed by 2.8318 standard deviations above the reference.

To quantify the prevalence of overexpression of HSF1-CanSig genes among cancer cases, we devised the following scoring scheme to assess the magnitude of a gene's overexpression as:

$$Overexpression\ Score = Number\ of\ overexpressed\ cases/Total\ number\ of\ cases$$

A gene is considered overexpressed if its cBioPortal's expression z-score is ≥ 2, the same threshold used in cBioPortal website. For instance, the Adrenocortical Carcinoma study consists of 79 cancer cases (see Table 3), UBE2B gene was detected to overexpress in 33 cases. The overexpression score of UBE2B is 33/79 = .4177. The full list of genes' overexpression scores by primary site can be found in Additional file 1: Table S4.

Chromosome localization of top 100 HSF1-CanSig genes

When expression data of different primary tumor sites was combined for analysis, the overexpression score of an HSF1-CanSig gene was calculated by adding the overexpression scores of the gene in all primary sites. The top 100 highest scoring genes were used for the chromosome localization analysis. The complete list of the top 100 HSF1-CanSig genes can be found in Additional file 1: Table S5. Two sets of genes were chosen as the reference or null model: all human protein-coding genes based on HuGO [48] and genes implicated in cancer when mutated according to the COSMIC Cancer Gene Census [49]. In total, 19,073 and 633 of protein-coding genes and cancer census genes were used as references, respectively.

A hypergeometric model was used to assess the probability of localization. $P(i \geq k) = 1-\Sigma_{i=0}^{i=k-1}\binom{K}{i}\binom{N-K}{n-i}/\binom{N}{n}$, where K is the number of genes encoded in the chromosome 8q, k is the number of 8q genes among the top 100 high-scoring HSF1-CanSig genes, n is the sample size, and N is the total number of protein-coding genes. For $K = 401$, $k = 27$, $n = 100$, and $N = 19{,}073$, the probability of observing 27 or more HSF1-CanSig 8q genes in a random sample of 100 genes by chance is 1.02×10^{-22}.

There are 29 HSF1-CanSig genes in 8q. The probability of finding 27 out of 29 HSF1-CanSig 8q genes in a sample of 100 HSF1-CanSig genes can be determined by hypergeometric model. Using the same formula above: K (= 29) is the number of HSF1-CanSig genes encoded in 8q, k (= 27) is the number of 8q genes in the top 100, n (= 100) is the sample size, and N (= 475) is the total number of HSF1-CanSig genes. The probability is 6.85×10^{-18}.

λ value analysis was performed by fitting of the linear form of the exponential distribution, i.e., $\ln p_i = -\lambda i + \ln \lambda$, to the rank data in Additional file 1: Table S5. Only the percentages of the top 10 high-ranking chromosome arms were used for fitting. Fitting was done by lm() function in *R*.

Synteny analysis

The genomic segment encoding human HSF1-CanSig 8q genes were analyzed for syntenic conservation. This segment spans from 80,034,869 (TPD52) to 144,901,461 (ZNF250) in chromosome 8 of human. By using the homology information from NCBI HomoloGene database (build 68) [50], 267, 165, 237, and 199 homologous genes were identified with genomic coordinates in human (hg38), bovine (bosTau8), mouse (mm10), and rat (rn6), respectively. Their genomic locations were retrieved automatically from the UCSC Genome Browser [51] through the Python package CruzDb [52]. For genomic locations that cannot be obtained by this approach, they were either determined manually by aligning the cDNA sequences on the genome by BLAT [53] or discarded. Genomic coordinates of the genes can be found in Additional file 1: Table S6.

Coexpression analysis

Ten genes immediately flanking the upstream and downstream regions of HSF1 were identified in the human genome (hg38) using the UCSC Genome Browser [51]. This region spans about 365 kbps. The ten immediate upstream genes of HSF1 are EXOSC4, GPAA1, CYC1, SHARPIN*, MAF1*, WDR97, HGH1, MROH1, BOP1, and SCX. The ten downstream genes are DGAT1, SCRT1, TMEM249, FBXL6, SLC52A2, ADCK5, CPSF1*, SLC39A4, VPS28, and TONSL (HSF1-CanSig genes are suffixed by an asterisk). Genomic coordinates of them can be found in Additional file 1: Table S7. Expressions (in fold changes) of these 21 genes, including HSF1, were retrieved from cBioPortal if HSF1's expression of a cancer case is ≥ 2 standard deviations higher than the reference. Correlation of expression fold change was computed between each of the 20 genes and HSF1 using the function cor.test in *R* where the method was Pearson.

Student's *t* test and hierarchical clustering

Our goal is to assess the statistical significance of the average rank of HSF1-CanSig 8q genes per primary site (listed in the second column from the right in Table 2). By assuming ranks are independent and uniformly distributed, the average rank of a sample consisting of 29 ranks randomly drawn from 1 to 466 without replacement does distribute normally with mean 233. (Note that the largest rank is 466 instead of 475 because of ties.) Thus, *t* test is suitable for this analysis. *R*'s t.test() function was used with mean 233 (null hypothesis). The mean was 233 as the range of rank is 1 to 466. *p* values of the t test can be found in the rightmost column in Table 2.

Hierarchical clustering was performed using *R*'s package pvclust [54]. One distinct feature offered by pvclust is the assessment of cluster subtrees by resampling bootstrap. The input to pvclust was the gene ranks in Table 2. The cluster method and the number of bootstrapping were "Ward" and 5000, respectively. Two distance calculation methods were used for cross-validation purpose: Euclidean distance and correlation.

WebGestalt analysis

We used WebGestalt to uncover possible gene networks commonly perturbed by HSF1-CanSig 8q genes [55]. At WebGestalt website [56], we selected "hsapiens" as the organism, "Network Topology-based Analysis (NTA)" as the method of interest, "network" as the functional database, and "genesymbol" as gene ID type. Based on these parameters, WebGestalt automatically shortlisted 33 cancer studies from The Cancer Genome Atlas (TCGA) that were available for searching. We used 27 HSF1-CanSig 8q genes, including HSF1, identified from the top 100 most frequently overexpressed genes to query WebGestalt while values of other parameters remained in default settings. We repeated the search for all 33 TCGA cancer studies (Additional file 1: Table S8).

Additional files

Additional file 1: Table S1. Statistical tests of observing HSF1-CanSig genes by chromosome arm. **Table S2.** List of 475 HSF1-CanSig genes. **Table S3.** List of 29 primary tumor sites. **Table S4.** Overexpression scores of HSF1-CanSig genes in each primary site. **Table S5.** Top 100 most frequently overexpressed HSF1-CanSig genes. **Table S6.** Genomic coordinates of syntenic genes. **Table S7.** Genomic coordinates of HSF1's flanking genes. **Table S8.** List of TCGA

Additional file 2: Percentage distribution of HSF1-CanSig genes by chromosome arm for each primary tumor site. For each primary site, two plots are included, one using all protein-coding genes and cancer census genes as references. The other uses HSF1-CanSig genes as the reference.

Additional file 3: Rank of HSF1 among primary sites. Syntenty visualization by Cinteny. An example showing the output web page of

Additional file 4: Expression correlation analysis of syntenic genes for

Abbreviations

GO: Gene Ontology; HSF1-CanSig Gene: Heat Shock Factor 1 Cancer Signature Gene; HuGO: Human Genome Organization; MYA: Million years ago; TCGA: The Cancer Genome Atlas; UTR: Untranslated region

Acknowledgements

The authors thank the patient participants in TCGA and the cBioPortal support team at the Memorial Sloan Kettering Cancer Center.

Funding

ESH is kindly supposed by the Biology Department at Lafayette College. CQZ is supported by the Weis Center for Research. TLP and HW are supported by Mowad Endowment for New Discoveries, Department of Urology, Geisinger Clinic.

Authors' contributions

All authors conceived the study. CQZ, TLP, and ESH conducted the data analysis. ESH performed the statistical analysis and programming. CQZ, HW, TLP, and ESH wrote the manuscript. All authors read and approved the final manuscript.

Competing interests

The authors declare that they have no competing interests.

Author details

[1]Department of Biology, Lafayette College, Easton, PA 18042, USA.
[2]Department of Computer Science, Lafayette College, Easton, PA 18042, USA.
[3]Urology Department, Geisinger Medical Center, Danville, PA 17822, USA.
[4]Weis Research Center, Geisinger Medical Center, Danville, PA 17822, USA.

References

1. Mendillo ML, Santagata S, Koeva M, Bell GW, Hu R, Tamimi RM, Fraenkel E, Ince TA, Whitesell L, Lindquist S. HSF1 drives a transcriptional program distinct from heat shock to support highly malignant human cancers. Cell. 2012;150(3):549–62.
2. Scherz-Shouval R, Santagata S, Mendillo ML, Sholl LM, Ben-Aharon I, Beck AH, Dias-Santagata D, Koeva M, Stemmer SM, Whitesell L, et al. The reprogramming of tumor stroma by HSF1 is a potent enabler of malignancy. Cell. 2014;158(3):564–78.
3. Liao Y, Xue Y, Zhang L, Feng X, Liu W, Zhang G. Higher heat shock factor 1 expression in tumor stroma predicts poor prognosis in esophageal squamous cell carcinoma patients. J Transl Med. 2015;13:338.
4. Engerud H, Tangen IL, Berg A, Kusonmano K, Halle MK, Oyan AM, Kalland KH, Stefansson I, Trovik J, Salvesen HB, et al. High level of HSF1 associates with aggressive endometrial carcinoma and suggests potential for HSP90 inhibitors. Brit J Cancer. 2014;111(1):78–84.
5. Powell CD, Paullin TR, Aoisa C, Menzie CJ, Ubaldini A, Westerheide SD. The heat shock transcription factor HSF1 induces ovarian cancer epithelial-mesenchymal transition in a 3D spheroid growth model. PLoS One. 2016;11(12)
6. Santarius T, Shipley J, Brewer D, Stratton MR, Cooper CS. EPIGENETICS AND GENETICS: a census of amplified and overexpressed human cancer genes. Nat Rev Cancer. 2010;10(1):59–64.
7. cBioPortal Web API. http://www.cbioportal.org/web_api.jsp. Accessed 1 May 2017.
8. Gao J, Aksoy BA, Dogrusoz U, Dresdner G, Gross B, Sumer SO, Sun Y, Jacobsen A, Sinha R, Larsson E, et al. Integrative analysis of complex cancer genomics and clinical profiles using the cBioPortal. Sci Signal. 2013;6(269):pl1.
9. Donoghue PC, Benton MJ. Rocks and clocks: calibrating the tree of life using fossils and molecules. Trends Ecol Evol. 2007;22(8):424–31.
10. Lander ES, Consortium IHGS, Linton LM, Birren B, Nusbaum C, Zody MC, Baldwin J, Devon K, Dewar K, Doyle M, et al. Initial sequencing and analysis of the human genome. Nature. 2001;409(6822):860–921.
11. Gibbs RA, Weinstock GM, Metzker ML, Muzny DM, Sodergren EJ, Scherer S, Scott G, Steffen D, Worley KC, Burch PE, et al. Genome sequence of the Brown Norway rat yields insights into mammalian evolution. Nature. 2004; 428(6982):493–521.
12. Elsik CG, Tellam RL, Worley KC, Gibbs RA, Abatepaulo ARR, Abbey CA, Adelson DL, Aerts J, Ahola V, Alexander L, et al. The genome sequence of taurine cattle: a window to ruminant biology and evolution. Science. 2009; 324(5926):522–8.
13. Sinha AU, Meller J. Cinteny: flexible analysis and visualization of synteny and genome rearrangements in multiple organisms. BMC Bioinf. 2007;8
14. Zhou Z, Li Y, Jia Q, Wang Z, Wang X, Hu J, Xiao J. Heat shock transcription factor 1 promotes the proliferation, migration and invasion of osteosarcoma cells. Cell Prolif. 2017;
15. Ishiwata J, Kasamatsu A, Sakuma K, Iyoda M, Yamatoji M, Usukura K, Ishige S, Shimizu T, Yamano Y, Ogawara K, et al. State of heat shock factor 1 expression as a putative diagnostic marker for oral squamous cell carcinoma. Int J Oncol. 2012;40(1):47–52.

16. Fang F, Chang RM, Yang LY. Heat shock factor 1 promotes invasion and metastasis of hepatocellular carcinoma in vitro and in vivo. Cancer-Am Cancer Soc. 2012;118(7):1782–94.
17. Dudeja V, Chugh RK, Sangwan V, Skube SJ, Mujumdar NR, Antonoff MB, Dawra RK, Vickers SM, Saluja AK. Prosurvival role of heat shock factor 1 in the pathogenesis of pancreatobiliary tumors. Am J Physiol-Gastr L. 2011; 300(6):G948–55.
18. El Gammal AT, Bruchmann M, Zustin J, Isbarn H, Hellwinkel OJC, Kollermann J, Sauter G, Simon R, Wilczak W, Schwarz J, et al. Chromosome 8p deletions and 8q gains are associated with tumor progression and poor prognosis in prostate cancer. Clin Cancer Res. 2010;16(1):56–64.
19. Toma-Jonik A, Widlak W, Korfanty J, Cichon T, Smolarczyk R, Gogler-Piglowska A, Widlak P, Vydra N. Active heat shock transcription factor 1 supports migration of the melanoma cells via vinculin down-regulation. Cell Signal. 2015;27(2):394–401.
20. Dobzhansky T. Nothing in biology makes sense except in light of evolution. Am Biol Teach. 1973;35(3):125–9.
21. Ghanbarian AT, Hurst LD. Neighboring genes show correlated evolution in gene expression. Mol Biol Evol. 2015;32(7):1748–66.
22. Liao BY, Zhang JZ. Coexpression of linked genes in mammalian genomes is generally disadvantageous. Mol Biol Evol. 2008;25(8):1555–65.
23. van Duin M, van Marion R, Vissers K, Watson JEV, van Weerden WM, Schroder FH, Hop WCJ, van der Kwast TH, Collins C, van Dekken H. High-resolution array comparative genomic hybridization of chromosome arm 8q: evaluation of genetic progression markers for prostate cancer. Genes Chromosomes Cancer. 2005;44(4):438–49.
24. Salinas CA, Kwon E, Carlson CS, Koopmeiners JS, Feng Z, Karyadi DM, Ostrander EA, Stanford JL. Multiple independent genetic variants in the 8q24 region are associated with prostate cancer risk. Cancer Epidemiol Biomarkers. 2008;17(5):1203–13.
25. Haiman CA, Patterson N, Freedman ML, Myers SR, Pike MC, Waliszewska A, Neubauer J, Tandon A, Schirmer C, McDonald GJ, et al. Multiple regions within 8q24 independently affect risk for prostate cancer. Nat Genet. 2007; 39(5):638–44.
26. Di Giammartino DC, Shi YS, Manley JL. PARP1 represses PAP and inhibits polyadenylation during heat shock. Mol Cell. 2013;49(1):7–17.
27. Hollerer I, Curk T, Haase B, Benes V, Hauer C, Neu-Yilik G, Bhuvanagiri M, Hentze MW, Kulozik AE. The differential expression of alternatively polyadenylated transcripts is a common stress-induced response mechanism that modulates mammalian mRNA expression in a quantitative and qualitative fashion. RNA. 2016;22(9):1441–53.
28. Skaggs HS, Xing H, Wilkerson DC, Murphy LA, Hong Y, Mayhew CN, Sarge KD. HSF1-TPR interaction facilitates export of stress-induced HSP70 mRNA. J Biol Chem. 2007;282(47):33902–7.
29. Nagaike T, Manley JL. Transcriptional activators enhance polyadenylation of mRNA precursors. RNA Biol. 2011;8(6):964–7.
30. Xing HY, Mayhew CN, Cullen KE, Park-Sarge OK, Sarge KD. HSF1 modulation of hsp70 mRNA polyadenylation via interaction with symplekin. J Biol Chem. 2004;279(11):10551–5.
31. Beaudoing E, Gautheret D. Identification of alternate polyadenylation sites and analysis of their tissue distribution using EST data. Genome Res. 2001; 11(9):1520–6.
32. Zhang HB, Lee JY, Tian B. Biased alternative polyadenylation in human tissues. Genome Biol. 2005;6(12)
33. Hoque M, Ji Z, Zheng DH, Luo WT, Li WC, You B, Park JY, Yehia G, Tian B. Analysis of alternative cleavage and polyadenylation by 3′ region extraction and deep sequencing. Nat Methods. 2013;10(2):133–9.
34. Xia Z, Donehower LA, Cooper TA, Neilson JR, Wheeler DA, Wagner EJ, Li W. Dynamic analyses of alternative polyadenylation from RNA-seq reveal a 3′-UTR landscape across seven tumour types. Nat Commun. 2014;5
35. Singh P, Alley TL, Wright SM, Kamdar S, Schott W, Wilpan RY, Mills KD, Graber JH. Global changes in processing of mRNA 3′ untranslated regions characterize clinically distinct cancer subtypes. Cancer Res. 2009;69(24): 9422–30.
36. Mayr C, Bartel DP. Widespread shortening of 3′ UTRs by alternative cleavage and polyadenylation activates oncogenes in cancer cells. Cell. 2009;138(4): 673–84.
37. Morris AR, Bos A, Diosdado B, Rooijers K, Elkon R, Bolijn AS, Carvalho B, Meijer GA, Agami R. Alternative cleavage and polyadenylation during colorectal cancer development. Clin Cancer Res. 2012;18(19):5256–66.
38. Masamha CP, Xia Z, Yang JX, Albrecht TR, Li M, Shyu AB, Li W, Wagner EJ. CFIm25 links alternative polyadenylation to glioblastoma tumour suppression. Nature. 2014;510(7505):412-+.
39. YG F, Sun Y, Li YX, Li J, Rao XQ, Chen C, AL X. Differential genome-wide profiling of tandem 3′ UTRs among human breast cancer and normal cells by high-throughput sequencing. Genome Res. 2011;21(5):741–7.
40. Liaw HH, Lin CC, Juan HF, Huang HC. Differential MicroRNA regulation correlates with alternative polyadenylation pattern between breast cancer and normal cells. PLoS One. 2013;8(2)
41. Elkon R, Drost J, van Haaften G, Jenal M, Schrier M, Vrielink JAFO, Agami R. E2F mediates enhanced alternative polyadenylation in proliferation. Genome Biol. 2012;13(7)
42. Sandberg R, Neilson JR, Sarma A, Sharp PA, Burge CB. Proliferating cells express mRNAs with shortened 3′ untranslated regions and fewer microRNA target sites. Science. 2008;320(5883):1643–7.
43. Buchert M, Papin M, Bonnans C, Darido C, Raye WS, Garambois V, Pelegrine A, Bourgaux JF, Pannequin J, Joubert D, et al. Symplekin promotes tumorigenicity by up-regulating claudin-2 expression. Proc Natl Acad Sci U S A. 2010;107(6):2628–33.
44. Amara SG, Jonas V, Rosenfeld MG, Ong ES, Evans RM. Alternative RNA processing in calcitonin gene-expression generates messenger-RNAs encoding different polypeptide products. Nature. 1982;298(5871):240–4.
45. Alt FW, Bothwell ALM, Knapp M, Siden E, Mather E, Koshland M, Baltimore D. Synthesis of secreted and membrane-bound immunoglobulin-mu heavy-chains is directed by messenger-RNAs that differ at their 3′ ends. Cell. 1980; 20(2):293–301.
46. Wu XB, Bartel DP. Widespread influence of 3′-end structures on mammalian mRNA processing and stability. Cell. 2017;169(5):905-+.
47. Shi YS, Di Giammartino DC, Taylor D, Sarkeshik A, Rice WJ, Yates JR, Frank J, Manley JL. Molecular architecture of the human pre-mRNA 3′ processing complex. Mol Cell. 2009;33(3):365–76.
48. HuGO Gene Nomenclature Committee. ftp://ftp.ebi.ac.uk/pub/databases/genenames/new/tsv/hgnc_complete_set.txt. Accessed 26 Apr 2017.
49. COSMIC Cancer Gene Census. http://cancer.sanger.ac.uk/census. Accessed 1 May 2017.
50. NCBI HomoloGene. ftp://ftp.ncbi.nih.gov/pub/HomoloGene/build68/. Accessed 1 May 2017.
51. UCSC Genome Browser. http://genome.ucsc.edu. Accessed 1 May 2017.
52. Pedersen BS, Yang IV, De S. CruzDB: software for annotation of genomic intervals with UCSC genome-browser database. Bioinformatics. 2013;29(23): 3003–6.
53. Kent WJ. BLAT—the BLAST-like alignment tool. Genome Res. 2002;12(4): 656–64.
54. Suzuki R, Shimodaira H. Pvclust: an *R* package for assessing the uncertainty in hierarchical clustering. Bioinformatics. 2006;22(12):1540–2.
55. Wang J, Vasaikar S, Shi Z, Greer M, Zhang B. WebGestalt 2017: a more comprehensive, powerful, flexible and interactive gene set enrichment analysis toolkit. Nucleic Acids Res. 2017;
56. WebGestalt 2017. http://www.webgestalt.org/option.php. Accessed May 2017.

7

Development and validation of a variant detection workflow for *BRCA1* and *BRCA2* genes and its clinical application based on the Ion Torrent technology

Ana Lígia Buzolin, Caroline Mônaco Moreira, Patricia Rossi Sacramento, Andre Yuji Oku, Alexandre Ricardo dos Santos Fornari, David Santos Marco Antonio, Caio Robledo D Angioli Costa Quaio, Wagner Rosa Baratela and Miguel Mitne-Neto*

Abstract

Background: Breast cancer is the most common among women worldwide, and ovarian cancer is the most difficult gynecological tumor to diagnose and with the lowest chance of cure. Mutations in *BRCA1* and *BRCA2* genes increase the risk of ovarian cancer by 60% and breast cancer by up to 80% in women. Molecular tests allow a better orientation for patients carrying these mutations, affecting prophylaxis, treatment, and genetic counseling.

Results: Here, we evaluated the performance of a panel for *BRCA1* and *BRCA2*, using the Ion Torrent PGM (Life Technologies) platform in a customized workflow and multiplex ligation-dependent probe amplification for detection of mutations, insertions, and deletions in these genes. We validated the panel with 26 samples previously analyzed by Myriad Genetics Laboratory, and our workflow showed 95.6% sensitivity and 100% agreement with Myriad reports, with 85% sensitivity on the positive control sample from NIST. We also screened 68 clinical samples and found 22 distinct mutations.

Conclusions: The selection of a robust methodology for sample preparation and sequencing, together with bioinformatics tools optimized for the data analysis, enabled the development of a very sensitive test with high reproducibility. We also highlight the need to explore the limitations of the NGS technique and the strategies to overcome them in a clinically confident manner.

Keywords: Cancer, Breast, Ovarian, Ion Torrent, BRCA

Background

Breast cancer is the most common among women worldwide, accounting for about 25% of new cases each year. Overall, there were 1.67 million new cases of breast cancer in 2012 and 522,000 deaths, with most of them being women [1]. Ovarian cancer, although infrequent, is the most difficult gynecological tumor to diagnose with the lowest chance of cure, accounting for 239,000 cases and 152,000 deaths in 2012 [1, 2].

A family history of breast and ovarian cancer is an important risk factor for the onset of the disease. *BRCA1* and *BRCA2* are genes that produce tumor-suppressing proteins. These proteins help the repair of damaged DNA and therefore play an essential role in ensuring the stability of the genetic material of cells. Together, *BRCA1* and *BRCA2* account for about 20 to 25% of cases of hereditary breast cancer and 15% of cases of ovarian cancer [3]. Specific germline mutations in these genes increase the risk of breast and ovarian cancer in women and are associated with an increased risk to develop other types of cancers. Women carrying mutations in *BRCA1* or *BRCA2* show up to 80% of increased risk for developing breast cancer, while men present up to 6%. For ovarian cancer, the risk is up to 50% [4–6].

* Correspondence: miguel.mitne@grupofleury.com.br
Research and Development, Fleury Group, Av. General Valdomiro de Lima, 508, São Paulo/SP 04344-070, Brazil

Molecular tests that are able to identify such mutations have a great impact on healthcare, since they allow a better orientation for patients, affecting prophylaxis, treatment, and genetic counseling. Women who tested positive for any of these genes can take steps to prevent the disease, as the realization of screenings before the recommended age for the general population, increasing the chance of detecting cancer at an initial stage. It is also possible to carry out a prophylactic mastectomy for risk reduction and even chemopreventive treatment, consisting in the use of natural or synthetic chemical agents to reverse, suppress, or prevent carcinogenic progression [7, 8].

From the technical perspective, the challenges of *BRCA1* and *BRCA2* mutation identification are the long genic extension and the clinical interpretation for each of the identified mutations. To overcome the technical challenges in terms of efficiency and turnaround time, the use of next-generation sequencing techniques have been adopted by diagnostic laboratories worldwide [9–11]. Here, we evaluated the performance of a panel for detecting *BRCA1* and *BRCA2* mutations, using the Ion Torrent PGM platform (Life Technologies) in a customized workflow. Accuracy tests were performed by using 26 samples that were previously analyzed by Myriad Genetic Laboratory and a reference sample from the National Institute for Standards and Technology (NIST). The pipeline that we created was able to identify all the pathogenic and variant of unknown significance (VUS) variants in both genes, reported by the reference laboratory and 85% of the variants present in the NIST sample, but all of them were benign. Using this workflow, we screened 68 clinical samples and found 22 distinct variants. Our data show that the present workflow is robust and is reliable for diagnostic procedures. Additionally, the generation of distinct databases for admixed populations, as the one studied here, and its comparison with other cohorts is an important step for the correct variant pathogenicity interpretation. Moreover, we explore the limitations of the technique and present strategies to overcome them in a clinically confident manner.

Methods

Validation

Sample selection and DNA extraction

Twenty-six blood samples were collected in two ethylenediaminetetraacetic acid (EDTA) vials. For each of them, one vial was sent to Myriad Genetic Laboratories as part of our diagnostic routine and the other was kept in Fleury Group. Samples were renumbered and anonymized so the donor could not be tracked.

DNA extraction from the whole EDTA blood was performed on QiaSymphony (Qiagen). DNA and amplicon quantification was based on Qubit 2.0 fluorometer (Life Technologies) using dsDNA BR Assay kit.

The reference sample NA12878, purchased from National Institute for Standards and Technology (NIST), was also used for the validation.

Strategies for capture and library preparation

In order to capture the entire coding region of both genes, we tested two capture strategies. In the first one, we designed 100 pairs of primers to amplify the target region (Additional file 1: Table S1), containing a total of 18,947 base pairs. These primers contained universal tag sequences, which allowed the amplification of the target region and insertion of barcodes and adaptors in a single PCR reaction. The primer design also allowed their use in Sanger sequencing.

A second capture strategy was based on the Ion AmpliSeq BRCA1 and BRCA2 panel (Ion Torrent) and was used to generate target amplicon libraries. This panel contains 167 primer pairs in 3 primer pools and is designed for 100% amplicon coverage of all targeted coding exons and exon–intron boundaries. Briefly, 20 ng of DNA was amplified by PCR in three distinct reactions of 10 μL using the Ion AmpliSeq primer pools and Ion AmpliSeq HiFi master mix (Ion AmpliSeq kit version 2.0). The resulting amplicons were pooled, and 20 μL was transferred to a new tube and treated with FuPa reagent to partially digest primer sequences and phosphorylate the amplicons. The amplicons were then ligated to adapters from the Ion Xpress barcoded adapters 1–16 kit. After ligation, the libraries were purified using Agencourt Ampure XP Beads and equalized to 100 pM with the Ion Library Equalizer kit according to the manufacturer's instructions (Life Technologies).

Emulsion PCR and sequencing

Multiplexed barcoded libraries were amplified by emulsion PCR on ion sphere particles (ISPs) using the Ion PGM Hi-Q OT2 Kit according to the manufacturer's instructions (Life Technologies). Positive-templated ISPs were biotinylated during the emulsion PCR process followed by enrichment with Dynabeads MyOne streptavidin C1 beads (Life Technologies). Ion 314 and 316 chips were used to sequence four and eight samples, respectively. Sequencing was performed on an Ion PGM System (Ion Torrent) using the Ion PGM Hi-Q Sequencing kit according to the manufacturer's instructions.

Bioinformatics

Torrent Suite software version 4.4 was used to demultiplex barcoded reads and to generate run metrics, including chip loading efficiency, coverage analysis, total read counts, and quality. A visual quality assessment of reads was performed with FastQC. The FASTQ files were used either in the Variant Caller plugin from the Torrent Suite 4.4 package or in the CLC Genomics Workbench 8.0 (CLCbio, Boston, MA). We designed a pipeline optimized for the Ion AmpliSeq BRCA1 and BRCA2 panel (Fig. 1), consisting of six main steps:

1. Trimming of 5 bp from the reads' 3′ end to avoid mapping of low-quality regions and exclusion of short reads (<15 bp) and reads end with a Phred score (Q value) <20.
2. Read mapping against UCSC hg19 (http://hgdownload.soe.ucsc.edu/goldenPath/hg19/bigZips, last accessed April 04, 2016) using default cost values for mismatches (2) and indels (3) and minimum reference similarity (80%). A mapping report and a .bam file were generated as outputs.
3. Read mapping was also performed against a reference containing all the amplicon sequences from the panels, so that the mean coverage could be assessed for each amplicon individually.
4. Variant calling was performed restricted to the target regions defined in the bed file. Bidirectional presence of variant alleles was required in a concordance of at least 5% between forward and reverse reads. The minimum coverage cut off was 10× with variant allele frequencies (VAFs) of 20%. Variant calls were filtered with a minimum average base quality of 16 (Phred Score), which removed all variants having alleles with an average base quality of less than the given threshold, even if they are in a region within a high overall quality and passed the first trimming step. This threshold increases sensitivity and lowers the number of variants called in homopolymer regions.
5. The variants were annotated with the COSMIC database and the Variant Effect Predictor (VEP) from Ensembl (http://grch37.ensembl.org/Homo_sapiens/Tools/VEP). The clinical significance of the variants was annotated with ClinVar database (http://www.ncbi.nlm.nih.gov/clinvar/) which contains publicly available information of the Sharing Clinical Reports Project, an initiative of diagnosis centers worldwide that submitted the variants of BRCA1/2 reported by Myriad Genetics since 2006. ClinVar also contains the variants from Breast Cancer Information Core (BIC, NIH), so it is

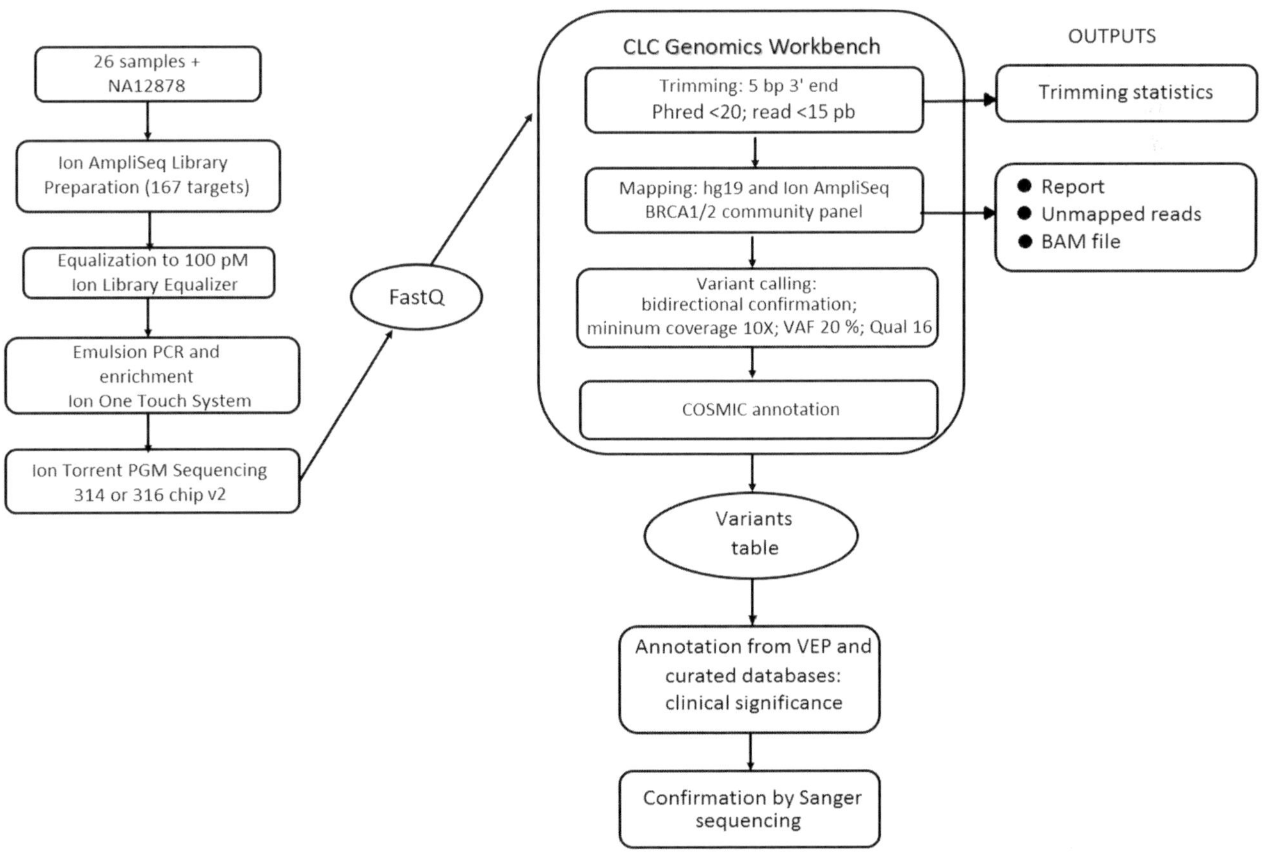

Fig 1 Workflow for processing and analysis of samples in the validation design. *PGM* personal genome machine, *VAF* variant allele frequency, *BAM* bam file, *VEP* variant effect predictor

the most complete public-curated database of BRCA1/2 variants. Fleury's database, consisting of past exams sent to Myriad, and Arup BRCA1/2 mutation database (http://arup.utah.edu/database/BRCA/) were also checked for variants not previously found.

A total of seven runs were performed in different days, accounting for 48 sequencings of the 26 samples. These assays comprehend inter- and intra-assay evaluations (Additional File 2: Table S2).

Confirmation by Sanger sequencing

All the identified variants were confirmed by bidirectional Sanger sequencing. The regions containing the variants were amplified using the above described primers for the first strategy. Amplification reactions were performed in a Veriti thermocycler (Applied Biosystems) using the enzyme AmpliTaq Gold DNA Polymerase (Applied Biosystems). PCR products were confirmed by 2% agarose gel and purified with the ExoSAP-IT enzyme (Affymetrix). The sequencing reactions were performed with BigDye Terminator v3.1 Cycle, and the capillary electrophoresis was carried out on ABI 3130xl equipment. Data analysis and comparison to reference was made in CLCbio Workbench software. The sensitivity of the sequencing by next-generation sequencing (NGS) was calculated by true positive ratio (confirmed by Sanger) and total positive.

MLPA

In order to follow the proper *BRCA1* and *BRCA2* evaluation workflow, we validated a multiplex ligation-dependent probe amplification (MLPA) assay, using 11 samples selected as described above. MLPA commercial kits from MRC-Holland for *BRCA1* and *BRCA2* were used here. Tests were performed in duplicate and at different days to evaluate the intra- and inter-assay reproducibility. We used 100 ng of DNA from each sample, three reference samples (which had no duplications and/or deletions), a negative control containing only ATE buffer (the same used in sample dilution), and a positive control for each gene. For the positive control of *BRCA1*, we used a sample purchased from Coriell Institute (USA), which presents the mutation 1294del40 in exon 11.

For the positive control of *BRCA2*, we amplified exon 9 and used the PCR product diluted proportionately in a sample without prior changes in order to simulate a duplication. The procedures were performed according to the manufacturer's instructions. The steps of denaturation, hybridization, binding, and PCR were performed in Veriti thermocycler (Applied Biosystems). The analysis of fragments was performed on ABI 3130xl sequencer and the data generated were imported and analyzed in Coffalyser.Net software.

Validation process and analytical assessment

Target regions containing variants detected in the Ion AmpliSeq panel were analyzed by Sanger sequencing. Thus, these variants were used for checking NGS accuracy on the patient's samples. Sensitivity was calculated as the relationship between true positive/total positives.

We also compared our results with Myriad reports to verify the agreement in the variant's classification between both exams. Myriad processes the test using HiSeq 2500 (Illumina) and classifies the variants through its proprietary pipeline (https://myriad.com/). Myriad's reports contain only VUS or pathogenic/likely pathogenic mutations, and other variants are not reported. For this reason, specificity could not be calculated.

To compare the NA12878 sample results obtained in our sequencing, we selected variants of the standard.vcf file for this sample (available at: ftp://ftp-trace.ncbi.nlm.nih.gov/giab/ftp/release/NA12878_HG001/NISTv3.2/) contained in the target intervals of Ion AmpliSeq panel BRCA1/2.

Additional sample evaluation

Based on the Ampliseq campture strategy, we analyzed 68 samples having a history of either mammary or ovarian cancer, which were sent to our service in order to evaluate the presence of *BRCA1* or *BRCA2* mutations. Variant classification followed the above described process. MLPA was performed for all the 68 samples. In order to guarantee the quality of the analysis, regions with <20× coverage were Sanger sequenced. Every pathogenic and VUS variants detected by the NGS workflow were also confirmed by Sanger sequencing.

The graphic of mutation distribution was built using the cBioPortal website (http://www.cbioportal.org/mutation_mapper.jsp).

Results

Development and validation process

The *in-house*-designed primer strategy presented a reduction of about 5× in the capture costs, when compared to the commercial available one. It was possible to cover the entire target region; however, there was a great coverage variability; while some amplicons presented 20× on average, others showed 1500× (data not shown). Since this variability could risk the following analysis, this method was set aside. Even being discarded for routine application, this strategy brought the advantage of creating a bank of validated primers, which can be used to sequence and confirm any *BRCA1* and *BRCA2* regions through Sanger sequencing.

The Ion Torrent PGM sequencings, based on the commercial available capture strategy, generated an average of 2.8 million reads with a mean size of 135 bp (based on the seven runs). The coverage analysis performed with the plugin Coverage Analysis from Torrent Suite v4.4 software showed that the target regions (167 amplicons) had 100% coverage (Fig. 2). Using 4 samples per 314 chips, the average coverage was 425×, with more than 95% of the bases with a coverage of at least 100× and 98.88% at least 20×. The template preparation showed values of polyclonal ranging from 28 to 42%.

Variant calling

During the validation process, we found 42 unique variants in the patients' samples (Table 1). Considering the complete sampling set, there were 574 variants, also accounting the reproducibility tests. The result obtained from the confirmation by capillary sequencing detected 25 false positives including 10 different variants with 8 in homopolymer regions (Additional File 3: Table S3). The variants reported by the reference laboratory (Myriad Genetics) were considered true positives variants and could be identified by our strategy, including a confirmation by Sanger.

Regarding the NA12878 sample from NIST, we identified 17 from the 20 variants (85%) contained in the vcf file filtered for Ion AmpliSeq regions. The three uncalled variants were present in endpoints of the target amplicons (5′ or 3′) located in exon–intron boundaries, and do not represent clinically significant variants.

Variant calling comparison

Using the in-house-developed bioinformatics pipeline, we could reach a variant calling sensitivity of 95.64%. The inter- and intra-assay evaluation, comprehended by 10 duplicates, 4 triplicates, and 1 quadruplicate showed high concordance in the variant calls, as demonstrated by the reproducibility of the test. The reproducibility rate within the NGS sequencing was 94.17%, but the errors only happened due to false positives. When we sequenced the target regions by Sanger, we excluded all the false positives and obtained 100% reproducibility for the true positive variants. The sensitivity observed separately for SNVs, insertions, and deletions using the in-house pipeline is summarized in Table 2.

As a comparison, we used the Variant Caller plugin available in the Torrent Suite v4.4 software (recommended by the supplier). The last one has a pipeline developed and optimized for the specific analysis of the Ion AmpliSeq panel *BRCA1*/*BRCA2*; however, the reached sensitivity was 94.03%, with the identification of 587 variants, with 35 of them being false positives (Table 3).

Regarding the reports from Myriad Genetic Laboratories, there was 100% agreement between the results *for mutation identification*. After comparing with databases, four mutations were classified as pathogenic and three as VUS (variants of unknown significance), as shown in Table 3.

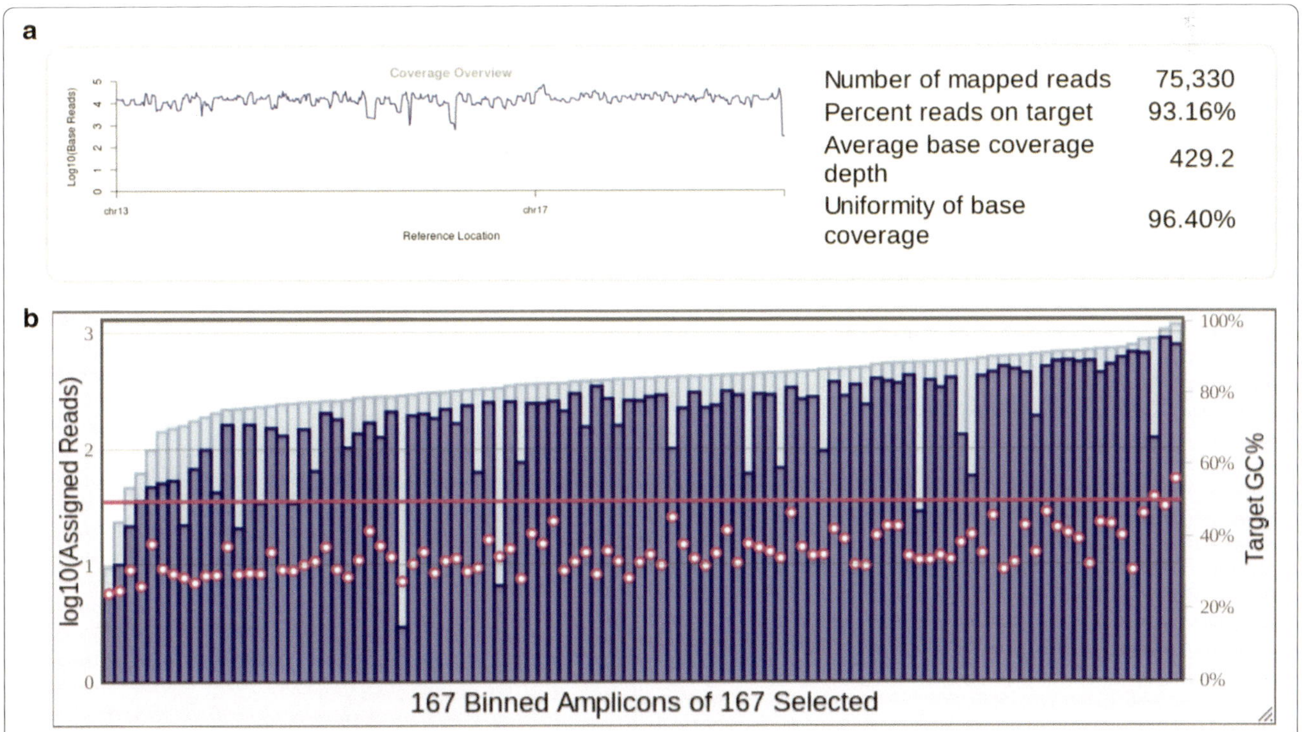

Fig 2 Coverage analysis report generated by Coverage Analysis plugin. **a** Coverage overview from the alignment regions of *BRCA1* (chr17) and *BRCA2* (chr13). **b** Reads distribution on the 167 targets of the Ion AmpliSeq *BRCA1/2* panel, overlayed with target GC content for each read. Representative data from one of the samples sequenced in this validation

Table 1 *BRCA1* and *BRCA2* variants in the 26 validation samples

Gene	HGVSc (hg19)	HGVSp
BRCA2	NM_000059.3:c.-26G>A	–
	NM_000059.3:c.425+67A>C	–
	NM_000059.3:c.681+56C>T	–
	NM_000059.3:c.865A>C	NP_000050.2:p.Asn289His
	NM_000059.3:c.1365A>G	NM_000059.3:c.1365A>G(p.Ser455=)
	NM_000059.3:c.1910-74T>C	–
	NM_000059.3:c.1910-51G>T	–
	NM_000059.3:c.2229T>C	NM_000059.3:c.2229T>C(p.His743=)
	NM_000059.3:c.2971A>G	NP_000050.2:p.Asn991Asp
	NM_000059.3:c.3396A>G	NM_000059.3:c.3396A>G(p.Lys1132=)
	NM_000059.3:c.3807T>C	NM_000059.3:c.3807T>C(p.Val1269=)
	NM_000059.3:c.4563A>G	NM_000059.3:c.4563ª>G(p.Leu1521=)
	NM_000059.3:c.4585G>A	NP_000050.2:p.Gly1529Arg
	NM_000059.3:c.5744C>T	NP_000050.2:p.Thr1915Met
	NM_000059.3:c.6100C>T	NP_000050.2:p.Arg2034Cys
	NM_000059.3:c.6322C>T	NP_000050.2:p.Arg2108Cys
	NM_000059.3:c.6513G>C	NM_000059.3:c.6513G>C(p.Val2171=)
	*NM_000059.3:c.6988A>G	NP_000050.2:p.Ile2330Val
	NM_000059.3:c.7008-62A>G	–
	NM_000059.3:c.7242A>G	NM_000059.3:c.7242A>G(p.Ser2414=)
	NM_000059.3:c.7397T>C	NP_000050.2:p.Val2466Ala
	NM_000059.3:c.7806-14T>C	–
	NM_000059.3:c.8482A>G	NP_000050.2:p.Ile2828Val
	NM_000059.3:c.8518A>G	NP_000050.2:p.Ile2840Val
	NM_000059.3:c.8755-66T>C	–
BRCA1	NM_007294.3:c.5266dupC	NP_009225.1:p.Gln1756ProfsTer74
	NM_007294.3:c.5095C>T	NP_009225.1:p.Arg1699Trp
	NM_007294.3:c.4837A>G	NP_009225.1:p.Ser1613Gly
	NM_007294.3:c.4535G>T	NP_009225.1:p.Ser1512Ile
	NM_007294.3:c.4308T>C	NM_007294.3:c.4308T>C(p.Ser1436)
	NM_007294.3:c.3916_3917delTT	NP_009225.1:p.Leu1306AspfsTer23
	NM_007294.3:c.3548A>G	NP_009225.1:p.Lys1183Arg
	NM_007294.3:c.3119G>A	NP_009225.1:p.Ser1040Asn
	NM_007294.3:c.3113A>G	NP_009225.1:p.Glu1038Gly
	NM_007294.3:c.2612C>T	NP_009225.1:p.Pro871Leu
	NM_007294.3:c.2311T>C	NM_007294.3:c.2311T>C(p.Leu771)
	NM_007294.3:c.2082C>T	NM_007294.3:c.2082C>T(p.Ser694)
	NM_007294.3:c.2077G>A	NP_009225.1:p.Asp693Asn
	NM_007294.3:c.1067A>G	NP_009225.1:p.Gln356Arg
	NM_007294.3:c.736T>G	NP_009225.1:p.Leu246Val
	NM_007294.3:c.442-34C>T	–
	NM_007294.3:c.-19-115T>C	–

Myriad did not send us the entire list of variants, with the report being composed solely by the pathogenic and VUS variants. For this reason, the specificity compared to Myriad results could not be calculated (Table 4).

Table 2 Comparison of the variant call sensitivity between SNVs, insertions, and deletions with the *in-house pipeline*

	SNVs	Insertion	Deletion
Variants found	539	22	13
False positives	0	15	10
Sensibility	100%	31.8%	23.07%

MLPA

All samples met the quality criteria evaluated in the Coffalyser.Net software including FRSS (fragment run separation score) and FMRS (fragment MLPA reaction score), and all expected probes were detected (48 for *BRCA1* and 44 for *BRCA2*). The samples analyzed showed no deletions and/or duplications detected by MLPA in the *BRCA1* and *BRCA2* genes, which is in agreement with the results of sequencing and the reports sent by Myriad. Interestingly, one of the samples showed a decrease in fluorescence referring to one of the *BRCA2* probes. By analyzing the sequence, we observe the presence of the mutation c.6988A>G, located exactly in the hybridization probe region, which explains the signal decrease.

Both the deletion of 40 bp in exon 11 of the *BRCA1* and the duplication of exon 9 in *BRCA2*, which were used as positive controls, were correctly identified. All results were 100% concordant between inter- and intra-assay repetitions, showing that the test is reproducible.

Evaluation of clinical samples

Based on the validation that we performed, we sought to analyze the *BRCA1* and *BRCA2* mutation status in 68 women that had their blood collected for our routine test.

In order to guarantee the detection of clinically significant variants, we Sanger sequenced the targeted regions that presented less than 20× coverage. Using this cutoff for the clinical cohort, we observed that the entire exon 20 and the final end of exon 23 from *BRCA2* had a similar poor performance and had to be confirmed by Sanger in 90% of our samples.

Table 3 Comparison of the variant call sensitivity between the Variant Caller plugin and the pipeline developed in-house

	In-house pipeline	Variant Caller Ion Torrent Suite
Variants found	574	587
False positives	25	35
Sensitivity	95.64%	94.03%
Reproducibility (NGS only)	94.17%	94.71%
Reproducibility (NGS+Sanger)	100%	100%

Table 4 Variants called in agreement with Myriad results

Variants	Clinical significance	Number of samples
BRCA1 c.5266dupC	Pathogenic	2
BRAC1 c.5095C>T	Pathogenic	1
BRCA1 c.3916_3917del	Pathogenic	1
BRCA2 c.6988A>G	VUS	1
BRCA2 c.8482A>G	VUS	1
BRCA2 c.8518A>G	VUS	1

Over these 68 samples, we found a total of 22 variants in the *BRCA1* and 49 in the *BRCA2* gene. No alterations on MLPA were found in any of the samples. Fifty-seven variants were classified as benign, and 14 were either pathogenic or VUS (Table 5), with great majority being identified in *BRCA2*. Mutations in *BRCA1* were mapped in the N- and C-terminal, while *BRCA2* variants had a more homogeneous distribution, with a slightly clusterization near the OB3 domain coding region (Fig. 3). All of 14 variants were tested by Sanger sequencing and confirmed by the orthogonal approach.

Discussion

Here, we evaluated strategies for *BRCA1* and *BRCA2* mutation detection, through Ion Torrent PGM NGS platform, and found that a commercial panel for capturing the coding *BRCA1* and *BRCA2* regions (Ampliseq BRCA1/BRCA2) is robust and meets the clinical requirements for diagnostic. This panel proved to be efficient, covering all exons and a part of the introns. However, there is a limitation in terms of performance, since there is great variability in amplification efficiency of the 167 targets, reflecting a variable final coverage of the sequencing run. Thus, a high value of mean coverage is essential to ensure that even regions of lower efficiency in the PCR are represented in a minimum cutoff in the sequencing data. This situation was especially evidenced in our clinical cohort, with the need of Sanger sequencing for some hot spot areas that consistently presented a poor coverage (<20×).

The comparison between the workflow that we designed on CLC Workbench software and the Variant Caller from Torrent Suite v4.4 software showed that the last one presents an increased amount of false positives, with reduced sensitivity. Even with the optimization of the bioinformatics parameters used in our pipeline, which improved the quality of mapping and variant calling, our in-house pipeline has a high false positive rate (4.3%), which is due mostly to homopolymers regions. This has been previously reported by other authors [12–14] and highlights the need for orthogonal confirmations. Having this scenario, we opted for the confirmation of every pathogenic or variant of unknown significance through Sanger sequencing in our clinical analysis test. Despite having a higher processing cost, this strategy reduces the chance of losing clinically important variants.

The accuracy tests were performed with basis in the Myriad Genetics Laboratory reports and the NA12878 (NIST) evaluation. The first comparison showed 100% accuracy, since all the mutations reported by Myriad could be identified in our test and were also validated by Sanger sequencing. This data shows that our test is reliable, since Myriad is a reference when dealing with mutations in *BRCA1* and *BRCA2*. Furthermore, intra- and inter-assays demonstrated that the test is reproducible. It was not possible to obtain specificity values for the test because we do not have information of all the

Table 5 Summary of the main variants found in this clinical cohort

Gene	Mutation	Classification	Type
BRCA1 (NM_007294.3)	c.441+2T>A	Pathogenic	Intronic (splice donor variant)
	c.68_69delAG: p.Glu23Valfs*17	Pathogenic	Frameshift
	c.5365G>T: p.Ala1789Ser	VUS	Missense
BRCA2 (NM_000059.3)	c.4965C>: p.Y1655*	Pathogenic	Nonsense
	c.8878C>T: p.Gln2960*	Pathogenic	Nonsense
	c.9382C>T: p.Arg3128*	Pathogenic	Nonsense
	c.1813dupA: p.Ile605Asnfs*11	Pathogenic	Frameshift
	c.9004G>A: p.Glu3002Lys	Pathogenic	Missense
	c.8850G>T: p.Lys2950Asn	VUS	Missense
	c.5729A>T: p.Asn1910Ile	VUS	Missense
	c.7469T>C: p.Ile2490Thr	VUS	Missense
	c.956A>C: p.Asn319Thr	VUS	Missense
	c.3262C>T: p.Pro1088Ser	VUS	Missense
	c.4183G>T: p.Ala1395Ser	VUS	Missense

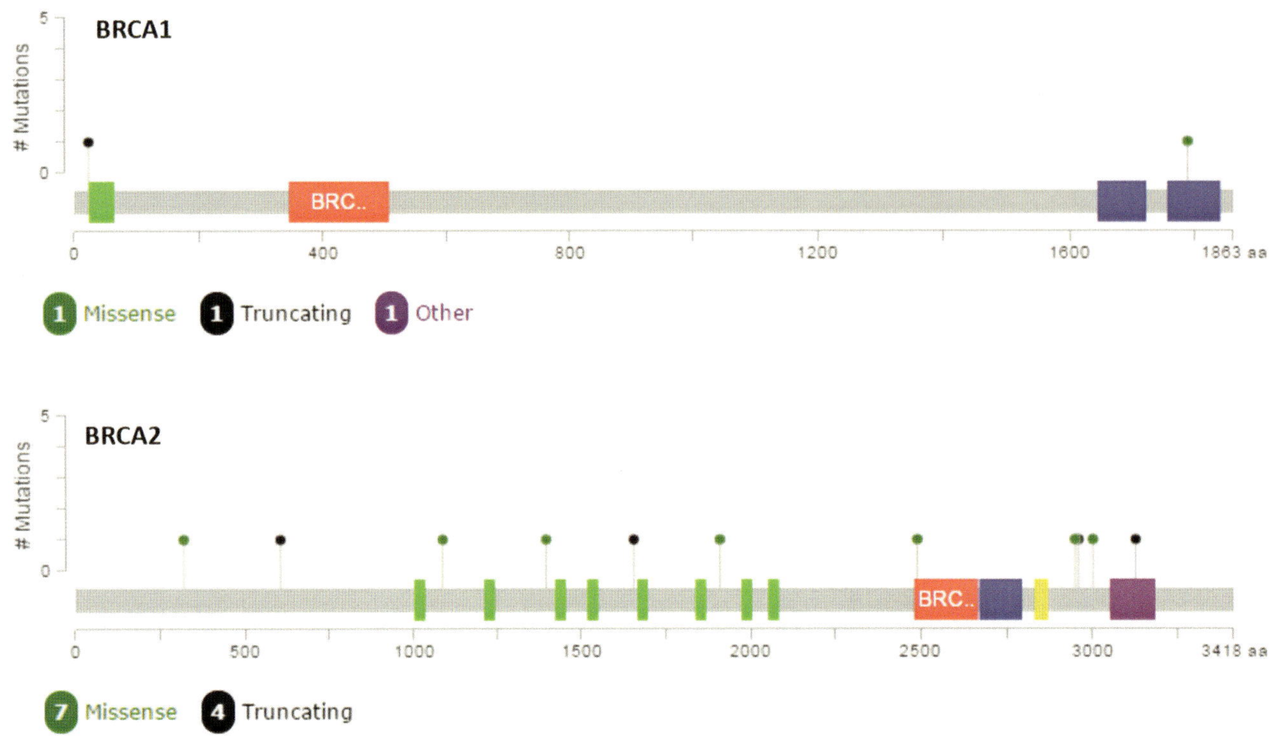

Fig 3 Distribution of the *BRCA1* and *BRCA2* mutations identified in the clinical cohort. The c.441+2T>A variant was not mapped, since it is an intronic variant.

variants in the samples that were sent to Myriad. Additionally, it is important to highlight that in the regions analyzed by Sanger sequencing for variants confirmation, we found no other changes than those observed by NGS.

The second comparison, using the sample NA12878 reference, found that our workflow failed to find three variants. However, when analyzing the read mappings, we observed that these variants are located in the endpoints of the target amplicons (5′ or 3′), regions usually with low-quality bases in exon–intron boundaries, with low mapping quality, and that do not contain clinically significant variants.

MLPA tests also showed high reproducibility, with concordant results between repetitions and the detection of any changes expected in the positive controls. One sample showed reduced fluorescence signal for one of the *BRCA2* probes, since this variant was present in the exact site of hybridization, which generated an equivocal result for the presence of a deletion. This observation is important to demonstrate that the results of sequencing and MLPA are complementary and that the thorough analysis and interpretation of data by qualified professionals is essential for diagnosis.

During this validation process and the evaluation of the 68 clinical samples, we were also able to join a huge amount of data from different databases. Using publicly available data and the insertion of *BRCA1* and *BRCA2* variants that were previously reported by Myriad Genetics Laboratory during our more than 10-year sent out test, turned possible to produce a very robust database with over 9000 variants that can be used for the interpretation of each identified variant. This is of special interest, since one of the most critical points of this workflow is the definition between a pathogenic mutation and a benign variant. Additionally, the generation of specific databases is important for populations like the one we have in Brazil due to its admixture, with different representations of African, European, and Native American variant frequencies [15]. It is interesting to note a slight clusterization of *BRCA2* variants near the OB3 domain.

Conclusion

The workflow for the complete analysis of *BRCA1* and *BRCA2* genes has proved to be highly efficient and accurate for the detection of point mutations and indels by NGS with the Ion Torrent PGM system, in addition to large insertions and deletions with MLPA technique. The selection of a robust methodology for sample preparation and sequencing, together with bioinformatics tools optimized for the data analysis, enabled the development of a very sensitive test with high reproducibility. We also highlight the need to explore the limitations of the NGS technique and the strategies to overcome them in a clinically confident manner.

Acknowledgements
We thank Fleury Group (São Paulo, Brazil) for supporting this research, including the materials and the development infrastructure.

Funding
Not applicable.

Authors' contributions
MMN conceived and designed the study and gave all the scientific assessment. ALB designed the primers, prepared the libraries, and performed the sequencings and data analysis. AYO and DSMA helped with the workflow design and development of a database search tool. ARSF helped with the NGS and Sanger sequencings. PRS and CMM did the DNA extractions and processed the clinical samples. WRB and CRDAC provided the medical assessment for the products' development. ALB and MMN prepared the manuscript. All authors read and approved the final manuscript.

Competing interests
The authors declare that they have no competing interests.

References

1. Ferlay J, Soerjomataram I, Dikshit R, Eser S, Mahters C, Rebelo M, Parkin D M, Forman D, Bray F. Cancer incidence and mortality worldwide: sources, methods and major patterns in GLOBOCAN 2012. International Journal Of Cancer. 2014; doi:10.1002/ijc.29210.
2. Cramer D W. The Epidemiology of Endometrial and Ovarian Cancer. Hematology/oncology Clinics Of North America. 2012; doi:10.1016/j.hoc.2011.10.009.
3. Pal T, Permuth-Wey J, Betts J A, Krischer J P, Fiorica J, Arango H, LaPolla J, Hoffman M, Martino M A, Wakeley K, Wilbanks G, Nicosia S, Cantor A, Stuphen R. BRCA1 and BRCA2 mutations account for a large proportion of ovarian carcinoma cases. Cancer. 2005; doi:10.1002/cncr.21536.
4. NIH, BRCA1 and BRCA2: Cancer Risk and Genetic Testing. 2016. http://www.cancer.gov/about-cancer/causes-prevention/genetics/brca-fact-sheet#r5. Accessed 04 Apr 2016.
5. O'Donovan P J, Livingston D M. BRCA1 and BRCA2: breast/ovarian cancer susceptibility gene products and participants in DNA double-strand break repair. Carcinogenesis. 2010; doi:10.1093/carcin/bgq069.
6. Roy R, Chun J, Powell S N. BRCA1 and BRCA2: different roles in a common pathway of genome protection. Nature Reviews Cancer. 2011; doi:10.1038/nrc3181.
7. Aebi S, Davidson T, Gruber G, Cardoso F, ESMO Guidelines Working Group. Primary breast cancer: ESMO Clinical Practice Guidelines for diagnosis, treatment and follow-up. Annals of Oncology. 2011; doi:10.1093/annonc/mdr371.
8. Bozovic-Spasojevic I, Azambuja E, McCaskill-Stevens W, Dinh P, Cardoso F. Chemoprevention for breast cancer. Cancer Treatment Reviews. 2012; doi:10.1016/j.ctrv.2011.07.005.
9. Feliubadaló L, Lopez-Doriga A, Castellsagué E, del Valle J, Menéndez M, Tornero E, Montes E, Cuesta R, Gómez C, Campos O, Pineda M, González S, Moreno V, Brunet J, Blanco I, Serra E, Capellá G, Lázaro C. Next-generation sequencing meets genetic diagnostics: development of a comprehensive workflow for the analysis of BRCA1 and BRCA2 genes. Eur J Hum Genet. 2012; doi:10.1038/ejhg.2012.270.
10. Spurdle A B, Healey S, Devereau A, Hogervorst F B L, Monteiro A N A, Nathanson K L, Radice P, Stoppa-Lyonnet D, Tavtigian S, Wappenschmidt B, Couch F J, Goldgar D E. ENIGMA-Evidence-based network for the interpretation of germline mutant alleles: an international initiative to evaluate risk and clinical significance associated with sequence variation in BRCA1 and BRCA2 genes. Human Mutation. 2011; doi:10.1002/humu.21628.
11. Tung N, Battelli C, Allen D, Kaldate R, Bhatnagar S, Bowles K, Timms K, Garber J E, Herold C, Ellisen L, Krejdovsky J, DeLeonardis K, Sedgwick K, Soltis K, Roa B, Wenstrup R J, Hartman A R. Frequency of mutations in individuals with breast cancer referred for BRCA 1 and BRCA 2 testing using next-generation sequencing with a 25-gene panel. Cancer. 2014; doi:10.1002/cncr.29010.
12. Bragg L M, Stone G, Butler M K, Hugenholtz P, Tyson G W. Shining a light on dark sequencing: characterising errors in Ion Torrent PGM data. Plos Comput Biol. 2013; doi:10.1371/journal.pcbi.1003031.
13. Quail M, Smith M, Coupland P, Otto T D, Harris S R, Connor T R, Bertoni A, Swerdlow H P, Gu Y. A tale of three next generation sequencing platforms: comparison of Ion torrent, Pacific Biosciences and Illumina MiSeq sequencers. Bmc Genomics. 2012; doi:10.1186/1471-2164-13-341.
14. Yeo Z, Wong J C L, Rozen S G, Lee A S G. Evaluation and optimization of indel detection workflows for ion torrent sequencing of the BRCA1 and BRCA2 genes. Bmc Genomics. 2014; doi:10.1186/1471-2164-15-516.
15. Naslavsky MS, Yamamoto GL, de Almeida TF, Ezquina SAM, Sunaga DY, Pho N, Bozoklian D, Sandberg TOM, Brito LA, Lazar M, Bernardo DV, Amaro E Jr, Duarte YAO, Lebrão ML, Passos-Bueno MR, Zatz M. Exomic variants of an elderly cohort of Brazilians in the ABraOM database. Hum Mutat. 2017 Mar 23. doi:10.1002/humu.23220.

8

Identification of compound heterozygous variants in the noncoding *RNU4ATAC* gene in a Chinese family with two successive foetuses with severe microcephaly

Ye Wang[1], Xueli Wu[2], Liu Du[3], Ju Zheng[3], Songqing Deng[1], Xin Bi[4], Qiuyan Chen[5], Hongning Xie[3], Claude Férec[6], David N. Cooper[7], Yanmin Luo[1*], Qun Fang[1*] and Jian-Min Chen[6,8*]

Abstract

Background: Whole-exome sequencing (WES) over the last few years has been increasingly employed for clinical diagnosis. However, one *caveat* with its use is that it inevitably fails to detect disease-causative variants that occur within noncoding RNA genes. Our experience in identifying pathogenic variants in the noncoding *RNU4ATAC* gene, in a Chinese family where two successive foetuses had been affected by severe microcephaly, is a case in point. These foetuses exhibited remarkably similar phenotypes in terms of their microcephaly and brain abnormalities; however, the paucity of other characteristic phenotypic features had made a precise diagnosis impossible. Given that no external causative factors had been reported/identified during the pregnancies, we sought a genetic cause for the phenotype in the proband, the second affected foetus.

Results: A search for chromosomal abnormalities and pathogenic copy number variants proved negative. WES was also negative. These initial failures prompted us to consider the potential role of *RNU4ATAC*, a noncoding gene implicated in microcephalic osteodysplastic primordial dwarfism type-1 (MOPD1), a severe autosomal recessive disease characterised by dwarfism, severe microcephaly and neurological abnormalities. Subsequent targeted sequencing of *RNU4ATAC* resulted in the identification of compound heterozygous variants, one being the most frequently reported MOPD1-causative mutation (51G>A), whereas the other was a novel 29T>A variant. Four distinct lines of evidence (allele frequency in normal populations, evolutionary conservation of the affected nucleotide, occurrence within a known mutational hotspot for MOPD1-causative variants and predicted effect on RNA secondary structure) allowed us to conclude that 29T>A is a new causative variant for MOPD1.

Conclusions: Our findings highlight the limitations of WES in failing to detect variants within noncoding RNA genes and provide support for a role for whole-genome sequencing as a first-tier genetic test in paediatric medicine. Additionally, the identification of a novel *RNU4ATAC* variant within the mutational hotspot for MOPD1-causative variants further strengthens the critical role of the 5′ stem-loop structure of U4atac in health and disease. Finally, this analysis enabled us to provide prenatal diagnosis and genetic counselling for the mother's third pregnancy, the first report of its kind in the context of inherited *RNU4ATAC* variants.

(Continued on next page)

* Correspondence: luoyanm@mail.sysu.edu.cn; fang_qun@163.com; jian-min.chen@univ-brest.fr
[1]Fetal Medicine Centre, Department of Obstetrics and Gynaecology, The First Affiliated Hospital of Sun Yat-Sen University, Guangzhou, China
[6]UMR1078 "Génétique, Génomique Fonctionnelle et Biotechnologies", INSERM, EFS - Bretagne, Université de Brest, CHRU Brest, Brest, France
Full list of author information is available at the end of the article

(Continued from previous page)
Keywords: Genetic counselling, Microcephalic osteodysplastic primordial dwarfism type 1, MOPD1, Noncoding *RNU4ATAC* gene, Prenatal diagnosis, RNA secondary structure, Small nuclear RNA, Taybi-Linder syndrome, WES, Whole-exome sequencing

Background

Microcephaly is usually defined in terms of a head circumference more than two standard deviations below the mean for age and sex; it can occur in the womb or may develop during the first few years of life [1, 2]. Abnormal growth of the head may occur as a consequence of a number of factors, both genetic and environmental (e.g. exposure to certain viruses such as rubella, drugs and alcohol during pregnancy) [3]. The genetic causes are highly heterogeneous; thus, a search for microcephaly in the Human Phenotype Ontology database [4] yielded 652 genes. Depending on the precise nature of the condition involved, microcephaly may be associated with seizures, developmental delay, intellectual disability or other problems. It may even be associated with substantial physical disability and premature death; there is no treatment for microcephaly. Therefore, it is extremely important to identify the genetic causes of severe microcephaly in affected families with a view to providing prenatal diagnosis and genetic counselling in subsequent pregnancies.

With the decreased cost of next-generation sequencing, whole-exome sequencing (WES) has rapidly evolved from its original application as a tool for gene discovery in research settings to an important diagnostic tool in a clinical context [5–7], especially for diseases that are characterised by a significant level of genetic heterogeneity [8]. However, one *caveat* with WES is that disease-causative variants which occur within noncoding RNA genes will invariably be missed [9, 10]. Here, we highlight this issue by describing our experience of identifying novel compound heterozygous variants in the noncoding *RNU4ATAC* gene (OMIM #601428), in a Chinese family with two successive foetuses affected by severe microcephaly.

Results

Family description

A 30-year-old woman was referred to our centre at the First Affiliated Hospital of Sun Yat-Sen University after her second foetus (II:2) had been found to have severe microcephaly at 24 gestational weeks (GW), just as her first one (II:1; Fig. 1a) had previously. Clinical findings in the two affected foetuses, who were terminated at 36 GW (II:1) and 30 GW (II:2) respectively, are illustrated in Fig. 2 and summarised in Table 1. However, no precise diagnosis of the underlying abnormality could be made based upon these clinical findings owing to the paucity of characteristic features beyond severe microcephaly. In the case of II:1, standard G-banding karyotyping using cord blood cells taken at 35 GW revealed a normal karyotype, whereas chromosomal microarray analysis failed to detect any pathogenic copy number variations; no further analyses were performed at the time.

The parents were of North Chinese origin, healthy and nonconsanguineous. Exposure to known causative environmental factors during pregnancy was neither reported nor identified. Taken together with the remarkably similar clinical phenotypes in the two affected foetuses (Fig. 2; Table 1), a genetic cause was considered to be likely. An extensive molecular genetic analysis was therefore performed on foetus II:2.

Extensive karyotyping and chromosomal microarray analysis failed to identify any chromosomal abnormality or pathogenic copy number variations in II:2

We first performed standard G-banding karyotyping using cord blood cells from II:2 (taken at 29 GW), but no chromosomal abnormalities were found. In the meantime, we also performed chromosomal microarray analysis using genomic DNA prepared from the cord blood cells taken from II:2. No pathogenic copy number variants were identified by reference to data available in OMIM [11], DGV [12] and DECIPHER [13].

WES also failed to reveal a genetic cause of the microcephaly in II:2

We further employed WES to search for putative causal variants in an unbiased and hypothesis-free manner. The resulting single-nucleotide variants (SNVs) and small insertions or deletions (indels) were subjected to the following prioritizations: (i) variants that cause nonsynonymous, frameshift and in-frame changes and variants that occurred at splice sites; (ii) variants with a minor allele frequency of less than 5% according to either the 1000 Genomes Project [14] or the ESP5400 data of the National Heart, Lung, and Blood Institute GO Exome Sequencing Project [15]; (iii) in case of missense variants, those predicted to be deleterious using the programs of PolyPhen-2 [16], SIFT [17] and Mutation Taster [18] and (iv) variants occurring in known microcephaly-causing or microcephaly-associated genes as well as in candidate genes selected on the basis of known biological, physiological or functional relevance

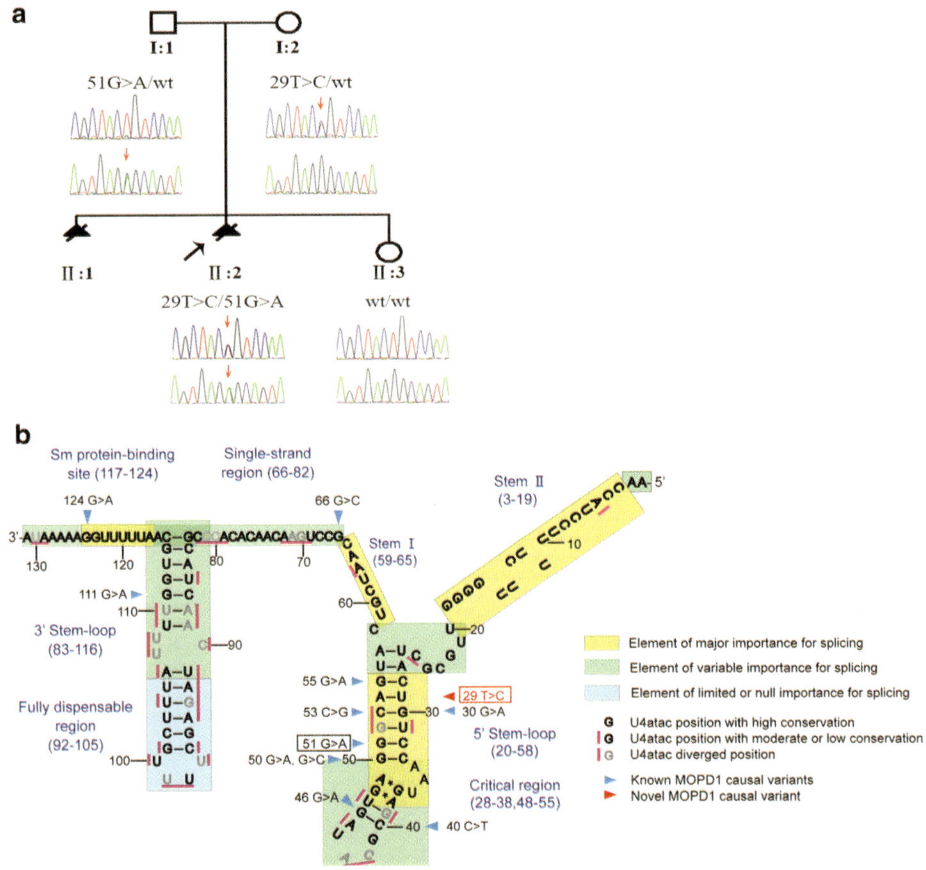

Fig. 1 Identification of the genetic cause of severe microcephaly in a Chinese family. **a** Family pedigree. Filled triangles with oblique lines indicate the two successive foetuses affected with severe microcephaly and terminated by therapeutic abortion. Arrow indicates the proband. Open symbols indicate clinically unaffected family members. Genotypes with respect to the *RNU4ATAC* gene are also provided where it was possible to determine them. wt, wild-type. **b** U4atac snRNA secondary structure elements, evolutionary conservation status of each nucleotide position and MOPD1-causative SNVs (adapted from [46]). The novel variant found in the present study, 29T>C, is highlighted in red and boxed. For a detailed description of the structure and function of U4atac, see Merico et al. [46] and references therein

to microcephaly. However, no variants survived this process of prioritisation.

Targeted sequencing of the noncoding *RNU4ATAC* gene identified causal variants in II:2

After failing to detect any pathogenic lesion by karyotyping, chromosomal microarray analysis and WES, we began to consider the potential involvement of noncoding RNA genes in the aetiology of microcephaly. An extensive literature research resulted in the recognition of two such genes. The first was the miR-17-92a-1 cluster host gene (*MIR17HG*; OMIM #609415). Large-scale copy number variants that serve either to delete or duplicate the entire *MIR17HG* locus cause Feingold syndrome 2 (OMIM #614326), a rare autosomal dominant disorder characterised by variable combinations of microcephaly, limb malformations, oesophageal and duodenal atresias and learning disability [19–26]. Although the disease entity under study here is most consistent with a model of autosomal recessive inheritance, we nevertheless revisited our chromosomal microarray analysis data and confirmed the absence of large deletions or duplications involving the *MIR17HG* locus.

The second noncoding gene emerging from our literature search was *RNU4ATAC*, in which homozygous or compound heterozygous variants have been reported to cause microcephalic osteodysplastic primordial dwarfism type-1 (MOPD1; OMIM #210710) in two simultaneous papers in 2011 [27, 28]. MOPD1, also known as Taybi-Linder syndrome [29], is a severe autosomal recessive disease characterised by dwarfism, microcephaly and neurologic abnormalities; patients usually die within the first year of life [30]. *RNU4ATAC* is located on chromosome 2q14.2 and encodes the highly conserved, 130-bp small nuclear RNA (snRNA) U4atac (RefSeq NR_023343.1). U4atac is a component of the minor spliceosome that is responsible for the correct splicing of the U12-dependent class of introns [31–35]. To date, a

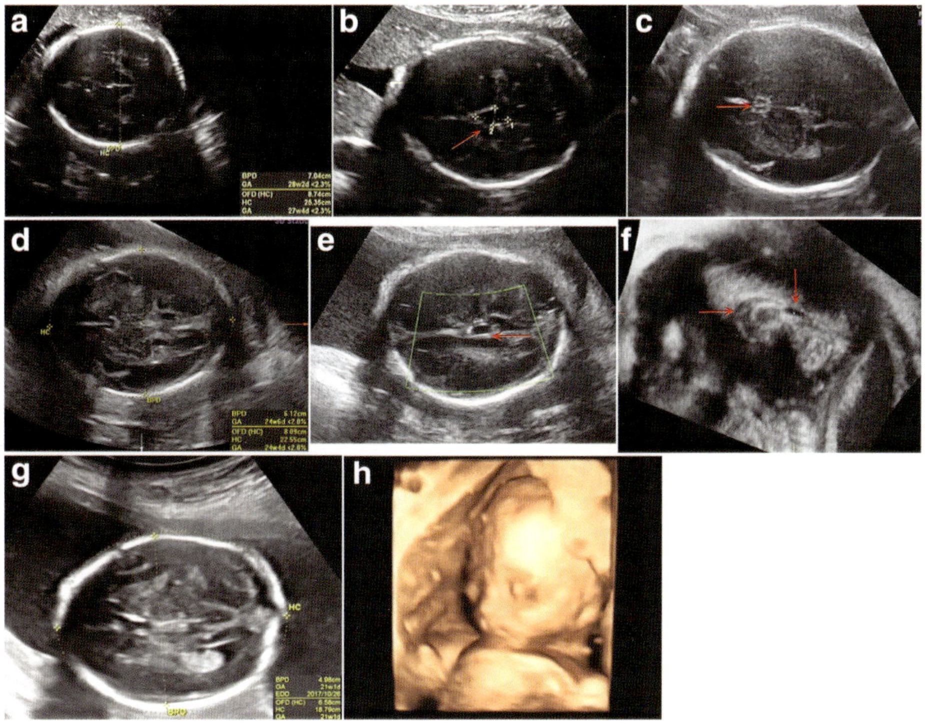

Fig. 2 Ultrasound images of the three foetuses. **a** Biparietal diameter (BPD) and head circumference (HC) of foetus II:1 measured at 35 GW indicating severe microcephaly. **b** Cross-section plane of the skull displaying arachnoid cysts (arrow) in foetus II:1. **c–f** Ultrasound images of foetus II:2: BPD and HC measured at 29 GW indicating severe microcephaly (**d**); cross-section and three-dimensional sagittal plane of the skull showing the absence of the septum pellucidum cavity (arrow; **c**), presence of intracranial cyst (arrows; **e**, **f**) and agenesis of corpus callosum (arrow; **f**). **g**, **h** Ultrasound images of the healthy foetus II:3: BPD and HC (measured at 21 GW) shown in cross-section plane (**g**) and three-dimensional rebuilt imaging for foetus face (**h**)

Table 1 Clinical data of the two affected foetuses

Case	Foetus 1 (II:1)			Foetus 2 (II:2)		
Growth (GW)	24	33	36	24	26	29
BPD (SD)	− 6.0	− 6.0	− 6.1	− 4.4	− 5.6	− 6.0
HC (SD)	− 4.0	− 5.6	− 7.5	− 3.7	− 4.2	− 5.5
FL (SD)	− 2.0	− 1.6	− 2.0	0	− 1.0	0
HL (SD)	− 1.5	/	− 1.0	0	0	0
AC (SD)	/	− 2.4	− 3.8	− 0.7	− 1.0	− 1.4
Weight	/			1.047 ± 0.153 kg (29 GW, < 50 centile)		
Brain anomalies						
Hypogenesis or agenesis of corpus callosum	−			−		
Absence of septum pellucidum cavity	−			+		
Intracranial cysts	+			+		
Small vermis	−			−		
Skeletal anomalies						
Short limb	+ (slightly short)			−		
Flexion contractures	−			−		
Cardiac abnormalities	−			−		
Skin and skin appendage	/			/		

BPD biparietal diameter, *HC* head circumference, *FL* femur length, *HL* humerus length, *AC* abdomen circumference, *GW* gestational week, *SD* standard deviation, / not evaluable, − negative, + positive

total of 12 *RNU4ATAC* variants including 11 SNVs (i.e. 30G>A, 40C>T, 46G>A, 50G>A, 50G>C, 51G>A, 53C>G, 55G>A, 66G>C, 111G>A and 124G>A) and 1 duplication variant (i.e. 16_100dup) have been reported to be causative for MOPD1 [27, 28, 36–41]. Six of the 11 SNVs (i.e. 30G>A, 50G>A, 50G>C, 51G>A, 53C>G and 55G>A) occurred within the critical canonical stem region (i.e. 28–33, 50–55) of a functionally indispensable element of U4atac, the 5′ stem-loop structure (Fig. 1b). In what follows, we shall term this critical canonical stem region the mutational hotspot region for MOPD1-causative variants.

We, therefore, speculated that variants in the *RNU4ATAC* gene, which would not have been detected by WES, might underlie the severe microcephaly in this family. Subsequent targeted testing of the *RNU4ATAC* gene by Sanger sequencing identified compound heterozygous variants, 29T>C (rs779143800) and 51G>A (rs188343279), in II:2. Carrier analysis confirmed that the two variants had been inherited from the mother and father, respectively (Fig. 1a). Although it was suspected that the affected foetus II:1 had also inherited these two variants, this could not be confirmed due to the non-availability of genetic material.

51G>A was among the first described MOPD1-causative variants [27, 28] and represents the most common MOPD1-causative variant so far reported. By contrast, 29T>C has not been previously reported in MOPD1 patients. It has however been reported at a very low frequency in normal populations; thus, it is present in heterozygous form in two individuals in the Genome Aggregation Database [42], corresponding to an allele frequency of 1.6×10^{-5}. Further, in common with all 11 previously reported MOPD1-causative *RNU4ATAC* SNVs, 29T>C affected one of the evolutionarily highly conserved positions of U4atac (Fig. 1b). Furthermore, and most importantly, 29T is located within the mutational hotspot region for MOPD1-causative variants (Fig. 1b). In this latter regard, our current understanding of the pathogenetic mechanism underlying the six known MOPD1-causing *RNU4ATAC* SNVs occurring within the mutational hotspot is that they abrogate U4atac snRNA function by disrupting the 5′ stem-loop structure [27, 28, 41]. Accordingly, we compared the potential effect of 29T>C on the 5′ stem-loop structure of U4atac with those of the aforementioned six known MOPD1-causative SNVs. To this end, wild-type and the seven mutant sequences spanning positions 20 to 58 (i.e. the sequence forming the 5′ stem-loop structure; Fig. 1b) of U4atac were separately subjected to Mfold analysis [43] under default conditions. All seven SNVs were predicted to significantly affect the 5′ stem-loop structure of U4atac as compared with the wild-type. In particular, 29T>C was predicted to alter the secondary structure in the same way as the pathogenic nucleotide substitutions 30G>A, 50G>A and 53C>G; it was also predicted to alter the secondary structure in a similar way to the most common pathogenic 51G>A variant (Fig. 3). These observations, taken together, strongly suggest that 29T>C constitutes a novel causative variant for MOPD1.

Prenatal diagnosis of the third pregnancy

Prenatal diagnosis was performed on the third foetus (II:3) (Fig. 1a). Genomic DNA was prepared from amniotic fluid cells taken by ultrasound-mediated amniocentesis at 16 GW. However, neither the *RNU4ATAC* 51G>A variant nor the 29T>C variant was detected. Normal foetal growth was confirmed by continual ultrasound monitoring during the whole period of pregnancy (Fig. 2g, h). The third foetus was born healthy after 40 GW.

Discussion

In this study, we relate our experience of how the genetic cause was finally identified in a Chinese family presenting with two successive foetuses with severe microcephaly. In brief, negative findings from karyotyping, chromosomal microarray analysis and WES in foetus II:2 prompted us to consider the potential role of noncoding genes in causing microcephaly in the family. Consequently, targeted sequencing of the noncoding *RNU4ATAC* gene resulted in the identification of compound heterozygous variants, one being the most frequently reported MOPD1-causative 51G>A, the other being a novel 29T>A variant. Based upon the four lines of evidence, namely allele frequency in normal populations, evolutionary conservation, occurrence within a known mutational hotspot for MOPD1-causative variants and predicted effect on the 5′ stem-loop structure, we were able to conclude with confidence that the newly found 29T>A variant represents a new causative variant for MOPD1. Here, we should like to make two additional points. First, in the context of in silico analysis, many algorithms have been designed to predict the functional consequences of intronic or missense variants found in protein-coding genes. However, these tools are inappropriate for use with the *RNU4ATAC* variants discussed here, whose functional consequences depend upon their potential effect on RNA secondary structure. Currently, Mfold analysis is the gold standard for performing RNA secondary structure predictions. Second, stringent standards and guidelines have been proposed for investigating the causality of sequence variants in human genetic disease [44, 45]. Apart from the aforementioned four lines of evidence supporting causality of the detected compound heterozygous *RNU4ATAC* variants, we would like to add a new consideration. The genomic

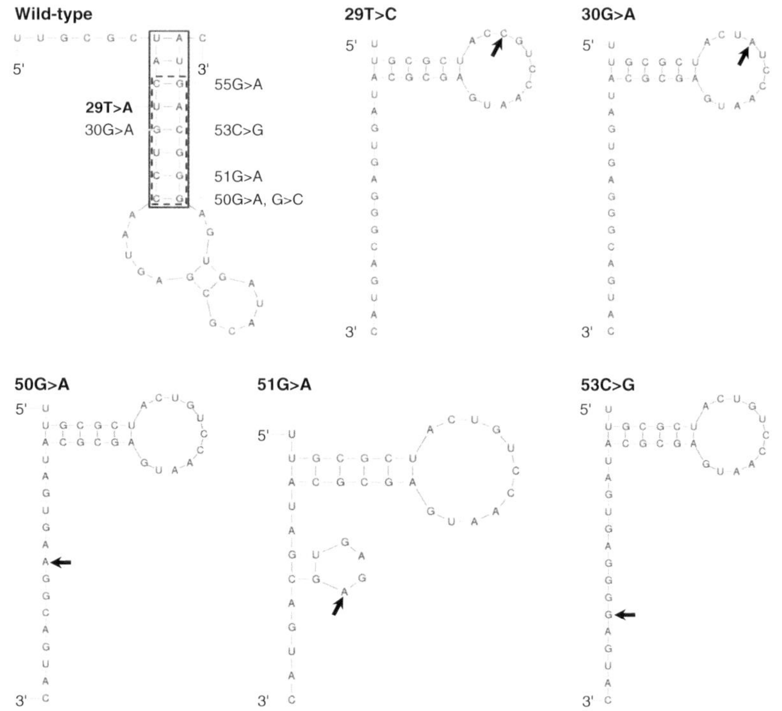

Fig. 3 Predicted effects of 29T>C, 30G>A, 50G>A, 51G>A and 53C>G on the 5′ stem-loop structure of U4atac. Secondary structures of the wild-type and corresponding mutant sequences between positions 20 and 58 of U4atac (see Fig. 2b) were predicted by Mfold under default parameters, with the lowest energy structures being shown. In the wild-type panel, the solid-boxed area indicates the canonical stem of the 5′ stem-loop structure in accordance with [53, 54]; the dotted-boxed area indicates the mutational hotspot region for MOPD1-causative variants; all six known MOPD1-causative SNVs as well as the newly found 29T>C variant occurring within the mutational hotspot region are also indicated. In the mutant panels, the respective variants are indicated by arrows

structure of *RNU4ATAC* is very simple, comprising only 130 nucleotides. All the so far reported MOPD1-causative *RNU4ATAC* variants were invariably located within the 130 nucleotides.

Most previous studies have reported homozygous or compound heterozygous *RNU4ATAC* variants in patients with a diagnosis, or suggestive diagnosis, of MOPD1 [27, 28, 36–40]. Only very recently have *RNU4ATAC* variants been described in foetuses [41]; all four foetuses (two of whom were twins) had severe microcephaly together with some other brain and skeletal abnormalities including corpus callosum agenesis, short limb, brachydactyly and ossification delay, suggestive of a diagnosis of MOPD1. By contrast, the two foetuses in the family under study here showed only severe microcephaly and corpus callosum agenesis. The identification of compound heterozygous *RNU4ATAC* variants in II:2, therefore, provided a definite diagnosis of the disease that could not otherwise have been made merely on the basis of clinical findings.

In a more general context, our study adds to the increasing appreciation that variants in noncoding RNA genes are an underestimated cause of human inherited disease. Here, we further emphasise this point by citing a recent finding concerning the *RNU4ATAC* gene. Compound heterozygous *RNU4ATAC* variants have also been reported to cause Roifman syndrome (OMIM #300258) [10, 46], a rare congenital association of antibody deficiency, spondyloepiphyseal chondro-osseous dysplasia, retinal dystrophy, poor pre- and postnatal growth and cognitive delay, which is phenotypically quite different from MOPD1. It should be noted that Roifman syndrome-causative compound heterozygous *RNU4ATAC* variants comprise one variant that is located within MOPD1-implicated structural elements and one variant that is located outside of MOPD1-implicated structural elements [10, 46].

Conclusions

In a general context, our findings highlight one key limitation of WES, namely that it fails to detect disease causative variants within noncoding RNA genes. This provides support for a role for whole-genome sequencing as a first-tier genetic test in paediatric medicine [9]. This is also the first report of MOPD1-causative *RNU4ATAC* variants in the Chinese population and the first report of prenatal diagnosis and genetic counselling provided for a subsequent pregnancy once *RNU4ATAC* variants had been identified as a cause of MOPD1. Finally, the identification of a novel *RNU4ATAC* variant within the mutational hotspot for MOPD1-causative variants further strengthens the critical role of the 5′ stem-loop structure of U4atac in health and disease.

Methods

Karyotyping and chromosomal microarray analysis

Standard G-banding karyotyping was performed. The array experiments were performed using the high-resolution Affymetrix CytoScan HD microarray (Affymetrix Inc., Santa Clara, CA) in accordance with the manufacturer's protocols. The results were analysed using the Chromosome Analysis Suite software version 1.2.2; the reporting threshold of the copy number was set at 10 kb, with marker count at ≥ 50, as previously reported [47].

WES

Genomic DNA was fragmented randomly and then purified by means of the magnetic particle method. Sequences were captured by Agilent SureSelect version 4 (Agilent Technologies, Santa Clara, CA) according to the manufacturer's protocols. The DNA libraries, after enrichment and purification, were sequenced on the NextSeq500 sequencer according to the manufacturer's instructions (Illumina, San Diego). The sequencing reads were aligned to GRCh37.p10 using Burrows-Wheeler Aligner software (version 0.59) [48]. Local realignment and base quality recalibration of the Burrows-Wheeler aligned reads were then performed using the GATK IndelRealigner [49] and GATK BaseRecalibrator [50], respectively. SNVs and small indels were identified by the GATK UnifiedGenotyper [51]. Variants were annotated using the Consensus Coding Sequences Database at the National Centre for Biotechnology Information [52].

Targeted sequencing of the *RNU4ATAC* gene

Primer sequences and PCR conditions are available upon request.

RNA secondary structure prediction

This was performed by means of Mfold analysis under default conditions [43].

Abbreviations

BPD: Biparietal diameter; GW: Gestational weeks; HC: Head circumference; indels: Insertions or deletions; MOPD1: Microcephalic osteodysplastic primordial dwarfism type 1; snRNA: Small nuclear RNA; SNVs: Single-nucleotide variants; WES: Whole-exome sequencing

Acknowledgements

Not applicable.

Funding

This work was supported in part by the National Natural Science Foundation of China (nos. 81270705 and 81671464) and the Science and Technology Project of Guangdong, China (2017A020214013).

Authors' contributions

YW, YL and QF designed the study with the assistance of JMC. YW, XW and XB performed the genetic analysis. YL, LD, JZ, SD, QC and HX conducted the clinical and ultrasound evaluations. CF and JMC interpreted the pathogenic relevance of the novel *RNU4ATAC* variant. YW and JMC drafted the manuscript. DNC critically revised the manuscript. All authors analysed the data and approved the final manuscript.

Competing interests

The authors declare that they have no competing interests.

Author details

Fetal Medicine Centre, Department of Obstetrics and Gynaecology, The First Affiliated Hospital of Sun Yat-Sen University, Guangzhou, China. [2]Department of Dermatology, Guangzhou Institute of Dermatology, Guangzhou, China. [3]Department of Ultrasonic Medicine, The First Affiliated Hospital of Sun Yat-Sen University, Guangzhou, China. [4]Guangzhou KingMed Center for Clinical Laboratory, Guangzhou, China. [5]Dongguan Women and Children's Hospital, Dongguan, China. [6]UMR1078 "Génétique, Génomique Fonctionnelle et Biotechnologies", INSERM, EFS - Bretagne, Université de Brest, CHRU Brest, Brest, France. [7]Institute of Medical Genetics, School of Medicine, Cardiff University, Cardiff, UK. [8]INSERM UMR1078, EFS, UBO, 22 avenue Camille Desmoulins, 29238 Brest, France.

References

1. Leviton A, Holmes LB, Allred EN, Vargas J. Methodologic issues in epidemiologic studies of congenital microcephaly. Early Hum Dev. 2002;69:91–105.
2. Opitz JM, Holt MC. Microcephaly: general considerations and aids to nosology. J Craniofac Genet Dev Biol. 1990;10:175–204.
3. Duerinckx S, Abramowicz M. The genetics of congenitally small brains. Semin Cell Dev Biol. 2017. https://doi.org/10.1016/j.semcdb.2017.09.015. [Epub ahead of print]
4. The Human Phenotype Ontology database. http://compbio.charite.de/hpoweb/showterm?id=HP:0000252. Accessed 23 Nov 2017.
5. Boycott KM, Vanstone MR, Bulman DE, MacKenzie AE. Rare-disease genetics in the era of next-generation sequencing: discovery to translation. Nat Rev Genet. 2013;14:681–91.
6. Lee H, Deignan JL, Dorrani N, Strom SP, Kantarci S, Quintero-Rivera F, et al. Clinical exome sequencing for genetic identification of rare Mendelian disorders. JAMA. 2014;312:1880–7.
7. Posey JE, Harel T, Liu P, Rosenfeld JA, James RA, Coban Akdemir ZH, et al. Resolution of disease phenotypes resulting from multilocus genomic variation. N Engl J Med. 2017;376:21–31.
8. Ku CS, Cooper DN, Polychronakos C, Naidoo N, Wu M, Soong R. Exome sequencing: dual role as a discovery and diagnostic tool. Ann Neurol. 2012;71:5–14.
9. Lionel AC, Costain G, Monfared N, Walker S, Reuter MS, Hosseini SM, et al. Improved diagnostic yield compared with targeted gene sequencing panels suggests a role for whole-genome sequencing as a first-tier genetic test. Genet Med. 2017. https://doi.org/10.1038/gim.2017.119. [Epub ahead of print]
10. Bogaert DJ, Dullaers M, Kuehn HS, Leroy BP, Niemela JE, De Wilde H, et al. Early-onset primary antibody deficiency resembling common variable immunodeficiency challenges the diagnosis of Wiedeman-Steiner and Roifman syndromes. Sci Rep. 2017;7:3702.
11. Online Mendelian Inheritance in Man. https://www.omim.org/. Accessed 23 Nov 2017.
12. Database of Genomic Variants; http://dgv.tcag.ca/dgv/app/home. Accessed 23 Nov 2017.
13. DatabasE of genomiC varIation and Phenotype in Humans using Ensembl Resources; https://decipher.sanger.ac.uk. Accessed 23 Nov 2017.
14. Abecasis GR, Altshuler D, Auton A, Brooks LD, Durbin RM, Gibbs RA, et al. A map of human genome variation from population-scale sequencing. Nature. 2010;467:1061–73.
15. The ESP5400 data of the National Heart, Lung and Blood Institute GO Exome Sequencing Project. http://evs.gs.washington.edu/EVS. Accessed 23 Nov 2017.
16. PolyPhen-2. http://genetics.bwh.harvard.edu/pph2/. Accessed 23 Nov 2017.
17. SIFT. http://sift.jcvi.org/www/SIFT_chr_coords_submit.html. Accessed 23 Nov 2017.

18. Mutation Taster. http://www.mutationtaster.org/. Accessed 23 Nov 2017.
19. de Pontual L, Yao E, Callier P, Faivre L, Drouin V, Cariou S, et al. Germline deletion of the miR-17 approximately 92 cluster causes skeletal and growth defects in humans. Nat Genet. 2011;43:1026–30.
20. Sharaidin HS, Knipe S, Bain N, Goel H. Clinical features associated with a 15.41 Mb deletion of chromosome 13q encompassing the *MIR17HG* locus. Clin Dysmorphol. 2013;22:68–70.
21. Valdes-Miranda JM, Soto-Alvarez JR, Toral-Lopez J, Gonzalez-Huerta L, Perez-Cabrera A, Gonzalez-Monfil G, et al. A novel microdeletion involving the 13q31.3-q32.1 region in a patient with normal intelligence. Eur J Med Genet. 2014;57:60–4.
22. Ganjavi H, Siu VM, Speevak M, MacDonald PA. A fourth case of Feingold syndrome type 2: psychiatric presentation and management. BMJ Case Rep. 2014. https://doi.org/10.1136/bcr-2014-207501.
23. Low KJ, Buxton CC, Newbury-Ecob RA. Tetralogy of Fallot, microcephaly, short stature and brachymesophalangy is associated with hemizygous loss of noncoding *MIR17HG* and coding *GPC5*. Clin Dysmorphol. 2015; 24:113–4.
24. Grote LE, Repnikova EA, Amudhavalli SM. Expanding the phenotype of feingold syndrome-2. Am J Med Genet A. 2015;167A:3219–25.
25. Sirchia F, Di Gregorio E, Restagno G, Grosso E, Pappi P, Talarico F, et al. A case of Feingold type 2 syndrome associated with keratoconus refines keratoconus type 7 locus on chromosome 13q. Eur J Med Genet. 2017;60: 224–7.
26. Hemmat M, Rumple MJ, Mahon LW, Strom CM, Anguiano A, Talai M, et al. Short stature, digit anomalies and dysmorphic facial features are associated with the duplication of miR-17 ~ 92 cluster. Mol Cytogenet. 2014;7:27.
27. Edery P, Marcaillou C, Sahbatou M, Labalme A, Chastang J, Touraine R, et al. Association of TALS developmental disorder with defect in minor splicing component U4atac snRNA. Science. 2011;332:240–3.
28. He H, Liyanarachchi S, Akagi K, Nagy R, Li J, Dietrich RC, et al. Mutations in U4atac snRNA, a component of the minor spliceosome, in the developmental disorder MOPD I. Science. 2011;332:238–40.
29. Taybi H, Linder D. Congenital familial dwarfism with cephaloskeletal dysplasia. Radiology. 1967;89:275–81.
30. Pierce MJ, Morse RP. The neurologic findings in Taybi-Linder syndrome (MOPD I/III): case report and review of the literature. Am J Med Genet A. 2012;158A:606–10.
31. Hall SL, Padgett RA. Requirement of U12 snRNA for in vivo splicing of a minor class of eukaryotic nuclear pre-mRNA introns. Science. 1996;271: 1716–8.
32. Tarn WY, Steitz JA. Highly diverged U4 and U6 small nuclear RNAs required for splicing rare AT-AC introns. Science. 1996;273:1824–32.
33. Sharp PA, Burge CB. Classification of introns: U2-type or U12-type. Cell. 1997; 91:875–9.
34. Nilsen TW. The spliceosome: the most complex macromolecular machine in the cell? BioEssays. 2003;25:1147–9.
35. Will CL, Luhrmann R. Splicing of a rare class of introns by the U12-dependent spliceosome. Biol Chem. 2005;386:713–24.
36. Kilic E, Yigit G, Utine GE, Wollnik B, Mihci E, Nur BG, et al. A novel mutation in *RNU4ATAC* in a patient with microcephalic osteodysplastic primordial dwarfism type I. Am J Med Genet A. 2015;167A:919–21.
37. Abdel-Salam GM, Abdel-Hamid MS, Issa M, Magdy A, El-Kotoury A, Amr K. Expanding the phenotypic and mutational spectrum in microcephalic osteodysplastic primordial dwarfism type I. Am J Med Genet A. 2012;158A: 1455–61.
38. Nagy R, Wang H, Albrecht B, Wieczorek D, Gillessen-Kaesbach G, Haan E, et al. Microcephalic osteodysplastic primordial dwarfism type I with biallelic mutations in the *RNU4ATAC* gene. Clin Genet. 2012;82:140–6.
39. Abdel-Salam GM, Miyake N, Eid MM, Abdel-Hamid MS, Hassan NA, Eid OM, et al. A homozygous mutation in *RNU4ATAC* as a cause of microcephalic osteodysplastic primordial dwarfism type I (MOPD I) with associated pigmentary disorder. Am J Med Genet A. 2011;155A:2885–96.
40. Kroigard AB, Jackson AP, Bicknell LS, Baple E, Brusgaard K, Hansen LK, et al. Two novel mutations in *RNU4ATAC* in two siblings with an atypical mild phenotype of microcephalic osteodysplastic primordial dwarfism type 1. Clin Dysmorphol. 2016;25:68–72.
41. Putoux A, Alqahtani A, Pinson L, Paulussen AD, Michel J, Besson A, et al. Refining the phenotypical and mutational spectrum of Taybi-Linder syndrome. Clin Genet. 2016;90:550–5.
42. The Genome Aggregation Database (gnomAD). http://gnomad.broadinstitute.org/. Accessed 23 Nov 2017.
43. Mfold. http://unafold.rna.albany.edu/?q=mfold/rna-folding-form. Accessed 23 Nov 2017.
44. MacArthur DG, Manolio TA, Dimmock DP, Rehm HL, Shendure J, Abecasis GR, et al. Guidelines for investigating causality of sequence variants in human disease. Nature. 2014;508:469–76.
45. Richards S, Aziz N, Bale S, Bick D, Das S, Gastier-Foster J, et al. Standards and guidelines for the interpretation of sequence variants: a joint consensus recommendation of the American College of Medical Genetics and Genomics and the Association for Molecular Pathology. Genet Med. 2015; 17:405–24.
46. Merico D, Roifman M, Braunschweig U, Yuen RK, Alexandrova R, Bates A, et al. Compound heterozygous mutations in the noncoding *RNU4ATAC* cause Roifman syndrome by disrupting minor intron splicing. Nat Commun. 2015;6:8718.
47. Wang Y, Su P, Hu B, Zhu W, Li Q, Yuan P, et al. Characterization of 26 deletion CNVs reveals the frequent occurrence of micro-mutations within the breakpoint-flanking regions and frequent repair of double-strand breaks by templated insertions derived from remote genomic regions. Hum Genet. 2015;134:589–603.
48. Li H, Durbin R. Fast and accurate short read alignment with Burrows-Wheeler transform. Bioinformatics. 2009;25:1754–60.
49. The GATK IndelRealigner. https://software.broadinstitute.org/gatk/documentation/tooldocs/current/org_broadinstitute_gatk_tools_walkers_indels_IndelRealigner.php. Accessed 23 Nov 2017.
50. The GATK BaseRecalibrator. https://software.broadinstitute.org/gatk/documentation/tooldocs/current/org_broadinstitute_gatk_tools_walkers_bqsr_BaseRecalibrator.php. Accessed 23 Nov 2017.
51. The GATK UnifiedGenotyper. https://software.broadinstitute.org/gatk/documentation/tooldocs/current/org_broadinstitute_gatk_tools_walkers_genotyper_UnifiedGenotyper.php. Accessed 23 Nov 2017.
52. The Consensus Coding Sequences Database at the National Centre for Biotechnology Information. https://www.ncbi.nlm.nih.gov/CCDS/. Accessed 23 Nov 2017.
53. Padgett RA, Shukla GC. A revised model for U4atac/U6atac snRNA base pairing. RNA. 2002;8:125–8.
54. Cojocaru V, Klement R, Jovin TM. Loss of G-A base pairs is insufficient for achieving a large opening of U4 snRNA K-turn motif. Nucleic Acids Res. 2005;33:3435–46.

9

Copy number variation of human *AMY1* is a minor contributor to variation in salivary amylase expression and activity

Danielle Carpenter, Laura M. Mitchell and John A. L. Armour*

Abstract

Background: Salivary amylase in humans is encoded by the copy variable gene *AMY1* in the amylase gene cluster on chromosome 1. Although the role of salivary amylase is well established, the consequences of the copy number variation (CNV) at *AMY1* on salivary amylase protein production are less well understood. The amylase gene cluster is highly structured with a fundamental difference between odd and even *AMY1* copy number haplotypes. In this study, we aimed to explore, in samples from 119 unrelated individuals, not only the effects of *AMY1* CNV on salivary amylase protein expression and amylase enzyme activity but also whether there is any evidence for underlying difference between the common haplotypes containing odd numbers of *AMY1* and even copy number haplotypes.

Results: *AMY1* copy number was significantly correlated with the variation observed in salivary amylase production (11.7% of variance, $P < 0.0005$) and enzyme activity (13.6% of variance, $P < 0.0005$) but did not explain the majority of observed variation between individuals. *AMY1*-odd and *AMY1*-even haplotypes showed a different relationship between copy number and expression levels, but the difference was not statistically significant ($P = 0.052$).

Conclusions: Production of salivary amylase is correlated with *AMY1* CNV, but the majority of interindividual variation comes from other sources. Long-range haplotype structure may affect expression, but this was not significant in our data.

Keywords: Genome instability, Amylase, CNV, Gene expression

Introduction

The enzyme amylase plays a major role in starch hydrolysis, which begins in the oral cavity and continues into the stomach and then small intestine. Amylase is the most abundant protein in saliva, accounting for at least 50% of salivary protein [1], but the quantity and enzyme activity of salivary amylase varies greatly among individuals. This variation in amylase production could be attributable to a number of factors including environmental factors, such as stress [2] and circadian rhythms [3], oral health [4] and the genetic background of an individual's amylase gene cluster. Whilst it has been suggested that quantitative variation in amylase protein patterns does not always reflect variation in the amylase gene cluster [5], some studies have shown a relationship between the observed copy number variation (CNV) at the salivary amylase gene (*AMY1*) and an increased level of amylase protein expression [6, 7]. Perry et al. [7], using immunoblotting to investigate amylase protein levels, identified a significant positive correlation ($R = 0.59$) between CNV at *AMY1* and levels of amylase protein in saliva. Mandel and colleagues [6], also using immunoblotting, observed a similar correlation ($R = 0.50$) with copy number at *AMY1* and amylase protein levels as well as a correlation ($R = 0.52$) between CNV at *AMY1* and salivary enzyme activity. These results suggest that approximately 20–35% of the variance in salivary amylase expression can be attributed to variation in *AMY1* copy number.

The human amylase genes form a cluster on chromosome 1 which contains both the salivary (*AMY1*) and pancreatic (*AMY2*) amylase genes, both of which vary in copy number [5, 8, 9]. The CNV at *AMY1* has an observed range of 2–18 copies per person [7, 10–12] and an average of 6 copies per person, whilst the CNV at *AMY2* has an observed range of 2–12 copies per person and an average

* Correspondence: john.armour@nottingham.ac.uk
School of Life Sciences, University of Nottingham, Nottingham NG7 2UH, UK

of 4 copies per person. The amylase gene cluster is highly structured [13–15], with a correlation between the CNV at *AMY1* and the CNV at *AMY2* [10, 12]. Recent observations have identified a fundamental difference in the underlying genomic structure across the amylase gene cluster between majority haplotypes containing an odd number of copies of *AMY1* and one copy each of *AMY2A* and *AMY2B*, and less common variant haplotypes containing even copy number haplotypes of *AMY1* and deletions or duplications of *AMY2* genes. Consequently, the majority of individuals (60–70%), with two *AMY1*-odd haplotypes, have an even copy number of *AMY1* and no CNV of *AMY2*, whereas those individuals with an odd copy number of *AMY1* (usually heterozygous for an *AMY1*-even haplotype) also display CNV of *AMY2* [10, 12].

Previous studies investigating the relationship between CNV at *AMY1* and salivary amylase protein expression have used qPCR to measure copy number. However, qPCR measurement of *AMY1* has since been shown to be subject to systematic error and, in one study, consistently underestimated the *AMY1* copy number [7, 10]. We aimed to re-evaluate the relationship between CNV at *AMY1* and salivary amylase protein expression using alternative copy number measurement methods that have been shown to be precise and reproducible [10]. Our experimental plan was designed to measure both the expression of salivary amylase total protein and amylase enzyme activity in saliva from a larger cohort of individuals than has been previously studied, in parallel with determination of copy number at *AMY1*. Knowledge of the haplotype structures also allows us to test whether all copies of *AMY1* are functionally equivalent or whether there is any evidence for context dependence of gene expression. Therefore, our aim is to explore the functional consequences of the multi-allelic copy variable gene *AMY1* on more ($N = 119$) samples than previously investigated and using novel methods of *AMY1* copy number measurement, capable of resolving single integer copy numbers.

Results

Variation in AMY1 and AMY2 copy numbers

Copy number measurement of both *AMY1* and *AMY2* was performed on all 119 independent UK samples (see "Methods"). The *AMY1* copy number distribution is shown in Fig. 1 and shows a predominance of even copy numbers (75%), with a range of 2–15 and a modal copy number of 6, consistent with prior studies of *AMY1* copy number [7, 10–12]. Variation in *AMY2* copy number was also observed with *AMY2A* copy variable in 24% of samples and *AMY2B* showing CNV in about 10% of samples (Table 1).

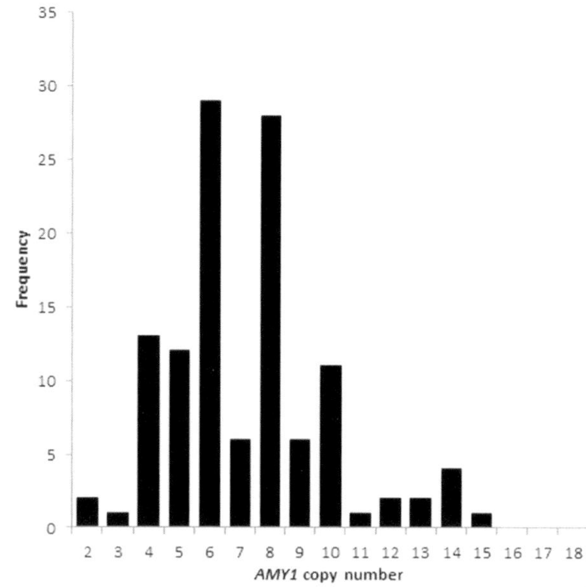

Fig. 1 Distribution histogram of *AMY1* copy number in 119 unrelated UK samples; a clear majority have even copy numbers (89 out of 119)

Correlation of AMY1 copy number with protein production and enzyme activity

We investigated both amylase protein levels and salivary amylase enzyme activity. Our data are consistent with previous studies in exhibiting considerable variation in protein expression [6, 7] and include some samples (across all copy numbers) with very low amounts of amylase protein (lowest value 0.48 mg/mL), as also detected by Mandel et al. [6].

The raw data for total protein (antigen) concentration (Fig. 2) and for enzyme activity (Fig. 3) did not show a strong relationship with copy number, and the residuals of the regression are far from normally distributed (Additional file 1: Figure S2). A linear regression was performed using $\log_{10}$ of protein and of enzyme activity giving residuals that follow a normal distribution (Additional file 1: Figure S2) and satisfy other assumptions of linear regression modelling, and therefore, all further analyses were performed with the transformed data.

Table 1 CNV of *AMY2* in 119 UK samples studied

Copy number	*AMY2A*	*AMY2B*
0	0	0
1	14	0
2	91	107
3	13	12
4	1	0
TOTAL	119	119

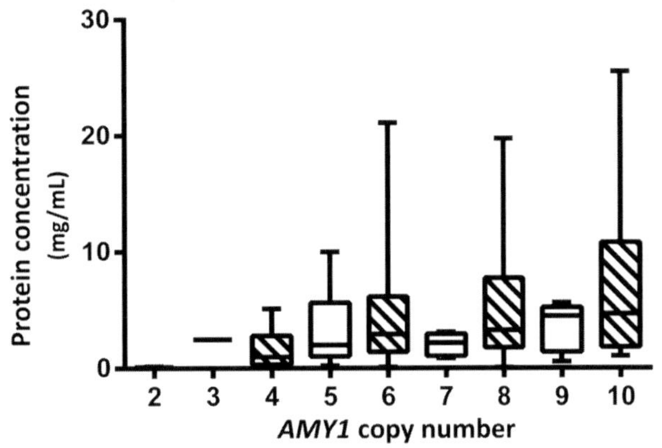

Fig. 2 A *box* and *whiskers plot* of amylase protein concentration by *AMY1* copy number, with mean for all samples at a given copy number shown as a *black bar*, the standard deviation as the *box*, and *whiskers* showing the observed full range of data. Each contributing data point is the mean of three experimental replicates, and further details of biological replicates from the same subjects can be found in the "Methods"

A significant correlation was observed between *AMY1* copy number and amylase protein ($R = 0.342$) ($P < 0.0005$). Our data suggests that *AMY1* copy number accounts for 11.7% of the variation observed in salivary amylase protein levels, much less than previous reports of 35% from a study of 50 European American individuals [7], and 25% in a study of 62 individuals of unspecified ancestry [6]. Our observation suggests that the CNV at *AMY1* plays much less of a role in the variation of salivary amylase protein levels than previously proposed. Furthermore, the great spread of observed levels of amylase protein production suggests that the genetic contribution of the CNV is not simply proportional to protein production.

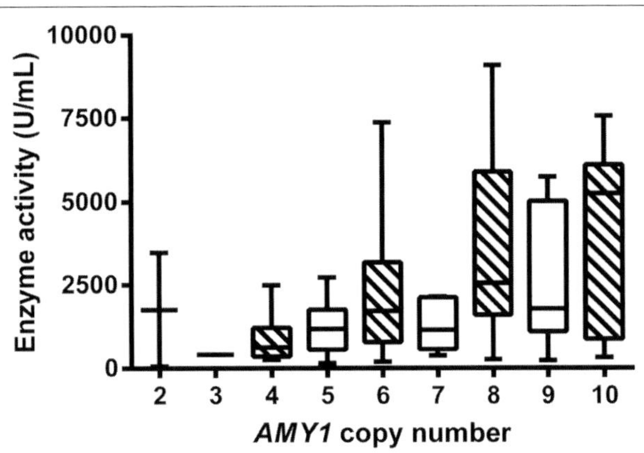

Fig. 3 A *box* and *whiskers plot* of amylase enzyme activity by *AMY1* copy number, with mean of all samples at each copy number shown as a *black bar*, and *whiskers* showing the observed range of data. The *boxes* indicate the standard deviation at each copy number. Each data point used in the analysis is the mean of two experimental replicates, and further details of biological replicates from the same subjects can be found in the "Methods"

A similar relationship was observed with salivary amylase enzyme activity. A significant correlation was observed between *AMY1* copy number and enzyme activity ($R = 0.369$) ($P < 0.0005$). Again, our data suggest that copy number plays less of a role than previously reported, with copy number accounting for 13.6% of the variation in enzyme activity observed in our study, rather than 27% as previously suggested [6]. A similar observation was reported in a Chinese population ($n = 92$) which found the gene copy number provided 12.2% of the observed salivary enzyme activity variation [16]. However, direct comparison between these studies is not straightforward, as Chinese populations do have a distinct *AMY1* distribution to Europeans [10, 12].

As our copy number measurement system is accurate enough to assign single integers, we were able to investigate whether there are differences in gene expression between those individuals that have even *AMY1* copy numbers and those with odd. We fitted a logistic regression model to protein and copy number data and used the model to predict protein expression from copy number to examine whether the odd or even number status was associated with a systematic difference in the relationship. This analysis gave marginally non-significant evidence ($P = 0.052$) for a difference between the regressions of log protein with even ($R = 0.168$) and odd ($R = 0.017$) copy numbers (Additional file 1: Figure S3), suggesting that the relationship between copy number and protein may be different for the odd and even copy numbers.

Discussion

This is only the second study to investigate both protein levels and enzyme activity in the same samples. There is a highly significant correlation between the two measures ($R = 0.66$; $P < 0.0001$) (Additional file 1: Figure S4); whilst this is not a strong relationship, it is consistent with previous observations between these two measures ($R = 0.61$) [6]. This observation does suggest that for a particular quantity of amylase protein, there are variations in measurable enzyme activity, and supports the proposal that the enzymatic functions of amylase may be affected by protein modifications or the formation of complexes [6, 17].

With the complex underlying structure at the amylase gene cluster, it is possible that longer-range structure, including the CNV at *AMY2*, may influence *AMY1* expression, but there was no significant correlation observed between CNV at either *AMY2A* or *AMY2B* with either salivary amylase protein production or enzyme activity.

Conclusions

To re-assess the relationship between copy number and salivary amylase protein expression and activity, our work used a more accurate and precise *AMY1* copy number measurement method than the qPCR methods previously employed. Our previous work demonstrated the reliability of PRT-based methods and the susceptibility of qPCR methods to measurement error [10]. Our data clearly show that copy number plays much less of a role in salivary amylase expression and activity than has been previously suggested, and that it is not possible to predict an individual's salivary amylase concentration or enzyme activity solely from their copy number, with implications for studies of the effects of *AMY1* copy number variation, such as with diet. It is interesting to speculate on possible reasons for the differences between our results and those of other researchers. In addition to the improved methodology for copy number measurement, there may also have been differences in the sampling regime for saliva; in our work, we specified the method and time of collection but did not examine or standardise other factors, such as the timing relative to meals. Because of the fundamental structural difference between haplotypes containing odd or even numbers of copies, we wanted to test the possibility that odd or even number haplotypes might have different relationships between copy number and gene expression. Our data neither confirm nor exclude functional differences that arise from the underlying genomic structure across the amylase region between odd and even copy number haplotypes. Further studies would be needed to support the idea, but it does remain possible that the longer-range genomic structure, in addition to *AMY1* copy number itself, may have a role in determining variation in gene expression.

Methods

Study population

Our analysis utilised 120 independent volunteers from the University of Nottingham staff and student body, with 10 randomly selected to provide repeat samples. The blood, for DNA extraction, and saliva, for salivary amylase analysis, were taken with full consent from individuals and under local ethical approval (University of Nottingham Medical School Ethics Committee approval reference number BT10/02/2010). All samples were of the UK origin with no known clinical phenotype. DNA was extracted using isolated lymphocytes and a standard 'salting out' method for protein removal followed by phenol-chloroform extraction. DNA concentration was measured using a NanoDrop spectrophotometer, and DNA purity was assessed from the 260:280 nm absorbance ratio. All samples were diluted to a working concentration of 10 ng/mL. DNA was successfully extracted for all samples, except one, giving a total sample size of 119 independent individuals.

Sample preparation

The saliva samples were collected from each volunteer at approximately 9.30 am (+/−10 min). The volunteers chewed on a 4 cm piece of parafilm for 30 s to allow saliva to be produced and then collected into a 15 ml sterile polypropylene container. The tubes were centrifuged at 13 rpm for 5 min to remove any solids from the suspension, and the remaining saliva was stored at −80 ° C. For genotyping, 20 mL of the whole blood was taken from each volunteer from which genomic DNA was isolated and stored at −80 °C.

Measurement of AMY1 and AMY2 copy numbers

The copy number of *AMY1* was measured from genomic DNA using a paralogue ratio test (PRT) in combination with a TATC microsatellite assay, as previously described [10]. *AMY2* copy number was measured using an *AMY2A*:*AMY2B* ratio assay, an *AMY2A*:*AMY2A* pseudogene ratio assay and an *AMY2A/2B* duplication junction assay, as previously described [10].

PRT PCR reactions were performed using previously described primers PRT_ref12 [10] that amplify from each copy of *AMY1* and from a reference locus at hg19 chr12:9,867,565–9,867,813. PCR products were mixed with 10 µl HiDi formamide with ROX-500 marker (Applied Biosystems, Warrington, UK), and subsequent fragment analysis was carried out by electrophoresis on an ABI3130xl 36 cm capillary using POP-7 polymer with an injection time of 30 s at 1 kV. GeneMapper software (Applied Biosystems, Warrington, UK) was used to extract the peak areas for the PRT and calculate the ratio of test (244 bp) to reference (249 bp) products. Copy number values were calculated by calibrating the ratios using HapMap CEU samples [NA11930 with *AMY1* copy number (CN) = 2; NA06993 with CN = 6; NA10852 with CN = 6; NA10835 with CN = 8; NA12248 with CN = 8; NA11931 with CN = 8; NA11993 with CN = 10 and NA07347 with CN = 11], which were included in every experiment in duplicate.

For further confirmation of *AMY1* gene copy number, a TATC microsatellite PCR was performed for each sample [10]. A single PCR reaction was performed and the products were mixed with 10 µl HiDi formamide with ROX-500 marker (Applied Biosystems, Warrington, UK), and fragment analysis was carried out by electrophoresis on an ABI3130xl 36 cm capillary using POP-7 polymer with an injection time of 30 s at 1 kV. GeneMapper software (Applied Biosystems, Warrington, UK) was used to extract the peak areas.

The ratio of *AMY2A* copy number to *AMY2B* copy number and the ratio of *AMY2A* copy number to *AMY2A* pseudogene copy number were measured as previously described [10]. One microliter of PCR products from both assays were mixed and added to 10 µl

HiDi formamide with ROX-500 marker (Applied Biosystems, Warrington, UK), and fragment analysis was carried out by electrophoresis on an ABI3130xl 36 cm capillary using POP-7 polymer, injecting at 1 kV for 10 s. GeneMapper software (Applied Biosystems, Warrington, UK) was used to extract the peak areas and calculate the ratio of *AMY2A* (163 bp) to *AMY2B* (167 bp) and the ratio of *AMY2A* (197 bp) to *AMY2A* pseudogene (232 bp).

The *AMY2A/2B* duplication junction assay is a three-primer assay producing PCR amplicons of 424 bp in all samples and a specific 323 bp only from the duplication junction. The products were visualised on a 2% (*w*/*v*) agarose gel, as previously described [10].

Measurement of amylase protein

The concentration of amylase protein antigen present in the saliva was measured using a sandwich amylase ELISA with 1 μg/mL of anti-salivary amylase antibody (Abcam, Cambridge, UK) and 100 μg/mL of biotinylated detection antibody (Biorbyt, Cambridge, UK). Assays were performed using serial dilutions (1:5) of natural human salivary amylase protein of known concentration (200 μg/mL) (Sigma-Aldrich, Gillingham, Dorset, UK) to generate a standard curve. Assays were performed in duplicate for each unknown sample, and the standard curve was measured in triplicate.

Measurement of amylase enzyme activity

The amylase enzyme activity within saliva was measured using the EnzCheck® *Ultra* Amylase Assay Kit (Invitrogen, ThermoFisher, Paisley, UK) according to manufacturer's instructions. The saliva samples were added to the substrate solution, vortexed, and the fluorescence of the samples was measured after 10 min incubation at room temperature. Assays were performed using serial dilutions (1:5) of natural salivary amylase protein of known concentration (200 μg/mL) (Sigma-Aldrich, Gillingham, Dorset, UK) to generate a standard curve. Assays were performed in duplicate for each unknown sample, and the standard curve was measured in triplicate.

In order to deduce the variation in concentration for protein expression and enzyme activity within each individual, the repeat samples from an initial cohort of 10 individuals were investigated on four separate occasions (Additional file 1: Figure S1). These 10 repeat samples comprise samples with 2 (×1), 4 (×1), 6 (×4), 8 (×2) and 9 (×2) copies of *AMY1*. Analysis of repeat measures found that neither of the within-subject factors (time and measurement) was significant for measurement of salivary amylase protein expression or enzyme activity, and therefore, a single time point is suitable for comparing measurements of salivary amylase protein and enzyme activity between individuals.

Bradford assay for measurement of total protein concentration

The total protein concentration in the saliva samples was measured using Bradford Reagent (Sigma-Aldrich, Gillingham, Dorset, UK) according to manufacturer's instructions. Assays were performed using serial dilutions (1:2) of bovine serum albumin (BSA) protein of known concentration (1.4 mg/mL) (Sigma-Aldrich, Gillingham, Dorset, UK) to generate a standard curve. Assays were performed in duplicate for each unknown sample, and the standard curve measured in triplicate.

Statistical analysis

Correlations between groups of copy number data and either protein expression or enzyme activity were assessed using logistic regression in SPSS V22 (IBM, Armonk, New York, USA), and figures were drawn with the software GraphPad Prism (GraphPad Software, Inc., La Jolla, CA, USA). The repeat measures were analysed in SPSS using a general linear model with repeated measures, with the within-subject factors defined as time and measurement and the between-subject factor defined as copy number.

Abbreviations

BSA: Bovine serum albumin; CN: Copy number; CNV: Copy number variation/variant; ELISA: Enzyme-linked immunosorbent assay; HiDi: Highly deionised (formamide)

Acknowledgements

The authors would like to thank Dr David Sirl (University of Nottingham) for statistical guidance.

Funding

This work was supported by the Biotechnology and Biological Sciences Research Council [grant BB/I006370/1] (awarded to JALA). The funding body had no role in the design of the study, collection, analysis, interpretation of data or in writing the manuscript.

Authors' contributions

DC participated in the study design, coordinated the study, performed copy number typing, optimised the ELISA assay, performed statistical analysis and wrote the manuscript. LM recruited volunteers, performed copy number typing, optimised and performed ELISA assays, optimised and performed enzyme activity assays, performed Bradford assay and generated the DNA from the samples. JALA participated in the study design and wrote the manuscript. All authors read and approved the final manuscript.

Competing interests

The authors declare that they have no competing interests.

References

1. Noble RE. Salivary alpha-amylase and lysozyme levels: a non-invasive technique for measuring parotid vs submandibular/sublingual gland activity. J Oral Science. 2000;42:83–6.
2. Granger DA, Kivlighan KT, El-Sheikh M, Gordis EB, Stroud LR. Salivary α-amylase in biobehavioral research. Ann N Y Acad Sci. 2007;1098:122–44.
3. Nater UM, Hoppmann CA, Scott SB. Diurnal profiles of salivary cortisol and alpha-amylase change across the adult lifespan: evidence from repeated daily life assessments. Psychoneuroendocrinology. 2013;38:3167–71.

4. Lawrence HP. Salivary markers of systemic disease: noninvasive diagnosis of disease and monitoring of general health. J Canadian Dental Association. 2002;68:170–4.
5. Bank RA, Hettema EH, Muijs MA, Pals G, Arwert F, Boomsma DI, Pronk JC. Variation in gene copy number and polymorphism of the human salivary amylase isoenzyme system in Caucasians. Hum Genet. 1992;89:213–22.
6. Mandel AL, Peyrot des Gachons C, Plank KL, Alarcon S, Breslin PAS. Individual differences in *AMY1* gene copy number, salivary α-amylase levels, and the perception of oral starch. PLoS One. 2010;5:e13352.
7. Perry GH, Dominy NJ, Claw KG, Lee AS, Fiegler H, Redon R, et al. Diet and the evolution of human amylase gene copy number variation. Nat Genet. 2007;39:1256–60.
8. Pronk JC, Frants RR, Jansen W, Eriksson AW, Tonino GJM. Evidence for duplication of the human salivary amylase gene. Hum Genet. 1982;60:32–5.
9. Sudmant PH, Kitzman JO, Antonacci F, Alkan C, Malig M, Tsalenko A, et al. Diversity of human copy number variation and multicopy genes. Science. 2010;330:641–6.
10. Carpenter D, Dhar S, Mitchell L, Fu B, Tyson J, Shwan N, et al. Obesity, starch digestion and amylase: association between copy number variants at human salivary (AMY1) and pancreatic (AMY2) amylase genes. Hum Mol Genet. 2015;24:3472–80.
11. Falchi M, El-Sayed Moustafa JS, Takousis P, Pesce F, Bonnefond A, Andersson-Assarsson JC, et al. Low copy number of the salivary amylase gene predisposes to obesity. Nat Genet. 2014;46:492–7.
12. Usher CL, Handsaker RE, Esko T, Tuke MA, Weedon MN, Hastie AR, et al. Structural forms of the human amylase locus and their relationships to SNPs, haplotypes and obesity. Nat Genet. 2015;47:921–5.
13. Groot PC, Bleeker MJ, Pronk JC, Arwert F, Mager WH, Planta RJ, et al. The human α-amylase multigene family consists of haplotypes with variable numbers of genes. Genomics. 1989;5:29–42.
14. Groot PC, Mager WH, Frants RR. Interpretation of polymorphic DNA patterns in the human α-amylase multigene family. Genomics. 1991;10:779–85.
15. Groot PC, Mager WH, Henriquez NV, Pronk JC, Arwert F, Planta RJ, et al. Evolution of the human alpha-amylase multigene family through unequal, homologous, and interchromosomal and intrachromosomal crossovers. Genomics. 1990;8:97–105.
16. Yang Z-M, Lin J, Chen L-H, Zhang M, Chen W-W, Yang X-R. The roles of AMY1 copies and protein expression in human salivary α-amylase activity. Physiol Behav. 2015;138:173–8.
17. Iontcheva I, Oppenheim FG, Troxler RF. Human salivary mucin MG1 selectively forms heterotypic complexes with amylase, proline-rich proteins, statherin, and histatins. J Dent Res. 1997;76:734–43.

10

MicroRNAs in acute kidney injury

Pei-Chun Fan[1,2], Chia-Chun Chen[3], Yung-Chang Chen[1], Yu-Sun Chang[3] and Pao-Hsien Chu[4,5,6,7*]

Abstract

Acute kidney injury (AKI) is an important clinical issue that is associated with significant morbidity and mortality. Despite research advances over the past decades, the complex pathophysiology of AKI is not fully understood. The regulatory mechanisms underlying post-AKI repair and fibrosis have not been clarified either. Furthermore, there is no definitively effective treatment for AKI. MicroRNAs (miRNAs) are endogenous single-stranded noncoding RNAs of 19~23 nucleotides that have been shown to be crucial to the post-transcriptional regulation of various cellular biological functions, including proliferation, differentiation, metabolism, and apoptosis. In addition to being fundamental to normal development and physiology, miRNAs also play important roles in various human diseases. In AKI, some miRNAs appear to act pathogenically by promoting inflammation, apoptosis, and fibrosis, while others may act protectively by exerting anti-inflammatory, anti-apoptotic, anti-fibrotic, and pro-angiogenic effects. Thus, miRNAs have not only emerged as novel biomarkers for AKI; they also hold promise to be potential therapeutic targets.

Keywords: MicroRNAs, Acute kidney injury, Renal fibrosis

Abbreviations: AA, aristolochic acid; ADIPOR2, adiponectin receptor 2; AGO, argonaute; AKI, acute kidney injury; ATF3, activating transcription factor 3; B, blood; BCL-2, B cell lymphoma 2; BUMPT-306 cell, Boston University mouse proximal tubule cell clone 306; $CdCl_2$, cadmium chloride; CRL-2753 cell, rat mesangial cell line; CKD, chronic kidney disease; CXCR4, chemokine receptor type 4; DGCR8, Di-George syndrome critical region gene 8 or Pasha; DM, diabetes mellitus; EMT, epithelial-to-mesenchymal transition; ER, endoplasmic reticulum; ERK-2, extracellular signal-regulated kinase 2; FGF-2, fibroblast growth factor 2; Foxo3, forkhead box O3; FSGS, focal segmental glomerulosclerosis; H2A. X, H2A histone family member X; HEK cell, human embryonic kidney cell; HepG2 cell, human hepatocellular liver carcinoma cell line; HIF-1α, hypoxia-inducible factor 1 alpha, HK-2 cell, human kidney 2 cell; HO-1, heme oxygenase-1; HPTEC, human proximal tubular epithelial cell; HUVEC, human umbilical vein endothelial cell; ICU, intensive care units; IGF1R, insulin-like growth factor 1 receptor; IL, interleukin; IKKb, inhibitor of NF-kB kinases b; IRAK-1, interleukin-1 receptor-associated kinase 1; IRI, ischemia-reperfusion injury; $K_2Cr_2O_7$, potassium dichromate; LC3-II, light chain 3-II; MCP-1, monocyte chemoattractant protein-1; MDM2, murine double-minute 2; miRNA, microRNA; mRNA, messenger RNA; NF-kB, nuclear factor-kappaB; NRK-52E cell, rat renal proximal tubular cell line; PDCD4, programmed cell death protein 4; Pparα, peroxisome proliferator activated receptor alpha; PTC, proximal tubular cell; PTEN, phosphatase and tensin homolog; Rab-11a, Ras-related proteins in brain 11 a; RISC, RNA-induced silencing complex; ROS, reactive oxygen species; S1PR1, sphingosine-1-phosphate receptor 1; SHRSP, stroke-prone spontaneously hypertensive rat; STZ, streptozocin; T, tissue; TEC, tubular epithelial cell; TEnC, tubular endothelial cell; TEpC, tubular epithelial cell; TNF, tumor necrosis factor; TGF-β, transforming growth factor beta; TRAF-6, TNF receptor-associated factor 6; Treg, regulator T cell; U, urine; UTR, untranslated region; UUO, unilateral ureteral obstruction; VEGF, vascular endothelial growth factor; VEGFR2, vascular endothelial growth factor receptor 2; ZEB1/ZEB2, zinc finger E-box-binding homeobox

* Correspondence: taipei.chu@gmail.com
[4]Division of Cardiology, Department of Internal Medicine, Chang Gung Memorial Hospital, College of Medicine, Chang Gung University, Taipei, Taiwan
[5]Healthcare Center, Chang Gung Memorial Hospital, College of Medicine, Chang Gung University, Taipei, Taiwan
Full list of author information is available at the end of the article

Background

Acute kidney injury

Acute kidney injury (AKI) is a complex syndrome that occurs in a variety of settings with clinical manifestations ranging from a minimal elevation in serum creatinine to anuric renal failure. AKI conveys significant morbidity and mortality, is a major risk factor of chronic kidney disease, and is thus associated with huge health and socioeconomic burdens [1, 2]. Despite research advances in the past decades, however, the complex pathophysiology of AKI is not fully understood. The regulatory mechanisms underlying post-AKI repair and fibrosis remain to be clarified. Furthermore, there is no definitively effective treatment for AKI.

MicroRNA biogenesis and function

MicroRNAs (miRNAs) are endogenous single-stranded noncoding mRNAs of 19~23 nucleotides. They were first discovered in *Caenorhabditis elegans* by Ambros's group in 1993 [3] and show surprisingly high conservation across species. The evidence accumulated over the past two decades shows that miRNAs play a critical role in the post-transcriptional regulation of almost all biological cell functions, including proliferation, differentiation, metabolism, and apoptosis [4]. miRNAs, which are expressed in a tissue-specific manner, are fundamental to normal development and physiology [4] and are involved in the pathologic pathways of many disease models.

To date, more than 2000 miRNAs have been discovered in the human genome. The miRNA-encoded genes are found as either independent genes having their own promoters, or as sequences in the introns of protein-coding genes [5]. RNA polymerase II transcribes an miRNA gene into a primary transcript (called a pri-miRNA) of several kilobases that can encode either an individual miRNA or a polycistronic cluster of two or more miRNAs. The RNase III enzyme, DROSHA, and its cofactor DGCR8 (Di-George syndrome critical region gene 8 or Pasha), cleave a pri-miRNA at its stem-loop structure, generating an approximately 70-nucleotide intermediate called the pre-miRNA. Exportin-5 exports the pre-miRNA from the nucleus to the cytoplasm, and the RNase III enzyme, DICER, further cleaves it to yield a single-stranded mature miRNA. To perform its function, an miRNA is incorporated along with the argonaute (AGO) protein to form an effector complex called the RNA-induced silencing complex (RISC). RISC binds to the 3′-untranslated region (UTR) of a target messenger RNA (mRNA), leading to the repression of either protein translation or mRNA degradation. Unlike small interfering RNAs in plants, miRNAs do not require complete complementarity to bind their targets. Instead, the evidence suggests that the "seed sequence" (nucleotides 2 through 8 of the miRNA) is the most important region for the ability of an miRNA to bind and regulate its target gene(s). Once bound, miRNAs induce repression by blocking the initiation or elongation of translation or de-adenylating the mRNA transcripts. Because miRNAs do not require complete complementarity to repress gene expression, a given miRNA can regulate multiple mRNA transcripts and a given mRNA transcript can be repressed by multiple miRNAs. It is estimated that miRNAs regulate more than half of the protein-coding genes in human [6]. Moreover, miRNAs have been implicated in various human diseases [7, 8], including kidney diseases, such as polycystic kidney disease [9], renal cell carcinoma [10], diabetic nephropathy [11], lupus nephritis, [12] and renal allograft rejection [13]. In the past few years, researchers have begun to address the relevance of miRNAs to AKI.

miRNAs in acute kidney injury

The miRNAs that have been implicated in AKI are summarized in Tables 1 and 2, and those with potential pathological or protective roles are summarized in Table 3. The first evidence of miRNAs having pathological roles in AKI was reported by Wei et al. who developed a *Dicer*-knockout mouse model, in which *Dicer* was specifically deleted from proximal tubular cells. These mice exhibit a global down-regulation of microRNAs in the renal cortex. They have normal renal function and histology under control conditions but show resistance to the AKI that follows bilateral renal ischemia-reperfusion (IRI). Under the latter conditions, *Dicer*-null mice show significantly better renal function, less tissue damage, less tubular apoptosis, and better survival than their wild-type counterparts [14].

miR-10a is renal tubule-specific miRNA that is released from kidney tissues upon injury. In rodent models of renal IRI and streptozocin (STZ)-induced diabetic nephropathy, the levels of miR-10a are increased decreased in urine and kidney tissue, respectively [15, 16]. miR-10a is thought to exert protective actions during injury by targeting IL-12/IL-23p40 and the pro-apoptotic protein BIM [17]. In humans, decreased plasma levels of miR-10a have been shown to predict AKI in critical patients of intensive care units (ICUs) [18].

The members of the miR-17 family have been shown to be induced by pro-inflammatory cytokines, and their tissue expressions are increased in rodent models of renal IRI [19, 20].

miR-21 appears to play a dual role; on the one hand, it protects against injury by inhibiting apoptosis and inflammation; on the other hand, it may amplify the injury response and promote fibrosis. Studies have shown that miR-21 inhibits apoptosis by down-regulating programmed cell death protein 4 (PDCD4), down-regulating

Table 1 miRNAs implicated in acute kidney injury

miRNA	Samples	Species	Model	Expression	Reference
k12-3	In vitro	HK-2 cells	Oxidative stress	Down then up	[51]
let-7a	T, B	Rat, human	Contrast nephropathy, contrast nephropathy[a]	Down	[52]
let-7a-1-3p	T, U	Rat	Cisplatin nephropathy	Up (urine), down (tissue)	[33]
let-7a-2*	In vitro	HK-2 cells, primary PTCs	AA nephropathy	Up	[38]
let-7b	B	Human	ICU AKI[a]	Down	[46]
let-7d	U	Rat	Gentamicin nephropathy	Down	[53]
let-7e	T, in vitro	Mouse, HK-2 cells	IRI	Up, down	[23, 54]
let-7f	B, T	Human, mouse	ICU AKI[a], IRI	Down	[34, 46]
let-7g	T, U	Mouse, rat	Cisplatin nephropathy	Up, down	[33, 35]
miR-7	T, in vitro	Mouse, HK-2 cells	IRI, oxidative stress	Up	[14, 51]
miR-7a-1-3p	T, U	Rat	Cisplatin nephropathy	Up (urine), down (tissue)	[33]
miR-10a	T, U, B	Mouse, human, rat	IRI, DM-CKD (STZ), FSGS[a], ICU AKI[a]	Up, down	[15, 16, 18]
miR-10b*	T	Mouse	Cisplatin nephropathy	Down	[35]
miR-15	U	Rat	Cisplatin nephropathy	Up	[55]
miR-15b-5p	T, in vitro	Mouse, HK-2 cells	IRI	Down	[54]
miR-16	B, U	Human, rat	ICU AKI[a], cisplatin nephropathy	Up, down	[46, 55]
miR-17-3p	T	Mouse	IRI	Up	[14, 49]
miR-17-5p	T, U	Mouse, rat	IRI, cisplatin nephropathy	Up, down	[19, 20, 33]
miR-18a	T, B, U, in vitro	Mouse, rat, human, HPTECs	IRI, gentamicin nephropathy, folic acid, $CdCl_2$, arsenic trioxide, AA, $K_2Cr_2O_7$, cisplatin, UUO, allograft rejection[a], renal fibrosis[a]	Up, down	[14, 34, 47, 56, 57]
miR-19a	T	Mouse	IRI	Up	[34]
miR-20a	T, in vitro, U	Mouse, TECs, rat, HK-2 cells	Cisplatin nephropathy, IRI	Up, down	[37, 54, 55]
miR-20b-5p	T, U, in vitro	Rat, mouse, HK-2 cells	Cisplatin nephropathy, IRI	Up (urine), down (tissue)	[33, 54]
miR-21	B, U, T, in vitro	Human, rat, mouse, TEC, CRL-2753 cells, NRK52E cells, HK-2 cells	IRI, TGF-β, anti-Thy 1.1, UUO, SHRSP, gentamicin nephropathy, folic acid, $CdCl_2$, arsenic trioxide, AA, $K_2Cr_2O_7$, allograft rejection[a], renal fibrosis[a], AKI[a]	Up, down	[19–30, 34, 37, 45, 56–58]
miR-24	B, T, in vitro	Human, rat, CRL-2753 cells, NRK52E cells, HK-2 cells, HUVECs	ICU AKI[a], transplantation[a], UUO, IRI	Up, down	[31, 45, 46]
miR-24-2	T	Mouse	IRI	Up	[34]
miR-25-3p	T, U	Rat	Cisplatin nephropathy	Up (urine), down (tissue)	[33]
miR-26a	In vitro, T	HK-2 cells, mouse	IRI, oxidative stress, cisplatin nephropathy	Down	[32, 35, 51]
miR-26b	T, in vitro, U, B	Rat, CRL-2753 cells, NRK52E cells, human	UUO, cisplatin nephropathy, ICU AKI[a]	Down (tissue, blood), up (urine)	[18, 33, 45]
miR-27a-3p	B	Human	ICU AKI[a]	Down	[18]
miR-29a	T, in vitro, B	HK-2 cells, human	Oxidative stress, ICU AKI[a]	Up, down	[18, 51, 59]
miR-29b	T, in vitro	Rat, HK-2 cells	Oxidative stress	Up	[51, 59]
miR-29c	T	Mouse	IRI	Up	[34, 59]

Table 1 miRNAs implicated in acute kidney injury *(Continued)*

miR-30a-5p	T, U, in vitro, B	Rat, mouse, HK-2 cells, human	Cisplatin nephropathy, IRI, contrast-induced nephropathy, contrast-induced nephropathy[a]	Up (urine, blood, tissue), down (tissue)	[33, 52, 54]
miR-30c	T, in vitro, B	Rat, CRL-2753 cells, NRK52E cells, mouse, human	TGF-β, UUO, SHRSP, contrast-induced nephropathy, contrast-induced nephropathy[a]	Up, down	[34, 45, 52]
miR-30c-1	T	Mouse	IRI	Up	[34]
miR-30c-2*	In vitro	HK-2 cells	Oxidative stress	Down	[51]
miR-30d	T, U, B	Mouse, human	IRI, DM-CKD (STZ), FSGS[a]	Up, down, unchanged	[16]
miR-30d*	B	Human	ICU AKI[a]	Down	[46]
miR-30e	T, B	Mouse, rat, human	Cisplatin nephropathy, contrast-induced nephropathy, contrast-induced nephropathy[a]	Up, down	[35, 52]
miR-34a	T, in vitro	Mouse, BUMPT-306 cells, NRK-52E cells, RTECs	Cisplatin nephropathy, IRI	Up	[35, 60, 61]
miR-34b	T	Mouse	IRI	Up	[47]
miR-92a	T	Mouse	IRI	Up	[34]
miR-92b*	B	Human	ICU AKI[a]	Up	[46]
miR-93-3p	B	Human	ICU AKI[a], AKI post-cardiac surgery[a]	Down	[18]
miR-93-5p	T, U	Rat	Cisplatin nephropathy	Up (urine), down (tissue)	[33]
miR-99b	In vitro, T	HK-2 cells, mouse	ER stress, IRI	Down	[51, 54]
miR-101-3p	B	Human	ICU AKI[a]	Down	[18]
miR-101a	T, in vitro	Mouse, HK-2 cells	UUO	Down	[25]
miR-106a-5p	T, in vitro	Mouse, HK-2 cells, primary PTCs, rat	IRI, AA nephropathy	Up, down	[19, 20, 38]
miR-122	T	Mouse	Cisplatin nephropathy, IRI	Down	[35, 49]
miR-123	T	Mouse	IRI	Up	[49]
miR-125a-5p	T, in vitro	Mouse, HK-2 cells	IRI	Down	[54]
miR-125b	T, in vitro	Mouse, HepG2 cells, HEK293 cells, NRK52E cells	Cisplatin nephropathy		[62]
miR-126-3p	B	Human	ICU AKI[a]	Down	[18]
miR-126-5p	T, in vitro	Mouse, rat, TEnCs, TEpCs	IRI	Up	[34, 43, 44, 63]
miR-127-3p	T, in vitro, B	Rat, mouse, NRK-52E cells, HK-2 cells, human	IRI, ICU AKI[a], AKI post-cardiac surgery[a]	Up, down	[14, 18, 36, 49]
miR-129-3p	T	Mouse	IRI	Up	[34]
miR-129-5p	In vitro	HK-2 cells, primary PTCs	AA nephropathy	Down	[38]
miR-130b-3p	T, U	Rat	Cisplatin nephropathy	Up (urine), down (tissue)	[33]
miR-132	T, in vitro	Mouse, human, HPTECs	IRI, folic acid, $CdCl_2$, arsenic trioxide, AA, $K_2Cr_2O_7$, cisplatin, UUO, allograft rejection[a], renal fibrosis[a]	Up	[14, 57]
miR-133a	In vitro	HK-2 cells	ER stress	Down	[51]
miR-134	T	Mouse	IRI	Up	[47]
miR-135b	T	Mouse	IRI	Down	[14, 49]
miR-140-3p	T, U	Rat	Cisplatin nephropathy	Up (urine), down (tissue)	[33]
miR-141	T	Mouse	IRI	Up	[34]
miR-142-3p	T, in vitro	Mouse, HK-2 cells	UUO	Up	[25]

Table 1 miRNAs implicated in acute kidney injury *(Continued)*

miR-142-5p	T, in vitro	Mouse, HK-2 cells	UUO	Up	[25]
miR-145	T, in vitro	Rat, mouse, CRL-2753 cells, NRK52E cells, CD133+ renal medullary progenitor cells	TGF-β, SHRSP salt challenge	Up, down	[39, 45, 64]
miR-146a	T, in vitro, B	Mouse, TECs, human	IRI, ICU AKI[a]	Down (blood), up (tissue)	[18, 37]
miR-146b-5p	T, in vitro	Mouse, human, HPTECs	IRI, folic acid, $CdCl_2$, arsenic trioxide, AA, $K_2Cr_2O_7$, cisplatin, UUO, allograft rejection[a], renal fibrosis[a]	Up	[57]
miR-149	T	Mouse	IRI	Down	[34]
miR-150	T, in vitro	Mouse, immortalized mouse cardiac endothelial cell lines	IRI, AMI using LAD ligation	Down	[65]
miR-155	B, U, T, in vitro	Rat, human, mouse, HK-2 cells	IRI, gentamicin nephropathy, Cisplatin nephropathy, AKI[a]	Up, down	[54, 56, 66]
miR-181a*	In vitro	HK-2 cells	ER stress	Up	[51]
miR-181a-2*	In vitro	HK-2 cells	ER stress	Down	[51]
miR-181d	T	Mouse	IRI	Down	[34]
miR-182	T	Mouse	IRI	Up	[47]
miR-183-5p	T, U	Rat	Cisplatin nephropathy	Up (urine), down (tissue)	[33]
miR-187	T, in vitro	Mouse, TECs	IRI	Down	[37]
miR-188-5p	T	Mouse	IRI	Up	[34]
miR-191a-5p	T, U	Rat	Cisplatin nephropathy	Up (urine), down (tissue)	[33]
miR-192	T, in vitro, B, U	Mouse, rat, CRL-2753 cells, NRK52E cells, TECs, HK-2 cells, primary PTCs	IRI, UUO, SHRSP, AA nephropathy, cisplatin nephropathy, contact freezing, Dahl salt-sensitive rat with high salt administration	Up, down	[15, 33, 45, 55]
miR-193	T, in vitro, U	Mouse, HK-2 cells, Rat	UUO, cisplatin nephropathy	Down (tissue), up (urine)	[25, 33, 35, 55]
miR-194	T, in vitro, B, U	Mouse, rat, TECs, HK-2 cells, primary PTCs	IRI, AA nephropathy, contact freezing, Dahl salt-sensitive rat with high salt administration	Up, down	[15, 37–39]
miR-197	T	Mouse	IRI	Down	[34]
miR-199a-3p	T, in vitro	Mouse, TECs	IRI	Up	[37]
miR-200a	T, B, U	Human, Rat, mouse	Contact freezing, Dahl salt-sensitive rat with high salt administration, contrast-induced nephropathy, contrast-induced nephropathy[a]	Up, down	[39, 52]
miR-200b	T, in vitro, B, U	Rat, CRL-2753 cells, NRK52E cells, human	TGF-β, UUO, contact freezing, early CKD (Dahl salt-sensitive rat with high salt administration)	Up, down	[34, 39, 45]
miR-200c	T, in vitro, U, B	Rat, CRL-2753 cells, NRK52E cells, human	TGF-β, contact freezing, early CKD (Dahl salt-sensitive rat with high salt administration), ICU and transplant AKI[a]	Up, down	[29, 39, 45]
miR-202	In vitro	HK-2 cells	ER stress	Down	[51]
miR-203	U	Rat	Gentamicin nephropathy	Down	[53]
miR-205	In vitro	HK-2 cells, primary PTCs	Oxidative stress, ER stress, AA nephropathy	Down	[38, 51]
miR-207	T	Mouse	IRI	Up, down	[14, 34]
miR-210	B, T, in vitro, U	Human, mouse, HUVEC-12 cells, HK-2 cells, primary PTCs, rat	IRI, Oxidative stress, AA nephropathy, cisplatin nephropathy, ICU AKI[a]	Up, down	[18, 34, 38, 46, 47, 51, 55]

Table 1 miRNAs implicated in acute kidney injury *(Continued)*

miR-211	T	Mouse	IRI	Down	[34]
miR-212	T	Mouse, human, HPTECs	IRI, folic acid, $CdCl_2$, arsenic trioxide, AA, $K_2Cr_2O_7$, cisplatin, UUO, allograft rejection[a], renal fibrosis[a]	Up, down	[34, 57]
miR-214	T, in vitro	Mouse, rat, HK-2 cells, TECs, CRL-2753 cells, NRK52E cells, human	TGF-β, anti-Thy 1.1, UUO, SHRSP, IRI, diabetic nephropathy[a]	Up	[23–25, 37, 45, 47]
miR-215	In vitro	HK-2 cell	ER stress	Down	[51]
miR-218	T, in vitro	Mouse, HK-2 cells	UUO	Down	[25]
miR-218-1	T	Mouse	IRI	Up	[34]
miR-218a-5p	T, U	Rat	Cisplatin nephropathy	Up (urine),down (tissue)	[33]
miR-221*	In vitro	HK-2 cells	Oxidative stress	Up	[51]
miR-223	T, in vitro	Mouse, HK-2 cells	UUO	Up	[25]
miR-290-3p	T	Mouse	IRI	Up	[34]
miR-296	T, in vitro	Rat, mouse, TEnCs, TEpCs	IRI	Up, down	[14, 43]
miR-302b	T	Mouse	IRI	Up	[34]
miR-302c	T	Mouse	IRI	Up	[34]
miR-320	B, T, U	Human, mouse, rat	IRI, cisplatin nephropathy, gentamicin nephropathy, contrast-induced nephropathy, ICU AKI[a], contrast-induced nephropathy[a]	Up, down	[23, 33, 34, 46, 52, 53]
miR-322	T	Mouse	IRI	Down	[14]
miR-324-3p	T	Mouse	IRI	Down	[14]
miR-326	T	Mouse	IRI	Down	[34]
miR-328	T	Mouse	IRI	Down	[34]
miR-328a-3p	T, U	Rat	Cisplatin nephropathy	Up (urine),down (tissue)	[33]
miR-329	T, in vitro	Rat, CRL-2753 cells, NRK52E cells	UUO	Down	[45]
miR-335	T, U	Rat	Cisplatin nephropathy	Up (urine),down (tissue)	[33]
miR-340-5p	T, U	Rat	Cisplatin nephropathy	Up (urine),down (tissue)	[33]
miR-346	T	Mouse	IRI	Down	[34]
miR-362-5p	T	Mouse	IRI	Up	[14, 34]
miR-365*	In vitro	HK-2 cells, primary PTCs	AA nephropathy	Down	[38]
miR-378a-5p	T, U	Rat	Cisplatin nephropathy	Up (urine),down (tissue)	[33]
miR-379	T	Mouse	IRI	Down	[14, 49]
miR-382	In vitro	HK-2 cells, primary PTCs	AA nephropathy	Up	[38]
miR-423	U	Human	ICU and transplant AKI[a]	Up	[29]
miR-449	In vitro	NRK-52E cells	Cisplatin nephropathy	Up	[67]
miR-450a-3p	T, in vitro	Mouse, HK-2 cells, primary PTCs	IRI, AA nephropathy	Up, down	[34, 38]
miR-451	T	Mouse	IRI	Up	[34]
miR-455-3p	T	Mouse	IRI	Down	[14]
miR-466a-5p	T	Mouse	IRI	Up	[34]
miR-466b-5p	T	Mouse	IRI	Up	[34]

Table 1 miRNAs implicated in acute kidney injury *(Continued)*

miR-466c-5p	T	Mouse	IRI	Down	[34]
miR-466f-3p	T	Mouse	IRI	Down	[34]
miR-466g	T	Mouse	IRI	Down	[34]
miR-466i	T	Mouse	IRI	Down	[34]
miR-467	T	Mouse	IRI	Up	[14]
miR-467a	T	Mouse	IRI	Down	[34]
miR-467b	T	Mouse	IRI	Down	[34]
miR-467e	T	Mouse	IRI	Down	[34]
miR-467f	T	Mouse	IRI	Down	[34]
miR-467g	T	Mouse	IRI	Down	[34]
miR-468	T	Mouse	IRI	Down	[34]
miR-483	T	Mouse	IRI	Up, down?	[34]
miR-484	T	Mouse	IRI	Down	[34]
miR-486	T	Mouse	IRI	Up	[14]
miR-487b	T	Mouse	IRI	Down	[14]
miR-489	T	Mouse	IRI	Up	[14]
miR-491	T	Mouse	IRI	Down	[14]
miR-494	T, U, B	Mouse, human	IRI, ICU AKI[a]	Up, unchanged	[48]
miR-495	T	Mouse	IRI	Up	[14]
miR-503	In vitro	HK-2 cells	ER stress	Down	[51]
miR-532-3p	T, U	Mouse, rat	IRI, Cisplatin nephropathy	Up, down	[33, 34]
miR-542-3p	In vitro	HK-2 cells, primary PTCs	AA nephropathy	Up	[38]
miR-547-3p	T	Mouse	IRI	Down	[34]
miR-574-5p	In vitro	HK-2 cells, primary PTCs	AA nephropathy	Down	[38]
miR-617	B	Human	ICU AKI[a]	Up	[46]
miR-620	B	Human	ICU AKI[a]	Down	[46]
miR-625*	In vitro	HK-2 cells, primary PTCs	AA nephropathy	Down	[38]
miR-630	In vitro	HK-2 cells	Oxidative stress	Up	[51]
miR-638	B	Human	ICU AKI[a]	Up	[46]
miR-663b	B	Human	ICU AKI[a]	Up	[46]
miR-668	T	Mouse	IRI	Up	[14]
miR-669a	T	Mouse	IRI	Down	[34]
miR-669f	T	Mouse	IRI	Down	[34]
miR-669h-3p	T	Mouse	IRI	Down	[34]
miR-671-3p	In vitro	HK-2 cells, primary PTCs	AA nephropathy	Down	[38]
miR-671-5p	T	Mouse	IRI	Up	[34]
miR-674	T	Mouse	IRI	Down	[34]
miR-680	T	Mouse	IRI	Up	[34]
miR-684	T	Mouse	IRI	Up	[34]
miR-685	T	Mouse	IRI	Up	[14, 34, 49]
miR-687	T, in vitro	Mouse, BUMPT-306 cells, HEK cells	IRI	Up	[14, 49]
miR-689	T	Mouse	IRI	Up	[34]
miR-694	T	Mouse	IRI	Up	[14]

Table 1 miRNAs implicated in acute kidney injury *(Continued)*

miR-705	T	Mouse	IRI	Up	[34]
miR-708	T	Mouse	IRI	Up	[34]
miR-714	T, B	Mouse	IRI	Up	[68]
miR-718	T	Mouse	IRI	Down	[34]
miR-721	T	Mouse	IRI	Up	[34]
miR-744-5p	T, U	Rat	Cisplatin nephropathy	Up (urine),down (tissue)	[33]
miR-805	T, in vitro	Mouse, TECs	IRI	Down	[34, 37]
miR-875-5p	T	Mouse	IRI	Down	[34]
miR-876-5p	T	Mouse	IRI	Up	[34]
miR-877	T	Mouse	IRI	Up, down?	[34]
miR-877*	T, B	Mouse	IRI	Up	[68]
miR-1187	T	Mouse	IRI	Down	[34]
miR-1188	T, B	Mouse	IRI	Up	[68]
miR-1196	T	Mouse	IRI	Down	[34]
miR-1198	T	Mouse	IRI	Down	[34]
miR-1224	T, B	Mouse	IRI	Up	[68]
miR-1244	B	Human	ICU AKI[a]	Down	[46]
miR-1249	In vitro	HK-2 cells, primary PTCs	AA nephropathy	Up	[38]
miR-1839-5p	T, U	Rat	Cisplatin nephropathy	Up (urine),down (tissue)	[33]
miR-1892	T	Mouse	IRI	Up	[34]
miR-1894-3p	T	Mouse	IRI	Up	[34]
miR-1897-3p	T, B	Mouse	IRI	Up	[68]
miR-4521	In vitro	HK-2 cells, primary PTCs	AA nephropathy	Down	[38]
miR-4640	U	Human	ICU and transplant AKI[a]	Down	[29]
miR-4716-5p	In vitro	HK-2 cells, primary PTCs	AA nephropathy	Up	[38]
miR-4730	In vitro	HK-2 cells, primary PTCs	AA nephropathy	Up	[38]
miR-4747-3p	In vitro	HK-2 cells, primary PTCs	AA nephropathy	Up	[38]

[a]Human studies

phosphatase and tensin homolog (PTEN), activating the AKT pathway, up-regulating B cell lymphoma 2 (BCL-2), and decreasing the levels of active caspase-3 and caspase-8 proteins [21, 22]. Up-regulation of miR-21 also inhibits inflammation by decreasing nuclear factor-kappaB (NF-kB), tumor necrosis factor (TNF), interleukin 6 (IL-6), and IL-18, and by increasing IL-10 [21]. Experimental up-regulation of miR-21 provides morphologic and functional renoprotection in animal models of AKI [21–23]. miR-21 is induced by transforming growth factor beta (TGF-β)/Smad, hypoxia inducible factor 1 alpha (HIF-1α), TNF, and fibroblast growth factor 2 (FGF-2) [24, 25], and this miRNA promotes fibrosis by targeting peroxisome proliferator-activated receptor alpha (Pparα) and altering lipid metabolism [26]. miR-21 also targets Mpv17l, a mitochondria inhibitor of reactive oxygen species (ROS) [26]. miR-21 inhibits autophagy by targeting Ras-related proteins in brain 11 a (Rab-11a), decreasing light chain 3-II (LC3-II), decreasing beclin-1, and increasing p62 [27]. In vivo blockade of miR-21 reduces renal fibrosis and macrophage infiltration in animal models. Moreover, increased urinary and plasma levels of miR-21 have been observed in various clinical AKI settings [26, 28, 29]. For example, urine and plasma miR-21 levels were shown to correlate with AKI severity and hospital mortality and to predict the need for postoperative renal replacement therapy [28]. Interestingly, one study found decreased, but not increased, expression of miR-21 in AKI patients. Lower baseline plasma levels of miR-21 have been demonstrated to predict cardiac surgery-associated AKI [30].

miR-24 is up-regulated in mouse kidney after IRI and in patients after kidney transplantation. This miRNA enhances apoptosis by down-regulating sphingosine-1-phosphate receptor 1 (S1PR1), H2A histone family

Table 2 miRNAs implicated in human studies related to kidney injury

miRNA	Kidney injury	Expression		Reference
		Up	Down	
hsa-let-7b	AKI in ICU		Blood	[46]
hsa-let-7f	AKI in ICU		Blood	[46]
hsa-miR-10a	Focal segmental sclerosis	Urine		[16]
	AKI in ICU		Blood	[18]
hsa-miR-16	AKI in ICU		Blood	[46]
hsa-miR-21	AKI, chronic renal allograft dysfunction, renal allograft rejection, renal fibrosis	Tissue, blood, urine		[24, 26, 28, 29, 56]
	AKI after cardiac surgery		Blood	[30]
hsa-miR-24	AKI in ICU		Blood	[46]
	Transplanted renal graft with prolonged cold ischemia time	Tissue		[31]
hsa-miR-26b	AKI in ICU		Blood	[18]
hsa-miR-27a-3p	AKI in ICU		Blood	[18]
hsa-miR-29a	AKI in ICU		Blood	[18]
hsa-miR-30a-5p	Contrast-induced nephropathy	Blood		[52]
hsa-miR-30c	Contrast-induced nephropathy	Blood		[52]
hsa-miR-30d	Focal segmental sclerosis	Urine		[16]
hsa-miR-30d*	AKI in ICU		Blood	[46]
hsa-miR-30e	Contrast-induced nephropathy	Blood		[52]
hsa-miR-92b*	AKI in ICU	Blood		[46]
hsa-miR-93-3p	AKI in ICU, AKI post-cardiac surgery		Blood	[18]
hsa-miR-101-3p	AKI in ICU		Blood	[18]
hsa-miR-126-3p	AKI in ICU		Blood	[18]
hsa-miR-127-3p	AKI in ICU, AKI post-cardiac surgery		Blood	[18]
hsa-miR-146a	AKI in ICU		Blood	[18]
hsa-miR-155	AKI	Urine		[56]
hsa-miR-200c	AKI in ICU, AKI in renal transplant	Urine		[29]
hsa-miR-210	AKI in ICU	Blood		[46]
	AKI in ICU		Blood	[18]
hsa-miR-214	Diabetes related chronic kidney disease stage 4	Tissue		[24]
hsa-miR-320	AKI in ICU		Blood	[46]
hsa-miR-423	AKI in ICU, AKI in renal transplant	Urine		[29]
hsa-miR-494	AKI in ICU	Urine		[48]
hsa-miR-617	AKI in ICU	Blood		[46]
hsa-miR-620	AKI in ICU		Blood	[46]
hsa-miR-638	AKI in ICU	Blood		[46]
hsa-miR-663b	AKI in ICU	Blood		[46]
hsa-miR-1244	AKI in ICU		Blood	[46]
hsa-miR-4640	AKI in ICU, AKI in renal transplant		Urine	[29]

member X (H2A.X), and heme oxygenase-1 (HO-1). Inhibition of miR-24 was shown to prevent renal injury in animal models [31].

miR-26a represses IL-6 expression to promote the expansion of regulator T cells (Tregs). The tissue levels of miR-26a is down-regulated in animal models of AKI, and experimental overexpression attenuates renal IRI and improves renal recovery [32]. miR-26b is down-regulated in the tissue and blood, yet up-regulated in the urine [18, 33]. Decreased blood levels of miR-26a and miR-

Table 3 Functional roles of miRNAs in acute kidney injury

Protective		Pathogenic	Kidney enriched, released from injured kidney tissues
Anti-inflammation	Pro-angiogenesis	Pro-inflammation	miR-10a
miR-10a	miR-126	miR-21	miR-30c
miR-21	miR-210	miR-214	miR-30d
miR-26a	miR-296	miR-494	miR-200 family
miR-126	Enhancing tubular proliferation	Pro-apoptosis	
miR-146a	miR-126	miR-24	
miR-199a	miR-296	miR-192	
miR-296	Cytoskeleton, cell-matrix, cell-cell	miR-494	
Anti-apoptosis	adhesion, cell trafficking	miR-687	
miR-10a	miR-127a	Pro-fibrosis	
miR-21		miR-21	
miR-122		miR-192	
miR-126		miR-214	
miR-199a			
miR-296			
miR-494			
Anti-fibrosis			
miR-29a			
miR-200b			
miR-200c			

27a predict AKI in the ICU. Decreased blood levels of miR-26a and miR-27a prior to cardiac surgery also predict AKI later on [18].

miR-29a is highly expressed in the kidney, where it acts against fibrosis by suppressing collagen expression in tubular cells. Decreased serum levels of miR-29a have been shown to predict AKI in ICU patients, and correlate with AKI severity [18].

miR-30c, which is essential for normal kidney homoeostasis, targets several genes important for kidney structure and function. miR-30c is up-regulated in the tissue, blood, and urine obtained from animal models of contrast nephropathy and IRI [34].

miR-30d, which is released to the urine from kidney tissues following injury, down-regulates the apoptotic proteins, caspase 3 and p53, and may provide protective effects during IRI [16].

miR-101-3p is highly expressed in the kidney, and decreased serum levels of this miRNA have been shown to predict AKI in the ICU [18].

miR-122 is down-regulated in the mice kidneys of mice subjected to cisplatin-induced AKI [35]. It exerts anti-apoptotic effects by down-regulating forkhead box O3 (Foxo3).

miR-127a, which is induced by HIF-1α, participates in protecting the cytoskeleton protection (by preventing actin depolmerization), maintaining cell-matrix and cell-cell adhesion maintenance (by preventing focal adhesion complexes disassembly and tight junctions disorganization), and promoting intracellular trafficking (by targeting kinesin family member 3B) [36]. Decreased blood levels of miR-127a were shown to predict AKI in the ICU. Decreased blood levels of miR-127a prior to cardiac surgery were found be predict AKI later on [18].

miR-146a is down- and up-regulated in the blood and kidney, respectively, during AKI. Decreased blood levels have been shown to predict AKI in the ICU and correlate with the severity of AKI [18]. It is induced by NF-kB and exerts anti-inflammatory effect by down-regulating TNF receptor-associated factor 6 (TRAF-6) and interleukin-1 receptor-associated kinase 1 (IRAK-1) [37].

miR-192 is enriched in kidneys and the small intestine. It is induced by TGF-β during the stress response. It promotes fibrosis by down-regulating SIP1. It also down-regulates E3 ubiquitin ligase and murine double-minute 2 (MDM2) and results in de-repression of p53 and G2/M arrest [38]. miR-194 is also enriched in kidneys and small intestine. It is induced during the stress response, and its levels in tissue, blood, and urine levels are increased during AKI [15, 38, 39].

miR-199a exerts anti-inflammatory effect by down-regulating inhibitor of NF-kB kinases b (IKKb) [40], exhibits anti-proliferatory effect by down-regulating the proto-oncogene MET [41], and confers anti-apoptosis effect by down-regulating extracellular signal–regulated kinase 2 (ERK-2) and HIF-1α [41, 42]. Therefore, it may help limit kidney injury.

miR-126 and miR-296 have been identified in microvesicles from endothelial progenitor cells and are thought to exert renoprotective effects via their abilities to decrease apoptosis and leukocyte infiltration, while promotes angiogenesis and tubular cell proliferation [43]. Hematopoietic overexpression of miR-126 enhances stromal cell-derived factor 1/chemokine receptor type 4 (CXCR4) -dependent vasculogenic progenitor cell mobilization and promotes vascular integrity and supports renal recovery after IRI [44]. Decreased serum levels of miR-126 have been shown to predict AKI in ICU patients, and correlate with the severity of AKI [18].

Members of the miR-200 family are highly expressed in tubular structures such as renal tubules, lungs, the small intestine, and various exocrine glands. miR-200b and miR-200c have been proposed to be anti-fibrotic. They down-regulate TGFβR1 and zinc finger E-box-binding homeobox (ZEB1/ZEB2), which are transcriptional repressors of E-cadherin, and thereby prevent the epithelial-to-mesenchymal transition (EMT) induced by TGF-β [45].

miR-210 is induced by HIF1-α and released by renal endothelial cell. It regulates angiogenesis by down-regulating ephrin-A3 and up-regulating vascular endothelial growth factor (VEGF) and vascular endothelial growth factor receptor 2 (VEGFR2). It also regulates mitochondria ROS production. Increased blood levels of miR-210 was shown to predict post-AKI mortality in critically ill patients [46]. In another study, decreased blood levels of miR-210 were shown to predict AKI in the ICU and correlate with the severity of AKI [18].

miR-214 is induced by TGF-β and promotes fibrosis; it has been shown to down-regulate PTEN, up-regulate the AKT pathway and inhibit apoptosis of monocytes and macrophages. miR-214 is up-regulated in various models of AKI and renal fibrosis [24, 45, 47] as well as in monocytes of animal with chronic kidney disease. Experimental antagonism of miR-214 has been shown to ameliorate renal fibrosis [24].

miR-494 is up-regulated early in AKI, with increased urine levels detected in rodent models of renal IRI and patients with AKI. It has been reported to promote apoptosis and inflammation by down-regulating activating transcription factor 3 (ATF3) and increasing IL-6, monocyte chemoattractant protein-1 (MCP-1), p-selectin [48]. Pathway analysis has suggested that it also targets adiponectin receptor 2 (ADIPOR2), BCL-2 facilitator, and insulin-like growth factor 1 receptor (IGF1R), which would increase inflammation and lead to more damage. However, miR-494 also targets pro-apoptotic proteins in the AKT pathway, and to exert protective effects. The mechanism responsible for regulating the balance between these anti- and pro- apoptotic effects requires further study.

Finally, miR-687 is induced by HIF-1, and enhances apoptosis by down-regulating PTEN. Animal studies have shown that miR-687 blockade preserves PTEN expression and attenuates cell cycle activation and decreases apoptosis, resulting in protection against kidney injury [49].

Conclusions

Many miRNAs have been implicated in the AKI. Some of them contribute to the pathogenesis by regulating apoptosis and inflammation, to amplifying or reduce acute injury responses, while others regulate fibrosis and angiogenesis, to participate in renal recovery or the progression to fibrosis. The biological and pathological functions of many miRNAs in AKI are still not fully understood in AKI. Some studies have yielded inconsistent data regarding the expression pattern of miRNAs across different samples, species, disease models, and time points. These discrepancies warrant investigations.

In addition to their tissue expressions, miRNAs may be detected in various extracellular human body fluids, such as serum, urine, saliva, and cerebral spinal fluid. miRNAs are contained in exosomes and may remained stable over prolonged periods. They may be specifically up-regulated or down-regulated in response to injury signals and/or released into body fluids from resident tissues. Certain miRNAs have been investigated for their potential to serve as novel biomarkers for the early detection or prognostication of AKI. Given the complex pathophysiology and the dynamic nature of AKI, an miRNA panel may be more feasible rather than a single miRNA. Further validation studies are needed to evaluate the clinical utility of such a panel.

Some miRNAs may be potential therapeutic targets for AKI. Recently, an miRNA inhibitor has been proven to successfully suppress the replication of hepatitis C virus in a clinical trial [50]. Systemic or local administration of specific miRNAs mimics or antagonists in vivo could offer a strategy for preventing or ameliorating AKI or barring its progression to chronic kidney disease.

In the post-genome era, miRNAs are promising rising stars in translational medicine as they offer the potential to guide the individualized diagnosis and treatment of human diseases including AKI.

Acknowledgements
Not applicable.

Funding
This work was supported by the Chang Gung Memorial Hospital Research Program grant CMRPG3D1452, CMRPG 3F0561, CMRPG1B0581 and CIRPG3B0042.; Ministry of Science and Technology 104-2314-B-182A-131 and 105-2314-B-182A-121.

Authors' contributions
The manuscript was written by PCF. All authors critically revised the manuscript. All authors read and approved the final manuscript.

Competing interests
The authors declare that they have no competing interests.

Author details
[1]Kidney Research Center, Department of Nephrology, Chang Gung Memorial Hospital, Linkou Medical Center, Taoyuan, Taiwan. [2]Graduate Institute of Clinical Medical Sciences, Chang Gung University, Taoyuan, Taiwan. [3]Molecular Medicine Research Center, Chang Gung University, Taoyuan, Taiwan. [4]Division of Cardiology, Department of Internal Medicine, Chang Gung Memorial Hospital, College of Medicine, Chang Gung University, Taipei, Taiwan. [5]Healthcare Center, Chang Gung Memorial Hospital, College of Medicine, Chang Gung University, Taipei, Taiwan. [6]Heart Failure Center, Chang Gung Memorial Hospital, College of Medicine, Chang Gung University, Taipei, Taiwan. [7]Department of Cardiology, Chang Gung Memorial Hospital, College of Medicine, Chang Gung University, 199 Tung Hwa North Road, Taipei 105, Taiwan.

References

1. Schrier RW, Wang W, Poole B, Mitra A. Acute renal failure: definitions, diagnosis, pathogenesis, and therapy. J Clin Invest. 2004;114(1):5–14. doi:10.1172/jci22353.
2. Bellomo R, Ronco C, Kellum JA, Mehta RL, Palevsky P. Acute renal failure - definition, outcome measures, animal models, fluid therapy and information technology needs: the Second International Consensus Conference of the Acute Dialysis Quality Initiative (ADQI) Group. Crit Care (London, England). 2004;8(4):R204–12. doi:10.1186/cc2872.
3. Lee RC, Feinbaum RL, Ambros V. The C. elegans heterochronic gene lin-4 encodes small RNAs with antisense complementarity to lin-14. Cell. 1993; 75(5):843–54.
4. Krol J, Loedige I, Filipowicz W. The widespread regulation of microRNA biogenesis, function and decay. Nat Rev Genet. 2010;11(9):597–610. doi:10.1038/nrg2843.
5. Bhatt K, Mi QS, Dong Z. microRNAs in kidneys: biogenesis, regulation, and pathophysiological roles. Am J Physiol Renal Physiol. 2011;300(3):F602–10. doi:10.1152/ajprenal.00727.2010.
6. Bartel DP. MicroRNAs: target recognition and regulatory functions. Cell. 2009;136(2):215–33. doi:10.1016/j.cell.2009.01.002.
7. Huang JB, et al. MiR-196a2 rs11614913 T > C polymorphism is associated with an increased risk of Tetralogy of Fallot in a Chinese population. Acta Cardiol Sin. 2015;31(1):18–23.
8. Hsu A, Chen SJ, Chang YS, Chen HC, Chu PH. Systemic approach to identify serum microRNAs as potential biomarkers for acute myocardial infarction. Biomed Res Int. 2014;2014:418628. doi:10.1155/2014/418628.
9. Pandey P, et al. Microarray-based approach identifies microRNAs and their target functional patterns in polycystic kidney disease. BMC Genomics. 2008; 9:624. doi:10.1186/1471-2164-9-624.
10. Nakada C, et al. Genome-wide microRNA expression profiling in renal cell carcinoma: significant down-regulation of miR-141 and miR-200c. J Pathol. 2008;216(4):418–27. doi:10.1002/path.2437.
11. Kato M, Natarajan R. MicroRNA circuits in transforming growth factor-beta actions and diabetic nephropathy. Semin Nephrol. 2012;32(3):253–60. doi:10.1016/j.semnephrol.2012.04.004.
12. Dai Y, et al. Comprehensive analysis of microRNA expression patterns in renal biopsies of lupus nephritis patients. Rheumatol Int. 2009;29(7):749–54. doi:10.1007/s00296-008-0758-6.
13. Sui W, et al. Microarray analysis of MicroRNA expression in acute rejection after renal transplantation. Transpl Immunol. 2008;19(1):81–5. doi:10.1016/j.trim.2008.01.007.
14. Wei Q, et al. Targeted deletion of Dicer from proximal tubules protects against renal ischemia-reperfusion injury. J Am Soc Nephrol. 2010;21(5):756–61. doi:10.1681/asn.2009070718.
15. Wang JF, et al. Screening plasma miRNAs as biomarkers for renal ischemia-reperfusion injury in rats. Med Sci Monit. 2014;20:283–9. doi:10.12659/msm.889937.
16. Wang N, et al. Urinary microRNA-10a and microRNA-30d serve as novel, sensitive and specific biomarkers for kidney injury. PLoS One. 2012;7(12): e51140. doi:10.1371/journal.pone.0051140.
17. Ho J, et al. The pro-apoptotic protein Bim is a microRNA target in kidney progenitors. J Am Soc Nephrol. 2011;22(6):1053–63. doi:10.1681/asn.2010080841.
18. Aguado-Fraile E, et al. A pilot study identifying a set of microRNAs as precise diagnostic biomarkers of acute kidney injury. PLoS One. 2015;10(6): e0127175. doi:10.1371/journal.pone.0127175.
19. Kaucsar T, et al. Activation of the miR-17 family and miR-21 during murine kidney ischemia-reperfusion injury. Nucleic Acid Ther. 2013;23(5):344–54. doi:10.1089/nat.2013.0438.
20. Ma L, et al. Changes of miRNA-17-5p, miRNA-21 and miRNA-106a level during rat kidney ischemia-reperfusion injury. Zhonghua yi xue za zhi. 2015;95(19):1488–92.
21. Hu H, Jiang W, Xi X, Zou C, Ye Z. MicroRNA-21 attenuates renal ischemia reperfusion injury via targeting caspase signaling in mice. Am J Nephrol. 2014;40(3):215–23. doi:10.1159/000368202.
22. Jia P, et al. Xenon protects against septic acute kidney injury via miR-21 target signaling pathway. Crit Care Med. 2015;43(7):e250–9. doi:10.1097/ccm.0000000000001001.
23. Xu X, et al. Delayed ischemic preconditioning contributes to renal protection by upregulation of miR-21. Kidney Int. 2012;82(11):1167–75. doi: 10.1038/ki.2012.241.
24. Denby L, et al. MicroRNA-214 antagonism protects against renal fibrosis. J Am Soc Nephrol. 2014;25(1):65–80. doi:10.1681/asn.2013010072.
25. Zarjou A, Yang S, Abraham E, Agarwal A, Liu G. Identification of a microRNA signature in renal fibrosis: role of miR-21. Am J Physiol Renal Physiol. 2011; 301(4):F793–801. doi:10.1152/ajprenal.00273.2011.
26. Chau BN, et al. MicroRNA-21 promotes fibrosis of the kidney by silencing metabolic pathways. Sci Transl Med. 2012;4(121):121ra18. doi:10.1126/scitranslmed.3003205.
27. Liu X, et al. MiR-21 inhibits autophagy by targeting Rab11a in renal ischemia/reperfusion. Exp Cell Res. 2015;338(1):64–9. doi:10.1016/j.yexcr.2015.08.010.
28. Du J, et al. MicroRNA-21 and risk of severe acute kidney injury and poor outcomes after adult cardiac surgery. PLoS One. 2013;8(5):e63390. doi:10.1371/journal.pone.0063390.
29. Ramachandran K, et al. Human miRNome profiling identifies microRNAs differentially present in the urine after kidney injury. Clin Chem. 2013;59(12):1742–52. doi:10.1373/clinchem.2013.210245.
30. Gaede L, et al. Plasma microRNA-21 for the early prediction of acute kidney injury in patients undergoing major cardiac surgery. Nephrol Dial Transplant. 2016. doi:10.1093/ndt/gfw007
31. Lorenzen JM, et al. MicroRNA-24 antagonism prevents renal ischemia reperfusion injury. J Am Soc Nephrol. 2014;25(12):2717–29. doi:10.1681/asn.2013121329.
32. Liang S, Wang W, Gou X. MicroRNA 26a modulates regulatory T cells expansion and attenuates renal ischemia-reperfusion injury. Mol Immunol. 2015;65(2):321–7. doi:10.1016/j.molimm.2015.02.003.
33. Kanki M, et al. Identification of urinary miRNA biomarkers for detecting cisplatin-induced proximal tubular injury in rats. Toxicology. 2014;324:158–68. doi:10.1016/j.tox.2014.05.004.
34. Liu F, et al. Upregulation of microRNA-210 regulates renal angiogenesis mediated by activation of VEGF signaling pathway under ischemia/perfusion injury in vivo and in vitro. Kidney Blood Press Res. 2012;35(3):182–91. doi:10.1159/000331054.
35. Lee CG, et al. Discovery of an integrative network of microRNAs and transcriptomics changes for acute kidney injury. Kidney Int. 2014;86(5): 943–53. doi:10.1038/ki.2014.117.
36. Aguado-Fraile E, et al. miR-127 protects proximal tubule cells against ischemia/reperfusion: identification of kinesin family member 3B as miR-127 target. PLoS One. 2012;7(9):e44305. doi:10.1371/journal.pone.0044305.
37. Godwin JG, et al. Identification of a microRNA signature of renal ischemia reperfusion injury. Proc Natl Acad Sci U S A. 2010;107(32):14339–44. doi:10.1073/pnas.0912701107.
38. Jenkins RH, et al. miR-192 induces G2/M growth arrest in aristolochic acid nephropathy. Am J Pathol. 2014;184(4):996–1009. doi:10.1016/j.ajpath.2013.12.028.
39. Kito N, Endo K, Ikesue M, Weng H, Iwai N. miRNA profiles of tubular cells: diagnosis of kidney injury. Biomed Res Int. 2015;2015:465479. doi:10.1155/2015/465479.
40. Chen R, et al. Regulation of IKKbeta by miR-199a affects NF-kappaB activity in ovarian cancer cells. Oncogene. 2008;27(34):4712–23. doi:10.1038/onc.2008.112.
41. Kim S, et al. MicroRNA miR-199a* regulates the MET proto-oncogene and the downstream extracellular signal-regulated kinase 2 (ERK2). J Biol Chem. 2008;283(26):18158–66. doi:10.1074/jbc.M800186200.
42. Rane S, et al. Downregulation of miR-199a derepresses hypoxia-inducible factor-1 alpha and Sirtuin 1 and recapitulates hypoxia preconditioning in cardiac myocytes. Circ Res. 2009;104(7):879–86. doi:10.1161/circresaha.108.193102.
43. Cantaluppi V, et al. Microvesicles derived from endothelial progenitor cells protect the kidney from ischemia-reperfusion injury by microRNA-dependent

reprogramming of resident renal cells. Kidney Int. 2012;82(4):412–27. doi:10.1038/ki.2012.105.
44. Bijkerk R, et al. Hematopoietic microRNA-126 protects against renal ischemia/reperfusion injury by promoting vascular integrity. J Am Soc Nephrol. 2014;25(8):1710–22. doi:10.1681/asn.2013060640.
45. Denby L, et al. miR-21 and miR-214 are consistently modulated during renal injury in rodent models. Am J Pathol. 2011;179(2):661–72. doi:10.1016/j.ajpath.2011.04.021.
46. Lorenzen JM, et al. Circulating miR-210 predicts survival in critically ill patients with acute kidney injury. Clin J Am Soc Nephrol. 2011;6(7):1540–6. doi:10.2215/cjn.00430111.
47. Cui R, Xu J, Chen X, Zhu W. Global miRNA expression is temporally correlated with acute kidney injury in mice. PeerJ. 2016;4:e1729. doi:10.7717/peerj.1729.
48. Lan YF, et al. MicroRNA-494 reduces ATF3 expression and promotes AKI. J Am Soc Nephrol. 2012;23(12):2012–23. doi:10.1681/asn.2012050438.
49. Bhatt K, et al. MicroRNA-687 induced by hypoxia-inducible factor-1 targets phosphatase and tensin homolog in renal ischemia-reperfusion injury. J Am Soc Nephrol. 2015;26(7):1588–96. doi:10.1681/asn.2014050463.
50. Janssen HL, et al. Treatment of HCV infection by targeting microRNA. N Engl J Med. 2013;368(18):1685–94. doi:10.1056/NEJMoa1209026.
51. Muratsu-Ikeda S, et al. Downregulation of miR-205 modulates cell susceptibility to oxidative and endoplasmic reticulum stresses in renal tubular cells. PLoS One. 2012;7(7):e41462. doi:10.1371/journal.pone.0041462.
52. Gutierrez-Escolano A, Santacruz-Vazquez E, Gomez-Perez F. Dysregulated microRNAs involved in contrast-induced acute kidney injury in rat and human. Ren Fail. 2015;37(9):1498–506. doi:10.3109/0886022x.2015.1077322.
53. Nassirpour R, et al. Identification of tubular injury microRNA biomarkers in urine: comparison of next-generation sequencing and qPCR-based profiling platforms. BMC Genomics. 2014;15:485. doi:10.1186/1471-2164-15-485.
54. Wang IK, et al. MiR-20a-5p mediates hypoxia-induced autophagy by targeting ATG16L1 in ischemic kidney injury. Life Sci. 2015;136:133–41. doi:10.1016/j.lfs.2015.07.002.
55. Pavkovic M, Riefke B, Ellinger-Ziegelbauer H. Urinary microRNA profiling for identification of biomarkers after cisplatin-induced kidney injury. Toxicology. 2014;324:147–57. doi:10.1016/j.tox.2014.05.005.
56. Saikumar J, et al. Expression, circulation, and excretion profile of microRNA-21, -155, and -18a following acute kidney injury. Toxicol Sci. 2012;129(2):256–67. doi:10.1093/toxsci/kfs210.
57. Pellegrini KL, et al. Application of small RNA sequencing to identify microRNAs in acute kidney injury and fibrosis. Toxicol Appl Pharmacol. 2015. doi:10.1016/j.taap.2015.12.002.
58. Jia P, et al. miR-21 contributes to xenon-conferred amelioration of renal ischemia-reperfusion injury in mice. Anesthesiology. 2013;119(3):621–30. doi:10.1097/ALN.0b013e318298e5f1.
59. Shen B, et al. Revealing the underlying mechanism of ischemia reperfusion injury using bioinformatics approach. Kidney Blood Press Res. 2013;38(1):99–108. doi:10.1159/000355759.
60. Bhatt K, et al. MicroRNA-34a is induced via p53 during cisplatin nephrotoxicity and contributes to cell survival. Mol Med (Cambridge, Mass). 2010;16(9-10):409–16. doi:10.2119/molmed.2010.00002.
61. Liu XJ, et al. MicroRNA-34a suppresses autophagy in tubular epithelial cells in acute kidney injury. Am J Nephrol. 2015;42(2):168–75. doi:10.1159/000439185.
62. Joo MS, Lee CG, Koo JH, Kim SG. miR-125b transcriptionally increased by Nrf2 inhibits AhR repressor, which protects kidney from cisplatin-induced injury. Cell Death Dis. 2013;4:e899. doi:10.1038/cddis.2013.427.
63. Bijkerk R, et al. Silencing of miRNA-126 in kidney ischemia reperfusion is associated with elevated SDF-1 levels and mobilization of Sca-1+/Lin-progenitor cells. MicroRNA (Shariqah, United Arab Emirates). 2014;3(3):144–9.
64. Bussolati B, et al. Hypoxia modulates the undifferentiated phenotype of human renal inner medullary CD133+ progenitors through Oct4/miR-145 balance. Am J Physiol Renal Physiol. 2012;302(1):F116–28. doi:10.1152/ajprenal.00184.2011.
65. Ranganathan P, et al. MicroRNA-150 deletion in mice protects kidney from myocardial infarction-induced acute kidney injury. Am J Physiol Renal Physiol. 2015;309(6):F551–8. doi:10.1152/ajprenal.00076.2015.
66. Pellegrini KL, et al. MicroRNA-155 deficient mice experience heightened kidney toxicity when dosed with cisplatin. Toxicol Sci. 2014;141(2):484–92. doi:10.1093/toxsci/kfu143.
67. Qin W, Xie W, Yang X, Xia N, Yang K. Inhibiting microRNA-449 attenuates cisplatin-induced injury in NRK-52E cells possibly via regulating the SIRT1/P53/BAX pathway. Med Sci Monit. 2016;22:818–23.
68. Bellinger MA, et al. Concordant changes of plasma and kidney microRNA in the early stages of acute kidney injury: time course in a mouse model of bilateral renal ischemia-reperfusion. PLoS One. 2014;9(4):e93297. doi:10.1371/journal.pone.0093297.

11

Molecular characterization of exonic rearrangements and frame shifts in the *dystrophin* gene in Duchenne muscular dystrophy patients in a Saudi community

Nasser A. Elhawary[1,2*], Essam H. Jiffri[3], Samira Jambi[4], Ahmad H. Mufti[1], Anas Dannoun[1], Hassan Kordi[1], Asim Khogeer[5], Osama H. Jiffri[3], Abdelrahman N. Elhawary[6] and Mohammed T. Tayeb[1]

Abstract

Background: In individuals with Duchenne muscular dystrophy (DMD), exon skipping treatment to restore a wild-type phenotype or correct the frame shift of the mRNA transcript of the *dystrophin* (*DMD*) gene are mutation-specific. To explore the molecular characterization of *DMD* rearrangements and predict the reading frame, we simultaneously screened all 79 *DMD* gene exons of 45 unrelated male DMD patients using a multiplex ligation-dependent probe amplification (MLPA) assay for deletion/duplication patterns. Multiplex PCR was used to confirm single deletions detected by the MLPA.

Results: There was an obvious diagnostic delay, with an extremely statistically significant difference between the age at initial symptoms and the age of clinical evaluation of DMD cases (*t* value, 10.3; 95% confidence interval 5.95–8.80, $P < 0.0001$); the mean difference between the two groups was 7.4 years. Overall, we identified 147 intragenic rearrangements: 46.3% deletions and 53.7% duplications. Most of the deletions (92.5%) were between exons 44 and 56, with exon 50 being the most frequently involved (19.1%). Eight new rearrangements, including a mixed deletion/duplication and double duplications, were linked to seven cases with DMD. Of all the cases, 17.8% had duplications with no hot spots. In addition, confirmation of the reading frame hypothesis helped account for new *DMD* rearrangements in this study. We found that 81% of our Saudi patients would potentially benefit from exon skipping, of which 42.9% had a mutation amenable to skipping of exon 51.

Conclusions: Our study could generate considerable data on mutational rearrangements that may promote future experimental therapies in Saudi Arabia.

Keywords: Duchenne muscular dystrophy, *Dystrophin* gene, Large rearrangements, Frame shift, MLPA, Saudi community

Background

Dystrophinopathies are the most common form of muscular dystrophy in childhood. They are caused by mutations in the *dystrophin* gene (*DMD*; OMIM #300377) [1, 2]. Duchenne muscular dystrophy (DMD; OMIM #310200) is a severe form of muscular dystrophy, with an incidence of 1 in 3600–5000 male births [3]. Becker muscular dystrophy (BMD) is a milder form of DMD, with an incidence of 1 in 20,000 male births (BMD; OMIM # 300376) [4].

DMD is characterized by rapidly progressive degeneration and necrosis of the proximal muscles and calf pseudo-hypertrophy. Most *DMD* patients show muscle weakness at age 2 or 3, but it may be seen as early as infancy. Patients commonly lose independent ambulation by the age of 12 and die of dilated cardiomyopathy around the second or third decade. In comparison, patients with BMD exhibit relatively minor pathological

* Correspondence: naelhawary@uqu.edu.sa
[1]Department of Medical Genetics, Medicine College, Umm Al-Qura University, P.O. Box 57543, Mecca 21955, Saudi Arabia
[2]Department of Molecular Genetics, Faculty of Medicine, Ain Shams University, Cairo 11566, Egypt
Full list of author information is available at the end of the article

symptoms, slower progression, later onset, and longer survival. Patients with an intermediate form of the disease, intermediate muscular dystrophy (IMD), may continue to walk until they are 16 years of age [4, 5].

The *DMD* gene is one of the largest known genes in humans, with 79 exons (approximately 2.4 Mb of genomic DNA) [1] expressing a 427-kDa muscular protein that plays a fundamental role in stabilizing the sarcolemma. It does so by using a complex of glycoproteins associated with dystrophin to link actin filaments within the cytoskeleton and the extracellular matrix. Lack of dystrophin breaks these connections, altering the plasma membrane and finally producing myofiber degeneration and necrosis [6]. Thus, according to the reading frame hypothesis [7], *DMD* mutations that destroy the reading frame result in a truncated, non-functional dystrophin protein associated with a "DMD" phenotype. These mutations frequently generate a premature stop codon that activates nonsense-mediated mRNA decay [8]. On the other hand, mutations that maintain the reading frame can permit semi-functional dystrophin protein and thus give rise to a "BMD" phenotype [4, 9]. Together, these two phenotype-genotype correlations explain more than 92% of all cases [7].

Different types of mutations have been reported in patients with DMD and BMD. These are mainly large rearrangements (deletions in approximately 60–70% of patients and duplications in approximately 7–10%), with the remaining being point mutations (mainly nonsense mutations) and small deletions or insertions [10, 11]. Most gross deletions can be detected by multiplex PCR (mPCR) [12, 13] and are clustered in the proximal and central hot spot regions [14, 15]. Although a large proportion of the duplications were reported many years ago [16, 17], most laboratories do not systematically screen for these rearrangements. Duplication analysis and the determination of at-risk carrier status of the *DMD* gene require quantitative investigation, which is laborious and technically demanding [18, 19]. Previous studies have applied Southern blotting [16, 20], pulsed-field gel electrophoresis, quantitative mPCR [21–23], multiplex amplifiable probe hybridization [24], and comparative genomic hybridization microarray [25].

Given that deletions and duplications of one or more exons are found in the majority (70%) of patients, it is most cost-efficient and labor-efficient to check for these mutations first. A reliable and rapid technique, multiplex ligation-dependent probe amplification (MLPA), has been applied to cover the whole *DMD* gene to detect deletions and duplications and to identify exactly which exons are involved in deletions or duplications [18, 26–29]. This approach reveals whether a given exon is present and allows the copy number of each exon to be calculated by comparing relative peak heights. MLPA can detect both deletions and duplications in patients as well as in female carriers. Compared to array comparative genomic hybridization, MLPA is a low-cost and technically uncomplicated method.

Although several studies have investigated exonic deletions in different populations [11, 30–36], it is unknown where these deletions occur in the Saudi population. Although a few studies have described the molecular diagnosis of DMD in Saudi patients, the large deletions associated with disease were examined in only some exons, and the studies were limited by small sample sizes [37, 38]. Molecular characterization of the large *DMD* gene has been proposed to address large intragenic rearrangements in the whole exons of the *DMD* gene using an MLPA strategy covering nearly 75% of whole gene mutations. Thus, accurate molecular diagnosis may provide information on eligibility for mutation-specific treatments. A plausible frame shift hypothesis suggests how one might reduce disease severity via exon skipping, for example, by correcting the fidelity of the translational reading frame with large *DMD* deletions or restoring the wild type with large *DMD* duplications.

To our knowledge, the present study is the first study using the MLPA strategy to identify genotype-phenotype correlations in *DMD* patients in a Saudi community. Our results will add valuable data on de novo mutations in this population and to the databases of different DMD web pages as well.

Methods

Ethics statement and participants

All participants were enrolled under a protocol approved by the Institutional Biomedical Ethics Committee at Umm Al-Qura University (ref. #HAPO-02-K-012). Parents of all participants gave written consent after being informed about the aim of the study.

The study included 45 unrelated male patients with DMD selected from 65 families from the western region of the Kingdom of Saudi Arabia (KSA), including Jeddah, Mecca, Taif, and Hada. Twenty additional eligible male patients did not enroll because their parents refused to share their clinical data, their clinical profiles were incomplete, or their creatine phosphokinase assessments were missing. For each patient included in the study, a clinical data sheet was recorded in the database of the Molecular Genetics Laboratory in the Department of Medical Genetics at Umm Al-Qura University. Clinical information was independent of any molecular DNA data for the *DMD* gene or its protein. *Dystrophin* probands were diagnosed by clinical geneticists or pediatricians based on strict criteria including a clinical presentation expected for DMD, family history of X-linked muscular dystrophy, or muscle biopsy with a dystrophin analysis performed using immunohistochemistry. Clinical diagnosis of dystrophin probands included age at onset, age at clinical evaluation, calf pseudohypertrophy, age at wheelchair confinement, cardiac function, and motor function. A histopathological study was performed before molecular DNA analysis if muscle biopsies were available. To avoid bias, we included only one case for each family. We categorized patients according to age at loss of ambulation: DMD ≤ 12 years, IMD 12–16 years, and BMD > 16 years. Cases with a family history of autosomal recessive inheritance or with normal dystrophin protein were excluded.

DNA isolation

Genomic DNA was isolated from buccal cells using the Oragene DNA-OGR-575 kit (DNA Genotek Inc., Ottawa, ON, Canada) according to the manufacturer's protocol with some modifications. Briefly, the full buccal cells were collected within 30 min, and the Oragene tube was capped immediately. The cells were incubated with the OGR-lysis buffer in a water bath at 53 °C to release the DNA, which was then precipitated by ethanol and dissolved in elution buffer [39].

Multiplex polymerase chain reaction

The genomic DNA of all *DMD* patients was subjected to multiplex PCR (mPCR) to screen for *DMD* deletions using 15 primer sets (Additional file 1: Table S1). The oligonucleotides included flanking sequences of exons 4, 8, 12, 17, 19, 44, 45, 48, and 51 [12] and of exons 6, 13, 47, 50, 52, and 60 [13]. We made some modifications to Chamberlain's mPCR set by not adding dimethylsulfoxide, which could result in a lower PCR yield. However, PCR cycling was programmed as initial denaturing at 95 °C for 6 min (1 round), then 94 °C for 30 s, annealing at 53 °C for 30 s, 65 °C for 4 min (repeated for 23 rounds), and final elongation at 65 °C for 7 min [12]. Hot-start mPCR was performed using Beggs' PCR program [13]: 95 °C for 6 min (1 round) and 25 subsequent cycles including DNA denaturing at 95 °C for 30 s, annealing at 56 °C for 1 min, and elongation at 68 °C for 4 min. Amplification reactions were carried out on thermal cycler Engine Dyad (Bio-Rad Laboratories Inc., Hercules, CA). PCR products (10–15 μl) were separated on 3% NuSieve agarose (BMA Bioproducts, Rockland, ME). The gels were viewed using the Gel Documentation and Analysis System (G-Box, SynGene, Frederick, MD, USA).

Multiplex ligation-dependent probe amplification

We analyzed all DMD cases for large deletions and large duplications using MLPA SALSA P034/P035 DMD kits (http://www.mrc-holland.com) following the manufacturer's instructions. In brief, denaturation, hybridization, ligation, and amplification steps were performed on a DNA Engine Dyad thermal cycler (Bio-Rad Laboratories Inc., Hercules, CA). Finally, PCR amplification was performed using SALSA MLPA PCR primers labeled with the FAM dye. A mixture of 0.7 μl of PCR product, 0.2 μl of 600 LIZ GS size-standard, and 9.0 μl of Hi-Di formamide was incubated for 3 min at 86 °C and cooled at 4 °C for 2 min. The MLPA product mix was separated on a POP7 polymer (Applied Biosystems Inc., Life Technologies, Foster City, CA) at 60 °C with the setting of 1.6 kV for injection voltage, 18 s for injection time, 15 kV for run voltage, and 1800 s for run time.

Data analysis

The raw data were analyzed using GeneMapper Software 5 (Applied Biosystems Inc., Life Technologies, Foster City, CA). The DNA of cases with single-exon deletions were re-examined using conventional PCR. Initial analysis was performed with the naked eye to look for missed exon-specific peaks. For the remaining samples, the peak height of each exon was divided by the two nearest control peaks. The median ratio across all samples for each peak was calculated and used as a reference for one copy. For the sake of accuracy, any normalized ratio below 0.3 was considered a possible deletion. A duplication was considered if a normalized ratio was 1.8–2.0. If any single-exon deletion was identified, conventional PCR amplification was carried out to validate this deletion using primer sets and PCR conditions given in the Leiden Muscular Dystrophy pages (http://www.dmd.nl).

Databases and confirming mutations for the DMD gene

We checked all mutations recorded in this study according to available databases established by the Leiden Muscular Dystrophy pages (http://www.dmd.nl) [40], the Leiden Open Variation Database 3.0 (http://www.lovd.nl/3.0/home) [41], and UMD-DMD (http://www.umd.be/DMD/) [31, 32]. Databases for exon skipping to restore the DMD reading frame were found on sites developed by Leiden University Medical Center (http://www.exonskipping.nl/?s=exon+skipping&submit=Go) and CureDuchenne (https://www.cureduchenne.org/cure/edystrophin/).

Statistical analysis

Hardy-Weinberg equilibrium (HWE) deviation was examined for X-linked *DMD* cases in this study using the Online Encyclopedia for Genetic Epidemiology studies software (http://www.oege.org/software/hwe-mr-calc.shtml). We used the G*Power Software (http://www.psycho.uni-duesseldorf.de/abteilungen/aap/gpower3/download-and-register/) to estimate power analysis to determine adequate sample sizes to achieve an 80% power for t testing of point biserial model. "*Priori*" sample size and "*post hoc*" power estimations were tested knowing our DMD sample size, a probability of $\alpha = 0.05$, and the effect size index "r" (the absolute value of the correlation coefficient in the population, $0 < "r" < 1$). We used paired t test analysis to compare the significant difference between the age at onset and the age of clinical evaluation for each *DMD* case. A two-sided P value less than 0.05 was considered to indicate statistical significance and 95% confidence interval (CI) for all analyses.

Results

Clinical profile

Among 45 unrelated patients, 21 were diagnosed with DMD, 10 with IMD, and 5 with BMD. The unassigned patients were defined as not determined (ND), as they were too young to permit a definitive diagnosis ($n = 9$). The median age at onset was 3.5 years (range 1.0–7. 0 years), while the median presenting age was 11.5 years (1.5–20 years) (Fig. 1). Most of the patients reported initial symptoms between 1 and 3 years of age (71.1%, 32/45), followed by those reporting symptoms at 4–5 years (24.4%, 11/45). The age at clinical evaluation was most frequently between 10 and 12 years (35.6%, 16/45). We found an extremely statistically significant difference between the age at initial symptoms and the age at clinical evaluation of DMD cases (t value, 10.3; 95% CI 5.95–8.8, $P < 0.0001$). The mean difference in age between the two groups was 7.4 years.

Hardy-Weinberg equilibrium

All affected males were in HWE at the *DMD* gene deletions/duplications ($\chi^2 = 1.00$, $P = 0.317$), where the heterozygotes were absent in such X-linked recessive mode of inheritance.

Large-scale rearrangements

Using mPCR, we identified 55 large deletions in the 45 unrelated *DMD* patients. MLPA detected 147 intragenic rearrangements, 68 (46.3%) of which were large deletions and 79 (53.7%) of which were large duplications. All deletions identified by mPCR were confirmed by the MLPA-based screening. The utility of MLPA assay for all exons is clear, as 13 (19%) of 68 deletions were detected using MLPA but were not detected by conventional mPCR analysis. The percentage of cases with deletions and duplications were 46.7% (21/45) and 17.8% (8/45), respectively. Table 1 includes the large rearrangements that were identified in the present study and had been previously described.

New mutations in the *DMD* gene

We also identified seven previously undescribed large *DMD* rearrangements from eight Saudi cases. These new mutations, based on the *DMD* databases [31, 32, 40, 41], included one mixed rearrangement (del 45–52 + dup 21–23), one large deletion (del 45–56), two large duplications (8–30 and 17–24), and three double duplications (dup 2–4 + dup 18–19, dup 13 + dup 21–24, and dup 56–58 + dup 62–64). These large mutations were from eight (17.8%) of the Saudi patients (Table 2).

Distribution of rearrangements

In this study, deletions did not have a random distribution. We found that 92.5% (63/68) of hot spot deletions were linked to exons 44–56 (central region), whereas 7. 5% (5/68) of deletions were related to exons 10–20. Exon 50 was most frequently involved in deletions (19. 1%, 13/68), followed by exons 48 and 49 (each 11.8%, 8/68). The rate of deletions increased from a minimum in exon 44 to a maximum in exon 50 and then decreased until the 3′ end of the *DMD* gene, with no deletion in exons 57–79 (distal region) (Fig. 2). Moreover, we found that the number of cases with a deletion of *only* one exon was lower than the number with deletions of more than one exon (9/21, 42.8% versus 12/21, 57.1%). About half of the deletions (44.4%) were detected only once, in

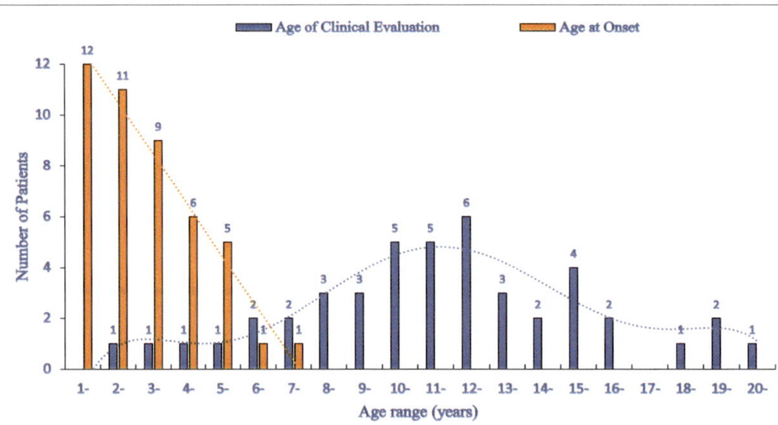

Fig. 1 The age at onset and the age of clinical evaluation of DMD patients in this study. The analysis of DMD cases showed an apparent diagnostic delay

Table 1 Previously described large rearrangements identified in this study and their reading frame shifts

Family no.	Phenotype	Multiplex PCR	MLPA del/dup	Exon(s) del/dup	Codons del/dup	Frame shift	Amino acid change[a]	cDNA[a]
DS-23	DMD	No del	Del 10–11	371	123 2/3	Stop at 323	p.His321PhefsX3	c.961_1331del
DS-1	DMD	Del 19	Del 18–20	454	151 1/3	− 1	p.Arg723Lys874	c.2169_2622del
DS-37	IMD	Del 44	Del 44	148	49 1/3	Stop at 2113	p.Arg2098AsnfsX16	c.6291_6438del
DS-34	ND	Del 44–48	Del 44–48	808	269 1/3	− 1	p.Arg2098Gln2366del	c.6291_7098del
DS-24	DMD	Del 45	Del 45	176	58 2/3	Stop at 2163	p.Glu2147AlafsX17	c.6439_6614del
DS-8	IMD	Del 45–50	Del 45–50	871	290 1/3	Stop at 2155	p.Glu2147LeufsX9	c.6439_7309del
DS-38	IMD	Del 45–52	Del 45–52	1222	407 1/3	Stop at 2168	p.Glu2147LeufsX22	c.6439_7660del
DS-29	DMD	Del 47–50	Del 47–50	547	182 1/3	Stop at 2263	p.Val2257LeufsX7	c.6763_7309del
DS-20	ND	Del 47–50	Del 47–50	547	182 1/3	Stop at 2263	p.Val2257LeufsX7	c.6763_7309del
DS-48	BMD	Del 48	Del 48	186	62	*In-frame*	p.Val2305Gln2366del	c.6913_7098del
DS-30	DMD	Del 50	Del 49–50	211	70 1/3	Stop at 2375	p.Glu2367LeufsX9	c.7099_7309del
DS-31	IMD	Del 50	Del 49–50	211	70 1/3	Stop at 2375	p.Glu2367LeufsX9	c.7099_7309del
DS-36	DMD	Del 50	Del 50	109	36 1/3	Stop at 2409	p.Arg2401LeufsX9	c.7201_7309del
DS-32	IMD	Del 50	Del 50	109	36 1/3	Stop at 2409	p.Arg2401LeufsX9	c.7201_7309del
DS-33	ND	Del 50	Del 50	109	36 1/3	Stop at 2409	p.Arg2401LeufsX9	c.7201_7309del
DS-35	ND	Del 50	Del 50	109	36 1/3	Stop at 2409	p.Arg2401LeufsX9	c.7201_7309del
DS-27	ND	Del 50–52	Del 50–52	460	153 1/3	Stop at 2422	p.Arg2401LeufsX22	c.7201_7660del
DS-12	DMD	Del 51	Del 51	233	77 2/3	Stop at 2469	p.Ser2437CysfsX33	c.7310_7542del
DS-18	DMD	No del	Del 55	190	63 1/3	Stop at 2700	p.Val2677ThrfsX24	c.8028_8217del
DS-11	ND	No del	Dup 50–51	343	114	*In-frame*	p.Arg2401Lys2514dup	c.7201-?_7542+?dup

DMD Duchenne muscular dystrophy, *IMD* intermediate muscular dystrophy, *BMD* Becker muscular dystrophy, *ND* not determined
[a]These data are based on the Leiden Muscular Dystrophy Pages (http://www.dmd.nl/) and the UMD-DMD (http://www.umd.be/DMD/)

agreement with the high allelic heterogeneity of the *DMD* gene.

Duplications were distributed in the proximal (68/79, 86.1%), central (5/79, 6.3%), and distal regions (6/79, 7.6%) (Fig. 2). Unlike deletions, duplicated exons were more frequent in the proximal region (26 duplications) than in the central and distal regions (13 duplications). The most frequent duplications were of exons 21, 22, and 23 (7.6%, 6/79 each), followed by exons 18 and 19 (5.1%, 4/79 each). We did not find any duplications in exons 31–49 (central region) or exons 69–79 (distal region) within our cases (Fig. 2). Similar to deletions, 42.5% of exonic duplications (17/40) were observed only once, revealing a considerable heterogeneity of duplications.

Reading frame shift and phenotype correlation

Gene rearrangements (deletions and duplications) were correlated with clinical phenotypes in 28 unrelated cases: 11 (39.3%) with DMD, 7 (25%) with IMD, 3 (10.7%) with BMD, and 7 (25%) with ND. We also predicted the translational reading frame in 28 DMD cases with rearrangements identified in this study, using the Leiden Muscular Dystrophy pages (http://www.dmd.nl). Applying the reading frame rule revealed consistency with the frame shift rule for 90.9% (10/11) of the individuals with

Table 2 New *DMD* mutational rearrangements identified in this study and their predicted reading frame shifts

Case no.	Phenotype	Multiplex PCR	MLPA del/dup	Exon(s) del/dup	Codons del/dup	Frame shift	Amino acid change[a]
DS-2	DMD	No del	dup 2–4 and dup 18–19	233; 212	77 $^{2/3}$ 70 $^{2/3}$	+ 2 + 2	p.Val89MetfsX15 [b] p.Lys724Gly795fsX1
DS-14	DMD	No del	dup 8–30	3679	1226 $^{1/3}$	+ 1	p.Val218K1412fsX
DS-15	ND	No del	dup 8–30	3679	1226 $^{1/3}$	+ 1	p.Val218K1412fsX
DS-52	BMD	No del	dup 13 and dup 21–24	120 654	40 218	0 0	p.Val495Val535dup p.Asp875Lys1093dup
DS-50	BMD	No del	dup 17–24	1248	428	0	p.Ile665Lys1093dup
DS-53	IMD	del 45–51	del 45–52 and dup 21–23	1222; 540	407 $^{1/3}$ 180	– 1[c] 0	p.Glu2147LeufsX22 [C] p.Asp875Asn1055dup
DS-25	IMD	del 45–51	del 45–56	1952	650 $^{2/3}$	– 2	p.Glu2147Ser2798
DS-22	DMD	No del	dup 56–58 and dup 62–64	451 198	150 $^{1/3}$ 66	+ 1 0	p.Ser2798Lys2891fsX4 p.Ser3056Asp3122

DMD Duchenne muscular dystrophy, *IMD* intermediate muscular dystrophy, *BMD* Becker muscular dystrophy, *ND* not determined
[a]Theoretical amino acid change based on the database of the Leiden Muscular Dystrophy Pages (http://www.dmd.nl/)
[b]Previously described duplication at cDNA (c.6439_7660del) showing amino acid change (p.Glu2147LeufsX22) resulting in a termination transcript at codon 2168
[c]Previously described deletion at cDNA (c.32_265dup) showing amino acid change (p.Val89MetfsX15) resulting in a termination transcript at codon 103

DMD phenotypes and 100% (7/7) of the individuals with IMD phenotypes. Likewise, the *DMD* genes in all cases with BMD phenotypes had in-frame functional effects on the DMD protein (cases #DS-48, #DS-50, and #DS-52) (Tables 1 and 2). All previously described rearrangements we detected gave rise to a stop codon and thus a truncated protein, except for case #DS-48 with a BMD phenotype and case #DS-11 with ND, which gave rise to in-frame predictions (Table 2). Two cases identified in this study (#DS-53 and #DS-22) reflected both in-frame and reading frame shift predictions (Fig. 3). The complex rearrangement of case #DS-53 (del 45–52 + dup 21–23) was associated with an IMD phenotype, with translational reading frame predictions with in-frame and frame shift patterns (Fig. 3). This phenotype may have occurred from the addition of exons 21–23 to the mRNA transcript lessening the damaging effect of del 45–52 on the functional protein. On the contrary, case #DS-22 could not have corrected for the harmful dup 56–58, giving rise to a DMD phenotype (Table 2).

Discussion

The present study used a facile, reliable, and time-consuming MLPA strategy to identify large rearrangements covering all 79 exons of the *DMD* gene. Our results showed the prevalence of 46.7 and 17.8%, respectively, for large deletions and large duplications in 45 Saudi patients with DMD. Unlike the hot spot deletions in exons 44–56 (92.5%), the hot spot deletions near the 5′ end of the gene were not distinctive, and no large hot spot duplications were found anywhere along the *DMD* gene. The presence of an unusual MLPA pattern in our Saudi sample, including non-contiguous duplications as well as contiguous deletions combined with

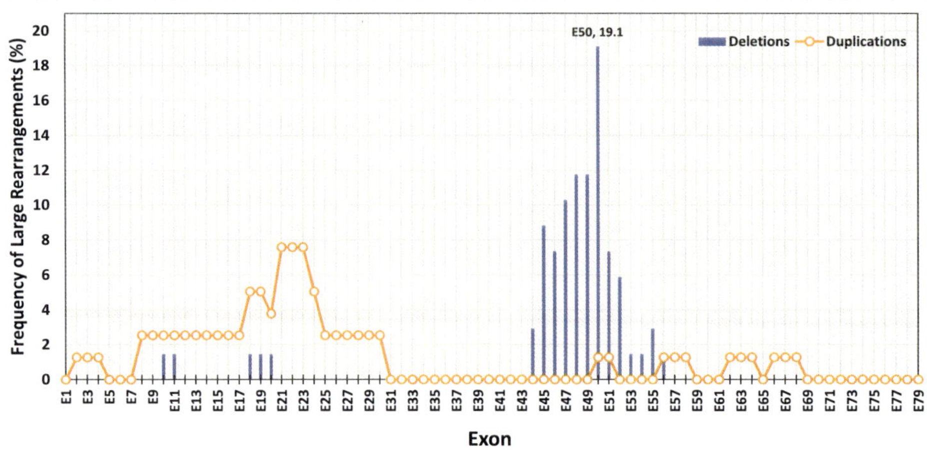

Fig. 2 The frequency of large mutational rearrangements for each exon of the *DMD* gene. A region with a high frequency of deletions was found in exons 44–56. No such region of frequency was detected for large duplications

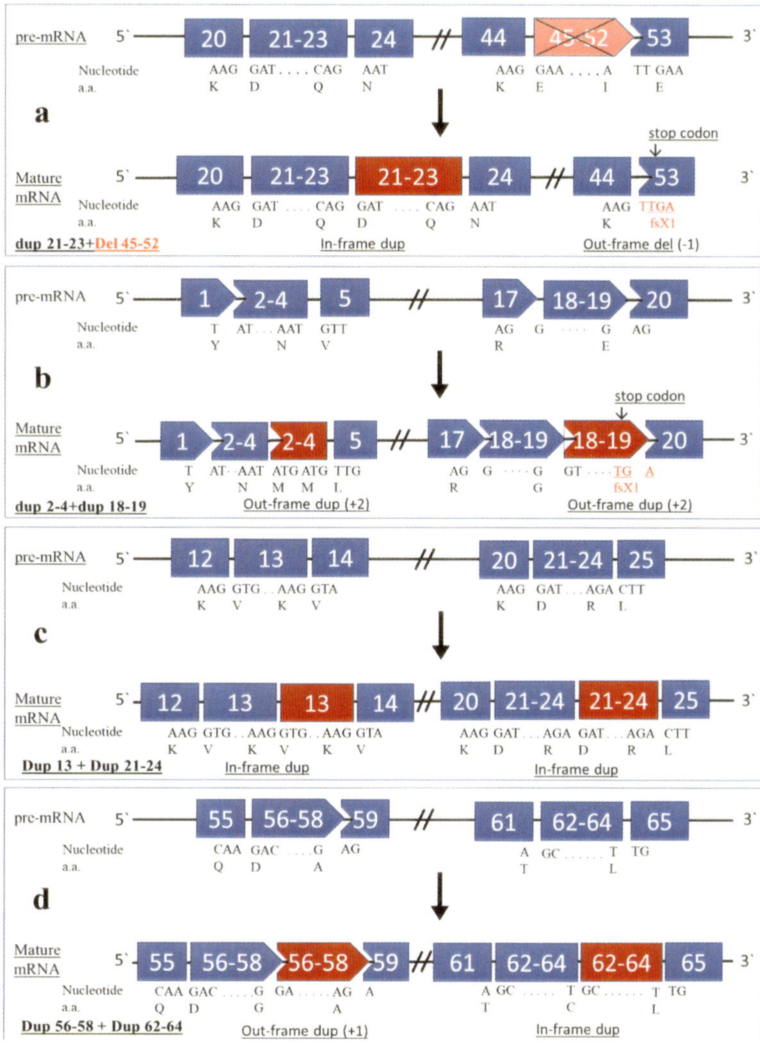

Fig. 3 A schematic overview of new complex large rearrangements in the *DMD* gene. **a** The case #DS-53 with an unusual mixed rearrangement (dup 21–23 + del 45–52) leads to an out-of-frame shift giving rise to a severe DMD phenotype. **b** The case #DS2 with a double duplication (dup 2–4 + dup 18–19) results in out-of-frame shifts with a DMD phenotype. **c** The case #DS-52 with two *in-frame* shift due to double duplications (dup 13 + dup 21–24) giving rise to a BMD phenotype. **d** The case #DS-22 showed two double duplications within the mature mRNA giving an out-frame (dup 56–58), in-frame (dup 62–64) mutations giving rise to a DMD phenotype

non-contiguous duplications, suggests complex rearrangements. Our findings regarding double, separate duplications and complex rearrangements are consistent with some previous reports in Serbian and South African patients [18, 42].

Results from MLPA-related studies among different ethnic populations are conflicting in terms of rates of large rearrangements within the *DMD* gene. Studies have found rates of deletions (and duplications) of 71.8–79.0% (16.4–19.8%) in Chinese [29], 79.5% (6.5%) in Indian [43], 60% (10.0%) in Japanese [44], 45.5–71.8% (16.7%) in Korean [35], and 28.2% (20.5%) in Taiwanese [45] populations. When compared with our sample, a Turkish sample has also been shown to have a relatively higher rate of deletions within the *DMD* gene (63.7%) [46], likely because of admixture with other European ethnicities. Rates of *DMD* deletions and duplications in some other Middle Eastern populations are more similar to what we found: Egyptian (51.3% deletions) [47], Iranian (51% deletions) [48], Moroccan (51% deletions) [49], and Syrian (49.0% deletions; 9.8% duplications) [50]. The majority of the reported *DMD* gene mutations in our Saudi data showed translational reading frame shifts (94.4%), while 5.6% of the mutations did not follow the reading frame rule. This latter outcome is relatively consistent with the corresponding values in the TREAT-NMD DMD Global database (7%) [11], the UMD-DMD database (4%) [32], and the Leiden database (9%) [41].

The overall rate of consanguinity in KSA is 57.7%, ranging from 34 to 80.6% [51], with lower rates in Mecca

(North Western region) than in Riyadh (Central region) (44.1% versus 62.8%) [51]. This may account for the increased deletions in patients of Riyadh (21/27, 77.8%) when compared with those in our study [37]. During Muslim immigration from the Levant, Africa, in Ancient Islamic times, much intermarriage reinforced gene flow of the *DMD* gene to the Saudi people. This has likely influenced the prevalence of different Mendelian patterns, particularly X-linked types, exemplified by the consistency of data for *DMD* rearrangements between our study and a recent Spanish cohort study (46.1%, 131/284 for deletions and 56/284, 19.7% for duplications) [52].

It is noteworthy that some populations have inherent reproductive barriers that prevent interbreeding, which keeps them at native levels without merging (i.e., cryptic taxa). Other populations may lack inherent reproductive isolation. Therefore, admixture among different geographical populations might increase genetic variations and perhaps create new genotypic combinations within non-isolated (or non-native) populations [53]. Thus, genetic variations among Gulf Arabs and some Middle Eastern individuals (e.g., Barbarians in North Africa, Kurdish, Upper Egyptian) [54, 55] should be handled with caution, as increased consanguinity, extensive reproductive isolation, and admixture with native source populations (e.g., Black Africans, South Eastern Asians, Caucasians) have had substantial roles in gene flow or founder effects in these populations.

In our study, the analysis of *DMD* cases showed an apparent diagnostic delay, as 69.8% of our patients showed their first symptoms at an early age (1–3 years), but 44% of these patients were 9–12 years old at first clinical examination. Other countries have also reported long delays in diagnosis of the disease, with a mean delay between 1.6 and 2.5 years [56, 57]. In south China, the first symptoms occurred by 3 years of age, but the age at clinical evaluation was 6–8 years [36]. Numerous studies have advocated raising public awareness to identify early symptoms in DMD patients [47, 57, 58], as parents are usually the first to notice symptoms, which prompt them to visit a health professional. To further reduce diagnostic delay, creatine phosphokinase (CPK) testing should be emphasized in primary care and performed as a routine test in children's physical examinations.

Earlier clinical trials reported the safety and biochemical efficacy of intravenous or intramuscular administration of antisense oligonucleotides (20-30 mer) to bring hope to DMD patients with large deletions [59]. Therefore, inducing exon 51 skipping to restore the open reading frame is an attractive therapeutic strategy that can be achieved with splice-switching oligomers. After the US Food and Drug Administration (FDA) accelerated approval of AVI-4658/eteplirsen (Exondys 51; Sarepta Therapeutics Inc., Cambridge, MA, USA), targeting *DMD* exon 51 skipping, *eteplirsen* was approved and introduced in some countries [60–63]. Eteplirsen is useful for patients with amenable *DMD* deletions, ending at exon 50 and starting at exon 52 [64]. To date, eteplirsen has not been approved by the Saudi FDA (https://www.sfda.gov.sa). Hence, numerous efforts have used antisense oligomers to target exon skipping of exon 53 (SRP4053, PRO053), exon 45 (DS-514b, SRP4045), and exon 44 (PRO044) (https://www.clinicaltrials.gov/beta/home) [62, 65]. Based on our data for deletions, exon skipping could eventually apply to 81% (17/21) of DMD cases with large deletions. Among our Saudi patients with *DMD* gene deletions, the exons most frequently skipped were exons 51 (42.9%, 9/21), 53 (14.3%, 3/21), 44 (9.5%, 2/21), 45 (4.8%, 1/21), 43 (4.8%, 1/21), and 50 (4.8%, 1/21). Wein et al. have recently reported the efficiency of exon skipping in the *DMD* gene, with each duplicated exon expressing a wild-type, full-length mRNA [66]. For more than one duplicated exon, several antisense oligomers can be delivered as a cocktail of drugs to skip larger regions of the transcript. Thus, for duplications in exons 45–55, therapeutic skipping can be applied to more than 60% of all DMD patients [67].

Although the power is conventionally utilized for polygenic disorders, the power under different monogenic model of inheritance has not been systematically considered. This issue could be explained because of wide issues, for example, rate of background variation in disease-associated genes, mode of inheritance, extent of penetrance, and locus heterogeneity.

In contrast to dominant model of inheritance, the incomplete penetrance does not hold for the recessive model, and in consequence, much smaller sample sizes are needed under a recessive model, even in the presence of high locus heterogeneity [68]. According to our *priori* sample size estimations at the effect size "r" = 0.3 (medium effect), or "r" = 0.5 (strong effect), we would need 64 or 21 sample sizes, respectively, to ensure a power detection of 80%. Thus, post hoc analysis using our DMD sample size data in this study ($n = 45$ cases) could achieve the power of 66.7% ($r = 0.3$) and 98.5% ($r = 0.5$).

Pinning down the spectrum of mutations for *DMD* has been difficult because of poor replication of studies. First, when compared with our study, some studies have had populations with admixed ethnicities, conflicted outcomes, or small sample sizes, which lessen the strength of the overall results. Second, various molecular technologies have been utilized to examine *DMD* patients, resulting in a broad range of false-positive or false-negative results regarding rearrangements. Our study mainly used the *DMD* MLPA test, providing a cheap and straightforward DNA-based test that can screen for deletions and duplications and be performed in any

DNA laboratory. Third, insufficient communication between clinicians and geneticists, because of difficulty accessing hospitals of interest, may result in underdiagnosis of critical cases. However, precise coordination between clinicians and geneticists may help promote and improve the genetic diagnosis of dystrophinopathies and ameliorate potential therapies in these cases.

Conclusions

We detected nine previously undescribed exonic rearrangements within the *DMD* gene, including one unusual mixed rearrangement. MLPA or mPCR can be used to define the molecular characteristics of *DMD* rearrangements and hence the effects of the frame shifts on genotype-phenotype correlations in Saudi patients. This information will also be important for future gene therapy targeting exon skipping of the *DMD* gene. Our clinical characteristics revealed a diagnostic delay, suggesting the need for more public awareness about early symptoms of disease. However, CPK testing should also be performed as a routine test in children's hospitals and in primary care settings. In KSA, molecular testing of DMD patients should be covered by medical insurance, at least once in a lifetime. This single test could lead to genetic diagnosis of more patients. The large deletions and duplications we identified are predictive and intriguing, but the study needs to be replicated in different ethnic populations of the Middle East, as well as in other Saudi governorates. Though the sample size for this study might not have been large enough to explore the *DMD* mutational mechanisms, extensive sequencing analyses will be needed to discover the *DMD* breakpoints at the nucleotide level. Ongoing analyses of whole-exome sequences for Saudi patients with DMD are being carried out to identify the small breakpoints within the *DMD* gene.

Abbreviations

BMD: Becker muscular dystrophy; CPK: Creatine phosphokinase; DMD: Duchenne muscular dystrophy; FDA: Food and Drug Administration; IMD: Intermediate muscular dystrophy; KSA: Kingdom of Saudi Arabia; MLPA: Multiplex ligation-probe dependent amplification; ND: Not determined

Acknowledgements

The authors would like to thank the parents of the cases for their participation in this study. The authors also thank the Institute of Scientific Research at Umm Al-Qura University (Project #43309030) for financial support and the Faculty of Medicine, Cairo University-Giza, Egypt, for allowing ANE to assist the following up the clinical phenotypes of the *DMD* cases.

Funding

This work was funded through grants from the Institute of Scientific Research at Umm Al-Qura University (Project #43309030).

Authors' contributions

NAE and MTT designed the research; NAE, MTT, SJ, AD, EHJ, ANE, HK, and AK performed the research; NAE, MTT, and AHM analyzed the data; NAE, MTT, NB, KFA, and MR wrote the paper. Also, NAE and MTT initiated the grant funding through a contract with the Institute of Scientific Research at Umm Al-Qura University. All authors read and approved the final manuscript.

Competing interests

The authors declare that they have no competing interests.

Author details

[1]Department of Medical Genetics, Medicine College, Umm Al-Qura University, P.O. Box 57543, Mecca 21955, Saudi Arabia. [2]Department of Molecular Genetics, Faculty of Medicine, Ain Shams University, Cairo 11566, Egypt. [3]Department of Medical Laboratory Technology, Faculty of Applied Medical Sciences, King Abdul-Aziz University, Jeddah, Saudi Arabia. [4]Department of Pediatrics, Al Hada Military Hospital, Al Hada, Saudi Arabia. [5]Department of Plan and Research, General Directorate of Health Affairs, Mecca Region, Ministry of Health, Mecca, Saudi Arabia. [6]Department of Pediatrics, Faculty of Medicine, Cairo University, Giza, Egypt.

References

1. Hoffman EP, Brown RH Jr, Kunkel LM. Dystrophin: the protein product of the Duchenne muscular dystrophy locus. Cell. 1987;51(6):919–28.
2. Koenig M, Monaco AP, Kunkel LM. The complete sequence of dystrophin predicts a rod-shaped cytoskeletal protein. Cell. 1988;53(2):219–28.
3. Emery AE. Population frequencies of inherited neuromuscular diseases—a world survey. Neuromuscul Disord. 1991;1(1):19–29.
4. Bushby K, Finkel R, Birnkrant DJ, Case LE, Clemens PR, Cripe L, Kaul A, Kinnett K, McDonald C, Pandya S, et al. Diagnosis and management of Duchenne muscular dystrophy, part 1: diagnosis, and pharmacological and psychosocial management. Lancet Neurol. 2010;9(1):77–93.
5. Jarmin S, Kymalainen H, Popplewell L, Dickson G. New developments in the use of gene therapy to treat Duchenne muscular dystrophy. Expert Opin Biol Ther. 2014;14(2):209–30.
6. Durbeej M, Campbell KP. Muscular dystrophies involving the dystrophin-glycoprotein complex: an overview of current mouse models. Curr Opin Genet Dev. 2002;12(3):349–61.
7. Monaco AP, Bertelson CJ, Liechti-Gallati S, Moser H, Kunkel LM. An explanation for the phenotypic differences between patients bearing partial deletions of the DMD locus. Genomics. 1988;2(1):90–5.
8. Hentze MW, Kulozik AE. A perfect message: RNA surveillance and nonsense-mediated decay. Cell. 1999;96(3):307–10.
9. Muntoni F, Torelli S, Ferlini A. Dystrophin and mutations: one gene, several proteins, multiple phenotypes. Lancet Neurol. 2003;2(12):731–40.
10. Flanigan KM, Dunn DM, von Niederhausern A, Howard MT, Mendell J, Connolly A, Saunders C, Modrcin A, Dasouki M, Comi GP, et al. DMD Trp3X nonsense mutation associated with a founder effect in North American families with mild Becker muscular dystrophy. Neuromuscul Disord. 2009; 19(11):743–8.
11. Bladen CL, Salgado D, Monges S, Foncuberta ME, Kekou K, Kosma K, Dawkins H, Lamont L, Roy AJ, Chamova T, et al. The TREAT-NMD DMD Global Database: analysis of more than 7,000 Duchenne muscular dystrophy mutations. Hum Mutat. 2015;36(4):395–402.
12. Chamberlain JS, Gibbs RA, Ranier JE, Nguyen PN, Caskey CT. Deletion screening of the Duchenne muscular dystrophy locus via multiplex DNA amplification. Nucleic Acids Res. 1988;16(23):11141–56.
13. Beggs AH, Koenig M, Boyce FM, Kunkel LM. Detection of 98% of DMD/BMD gene deletions by polymerase chain reaction. Hum Genet. 1990;86(1):45–8.
14. Forrest SM, Cross GS, Speer A, Gardner-Medwin D, Burn J, Davies KE. Preferential deletion of exons in Duchenne and Becker muscular dystrophies. Nature. 1987;329(6140):638–40.
15. Oudet C, Hanauer A, Clemens P, Caskey T, Mandel JL. Two hot spots of recombination in the DMD gene correlate with the deletion prone regions. Hum Mol Genet. 1992;1(8):599–603.
16. Den Dunnen JT, Grootscholten PM, Bakker E, Blonden LA, Ginjaar HB, Wapenaar MC, van Paassen HM, van Broeckhoven C, Pearson PL, van Ommen GJ. Topography of the Duchenne muscular dystrophy (DMD) gene: FIGE and cDNA analysis of 194 cases reveals 115 deletions and 13 duplications. Am J Hum Genet. 1989;45(6):835–47.

17. Hu XY, Ray PN, Murphy EG, Thompson MW, Worton RG. Duplicational mutation at the Duchenne muscular dystrophy locus: its frequency, distribution, origin, and phenotypegenotype correlation. Am J Hum Genet. 1990;46(4):682–95.
18. Lalic T, Vossen RH, Coffa J, Schouten JP, Guc-Scekic M, Radivojevic D, Djurisic M, Breuning MH, White SJ, den Dunnen JT. Deletion and duplication screening in the DMD gene using MLPA. Eur J Hum Genet. 2005;13(11):1231–4.
19. Elhawary NA, Shawky RM, Elsayed N. High-precision DNA microsatellite genotyping in Duchenne muscular dystrophy families using ion-pair reversed-phase high performance liquid chromatography. Clin Biochem. 2006;39(7):758–61.
20. Koenig M, Hoffman EP, Bertelson CJ, Monaco AP, Feener C, Kunkel LM. Complete cloning of the Duchenne muscular dystrophy (DMD) cDNA and preliminary genomic organization of the DMD gene in normal and affected individuals. Cell. 1987;50(3):509–17.
21. Ioannou P, Christopoulos G, Panayides K, Kleanthous M, Middleton L. Detection of Duchenne and Becker muscular dystrophy carriers by quantitative multiplex polymerase chain reaction analysis. Neurol. 1992;42(9):1783–90.
22. Kodaira M, Hiyama K, Karakawa T, Kameo H, Satoh C. Duplication detection in Japanese Duchenne muscular dystrophy patients and identification of carriers with partial gene deletions using pulsed-field gel electrophoresis. Hum Genet. 1993;92(3):237–43.
23. Yau SC, Bobrow M, Mathew CG, Abbs SJ. Accurate diagnosis of carriers of deletions and duplications in Duchenne/Becker muscular dystrophy by fluorescent dosage analysis. J Med Genet. 1996;33(7):550–8.
24. White S, Kalf M, Liu Q, Villerius M, Engelsma D, Kriek M, Vollebregt E, Bakker B, van Ommen GJ, Breuning MH, et al. Comprehensive detection of genomic duplications and deletions in the DMD gene, by use of multiplex amplifiable probe hybridization. Am J Hum Genet. 2002;71(2):365–74.
25. del Gaudio D, Yang Y, Boggs BA, Schmitt ES, Lee JA, Sahoo T, Pham HT, Wiszniewska J, Chinault AC, Beaudet AL, et al. Molecular diagnosis of Duchenne/Becker muscular dystrophy: enhanced detection of dystrophin gene rearrangements by oligonucleotide array-comparative genomic hybridization. Hum Mutat. 2008;29(9):1100–7.
26. Schouten JP, McElgunn CJ, Waaijer R, Zwijnenburg D, Diepvens F, Pals G. Relative quantification of 40 nucleic acid sequences by multiplex ligation-dependent probe amplification. Nucleic Acids Res. 2002;30(12):e57.
27. Schwartz M, Duno M. Improved molecular diagnosis of dystrophin gene mutations using the multiplex ligation-dependent probe amplification method. Genet Test. 2004;8(4):361–7.
28. Janssen B, Hartmann C, Scholz V, Jauch A, Zschocke J. MLPA analysis for the detection of deletions, duplications and complex rearrangements in the dystrophin gene: potential and pitfalls. Neurogenetics. 2005;6(1):29–35.
29. Chen C, Ma H, Zhang F, Chen L, Xing X, Wang S, Zhang X, Luo Y. Screening of Duchenne muscular dystrophy (DMD) mutations and investigating its mutational mechanism in Chinese patients. PLoS One. 2014;9(9):e108038.
30. Nobile C, Toffolatti L, Rizzi F, Simionati B, Nigro V, Cardazzo B, Patarnello T, Valle G, Danieli GA. Analysis of 22 deletion breakpoints in dystrophin intron 49. Hum Genet. 2002;110(5):418–21.
31. Cotton RG, Auerbach AD, Beckmann JS, Blumenfeld OO, Brookes AJ, Brown AF, Carrera P, Cox DW, Gottlieb B, Greenblatt MS, et al. Recommendations for locus-specific databases and their curation. Hum Mutat. 2008;29(1):2–5.
32. Tuffery-Giraud S, Beroud C, Leturcq F, Yaou RB, Hamroun D, Michel-Calemard L, Moizard MP, Bernard R, Cossee M, Boisseau P, et al. Genotype-phenotype analysis in 2,405 patients with a dystrophinopathy using the UMD-DMD database: a model of nationwide knowledgebase. Hum Mutat. 2009;30(6):934–45.
33. Mitsui J, Takahashi Y, Goto J, Tomiyama H, Ishikawa S, Yoshino H, Minami N, Smith DI, Lesage S, Aburatani H, et al. Mechanisms of genomic instabilities underlying two common fragile-site-associated loci, PARK2 and DMD, in germ cell and cancer cell lines. Am J Hum Genet. 2010;87(1):75–89.
34. Ankala A, Kohn JN, Hegde A, Meka A, Ephrem CL, Askree SH, Bhide S, Hegde MR. Aberrant firing of replication origins potentially explains intragenic nonrecurrent rearrangements within genes, including the human DMD gene. Genome Res. 2012;22(1):25–34.
35. Suh MR, Lee KA, Kim EY, Jung J, Choi WA, Kang SW. Multiplex ligation-dependent probe amplification in X-linked recessive muscular dystrophy in Korean subjects. Yonsei Med J. 2017;58(3):613 8.
36. Wang DN, Wang ZQ, Yan L, He J, Lin MT, Chen WJ, Wang N. Clinical and mutational characteristics of Duchenne muscular dystrophy patients based on a comprehensive database in South China. Neuromuscul Disord. 2017; 27(8):715–22.
37. Al-Jumah M, Majumdar R, Al-Rajeh S, Chaves-Carballo E, Salih MM, Awada A, Al-Shahwan S, Al-Uthaim S. Deletion mutations in the dystrophin gene of Saudi patients with Duchenne and Becker muscular dystrophy. Saudi Med J. 2002;23(12):1478–82.
38. Tayeb MT. Deletion mutations in Duchenne muscular dystrophy (DMD) in Western Saudi children. Saudi J Biol Sci. 2010;17(3):237–40.
39. Elhawary NA, Nassir A, Saada H, Dannoun A, Qoqandi O, Alsharif A, Tayeb MT. Combined genetic biomarkers confer susceptibility to risk of urothelial bladder carcinoma in a Saudi population. Dis Markers. 2017;2017:1474560.
40. Aartsma-Rus A, Van Deutekom JC, Fokkema IF, Van Ommen GJ, Den Dunnen JT. Entries in the Leiden Duchenne muscular dystrophy mutation database: an overview of mutation types and paradoxical cases that confirm the reading-frame rule. Muscle Nerve. 2006;34(2):135–44.
41. White SJ, den Dunnen JT. Copy number variation in the genome; the human DMD gene as an example. Cytogenet Genome Res. 2006;115(3–4):240–6.
42. Kerr R, Robinson C, Essop FB, Krause A. Genetic testing for Duchenne/Becker muscular dystrophy in Johannesburg. South Africa S Afr Med J. 2013;103(12 Suppl 1):999–1004.
43. Manjunath M, Kiran P, Preethish-Kumar V, Nalini A, Singh RJ, Gayathri N. A comparative study of mPCR, MLPA, and muscle biopsy results in a cohort of children with Duchenne muscular dystrophy: a first study. Neurol India. 2015;63(1):58–62.
44. Okubo M, Minami N, Goto K, Goto Y, Noguchi S, Mitsuhashi S, Nishino I. Genetic diagnosis of Duchenne/Becker muscular dystrophy using next-generation sequencing: validation analysis of DMD mutations. J Hum Genet. 2016;61(6):483–9.
45. Liang WC, Wang CH, Chou PC, Chen WZ, Jong YJ. The natural history of the patients with Duchenne muscular dystrophy in Taiwan: a medical center experience. Pediatr Neonatol. 2017.
46. Ulgenalp A, Giray O, Bora E, Hizli T, Kurul S, Sagin-Saylam G, Karasoy H, Uran N, Dizdarer G, Tutuncuoglu S, et al. Deletion analysis and clinical correlations in patients with Xp21 linked muscular dystrophy. Turk J Pediatr. 2004;46(4):333–8.
47. Elhawary NA, Shawky RM, Hashem N. Frameshift deletion mechanisms in Egyptian Duchenne and Becker muscular dystrophy families. Mol Cells. 2004;18(2):141–9.
48. Nouri N, Fazel-Najafabadi E, Salehi M, Hosseinzadeh M, Behnam M, Ghazavi MR, Sedghi M. Evaluation of multiplex ligation-dependent probe amplification analysis versus multiplex polymerase chain reaction assays in the detection of dystrophin gene rearrangements in an Iranian population subset. Adv Biomed Res. 2014;3:72.
49. Sbiti A, El Kerch F, Sefiani A. Analysis of dystrophin gene deletions by multiplex PCR in Moroccan patients. J Biomed Biotechnol. 2002;2(3):158–60.
50. Madania A, Zarzour H, Jarjour RA, Ghoury I. Combination of conventional multiplex PCR and quantitative real-time PCR detects large rearrangements in the dystrophin gene in 59% of Syrian DMD/BMD patients. Clin Biochem. 2010;43(10–11):836–42.
51. el-Hazmi MA, al-Swailem AR, Warsy AS, al-Swailem AM, Sulaimani R, al-Meshari AA. Consanguinity among the Saudi Arabian population. J Med Genet. 1995;32(8):623–6.
52. Vieitez I, Gallano P, Gonzalez-Quereda L, Borrego S, Marcos I, Millan JM, Jairo T, Prior C, Molano J, Trujillo-Tiebas MJ, et al. Mutational spectrum of Duchenne muscular dystrophy in Spain: study of 284 cases. Neurologia. 2017;32(6):377–85.
53. Lavergne S, Molofsky J. Increased genetic variation and evolutionary potential drive the success of an invasive grass. Proc Natl Acad Sci U S A. 2007;104:3883–8.
54. Rund D, Cohen T, Filon D, Dowling CE, Warren TC, Barak I, Rachmilewitz E, Kazazian HH Jr, Oppenheim A. Evolution of a genetic disease in an ethnic isolate: beta-thalassemia in the Jews of Kurdistan. Proc Natl Acad Sci U S A. 1991;88(1):310–4.
55. Jiffri EH, Bogari N, Zidan KH, Teama S, Elhawary NA. Molecular updating of β-thalassemia mutations in the upper Egyptian population. Hemoglobin. 2010;34(6):538–47.

56. Ciafaloni E, Fox DJ, Pandya S, Westfield CP, Puzhankara S, Romitti PA, Mathews KD, Miller TM, Matthews DJ, Miller LA, et al. Delayed diagnosis in duchenne muscular dystrophy: data from the Muscular Dystrophy Surveillance, Tracking, and Research Network (MD STARnet). J Pediatr. 2009; 155(3):380–5.
57. van Ruiten HJ, Straub V, Bushby K, Guglieri M. Improving recognition of Duchenne muscular dystrophy: a retrospective case note review. Arch Dis Child. 2014;99(12):1074–7.
58. Li X, Zhao L, Zhou S, Hu C, Shi Y, Shi W, Li H, Liu F, Wu B, Wang Y. A comprehensive database of Duchenne and Becker muscular dystrophy patients (0–18 years old) in East China. Orphanet J Rare Dis. 2015;10:5.
59. Cirak S, Arechavala-Gomeza V, Guglieri M, Feng L, Torelli S, Anthony K, Abbs S, Garralda ME, Bourke J, Wells DJ, et al. Exon skipping and dystrophin restoration in patients with Duchenne muscular dystrophy after systemic phosphorodiamidate morpholino oligomer treatment: an open-label, phase 2, dose-escalation study. Lancet. 2011;378(9791):595–605.
60. Mendell JR, Goemans N, Lowes LP, Alfano LN, Berry K, Shao J, Kaye EM, Mercuri E, Eteplirsen Study G, Telethon Foundation DMDIN. Longitudinal effect of eteplirsen versus historical control on ambulation in Duchenne muscular dystrophy. Ann Neurol. 2016;79(2):257–71.
61. Shimizu-Motohashi Y, Miyatake S, Komaki H, Takeda S, Aoki Y. Recent advances in innovative therapeutic approaches for Duchenne muscular dystrophy: from discovery to clinical trials. Am J Transl Res. 2016;8(6):2471–89.
62. Lee BL, Nam SH, Lee JH, Ki CS, Lee M, Lee J. Genetic analysis of dystrophin gene for affected male and female carriers with Duchenne/Becker muscular dystrophy in Korea. J Korean Med Sci. 2012;27(3):274–80.
63. Lim KR, Maruyama R, Yokota T. Eteplirsen in the treatment of Duchenne muscular dystrophy. Drug Des Devel Ther. 2017;11:533–45.
64. van Deutekom JC, van Ommen GJ. Advances in Duchenne muscular dystrophy gene therapy. Nat Rev Genet. 2003;4(10):774–83.
65. Mah JK. Current and emerging treatment strategies for Duchenne muscular dystrophy. Neuropsychiatr Dis Treat. 2016;12:1795–807.
66. Wein N, Vulin A, Findlay AR, Gumienny F, Huang N, Wilton SD, Flanigan KM. Efficient skipping of single exon duplications in DMD patient-derived cell lines using an antisense oligonucleotide approach. J Neuromuscul Dis. 2017; 4(3):199–207.
67. Aoki Y, Yokota T, Nagata T, Nakamura A, Tanihata J, Saito T, Duguez SM, Nagaraju K, Hoffman EP, Partridge T, et al. Bodywide skipping of exons 45-55 in dystrophic mdx52 mice by systemic antisense delivery. Proc Natl Acad Sci U S A. 2012;109(34):13763–8.
68. Guo MH, Dauber A, Lippincott MF, Chan YM, Salem RM, Hirschhorn JN. Determinants of power in gene-based burden testing for monogenic disorders. Am J Hum Genet. 2016;99(3):527–39.

12

Transcriptome analysis of bronchoalveolar lavage fluid from children with severe *Mycoplasma pneumoniae* pneumonia reveals novel gene expression and immunodeficiency

Kuo Wang[1†], Man Gao[2†], Mingyue Yang[1], Fanzheng Meng[2], Deli Li[2], Ruihua Lu[2], Yan Wang[2], Huadong Zhuang[2], Mengyao Li[3], Genhong Cheng[1,4] and Xiaosong Wang[1*]

Abstract

Background: A growing number of severe *Mycoplasma pneumoniae* pneumonia (MPP) cases have been reported recently. However, the pathogenesis of severe MPP is not clear. In the current study, transcriptome sequencing was used to identify gene expression and alternative splicing profiles to provide insights into the pathogenesis of severe MPP.

Methods: RNAs of bronchoalveolar lavage fluid (BALF) samples from three severe MPP children and three mild MPP children were analyzed respectively by deep sequencing followed by computational annotation and quantification.

Results: The gene expression analysis revealed 14 up-regulated and 34 down-regulated genes in severe MPP children comparing to mild MPP children. The top 10 most up-regulated genes were *IGHV1-69*, *CH17-472G23.1*, *ATP1B2*, *FCER2*, *MUC21*, *IL13*, *FCRLB*, *CLEC5A*, *FAM124A*, and *INHBA*. The top 10 most down-regulated genes were *OSTN-AS1*, *IL22RA2*, *COL3A1*, *C1orf141*, *IGKV2-29*, *RP11-731F5.2*, *IGHV4-4*, *KIRREL*, *DNASE1L3*, and *COL6A2*. Clustering analysis revealed similar expression pattern of *CLEC5A*, *IL13*, *FCER2*, and *FLT1*. Kyoto Encyclopedia of Genes and Genomes (KEGG) pathway enrichment analyses revealed changes related to primary immunodeficiency in severe MPP children comparing to mild MPP children; the pathway involves *CD19*, *TNFRSF13C*, *CD79A*, and *AICDA* genes. Among the differentially expressed genes, significant alternative splicing events were found in *FCER2* and *FCRLA*.

Conclusions: The current study on RNA sequencing provides novel insights into the pathogenesis of severe MPP in terms of gene expression and alternative splicing. The up-regulation of *IL13*, *FCER2*, *FLT1*, and *CLEC5A* and the down-regulation of *CD79A*, *AICDA*, *CD19*, and *TNFRSF13C* may contribute to the pathogenesis of severe MPP. The differential expressions of *FCER2* and *FCRLA* could be due to their alternative splicing.

Keywords: Severe *Mycoplasma pneumoniae* pneumonia, Children, Bronchoalveolar lavage fluid, Transcriptome sequencing, Gene expression profile, Alternative splicing

* Correspondence: xiaosongwang@jlu.edu.cn
†Equal contributors
[1]Institute of Translational Medicine, the First Hospital of Jilin University, Changchun 130061, China
Full list of author information is available at the end of the article

Background

Mycoplasma pneumoniae pneumonia (MPP), as a common community-acquired pneumonia, counts for 20 to 40% of children pneumonia and may reach 50 to 80% during the time of local outbreak [1, 2]. MPP is usually described as mild and self-limited; however, more and more severe or even fatal cases of MPP with severe complications such as pulmonary necrosis and chronic interstitial fibrosis have been reported recently [3–5]. Macrolide-resistant and excessive immunological inflammation are also commonly found in severe MPP [6]. Therefore, it is essential for pediatricians to recognize severe MPP early, treat it promptly, and prevent the progression of the disease effectively. However, the mechanism and etiology of severe MPP are largely unknown.

Based on published hypotheses, severe MPP is considered as a hyper-immune response that originates from repeated or longer lasting childhood MP infections in the lung [7]; further, severe MPP can be an overactive innate immune response such as macrophage activation via heterodimerization of Toll-like receptors two and six of the bronchoepithelial cells to *M. pneumoniae* lipoproteins [8]. With ELISA and real-time quantitative PCR techniques, researchers have found that the cell-mediated immune response plays an important role in the pathogenesis of MPP [9–11] but the role of humoral-mediated immune response in mild and severe MPP is still unclear.

High-throughput RNA sequencing technology, so called next-generation sequencing, revolutionarily enhanced our understanding on the complexity of eukaryotic transcriptome [12, 13]. It has several key advantages including being independent on the predetermined genome sequences, highly accurate in detecting gene expression with very wide dynamic detection ranges with low background. Thus, RNA sequencing is not only useful to precisely determine gene expression profiles but also particularly powerful to detect novel transcription variants via alternative splicing [12].

In the present study, we observed the transcriptome of bronchoalveolar lavage fluid (BALF) from children with mild MPP and severe MPP. The large sum of novel information on the gene expression profiles as well as novel transcripts through alternative splicing would provide not only insights into the pathogenesis of severe MPP but also as basis for the development of biomarkers and therapeutic targets.

Methods

Study subjects

The current study was conducted at the First Hospital of Jilin University (Changchun City, Jilin Province, People's Republic of China). Six newly diagnosed children (three male and three female) with acute stage of MPP admitted to our hospital were recruited [see Additional file 1: Table S1]. All of the children enrolled in this study had no recurrent severe or unusual infections and had no inflammatory disorders or autoimmunity. Therefore, based on the published diagnostic criteria, they had no history of common variable immunodefiency (CVID) [14]. After admission to our hospital, the levels of immunoglobulins in the blood of these children had been examined; the levels of IgG, IgA, and IgM had been found within normal range published for children [see Additional file 2: Figure S1] [15]. Lymphocyte profiles in the peripheral blood of these children had also been examined, the cell numbers and percentage of T cells, B cells, and natural killer cells had been found within normal range [see Additional file 3: Table S2] [15]. Therefore, the enrolled children had been excluded from having CVID, autosomal recessive agammaglobulinemia [15], or high IgM syndrome [16]. All children did not have untreated metabolic/congenital systemic diseases. The diagnosis of pneumonia was based on clinical manifestations (cough, fever, dry or productive sputum, dyspnea, abnormal breath sound, radiological pulmonary abnormalities). The diagnosis of *Mycoplasma pneumoniae* (MP) infection was based on positive results of serologic test (MP-IgM test ≥1:40) and positive results of MP DNA (>500 copy/L) in BALF with real-time quantitative PCR. MP was the only pathogen identified in all the MPP subjects. The mild and severe community-acquired pneumonia was defined based on the criteria described [17, 18]. Mild group was defined as fever <38.5 °C at any age, tachypnea but respiratory rate <70 breaths/min at age <3 years old or <50 breaths/min at age ≥3 years old, normal food-intake, and no dehydration. Severe group was defined as fever ≥38.5 °C at any age, breathless with respiratory rate ≥70 breaths/min at age <3 years old or ≥50 breaths/min at age ≥3 years old (excluding the reasons of fever and cry), cyanosis, marked retractions, anorexia, and dehydration.

The written informed consents were obtained by care givers of all children. The study was approved by the Institutional Medical Ethics Review Board of the First Hospital of Jilin University in compliance with the Declaration of Helsinki.

Bronchoscopy and bronchoalveolar lavage

Following the guidelines described previously [17], flexible fiber optic bronchoscopy with bronchoalveolar lavage (BAL) was performed within 3 days after the admission. Both groups received similar supportive and symptomatic treatment, including sputum aspiration, nebulization, and fluid therapy. Corticosteroid and the other immune regulation agents were not permitted before bronchoscopy. A 2.8-mm pediatric flexible bronchoscope (Olympus BF-XP60, New Hyde Park, NY) or a

4.0-mm flexible bronchoscope (Olympus P-260, New Hyde Park, NY) was used for children depending on their age and body weight. All of the enrolled subjects had indications for bronchoscopy and BAL: radiologically proven large pulmonary lesions (including atelectasis and consolidation of lung fields). Supplemental oxygen was administered during the procedure. Transcutaneous oxygen saturation and pulse rate (Masimo Radical-7 pulse oximetry, Masimo, CA) were continuously monitored during the bronchoscopy.

Intravenous injection of midazolam (0.1–0.15 mg/kg) was used for sedation; aerosolized lidocaine spraying on the throat insertion was performed 5–10 min before bronchoscope for throat local anesthesia; dripping 2% lidocaine through flexible bronchoscopy was used for the topical anesthesia of the upper and lower airways. BAL was performed in an area most prominently affected based on the chest radiology (MPP groups) by gently wedging the tip of the Bronchoscope in a segmental or subsegmental bronchus. 1 ml/kg sterile saline was instilled through the instrumentation channel. The BALF was gently aspirated and collected in a sterile container and immediately centrifuged. The pallet was resuspended in TRIzol (Life Technologies, CA, USA) and stored in −80 °C freezer. The composition of the nucleated cells in the BALF was counted; results were shown in Additional file 4: Table S3.

RNA preparation and sequencing

Total RNA was extracted using TRIzol according to the manufacturer's instructions. RNA degradation and contamination were monitored on 1% agarose gels. RNA purity was checked using the NanoPhotometer spectrophotometer (IMPLEN, CA, USA). RNA concentration was measured using Qubit RNA Assay Kit in Qubit 2.0 Flurometer (Life Technologies, CA, USA). RNA integrity was assessed using the RNA Nano 6000 Assay Kit of the Bioanalyzer 2100 system (Agilent Technologies, CA, USA).

A total amount of 3 μg RNA per sample was used as input material for the RNA sample preparation. Sequencing libraries were generated using NEBNext® Ultra™ RNA Library Prep Kit for Illumina® (NEB, USA) following the manufacturer's recommendations, and index codes were added to attribute sequences to each sample. The clustering of the index-coded samples was performed on a cBot Cluster Generation System using TruSeq PE Cluster Kit v3-cBot-HS (Illumia) according to the manufacturer's instructions. After cluster generation, the library preparations were sequenced on an Illumina Hiseq platform and 125 bp/150 bp paired-end reads were generated.

Sequencing data analysis

Raw data (raw reads) of fastq format were firstly processed through in-house perl scripts, and clean data (clean reads) were obtained. Index of the reference genome was built using Bowtie v2.2.3, and paired-end clean reads were aligned to the reference genome using TopHat v2.0.12. Only uniquely and properly mapped read pairs were used for further analysis. The differentially expressed genes between BALF samples were identified using the DESeq R package (1.18.0) [19]. Differentially expressed genes were defined as those with changes of at least twofold between samples. The resulting p values were adjusted using the Benjamini and Hochberg approach for controlling the false discovery rate (FDR). Genes with an adjusted p value <0.05 found by DESeq were assigned as differentially expressed. Protein functional classification of differentially expressed genes was performed using the PANTHER classification system [20]. KOBAS software was used to test the statistical enrichment of differential expression genes in KEGG pathways. The significance of enriched KEGG pathways were determined by corrected p value <0.05. Cufflinks v2.1.1 Reference Annotation Based Transcript (RABT) assembly method was used to construct and identify both known and novel transcripts from TopHat alignment results. The analysis of alternative splicing events was performed using MATS and IGV software [21]; alternative splicing events were classified to five basic types by software Asprofile v1.0. The differences in alternative splicing of genes were considered significant with a cutoff of 5% FDR.

Results

RNA sequencing results

Total RNA was extracted from six BALF samples of children with severe MPP or mild MPP [see Additional file 1: Table S1]. Then, mRNAs from each sample were sequenced. After the removal of adaptor sequences, ambiguous reads and low-quality reads, about 40–70 million pairs of clean read, were generated for each sample (Table 1). The percentage of reads mapped to the forward chain was equal to that mapped to the reverse chain. When compared with the reference sequence of the Genome Reference Consortium GRCh37/hg19, more than 85% of total read pairs were uniquely mapped on the human genome (Table 1). A correlation matrix shown a high consistency of measurements within each group, $R^2 > 0.8$ [see Additional file 5: Figure S2A]. Principal component analysis (PCA) was carried out to assess the clustering nature of these samples. Samples of each group had been clustered together; data shown good repeatability and correlation [see Additional file 5: Figure S2B].

Identification and classification of differentially expressed genes between severe MPP and mild MPP

Totally, 48 differentially expressed genes were identified between the severe MPP group and mild MPP group

Table 1 Summary of RNA sequencing read mapping result

Sample number	Mild 202	Mild 224	Mild 247	Severe 177	Severe 223	Severe 324
Total reads	55492664	47186542	64792680	68897254	42136856	46318894
Total mapped	48535137 (87.46%)	40517410 (85.87%)	56013052 (86.45%)	60481397 (87.78%)	36565361 (86.78%)	40224088 (86.84%)
Multiple mapped	844736 (1.52%)	614681 (1.30%)	797662 (1.23%)	881129 (1.28%)	543196 (1.29%)	630869 (1.36%)
Uniquely mapped	47690401 (85.94%)	39902729 (84.56%)	55215390 (85.22%)	59600268 (86.51%)	36022165 (85.49%)	39593219 (85.48%)
Reads map to "+"	23844413 (42.97%)	19967766 (42.32%)	27594117 (42.59%)	29790936 (43.24%)	18008541 (42.74%)	19797319 (42.74%)
Reads map to "−"	23845988 (42.97%)	19934963 (42.25%)	27621273 (42.63%)	29809332 (43.27%)	18013624 (42.75%)	19795900 (42.74%)
Non-splice reads	30580304 (55.11%)	22475106 (47.63%)	34530918 (53.29%)	37577003 (54.54%)	20733762 (49.21%)	24205574 (52.26%)
Splice reads	17110097 (30.83%)	17427623 (36.93%)	20684472 (31.92%)	22023265 (31.97%)	15288403 (36.28%)	15387645 (33.22%)

Total reads: The number of sequence after sequencing data filtering
Total mapped: The number of sequence which can map to the genome
Multiple mapped: The number of sequence which have multiple location on the reference sequencing
Uniquely mapped: The number of sequence which have single location on the reference sequencing
Reads map to "+": The statistics of sequence that were mapped on the "+" chain of the genome
Reads map to "−": The statistics of sequence that were mapped on the "−" chain of the genome

(Fig. 1a). The 14 up-regulated genes listed in Table 2 were *IGHV1-69, CH17-472G23.1, ATP1B2, FCER2, MUC21, IL13, FCRLB, CLEC5A, FAM124A, INHBA, FLT1, APOL4,* and two novel transcripts. These 14 up-regulated genes included cytokine (*IL13*), immunoglobin Fc receptors (*FCER2* and *FCRLB*), and inflammatory response regulator (*CLEC5A*). The top 20 most down-regulated genes were *OSTN-AS1, IL22RA2, COL3A1, C1orf141, IGKV2-29, RP11-731F5.2, IGHV4-4, KIRREL, DNASE1L3, COL6A2, COL6A1, FCRL4, HTRA3, TCL1A, RP11-356K23.1, PLD4, DKK3, UBE2QL1, KLRB1,* and *MS4A1* (Table 3).

Protein functional classification of differentially expressed genes between severe MPP and mild MPP was performed. As a result, the 48 differentially expressed genes were divided into 13 different classes of protein (Fig. 1b). The expression levels of genes classified as signaling molecule (*CLEC5A, IL13, INHBA*), transporter (*ATP1B2*), and transfer/carrier protein (*APOL4*) significantly increased in the severe MPP group comparing to the mild MPP group [see Additional file 6: Table S4]. On the other hand, genes in the categories of nucleic acid binding molecule (*AICDA, PAX5, SPIB, TCF7*), genes encodes defense/immunity protein (*IL22RA2, CD79A*), hydrase (*PLA2G2D, HTRA3, AICDA*), receptor (*MS4A1, IL22RA2*), and transcription factor (*PAX5*), were predominantly expressed in the mild MPP group. Among the cell adhesion molecules, *FCER2* and *FCRLB* were up-regulated in the severe MPP group; *FCRLA* and *FCRL4* were up-regulated in the mild MPP group.

The clustering analysis of differentially expressed genes indicated that *FCER2, FLT1, IL13,* and *CLEC5A* were

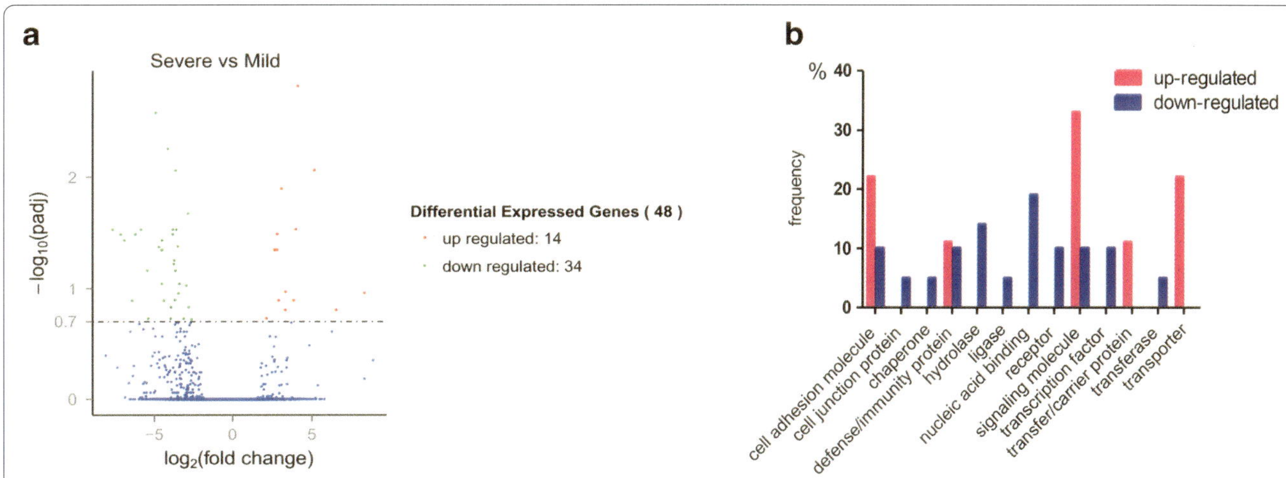

Fig. 1 Differentially expressed genes between the severe MPP group and mild MPP group in BALF. **a** Volcano plot of genes differentially expressed between the severe MPP group and mild MPP group. Each point represents one gene that is detectable in both groups. The *red points* represent significantly up-regulated genes; the *green points* represent significantly down-regulated genes. **b** Protein functional classification of differentially expressed genes has been performed using the PANTHER tool between the severe MPP group and mild MPP group. The protein category is shown on *x*-axis and the gene frequency is shown on *y*-axis

Table 2 Up-regulated genes of the severe MPP group comparing to the mild MPP group

Gene ID	Associated gene name	log_2foldchange	padj	Description
ENSG00000104921	*FCER2*	4.081288	0.001514	Fc fragment of IgE, low affinity II, receptor for (CD23)
ENSG00000129244	*ATP1B2*	5.123508	0.008687	ATPase, Na+/K+ transporting, beta 2 polypeptide
ENSG00000258227	*CLEC5A*	3.046087	0.012798	C-type lectin domain family 5 member A
Novel00326	–	3.957912	0.029750	–
ENSG00000122641	*INHBA*	2.792227	0.032804	Inhibin beta A
ENSG00000102755	*FLT1*	2.773680	0.044977	Fms-related tyrosine kinase 1
Novel00056	–	2.612021	0.044977	–
ENSG00000169194	*IL13*	3.320997	0.107345	Interleukin 13
ENSG00000211973	*IGHV1-69*	8.269132	0.110361	Immunoglobulin heavy variable 1–69
ENSG00000150510	*FAM124A*	2.878502	0.130273	Family with sequence similarity 124 member A
ENSG00000204544	*MUC21*	3.830138	0.130273	Mucin 21, cell surface associated
ENSG00000162746	*FCRLB*	3.307526	0.157765	Fc receptor-like B
ENSG00000274642	*CH17-472G23.1*	6.496741	0.157765	–
ENSG00000100336	*APOL4*	2.103424	0.186854	Apolipoprotein L4

log_2foldchange log_2 (severe MPP/mild MPP), *padj* adjusted *p* value, *Novel* novel gene

up-regulated in the severe MPP group comparing to the mild MPP group (Fig. 2). Similar up-regulation or down-regulation patterns among these genes were identified, which may indicate related local protein functions of these genes under MP infection in children.

Functional annotation of KEGG pathway enrichment analysis revealed changes related to primary immunodeficiency in the BALF of severe MPP children, which was associated with the down-regulation of *CD19, TNFRSF13C, CD79A*, and *AICDA* genes (Table 4). *CD19, TNFRSF13C, CD79A*, and *AICDA* were involved in the B cell differentiation process; down-regulation of these genes may restrain B cell maturation and antibody production (Fig. 3) [22]. Furthermore, *COL6A1, COL6A2, COL5A3, COL3A1*, and *COL1A2* genes were involved in the pathways including protein digestion and absorption, ECM-receptor interaction, P13K-Akt signaling, and focal adhesion; these molecules were found down-regulated in the severe MPP group comparing to the mild MPP group (Table 4). *COL6A1, COL6A2, COL5A3, COL3A1*, and *COL1A2* belong to the collagen super family, which play a role in maintaining the integrity of various tissues including the lung [23]. *FLT1*, which encoded a member of vascular endothelial growth factor receptor (VEGFR) family, was also found significantly increased in the severe MPP group comparing to the mild MPP group in the P13K-Akt signaling and focal adhesion pathways (Tables 2 and 4).

Alternative splicing events between severe MPP and mild MPP

More than 90% of human genes are alternatively spliced through different types of splicing [24]. MATS analysis of the RNA sequencing data significantly revealed 1500 differential alternative splicing events with a cutoff of 5% FDR (Table 5), more than half (50.5%) of them belong to the skipped exon type. Among the differentially expressed genes between the severe MPP group and mild MPP group, *FECR2* and *FCRLA* were identified to have significantly alternative splicing [see Additional file 7: Table S5, Additional file 8: Table S6, Additional file 9: Table S7, Additional file 10: Table S8, and Additional file 11: Table S9].

FCER2 locates on chromosome 19p13.2 (chr 19:7,688,758-7,702,146); its encoding protein is a B cell specific antigen, which is a low-affinity receptor for IgE. This protein plays essential roles in B cell growth, differentiation, and regulation of IgE production. It also exists as a soluble secreted form and acts as a potent mitogenic growth factor. Retained intron (RI) was identified in *FCER2* in some of the samples. RI lies on chr19: 7,698,355-7,698,854; the upstream exon locates on chr19: 7,698,355-7,698,409 and the downstream exon locates on chr19: 7,698,740-7,698,854 [see Additional file 8: Table S6]. Compared to the mild MPP group, the severe MPP group had less RI spliced transcript events of *FCER2*, which could be an explanation for the up-regulation of the *FCER2* in severe MPP children (Fig. 4a).

FCRLA locates on chromosome 1q23.3 (chr 1:161,706,972-161,714,352). This gene encodes a protein similar to Fc receptor of gamma immunoglobulin (IgG), which is selectively expressed in B cells and may be involved in their development. Alternatively, spliced transcript variants of *FCRLA* that encode different protein isoforms have been found in the current study. Two exons of *FCLRA* were involved in mutual exclusive exon (MEX), the first exon starts at 161,710,759 and ends at 161,710,912 and the second exon starts at 161,711,207 and ends at 161,711,474 [see

Table 3 Down-regulated genes of the severe MPP group comparing to the mild MPP group

Gene ID	Associated gene name	log_2foldchange	padj	Description
ENSG00000163687	*DNASE1L3*	−4.90655	0.002613	Deoxyribonuclease I-like 3
ENSG00000166428	*PLD4*	−4.12788	0.005539	Phospholipase D family member 4
ENSG00000269404	*SPIB*	−3.62528	0.008687	Spi-B transcription factor (Spi-1/PU.1 related)
ENSG00000081059	*TCF7*	−2.83313	0.021184	Transcription factor 7 (T cell specific, HMG-box)
ENSG00000156738	*MS4A1*	−3.80125	0.029750	Membrane-spanning 4-domains, subfamily A, member 1
ENSG00000159958	*TNFRSF13C*	−3.59110	0.029750	Tumor necrosis factor receptor superfamily member 13C
ENSG00000233308	*OSTN-AS1*	−7.65241	0.029750	OSTN antisense RNA 1
ENSG00000253364	*RP11-731F5.2*	−5.82530	0.029750	–
ENSG00000111796	*KLRB1*	−3.80851	0.032804	Killer cell lectin-like receptor subfamily B, member 1
ENSG00000164485	*IL22RA2*	−7.13138	0.032804	Interleukin 22 receptor subunit alpha 2
ENSG00000253998	*IGKV2-29*	−6.19209	0.032804	Immunoglobulin kappa variable 2–29 (gene/pseudogene)
ENSG00000168542	*COL3A1*	−6.89272	0.036862	Collagen, type III, alpha 1
ENSG00000170801	*HTRA3*	−4.50354	0.036862	HtrA serine peptidase 3
Novel00339	–	−3.48127	0.041780	–
ENSG00000142173	*COL6A2*	−4.69524	0.042554	Collagen, type VI, alpha 2
ENSG00000100721	*TCL1A*	−4.49274	0.044977	T cell leukemia/lymphoma 1A
ENSG00000142156	*COL6A1*	−4.52065	0.044977	Collagen, type VI, alpha 1
ENSG00000111732	*AICDA*	−3.71025	0.055876	Activation-induced cytidine deaminase
ENSG00000164692	*COL1A2*	−3.75418	0.059895	Collagen, type I, alpha 2
ENSG00000105369	*CD79A*	−3.63713	0.069048	CD79a molecule
ENSG00000276775	*IGHV4-4*	−5.43537	0.069048	Immunoglobulin heavy variable 4-4
ENSG00000080573	*COL5A3*	−3.37399	0.090838	Collagen, type V, alpha 3
ENSG00000163518	*FCRL4*	−4.51056	0.090838	Fc receptor-like 4
ENSG00000196092	*PAX5*	−2.93710	0.093937	Paired box 5
ENSG00000177455	*CD19*	−3.44060	0.110361	CD19 molecule
ENSG00000136573	*BLK*	−3.67317	0.128424	BLK proto-oncogene, Src family tyrosine kinase
ENSG00000203963	*C1orf141*	−6.39692	0.130273	Chromosome 1 open reading frame 141
ENSG00000258752	*RP11-356K23.1*	−4.39265	0.130273	–
ENSG00000167483	*FAM129C*	−2.78386	0.148367	Family with sequence similarity 129 member C
ENSG00000215218	*UBE2QL1*	−3.91473	0.149275	Ubiquitin conjugating enzyme E2Q family-like 1
ENSG00000050165	*DKK3*	−3.95056	0.186854	Dickkopf WNT signaling pathway inhibitor 3
ENSG00000132185	*FCRLA*	−3.11003	0.186854	Fc receptor-like A
ENSG00000183853	*KIRREL*	−5.37583	0.186854	Kin of IRRE like (drosophila)
ENSG00000117215	*PLA2G2D*	−2.60098	0.191201	Phospholipase A2 group IID

log_2foldchange log_2 (severe MPP/mild MPP), *padj* adjusted *p* value, *Novel* novel gene

Additional file 9: Table S7]. The analysis of alternative splicing events indicated that the MEX frequency of the first exon in the severe MPP group was significantly higher than that in the mild MPP group, which may result in the down-regulated expression of *FCRLA* in severe MPP children (Fig. 4b).

Discussion

Recent developments in RNA sequencing technology enabled elaborate analysis of gene expression in numerous human diseases. However, to our best knowledge, no report of RNA-sequencing study on human MPP has been published yet. The current study provides extensive information on gene expression and alternative splicing in the BALF of MPP children through transcriptome analysis, which is crucial for understanding the pathogenesis of severe MPP. The gene expression analysis revealed 14 up-regulated genes and 34 down-regulated genes in severe MPP children comparing to mild MPP children. The top 10 most up-regulated genes are *IGHV1-*

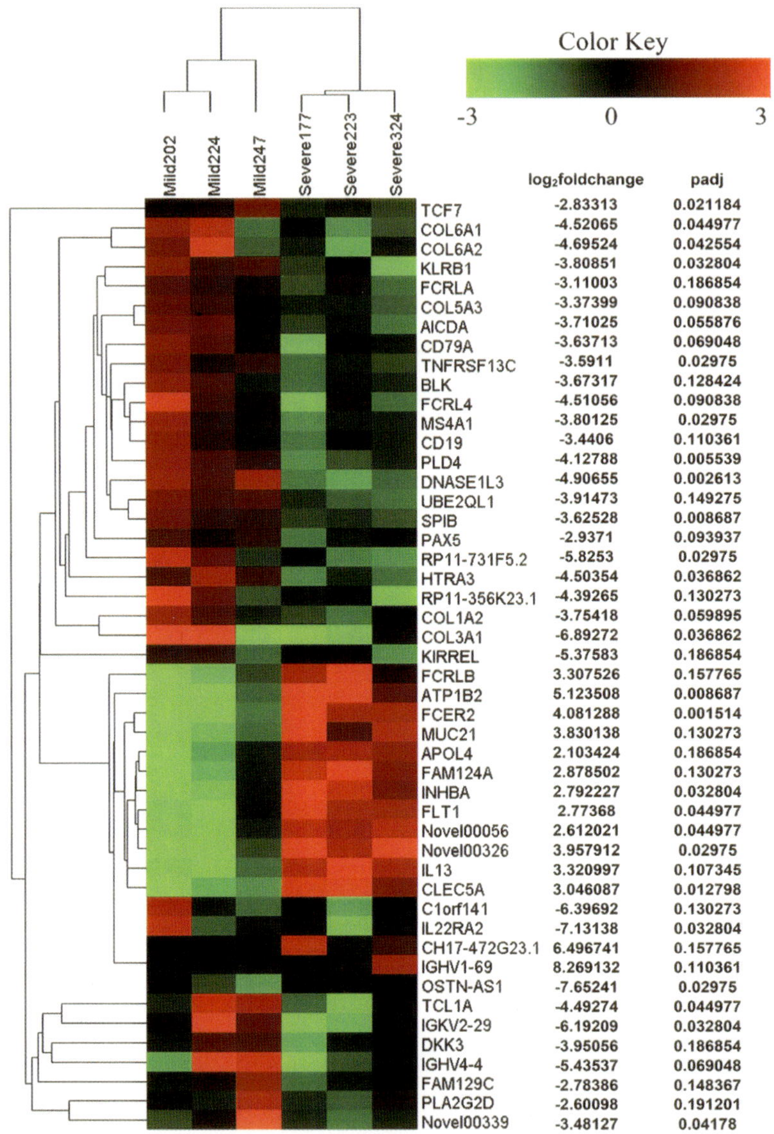

Fig. 2 Cluster of 48 genes showing representative expression patterns between the severe MPP group and mild MPP group. All of the genes that are differentially expressed between the severe MPP group and mild MPP group by $\log_2$ fold change >2 or <−2, adjusted p value <0.2, have been selected

Table 4 KEGG pathway enrichment

Term	ID	Adjusted p value	Input	KEGG_ID/KO
Protein digestion and absorption	hsa04974	0.000305	*COL6A1*| *COL6A2*| *ATP1B2*| *COL5A3* | *COL3A1*| *COL1A2*	hsa:1291|hsa:1292|hsa:482|hsa:50509 |hsa:1281|hsa:1278|
Primary immunodeficiency	hsa05340	0.001040	*CD19*| *TNFRSF13C*| *CD79A*| *AICDA*	hsa:930|hsa:115650|hsa:973|hsa:57379|
ECM-receptor interaction	hsa04512	0.001350	*COL6A2*| *COL5A3*| *COL6A1* | *COL1A2*| *COL3A1*	hsa:1292|hsa:50509|hsa:1291 |hsa:1278|hsa:1281|
PI3K-Akt signaling pathway	hsa04151	0.003493	*COL6A1*| *TCL1A*| *COL6A2*| *CD19*| *COL5A3* | *COL3A1*| *COL1A2*| *FLT1*	hsa:1291|hsa:8115|hsa:1292|hsa:930 |hsa:50509|hsa:1281|hsa:1278|hsa:2321|
Focal adhesion	hsa04510	0.005512	*COL6A1*| *COL6A2*| *COL5A3*| *COL3A1* | *COL1A2*| *FLT1*	hsa:1291|hsa:1292|hsa:50509|hsa:1281 |hsa:1278|hsa:2321|

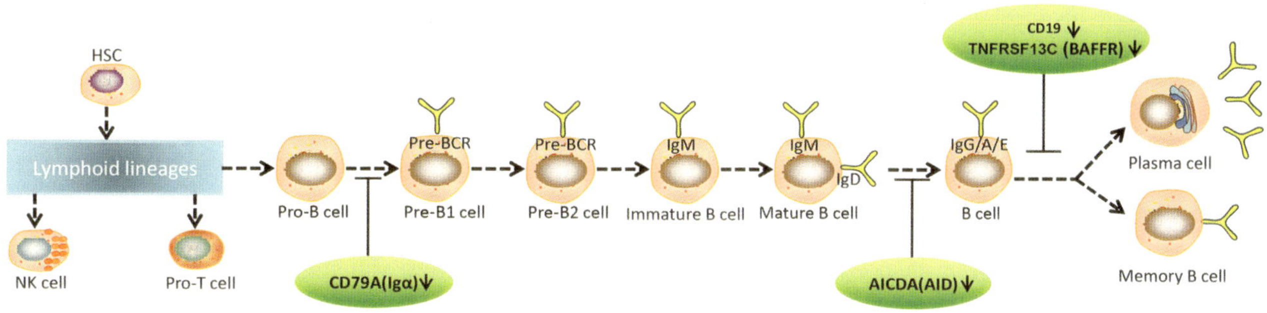

Fig. 3 Model diagram showing primary immunodeficiency. Hematopoietic stem cell (HSC)-derived lymphoid progenitor cells develop into progenitor (pro)-B cells, Pre-B1 cell, Pre-B2 cell, immature B cell, mature B cell, B cell, memory B cell, and plasma cell. The decreased expression of *CD79A* inhibits the differentiation of Pro-B cell into Pre-B1 cell; the decreased expression of *AICDA* inhibits the differentiation of mature B cell into B cell; the decreased expression of *CD19* and *TNFRSF13C* inhibits the differentiation of mature B cell into memory B cell and plasma B cell

69, CH17-472G23.1, ATP1B2, FCER2, MUC21, IL13, FCRLB, CLEC5A, FAM124A, and *INHBA* (Fig. 1a, Table 2). The top 10 most down-regulated genes are *OSTN-AS1, IL22RA2, COL3A1, C1orf141, IGKV2-29, RP11-731F5.2, IGHV4-4, KIRREL, DNASE1L3*, and *COL6A2* (Fig. 1a, Table 3).

Several key genes that are differentially expressed between severe MPP and mild MPP are associated with hyper-immune response and signaling. For example, IL13, a cytokine secreted by T helper type 2 (Th2) cells, can induce many features of allergic lung disease including airway hyper-responsiveness, goblet cell metaplasia, and mucus hyper-secretion, which all contribute to airway obstruction [25, 26]. IL13 is found to cause mucin overproduction through STAT6/EGFR-FOXA2 signaling and mucus plugging formation in MP infection, which results in pulmonary atelectasis or consolidation [27]. These results prove that IL13 play an important role in the airway obstruction of severe MPP. In addition, Wu Q et al. [26] have reported that IL13 can restrain MP clearance by the suppression of Toll-like receptor 2 in mice. Therefore, high levels of IL13 may make severe MPP children lose the ability to eradicate MP from the lung in primary infection, resulting in longer lasting MP infection and a hyper-immune response [7]. Another gene associated with hyper-immune response is *FCER2*. *FCER2* is a B cell specific antigen and a low-affinity receptor for IgE. It has essential roles in B cell growth, differentiation, and the regulation of IgE production. On the basis of study with animal models, *FCER2* has been implicated in IgE-mediated allergic diseases and bronchial hyper-reactivity [28]. It has been proved that *FCER2* is involved in the pharmacogenetic basis for severe exacerbations in children with asthma [29]. Up-regulated *FCER2* in severe MPP children has been discovered in the present study. Similarly, increased IgE levels in the serum of MPP patients have been reported [30]. Therefore, further study will be needed to prove that up-regulated *FCER2* causes the bronchial inflammation and hyper-immune reactivity. Among the up-regulated genes in severe MPP comparing to mild MPP, *FLT1* may also associate with hyper-immune response. *FLT1* (fms-like tyrosine kinase 1) encodes a member of the vascular endothelial growth factor receptor (VEGFR) family. Wu WK et al. demonstrate that Th2-related cytokines, such as IL4 and IL13, could drive the expression of *FLT1* [31]. Moreover, Th2-related cytokines can promote VEGF release in the airway, and VEGF has been proposed to be associated with severe MPP [32, 33]. Therefore, atopic children may be more prone to develop severe pneumonia [34]. We tentatively put forward the hypothesis that *IL13, FCER2*, and *FLT1* may be

Table 5 Summary of the differential alternative splicing event analysis

	Skipped exon	Retained intron	Mutual exclusive exon	Alternative 5′ splicing sites	Alternative 3′ splicing sites
Number of total alternative splicing events (genes)	44856 (11195)	3772 (2353)	6862 (3327)	2793 (2103)	4374 (2874)
Percentage of total alternative splicing event (%)	71.6	6.0	10.9	4.5	7.0
Number of differential alternative splicing events (up-regulation/down-regulation)	758 (398:360)	181 (107:74)	315 (193:122)	101 (74:27)	145 (86:59)
Percentage of total differential alternative splicing event (%)	50.5	12.1	21	6.7	9.7

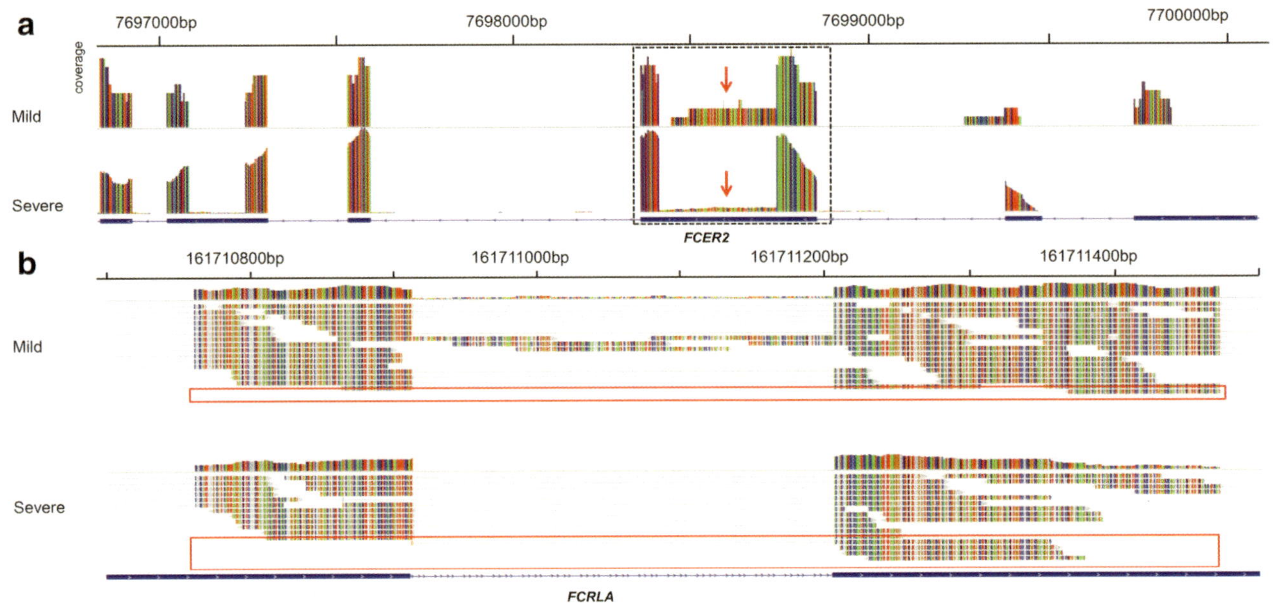

Fig. 4 Differential alternative splicing of *FCER2* and *FCRLA*. **a** Read distribution plot for *FCER2* with differential isoform expression due to retained intron in the mild MPP group is shown. The *black box* and *red arrows* indicated the location of the retained intron. **b** Read distribution plot for *FCRLA* with differential isoform expression due to mutually exclusive exon is shown. The ratio of mutually exclusive exon happened in the severe MPP group is compared with that in the mild MPP group

associated with each other and all of them are involved in the pathogenesis of severe MPP.

Based on our data [see Additional file 4: Table S3] and published results [35], more than half of the nucleated cells in BALF of MPP children without other pathogen infection are macrophages. But it is still unclear how macrophages are involved in the pathogenesis of severe MPP. Clustering analysis of the differentially expressed genes reveals that the expression patterns of *IL13*, *FCER2*, *FLT1*, and *CLEC5A* are similar in the severe MPP group (Fig. 2). One possible mechanism of severe MPP is the overactivation of macrophage in innate immune response [7]. *CLEC5A* (C-type lectin domain family 5, member A) is expressed on alveolar macrophages; it has been demonstrated to mediate macrophage response and play roles in pro-inflammatory cytokine expression and airspace enlargement in a mice model of chronic obstructive pulmonary disease (COPD) [36]. Muro S et al. suggested that MP infection could be an independent risk factor for COPD in the general population [37]. *CLEC5A* encodes a member of the CTL/CTLD (C-type lectin/C-type lectin-like domain) superfamily, which family members play roles in inflammation and immune responses. Teng O et al. have revealed that *CLEC5A*-mediated enhancement of the inflammatory response in myeloid cells contributes to influenza's pathogenicity in vivo [38]. We found significant higher expression levels of *CLEC5A* in the BALF of severe MPP comparing to that of mild MPP. Therefore, our results support the hypothesis that *CLEC5A* is involved in the pathogenesis of severe MPP through the overactivation of macrophage. Protein functional classification of the differentially expressed genes indicates that signaling molecules including *IL13*, *CLEC5A*, and *INHBA* are obviously increased in severe MPP comparing to mild MPP [see Fig. 1b, Additional file 6: Table S4]. *INHBA* (Inhibin beta A) encodes a member of the transforming growth factor superfamily. The encoded preproprotein is proteolytically processed to generate a subunit of the dimeric activin and inhibin protein complexes. Rheumatoid arthritis synovium fluid (RA-SF) promotes *INHBA* production as a pro-inflammatory cytokine from macrophages in vitro [39]. Similarly, *INHBA* is reported to be up-regulated in endometritis by Hoelker M et al. [40]. It is interesting that the current study finds increased levels of *INHBA* in severe MPP. The causal relationship between the up-regulation of *INHBA* and severe MPP requires further investigation.

It is still unclear how B cells are involved in the pathogenesis of severe MPP. In the current study, KEGG pathway enrichment analyses have revealed changes related to primary immunodeficiency in severe MPP patients, which involves *CD79A*, *AICDA*, *CD19*, and *TNFRSF13C* genes (Table 4, Fig. 3) [22]. *CD79A*, *AICDA*, *CD19*, and *TNFRSF13C* are related to the B cell antigen signaling pathway; lower expression of these genes can lead to the deficiency of B cell functions. *CD79A* encodes the Igα protein of the B cell antigen component, which is necessary for expression and function of the B cell antigen receptor. Defected *CD79A* has been discovered in immunodeficiency-related diseases [41]. Similarly, *AICDA* (activation-induced cytidine deaminase) encodes a RNA-editing deaminase, which is expressed in a B cell differentiation stage-specific fashion. *AICDA* is involved in somatic hyper-mutation, gene conversion, and class-switch recombination of immunoglobulin genes [42]. Defects in *AICDA* can cause autosomal recessive hyper-IgM immunodeficiency syndrome type 2 (HIGM2) [43]. *CD19* is a B cell-specific molecule, which serves as a major costimulatory molecule for amplifying B cell receptor (BCR) responses. Morbach H et al. have revealed that *CD19* is required for TLR9-induced B cell activation and CD19/PI3K/AKT/BTK is an essential axis integrating BCRs and TLR9 signaling in human B cells [44]. In addition, biallelic *CD19* gene mutations cause common variable immunodeficiency in human. BCR-induced B cell responses are impaired in most patients with common variable immunodeficiency. *TNFRSF13C* (tumor necrosis factor receptor superfamily member 13C) encodes a receptor for BAFF (B cell activating factor), which enhances B cell survival in vitro and regulates the peripheral B cell population. *TNFRSF13C* is a principal receptor required for BAFF-mediated mature B cell survival and it has been reported to be associated with common variable immunodeficiency [45]. In our study, significantly decreased expression levels of *CD79A*, *AICDA*, *CD19*, and *TNFRSF13C* have been observed in the BALF of the severe MPP group comparing to the mild MPP group. Comparing to the local reduction of *CD79A*, *AICDA*, *CD19*, and *TNFRSF13C* genes found in BALF, these patient's immunoglobulins and lymphocyte profiles in the peripheral blood are normal, which means they do not have any systemic immunodeficiency disease [see Additional file 2: Fig. S1, Additional file 3: Table S2]. We have found these local changes related to primary immunodeficiency in the bronchoalveolar of severe MPP. Local B cell-related immunodeficiency may be involved in the pathogenesis of severe MPP comparing with mild MPP. Figure 3 shows how these molecules are involved in the pathway of B cell differentiation and immunoglobulin gene class switch; down-regulation of these molecules may restrain antibody production and make the MPP children lose the ability to eradicate MP from the lung, which leads to happen of severe MPP [7].

Alternative splicing events of genes are involved in the diversity of proteome as well as genome evolution, control of developmental processes, and physiological regulation of various biological systems [46]. It could be deduced that dysregulation of alternative splicing event is often linked to various human diseases [47]. However, alternative splicing events in the context of MPP have rarely been investigated. The current study discovered significant differential alternative splicing events in *FCER2* and *FCRLA* which could be an explanation for the differential expression of these two genes between severe MPP and mild MPP. The alternative splicing type of *FCER2* is retained intron (RI), which can change the function and expression levels of a gene [48]. Therefore, lower rate of RI in the severe MPP group comparing to the mild MPP group may partly explain the significantly increased expression levels of *FCER2* in the severe MPP group. *FCRLA* is a soluble resident endoplasmic reticulum protein. It is capable of associating with multiple Ig isotypes including IgM, IgG, and IgA, which makes it unique among the large family of Fc receptors. The expression of *FCRLA* is restricted to B lineage and is most abundant in germinal center B lymphocytes [49]. In the present study, the alternative splicing type of *FCRLA* is MEX, which is significantly increased in the severe MPP group comparing to the mild MPP group. According to the literatures [50, 51], alternative splicing may be a causal explanation for the down-regulation of *FCRLA* in the severe MPP group.

Previous studies have found that cell-mediated immune response, specifically Th1-type cytokines such as IL8, IL18, and IFNγ, plays important roles in the mechanism of MPP [9–11, 52]. Most of these studies observed serum levels of Th1 cytokines, but we have chosen BALF to study the local differentially expressed genes. Cytokines may be expressed differently in BALF comparing to that in the peripheral blood; this could partly explain why significant difference of IL8, IL18, and IFNγ was not found in the current study. Additionally, our transcriptome analysis focused on comparing severe MPP with mild MPP in order to study the specific pathogenesis of severe MPP; similar results have been reported by Kang YM et al. group [53]. In their study, higher levels of IFNγ in BALF of MPP patients comparing with that of control children were discovered, but no significant difference of IFNγ was found between the severe MPP group and mild MPP group.

Some limitations of the current study should be discussed. First, this is a small size transcriptome analysis between mild MPP children and severe MPP children; bigger sized analysis would be preferred in future study to support solid conclusions. However, three samples in each group have been chosen carefully to receive next-generation sequencing separately; quality control analysis of the whole process has been greatly satisfied. Correlation matrix shows a high consistency of measurements within each group. Principal component analysis (PCA) shows good repeatability and correlation of these samples. Second, this is a preliminary study on the pathogenesis of severe MPP comparing to mild MPP. Further study will be needed to further prove the hypothesis that gene reduction related to primary immunodeficiency in bronchoalveolar is involved in the pathogenesis of severe MPP. Patient's primary cell culture and in vivo experiments using animal model may help to clarify how these genes and pathways are involved in the pathogenesis of severe MPP in the future.

Conclusions

The current study presented gene expression profiles as well as alternative splicing in BALF samples from MPP patients by next-generation RNA sequencing. This study clearly indicates that the up-regulation of *IL13, FCER2, FLT1,* and *CLEC5A* and the down-regulation of *CD79A, AICDA, CD19,* and *TNFRSF13C* may contribute to the pathogenesis of severe MPP or the progression from mild MPP to severe MPP. Furthermore, the differentially expression of *FCER2* and *FCRLA* may be due to the alternative splicing; further studies will be required to confirm this hypothesis.

Additional files

Additional file 1: Table S1. Summary of patients' information.

Additional file 2: Figure S1. The levels of immunoglobulins in the peripheral blood of MPP patients. A. The levels of IgG in each patients. Normal range of 5.09–14.17 g/L is shown as dotted lines. B. The levels of IgA in each patients. Normal range of 0.31–1.92 g/L is shown as dotted lines. C. The levels of IgM in each patient. Normal range of 0.98–2.56 g/L

Additional file 3: Table S2. Lymphocyte profiles in the peripheral

Additional file 4: Table S3. Nucleated cell count in the BALF of the

Additional file 5: Figure S2. Evaluation of each sample included in the current study. A. The correlation coefficient heat map. Correlation matrix shows a high consistency of measurements within each group. $R^2 \geq 0.8$ is needed for the up-coming analyzing. B. Principal component analysis (PCA) plot. PCA is conducted to evaluate the clustering nature of the samples. Each point represents one sample. The repeatability of the

Additional file 6: Table S4. Protein functional classification in differentially

Additional file 7: Table S5. Summary of the differential expressed

Additional file 8: Table S6. Summary of the differential expressed

Additional file 9: Table S7. Summary of the differential expressed

Additional file 10: Table S8. Summary of the differential expressed

Additional file 11: Table S9. Summary of the differential expressed

Abbreviations

AICDA: Activation-induced cytidine deaminase; BAFF: B cell activating factor; BAL: Bronchoalveolar lavage; BALF: Bronchoalveolar lavage fluid; BCR: B cell receptor; CAP: Community acquired pneumonia; CLEC5A: C-type lectin domain family 5, member A; COPD: Chronic obstructive pulmonary disease; CTL: C-type lectin; CTLD: C-type lectin-like domain; DNA: Deoxyribonucleic acid; ELISA: Enzyme-linked immunosorbent assay; FDR: False discovery rate; IgA: Immunoglobin A; IgG: Immunoglobin G; IgM: Immunoglobin M; IGV: Integrative Genomics Viewer; Igα: Immunoglobin α; KEGG: Kyoto Encyclopedia of Genes and Genomes; MEX: Mutual exclusive exon; MP: *Mycoplasma pneumoniae*; MPP: *Mycoplasma pneumoniae* pneumonia; PANTHER: Protein analysis through evolutionary relationships; PCR: Polymerase chain reaction; RA-SF: Rheumatoid arthritis synovium fluid; RI: Retained intron; RNA: Ribonucleic acid; Th2: T helper type 2; TNFRSF13C: Tumor necrosis factor receptor superfamily member 13C

Acknowledgements

The authors thank Dr. Aiping Wu from Suzhou Institute of Systems Medicine for the helpful discussions.

Funding

This work was supported by Starting Fund of the First Hospital, Jilin University (2011041).

Authors' contributions

KW collected the samples, performed the experiments, contributed to the interpretation of data, and made the figures and tables. MG determined the clinical status for the participation in the study, contributed to the interpretation of the data, and helped to draft the manuscript with the input from all authors. MY performed the statistical analysis, helped with the experiments, and made the tables. FM participated in the study design and coordination. DL, RL, YW, HZ, and ML provided the samples and collected the clinical information. GC participated in the study design and data analysis. XW designed the study, analyzed the data, finished the manuscript, and approved the final manuscript. All of the authors read and approved the manuscript.

Competing interests

The authors declare that they have no competing interests.

Author details

[1]Institute of Translational Medicine, the First Hospital of Jilin University, Changchun 130061, China. [2]Department of Pediatrics, the First Hospital of Jilin University, Changchun 130021, China. [3]Bethune Medical School of Jilin University, Changchun 130021, China. [4]Department of Microbiology, Immunology and Molecular Genetics, University of California Los Angeles, Los Angeles, CA 90095, USA.

References

1. Chaudhry R, Ghosh A, Chandolia A. Pathogenesis of Mycoplasma pneumoniae: an update. Indian J Med Microbiol. 2016;34(1):7–16.
2. Yan C, Sun H, Zhao H. Latest surveillance data on Mycoplasma pneumoniae infections in children, suggesting a new epidemic occurring in Beijing. J Clin Microbiol. 2016;54(5):1400–1.
3. Sawicki GS, Lu FL, Valim C, Cleveland RH, Colin AA. Necrotising pneumonia is an increasingly detected complication of pneumonia in children. Eur Respir J. 2008;31(6):1285–91.
4. Leonardi S, del Giudice MM, Spicuzza L, Saporito M, Nipitella G, La Rosa M. Lung abscess in a child with Mycoplasma pneumoniae infection. Eur J Pediatr. 2010;169(11):1413–5.
5. Hawkins S, Rausch CM, McCanta AC. Constrictive pericarditis secondary to infection with Mycoplasma pneumoniae. Curr Opin Pediatr. 2011;23(1):126–9.
6. Waites KB, Balish MF, Atkinson TP. New insights into the pathogenesis and detection of Mycoplasma pneumoniae infections. Future Microbiol. 2008;3(6):635–48.
7. Izumikawa K. Clinical features of severe or fatal Mycoplasma pneumoniae pneumonia. Front Microbiol. 2016;7:800.
8. Takeuchi O, Kawai T, Muhlradt PF, Morr M, Radolf JD, Zychlinsky A, Takeda K, Akira S. Discrimination of bacterial lipoproteins by Toll-like receptor 6. Int Immunol. 2001;13(7):933–40.

9. Tanaka H, Narita M, Teramoto S, Saikai T, Oashi K, Igarashi T, Abe S. Role of interleukin-18 and T-helper type 1 cytokines in the development of Mycoplasma pneumoniae pneumonia in adults. Chest. 2002;121(5):1493–7.
10. Zhang Y, Zhou Y, Li S, Yang D, Wu X, Chen Z. The clinical characteristics and predictors of refractory Mycoplasma pneumoniae pneumonia in children. PLoS One. 2016;11(5):e0156465.
11. Miyashita N, Kawai Y, Inamura N, Tanaka T, Akaike H, Teranishi H, Wakabayashi T, Nakano T, Ouchi K, Okimoto N. Setting a standard for the initiation of steroid therapy in refractory or severe Mycoplasma pneumoniae pneumonia in adolescents and adults. J Infect Chemother. 2015;21(3):153–60.
12. Wang Z, Gerstein M, Snyder M. RNA-Seq: a revolutionary tool for transcriptomics. Nat Rev Genet. 2009;10(1):57–63.
13. Garber M, Grabherr MG, Guttman M, Trapnell C. Computational methods for transcriptome annotation and quantification using RNA-seq. Nat Methods. 2011;8(6):469–77.
14. Ameratunga R, Woon ST, Gillis D, Koopmans W, Steele R. New diagnostic criteria for common variable immune deficiency (CVID), which may assist with decisions to treat with intravenous or subcutaneous immunoglobulin. Clin Exp Immunol. 2013;174(2):203–11.
15. Jiang YHZ. Zhu Futang's textbook of pediatrics. Beijing: People's Military Medical Publisher; 2003.
16. Qamar N, Fuleihan RL. The hyper IgM syndromes. Clinical reviews in allergy & immunology. 2014;46(2):120–30.
17. Chernick V, Kendig EL. Kendig's disorders of the respiratory tract in children. 7th ed. Philadelphia: Saunders/Elsevier; 2006.
18. Guo L, Liu F, Lu MP, Zheng Q, Chen ZM. Increased T cell activation in BALF from children with Mycoplasma pneumoniae pneumonia. Pediatr Pulmonol. 2015;50(8):814–9.
19. Anders S, Huber W. Differential expression analysis for sequence count data. Genome Biol. 2010;11(10):R106.
20. PANTHER classification system. http://pantherdb.org. Accessed 1 Nov 2016.
21. Shen S, Park JW, Huang J, Dittmar KA, Lu ZX, Zhou Q, Carstens RP, Xing Y. MATS: a Bayesian framework for flexible detection of differential alternative splicing from RNA-Seq data. Nucleic Acids Res. 2012;40(8), e61.
22. KEGG PATHWAY Database. http://www.genome.jp/kegg/pathway.html. Accessed 1 Jan 2017.
23. GeneCards. http://www.genecards.org/. Accessed 11 Nov 2016.
24. Wang ET, Sandberg R, Luo S, Khrebtukova I, Zhang L, Mayr C, Kingsmore SF, Schroth GP, Burge CB. Alternative isoform regulation in human tissue transcriptomes. Nature. 2008;456(7221):470–6.
25. Wills-Karp M, Luyimbazi J, Xu X, Schofield B, Neben TY, Karp CL, Donaldson DD. Interleukin-13: central mediator of allergic asthma. Science. 1998; 282(5397):2258–61.
26. Wu Q, Martin RJ, Lafasto S, Efaw BJ, Rino JG, Harbeck RJ, Chu HW. Toll-like receptor 2 down-regulation in established mouse allergic lungs contributes to decreased mycoplasma clearance. Am J Respir Crit Care Med. 2008; 177(7):720–9.
27. Hao Y, Kuang Z, Jing J, Miao J, Mei LY, Lee RJ, Kim S, Choe S, Krause DC, Lau GW. Mycoplasma pneumoniae modulates STAT3-STAT6/EGFR-FOXA2 signaling to induce overexpression of airway mucins. Infect Immun. 2014; 82(12):5246–55.
28. Sharma V, Michel S, Gaertner V, Franke A, Vogelberg C, von Berg A, Bufe A, Heinzmann A, Laub O, Rietschel E, et al. A role of FCER1A and FCER2 polymorphisms in IgE regulation. Allergy. 2014;69(2):231–6.
29. Tantisira KG, Silverman ES, Mariani TJ, Xu J, Richter BG, Klanderman BJ, Litonjua AA, Lazarus R, Rosenwasser LJ, Fuhlbrigge AL, et al. FCER2: a pharmacogenetic basis for severe exacerbations in children with asthma. J Allergy Clin Immunol. 2007;120(6):1285–91.
30. Ye Q, Xu XJ, Shao WX, Pan YX, Chen XJ. Mycoplasma pneumoniae infection in children is a risk factor for developing allergic diseases. Sci World J. 2014; 2014:986527.
31. Wu WK, Georgiadis A, Copland DA, Liyanage S, Luhmann UF, Robbie SJ, Liu J, Wu J, Bainbridge JW, Bates DO, et al. IL-4 regulates specific Arg-1(+) macrophage sFlt-1-mediated inhibition of angiogenesis. Am J Pathol. 2015; 185(8):2324–35.
32. Choi SH, Park EY, Jung HL, Shim JW, Kim DS, Park MS, Shim JY. Serum vascular endothelial growth factor in pediatric patients with community-acquired pneumonia and pleural effusion. J Korean Med Sci. 2006;21(4):608–13.
33. Shim JY, Park SW, Kim DS, Shim JW, Jung HL, Park MS. The effect of interleukin-4 and amphiregulin on the proliferation of human airway smooth muscle cells and cytokine release. J Korean Med Sci. 2008; 23(5):857–63.
34. Shin JE, Cheon BR, Shim JW, Kim DS, Jung HL, Park MS, Shim JY. Increased risk of refractory Mycoplasma pneumoniae pneumonia in children with atopic sensitization and asthma. Korean J Pediatr. 2014;57(6):271–7.
35. Tang LF, Shi YC, Xu YC, Wang CF, Yu ZS, Chen ZM. The change of asthma-associated immunological parameters in children with Mycoplasma pneumoniae infection. The Journal of asthma : official journal of the Association for the Care of Asthma. 2009;46(3):265–9.
36. Wortham BW, Eppert BL, Flury JL, Garcia SM, Donica WR, Osterburg A, Joyce-Shaikh B, Cua DJ, Borchers MT. Cutting edge: CLEC5A mediates macrophage function and chronic obstructive pulmonary disease pathologies. J Immunol. 2016;196(8):3227–31.
37. Muro S, Tabara Y, Matsumoto H, Setoh K, Kawaguchi T, Takahashi M, Ito I, Ito Y, Murase K, Terao C, et al. Relationship among chlamydia and Mycoplasma pneumoniae seropositivity, IKZF1 genotype and chronic obstructive pulmonary disease in a general Japanese population: the Nagahama study. Medicine (Baltimore). 2016;95(15), e3371.
38. Teng O, Chen ST, Hsu TL, Sia SF, Cole S, Valkenburg SA, Hsu TY, Zheng JT, Tu W, Bruzzone R et al. CLEC5A-mediated enhancement of the inflammatory response in myeloid cells contributes to influenza virus pathogenicity in vivo. J Virol. 2017;91(1):e01813-16.
39. Soler Palacios B, Estrada-Capetillo L, Izquierdo E, Criado G, Nieto C, Municio C, Gonzalez-Alvaro I, Sanchez-Mateos P, Pablos JL, Corbi AL, et al. Macrophages from the synovium of active rheumatoid arthritis exhibit an activin A-dependent pro-inflammatory profile. J Pathol. 2015;235(3):515–26.
40. Salilew-Wondim D, Ibrahim S, Gebremedhn S, Tesfaye D, Heppelmann M, Bollwein H, Pfarrer C, Tholen E, Neuhoff C, Schellander K, et al. Clinical and subclinical endometritis induced alterations in bovine endometrial transcriptome and miRNome profile. BMC Genomics. 2016;17:218.
41. Capello D, Gloghini A, Martini M, Spina M, Tirelli U, Bertoni F, Rinaldi A, Morra E, Rambaldi A, Sinigaglia F, et al. Mutations of CD79A, CD79B and EZH2 genes in immunodeficiency-related non-Hodgkin lymphomas. Br J Haematol. 2011;152(6):777–80.
42. Xu Z, Pone EJ, Al-Qahtani A, Park SR, Zan H, Casali P. Regulation of aicda expression and AID activity: relevance to somatic hypermutation and class switch DNA recombination. Crit Rev Immunol. 2007;27(4):367–97.
43. Trotta L, Hautala T, Hamalainen S, Syrjanen J, Viskari H, Almusa H, Lepisto M, Kaustio M, Porkka K, Palotie A, et al. Enrichment of rare variants in population isolates: single AICDA mutation responsible for hyper-IgM syndrome type 2 in Finland. Eur J Hum Genet. 2016;24(10):1473–8.
44. Morbach H, Schickel JN, Cunningham-Rundles C, Conley ME, Reisli I, Franco JL, Meffre E. CD19 controls Toll-like receptor 9 responses in human B cells. J Allergy Clin Immunol. 2016;137(3):889–98. e886.
45. Boqaert DJ, Dullaers M, Lambrecht BN, Vermaelen KY, De Baere E, Haerynck F. Gene associated with common variable immunodeficiency: one diagnosis to rule them all. J Med Genet. 2016;59:575–90.
46. Gamazon ER, Stranger BE. Genomics of alternative splicing: evolution, development and pathophysiology. Hum Genet. 2014;133(6):679–87.
47. Tazi J, Bakkour N, Stamm S. Alternative splicing and disease. Biochim Biophys Acta. 2009;1792(1):14–26.
48. Li Y, Bor YC, Fitzgerald MP, Lee KS, Rekosh D, Hammarskjold ML. An NXF1 mRNA with a retained intron is expressed in hippocampal and neocortical neurons and is translated into a protein that functions as an Nxf1 cofactor. Mol Biol Cell. 2016;27(24):3903–12.
49. Santiago T, Kulemzin SV, Reshetnikova ES, Chikaev NA, Volkova OY, Mechetina LV, Zhao M, Davis RS, Taranin AV, Najakshin AM, et al. FCRLA is a resident endoplasmic reticulum protein that associates with intracellular Igs, IgM, IgG and IgA. Int Immunol. 2011;23(1):43–53.
50. Kulemzin S, Chikaev N, Volkova O, Reshetnikova E, Taranin A, Najakshin A, Mechetina L. Characterization of human FCRLA isoforms. Immunol Lett. 2013;152(2):153–8.
51. Peng X, Li SS, Gilbert PB, Geraghty DE, Katze MG. FCGR2C polymorphisms associated with HIV-1 vaccine protection are linked to altered gene expression of Fc-gamma receptors in human B cells. PLoS One. 2016;11(3), e0152425.
52. Lee KE, Kim KW, Hong JY, Kim KE, Sohn MH. Modulation of IL-8 boosted by Mycoplasma pneumoniae lysate in human airway epithelial cells. J Clin Immunol. 2013;33(6):1117–25.
53. Kang YM, Ding MJ, Han YL, Wang SF, Ma X, Li H. Th1/Th2 immune response in bronchoalveolar lavage fluid in children with severe Mycoplasma pneumoniae pneumonia. Zhongguo Dang Dai Er Ke Za Zhi. 2011;13(3):188–90.

13

Major influence of repetitive elements on disease-associated copy number variants (CNVs)

Ana R. Cardoso[1,2,3], Manuela Oliveira[1,2,3], Antonio Amorim[1,2,3] and Luisa Azevedo[1,2,3*]

Abstract

Copy number variants (CNVs) are important contributors to the human pathogenic genetic diversity as demonstrated by a number of cases reported in the literature. The high homology between repetitive elements may guide genomic stability which will give rise to CNVs either by non-allelic homologous recombination (NAHR) or non-homologous end joining (NHEJ). Here, we present a short guide based on previously documented cases of disease-associated CNVs in order to provide a general view on the impact of repeated elements on the stability of the genomic sequence and consequently in the origin of the human pathogenic variome.

Keywords: Copy number variants (CNVs), Genetic diseases, Genomic structural variation, Low copy repeats, Retrotransposons, LINE, SINE, Non-allelic homologous recombination (NAHR)

Background

Copy number variants (CNVs) are structural genomic markers (insertions or deletions) ranging in size from 1 kb to several megabytes for each copy. They are categorized as copy number polymorphisms (CNPs) when multiple allelic states exist in the population or as rare copy number variants when they are found to be associated with genetic diseases (pathogenic copy number variants) [1, 2]. The origin of each repeated element of the CNV is influenced by the local genomic architecture which includes the presence of repetitive sequences within or flanking the repeated segment [3–7]. These repeated sequences drive non-allelic homologous recombination (NAHR) events which result in recurrent insertions and deletions with similar sequence sizes and clustered breakpoints [3, 6, 8] or non-homologous end joining (NHEJ) events that result in non-recurrent rearrangements that vary in terms of their size and breakpoint location [3, 6, 9]. Although several studies have been demonstrating the contribution of structural variants to the genome architecture, few have specifically focused the influence of repeated sequences at breakpoint locations. With the aim to draw attention to these unstable regions and to establish their role in CNVs, we collated a number of cases of CNV-associated disorders proven to have been generated by low and high copy number repeats which may have influenced the degree of stability of the genomic sequence.

* Correspondence: lazevedo@ipatimup.pt
[1]Instituto de Investigação e Inovação em Saúde, Universidade do Porto, Rua Alfredo Allen 208, 4200-135 Porto, Portugal
[2]IPATIMUP-Institute of Molecular Pathology and Immunology, University of Porto, Rua Júlio Amaral de Carvalho 45, 4200-135 Porto, Portugal
Full list of author information is available at the end of the article

Low copy repeats and their influence on pathogenic CNV formation

Low copy repeats (LCRs) are homologous sequences of ≥1 kb in length which are found in many copies throughout the genome since they are generated by duplication events [3, 10]. Large LCRs (>10 kb) with high sequence homology promote non-allelic homologous recombination (NAHR) [3–6, 10–12] and the misalignment of directly oriented sister chromatids carrying the LCR may promoted NAHR thereby generating both duplications and deletions [4, 5] which in turn give rise to copy number variation. A schematic representation of this process is shown in Fig. 1.

Certain properties of the LCRs such as homology length, sequence similarity, and distance, serve to influence the frequency of NAHR events [3, 6, 12] (Fig. 1). As recently reviewed by Carvalho and Lupski [3], the NAHR

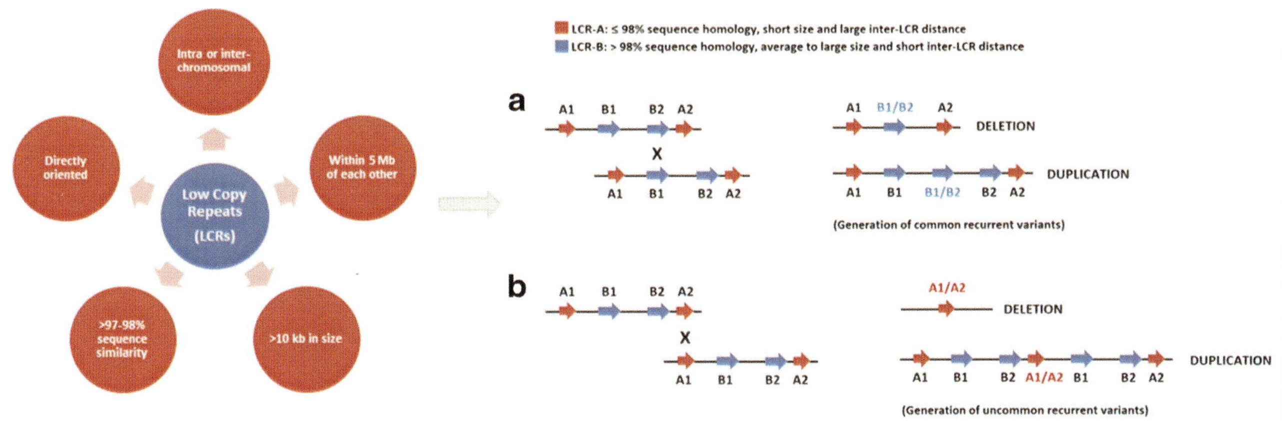

Fig. 1 Optimal LCRs features for the occurrence of NAHR events that result in CNV formation. Distinct LCR pairs with counter features such as homology, size, and inter-LCR distance influence NAHR rate and lead to the formation of common recurrent (**a**) or rare recurrent (**b**) copy number variants. Adapted from [3, 6, 12]

rate varies according to the length of the LCR sequence, the distance between distinct LCR sequences and the DNA sequence. The NAHR rate is, therefore, positively correlated with the LCR length but is inversely proportional to the distance between distinct LCRs [3, 9]. Since there is a high homology between distinct LCR sequences proximal to copy number variation regions; there is also an increased predisposition to NAHR events in these genomic regions [3, 4, 6, 9, 12].

A considerable number of disease-associated CNVs generated by LCRs have been documented and reviewed in previous works (e.g. [3, 6]), but for the purposes of this paper, we have only collated cases for which the specific repetitive element was found at the breakpoints of the structural variant and not those for which the causality of the repeats elements was only suggested. The resulting set is presented in Table 1. For example, a complex array of LCRs spanning a 4-Mb region around the X-linked *MECP2* gene was associated with unique duplications ranging in size from 200 kb to 2.2 Mb in developmentally delayed males [13]. Duplications and deletions affecting the *PLP1* gene causing Pelizaeus-Merzbacher disease (OMIM #312080) are also associated with a specific LCR (LCR-PMD A/B pair) within a 3-Mb region flanking the gene in which a multitude of LCRs are located [14]. LCRs are also frequent at the 2q11-q21.1 locus [11], where recurrent deletions of the *NPHP1* gene (2q13) have been associated with nephronophthisis 1 (OMIM #256100). A 0.3-Mb copy number gain was detected in three X-linked intellectual disability (XLID) families and one sporadic patient [15]. The region overlapped the *GDI1* gene, an important XLID-associated

Table 1 Repetitive elements detected at the breakpoints of CNVs associated with clinical phenotypes

Phenotype	Critical genes	Type of variant	Locus	Repetitive element involved	Ref.
MECP2 duplication syndrome	*MECP2, L1CAM*	Dup	Xq28	Several LCR-MECP2s pairs	[3, 6, 13, 44–46]
Rett syndrome	*MECP2*	Del	Xq28	Several LCR-MECP2 pairs	[6]
Neurofibromatosis type I	*NF1*	Del	17q11.2	NF1-REPs A/B/C	[3, 6]
Nephronophthisis	*NPHP1*	Del	2q13	Several LCR pairs	[11, 47–49]
Mental retardation, X-linked 41 (MRX41)	*GDI1*	Dup/Trip	Xq28	LCR-K1/L2 pair	[15]
Angelman and Prader-Willi syndromes	*UBE3A*	Del	15q11-q13	END-repeats (LCRs)	[6, 50]
Smith-Magenis syndrome	*RAI1* and *PMP22*	Del	17p11.2	SMS-REPs (LCRs)	[3, 6, 18]
Williams-Beuren syndrome	28 dosage-sensitive genes	Dup/Tripe/Del	7q11.23	A/B/C LCR blocks	[3, 6, 51]
15q13.1 microdeletion syndrome	*CHRNA7*	Dup/Trip	15q13.3	BP3/4/5	[3, 6, 52, 53]
3q29 microduplication or microdeletion syndrome	*DLG1, PAK2*	Dup/Del	3q29	A/B/C LCR blocks	[3, 54, 55]
Pelizaeus-Merzbacher disease	*PLP1*	Dup/Del	Xq22	LCR-PMD A/B pair	[3, 6, 14]
DiGeorge syndrome/velo-cardio facial syndrome	*COMT, TBX1*	Del	22q11.2	8 specific LCR22 repeats	[6, 17, 40]
Charcot-Marie-Tooth type 1A	*PMP22*	Dup	17p12	CMTA1-Reps (LCRs)	[3, 6, 37, 38]

gene highly expressed in the brain. The aberration was located in Xq28, a locus that includes other intellectual disability genes and that is frequently associated with recombination events caused by proximal LCRs (e.g., LCR K1/L2). The Angelman syndrome (AS) (OMIM #105830) and Prader-Willi syndrome (PWS) (OMIM #176270) are caused by recurrent 4-Mb deletions at the 15q11-q13 locus. The deleted region is flanked by LCRs [6] and accounts for 70 % of cases of AS and 70–75 % of cases of PWS [16]. The Smith-Magenis syndrome (SMS) (OMIM #182290) results from recurrent deletions of 3.7 Mb at 17p11.2 which account for more than 70 % of cases; about 25 % of affected individuals harbor deletions ranging from 1.5–9 Mb [6, 17]. The deletions are flanked by 200-kb highly homologous LCRs that play a role in generating meiotic NAHR events [16]. These deletions encompass the *RAI1* gene, which is critical in organ and neuronal development—patients with larger deletions manifest a more severe phenotype when the dosage-sensitive gene *PMP22* is deleted [18].

Retrotransposons (high copy repeats) and their influence on pathogenic CNVs

Interspersed repeats are the most common type of high copy repeats, covering about 44 % of the human genome [4]. Retrotransposons account for the majority of transposable elements [5, 7, 19]. These are mobile elements that through reverse transcription have the ability to integrate into different regions [7, 19]. Long interspersed nuclear elements (LINEs), short interspersed nuclear elements (SINEs), and retrovirus-like elements (LTR transposons) are the three major categories of mammalian retrotransposons (Table 2).

Among LINEs, L1 is the most abundant element, typically of 6–8 kb in length, with the ability to increase genomic instability through NAHR events [4]. It is known that about 83 % of the human genome is prone to LINE-LINE recombination events that contribute to genomic instability and can give rise to unbalanced structural variants [20].

Alu elements are the most common SINEs and have been associated with NAHR events that lead to pathogenic duplications and deletions [3, 4, 21, 22]. Table 3 presents examples of high copy repeats that have been detected at the breakpoints of disease-associated CNVs.

Borun and colleagues [23] reported the presence of CNV breakpoints within Alu elements in the *STK11* gene which lead to the Peutz-Jeghers syndrome (OMIM #175200), where CNVs account for 30 % of cases. The 17p13.3 locus is enriched in copy number variations associated with genomic disorders, such as the Miller-Dieker syndrome (17p13.3 deletion syndrome) (OMIM #247200) and its reciprocal 17p13.3 duplication syndrome (OMIM #613215) [24]. The breakpoints of the reported CNVs at this locus are highly enriched in Alu elements, which mediate these junctions through an Alu-Alu mechanism. About 70 % of CNVs found in the *SPAST* gene have been associated with Alu recombination events [25]. Local Alu-rich architecture predisposes to the formation of pathogenic structural rearrangements associated with spastic paraplegia (OMIM #182601). An extra copy of the *LMNB1* gene at the 5q23 locus has been previously associated with autosomal dominant adult-onset demyelinating leukodystrophy (ADLD) (OMIM #169500). The analysis of twenty ADLD-affected families revealed sixteen duplications ranging from 128 to 475 kb in size, all of them spanning the *LMNB1* gene [26]. The centromeric region of the critical gene is enriched with SINE elements, particularly Alus. Alu-mediated recombination events were also found to be linked to pathogenic deletions at the *OTC* gene [27], a urea cycle gene for which a significant number of structural variants are known [28]. NAHR events between Alu repeats are also strongly correlated with the birth of structural rearrangements at the Alu-rich *BRCA1* locus [29] which is associated with breast cancer. Duplications (220 to 394 kb) and a triplication (1.61 to 2.04 Mb) of the *SNCA* gene located at 4q21 locus have been implicated in autosomal dominant Parkinson's disease (PD1 and PD4) (OMIM #168601, #605543). The phenotypic severity is consistent with a gene dosage effect [6]. Regarding recessive PD (OMIM #600116), about one third of pathogenic variants associated with the *PRKN* gene are CNVs occurring between exon 2 and exon 5, which may therefore be considered to be a

Table 2 Main characteristics of the most abundant retrotransposons [4, 5, 7, 19]

	Retrotransposons (interspersed repeats)—44 % human genome		
	Non-long terminal repeat (LTR)		Long terminal repeat (LTR)
Repetitive element	Long interspersed nuclear repeats (LINEs)	Short interspersed nuclear repeats (SINEs)	Endogenous retroviruses (ERV)
Genomic coverage	20 %	11 %	8 %
Features	• L1 is the most abundant class • Autonomous transposons • Reverse transcriptase (RT) encoded by LINE-1	• Alu is the most abundant class • Dependent on LINEs transposable machinery • Mobile polymerase III promoter • 100–400 bp in length	• Reduced transposable activity • Presence of *gag* and *pol* viral genes

Table 3 High copy repeats detected at the breakpoints of CNVs associated with clinical phenotypes

Phenotype	Critical genes	Type of variant	Locus	Repetitive elements involved	Ref.
Peutz-Jeghers syndrome	*STK11*	Del	19p13.3	Several AluY/AluY pairs	[23]
Spastic paraplegia 4	*SPAST, SLC30A6*	Dup/Del	2p22.3	Several Alu pairs	[25]
OTC deficiency	*OTC*	Del	Xp11.4	AluSx/AluSq pair	[27, 56]
Miller-Dieker syndrome and 17p13.3 duplication syndrome	*LIS1*	Del	17p13.3	Several Alu pairs	[6, 24]
Breast cancer	*BRCA1*	Del	17q21.31	AluSx/AluSc pair	[29, 57]
Autosomal dominant adult-onset demyelinating leukodystrophy (ADLD)	*LMNB1*	Dup/Trip	5q23.2	LIPA3 LINE repeats AluYA/AluYB pair	[26]
Azoospermia	*AZFa*	Del	Yq11	HERV15 A/B proviruses	[34, 58]
Mental retardation, X-linked 60 (MRX60)	*OPHN1*	Del	Xq12	AluY/AluY pair	[35]
Pelizaeus-Merzbacher disease	*PLP1*	Del	Xq22	AluSq/AluSx pair	[3, 6, 59]
DiGeorge syndrome/velo-cardio facial syndrome	*COMT, TBX1*	Del	22q11.2	Unclassified Alu/Alu pair	[6, 17, 40]
Charcot-Marie-Tooth type 1A	*PMP22*	Dup	17p12	AluY/AluY pair AluSg/AluSg pair	[39]
Williams-Beuren syndrome	28 dosage-sensitive genes	Dup/Del	7q11.23	AluS subfamily elements	[36]
Parkinson's disease	*SNCA*	Dup/Trip	4q21	Several Alu pairs	[32]

recombination hotspot [30, 31]. Ross and colleagues [32] reported the presence of Alu and LINE1 elements at the *SNCA* locus that may contribute to the genomic instability at this locus.

Human endogenous retroviruses (HERVs) represent about 4.9 % of the human genome [4]. Sequences with about 95 % sequence similarity were previously associated with NAHR events and recurrent CNVs, some of which with pathogenic implications [3, 33]. For example, the occurrence of NAHR between a particular set of HERV elements flanking the male fertility *AZFa* locus in the Y chromosome is strongly associated with pathogenic deletions associated with male infertility (OMIM #400042, #415000) [4, 34].

Pathogenic copy number variants associated with both LCRs and retrotransposons

The breakpoints of some disease-associated CNVs have been reported to be caused by more than one type of repetitive elements which indicates that the same phenotype involves both low copy and high copy repeats that affect the stability of a target gene. Bergmann and colleagues [35] conducted a family study in which five brothers shared the same phenotypic pattern that included intellectual disability. The analysis of the OPHN1 locus (Xq12) revealed the presence of a 17.6-kb intronic deletion and the breakpoints spanning the deletion revealed two highly homologous Alu repeats and additional repetitive sequences (interspersed and simple repeats).

A recurrent deletion of 1.6 to 1.8 Mb (>95 % of the patients) at the 7q11.23 locus causes the Williams-Beuren syndrome (OMIM #194050) [6]. Genes within this region are dosage-sensitive and the recurrently deleted region encompasses a total of 28 genes. This locus is characterized by highly homologous flanking LCRs that contribute to NAHR events [6]. Antonell and colleagues [36] reported the presence of Alu elements at the junctions of large duplicated blocks in 7q11.23 suggesting the influence of these retrotransposons in the generation of large LCRs.

Heterozygous duplication and reciprocal deletions of a 1.4–1.5-Mb segment at the 17p12 locus have been previously linked with the Charcot-Marie-Tooth type 1A syndrome (CMT1A) (OMIM #118220). About 70 % of CMT1A patients have a recurrent duplication of the dosage-sensitive PMP22 locus and the NAHR event that gave rise to this copy number variation was mediated by LCRs [3, 6, 37, 38]. A study by Zhang and colleagues [39] revealed the presence of SINEs (Alu elements) and LINEs (L1 and L2) as well as LCRs within the breakpoints of rare non-recurrent deletions and duplications at the CMT1A locus.

About 96 % of the DiGeorge syndrome (DGS) (OMIM #188400)- and velo-cardio-facial syndrome (VCFS) (OMIM #192430)-affected patients harbor a 1.5–3 Mb deletion at the 22q11.2 locus that includes 24 to 30 genes [16]. The breakpoints of the common recurrent deletions at this locus are associated with LCRs [17] and one Alu sequence [40]. Both the deletions and duplications at this locus are generated by NAHR events between the repeated regions flanking the CNV, specifically the low copy repeat known as LCR22 [41]. Furthermore, 20–25 % of individuals who harbor this deletion also show signs of schizophrenia, mood disorders, and other behavioral alterations [41].

Conclusions

Although the majority of genetic diseases are caused by non-structural variants (e.g. [42, 43], an increasing number of causative mutations have been associated with CNVs and these cases were the focus of this short review. Low copy repeats and retrotransposons are the major contributors to CNV formation. Recurrent CNVs are mainly directed by NAHR events that occur between highly homologous LCR sequences. In terms of non-recurrent CNVs, NHEJ (among other molecular mechanisms [3]) generally occurs between sequences with a degree of homology lower than that observed between distinct LCRs. The diversity of breakpoint junctions of non-recurrent variants renders the establishment of phenotype-genotype relationships less reliable because the sequence that is deleted or duplicated in each patient is different and the affected region may also involve other genes. This review focused on disease-associated CNVs in order to show that although numerous cases of instability driven by repeated sequences around the affected locus (or loci) have been documented, we are still far from understanding all the phenotypic complexities associated with these unbalanced variants, mainly because the number of reported cases is still too small to draw general conclusions. Finally, it is important to mention that collated data, such as those presented in this paper, pertaining to the pathogenic structural variome are expected to drive future studies with the aim of establishing a map of unstable genomic hotspots which promises to be useful in the context of clinical genetic testing where the determination of the molecular basis of Mendelian and complex diseases (e.g., cancer) is of paramount importance.

Abbreviations

CNV: Copy number variant; LCR: Low copy repeat; CNP: Copy number polymorphism; LINE: Long interspersed nuclear repeat; SINE: Short interspersed nuclear repeat; LTR: Long terminal repeat; NAHR: Non-allelic homologous recombination; NHEJ: Non-homologous end joining; XLID: X-linked intellectual disability

Acknowledgements

Not applicable.

Funding

IPATIMUP integrates the i3S Research Unit, which is partially supported by FCT, the Portuguese Foundation for Science and Technology. This work is funded by FEDER funds through the Operational Programme for Competitiveness Factors - COMPETE and National Funds through the FCT-Foundation for Science and Technology, under the projects "PEst-C/SAU/LA0003/2013". M. Oliveira (SFRH/BPD/66071/2009) was supported by FCT fellowships funded by POPH-QREN - Promotion of Scientific Employment, the European Social Fund, and National Funds of the Ministry of Education and Science.

Authors' contributions

ARC performed literature search. ARC and LA drafted the manuscript. MO and AA discussed the data and performed critical revisions to the manuscript. All authors read and approved the final manuscript.

Competing interests

The authors declare that they have no competing interests.

Author details

[1]Instituto de Investigação e Inovação em Saúde, Universidade do Porto, Rua Alfredo Allen 208, 4200-135 Porto, Portugal. [2]IPATIMUP-Institute of Molecular Pathology and Immunology, University of Porto, Rua Júlio Amaral de Carvalho 45, 4200-135 Porto, Portugal. [3]Department of Biology, Faculty of Sciences, University of Porto, Rua do Campo Alegre S/N, 4169-007 Porto, Portugal.

References

1. Itsara A, Cooper GM, Baker C, Girirajan S, Li J, Absher D, et al. Population analysis of large copy number variants and hotspots of human genetic disease. Am J Hum Genet. 2009;84(2):148–61.
2. Henrichsen CN, Chaignat E, Reymond A. Copy number variants, diseases and gene expression. Hum Mol Genet. 2009;18(R1):R1–8.
3. Carvalho CM, Lupski JR. Mechanisms underlying structural variant formation in genomic disorders. Nat Rev Genet. 2016;17(4):224–38.
4. Chen L, Zhou W, Zhang L, Zhang F. Genome architecture and its roles in human copy number variation. Genomics Inform. 2014;12(4):136–44.
5. Jobling MA, Hollox E, Hurles M, Kivisild T, Tyler-Smith C. Human evolutionary genetics: origins, peoples and disease. 2nd ed. New York: Garland Science; 2014.
6. Lee JA, Lupski JR. Genomic rearrangements and gene copy-number alterations as a cause of nervous system disorders. Neuron. 2006;52(1):103–21.
7. Strachan T, Read A. Human Molecular Genetics. 4th ed. New York:Garland Science; 2011.
8. Gu W, Zhang F, Lupski JR. Mechanisms for human genomic rearrangements. Pathogenetics. 2008;1(1):4.
9. Liu P, Lacaria M, Zhang F, Withers M, Hastings PJ, Lupski JR. Frequency of nonallelic homologous recombination is correlated with length of homology: evidence that ectopic synapsis precedes ectopic crossing-over. Am J Hum Genet. 2011;89(4):580–8.
10. Potier MC, Golfier G, Eichler EE. Chromosome-specific repeats (Low-copy Repeats). In:eLS. Chichester: Wiley; 2007.
11. Dittwald P, Gambin T, Szafranski P, Li J, Amato S, Divon MY, et al. NAHR-mediated copy-number variants in a clinical population: mechanistic insights into both genomic disorders and Mendelizing traits. Genome Res. 2013;23(9):1395–409.
12. Peng Z, Zhou W, Fu W, Du R, Jin L, Zhang F. Correlation between frequency of non-allelic homologous recombination and homology properties: evidence from homology-mediated CNV mutations in the human genome. Hum Mol Genet. 2015;24(5):1225–33.
13. del Gaudio D, Fang P, Scaglia F, Ward PA, Craigen WJ, Glaze DG, et al. Increased MECP2 gene copy number as the result of genomic duplication in neurodevelopmentally delayed males. Genet Med. 2006;8(12):784–92.
14. Lee JA, Inoue K, Cheung SW, Shaw CA, Stankiewicz P, Lupski JR. Role of genomic architecture in PLP1 duplication causing Pelizaeus-Merzbacher disease. Hum Mol Genet. 2006;15(14):2250–65.

15. Vandewalle J, Van Esch H, Govaerts K, Verbeeck J, Zweier C, Madrigal I, et al. Dosage-dependent severity of the phenotype in patients with mental retardation due to a recurrent copy-number gain at Xq28 mediated by an unusual recombination. Am J Hum Genet. 2009;85(6):809–22.
16. Firth HV, Richards SM, Bevan AP, Clayton S, Corpas M, Rajan D, et al. DECIPHER: Database of Chromosomal Imbalance and Phenotype in Humans Using Ensembl Resources. Am J Hum Genet. 2009;84(4):524–33.
17. Shaikh TH, Kurahashi H, Saitta SC, O'Hare AM, Hu P, Roe BA, et al. Chromosome 22-specific low copy repeats and the 22q11.2 deletion syndrome: genomic organization and deletion endpoint analysis. Hum Mol Genet. 2000;9(4):489–501.
18. Madduri N, Peters SU, Voigt RG, Llorente AM, Lupski JR, Potocki L. Cognitive and adaptive behavior profiles in Smith-Magenis syndrome. J Dev Behav Pediatr. 2006;27(3):188–92.
19. Smit AF. The origin of interspersed repeats in the human genome. Curr Opin Genet Dev. 1996;6(6):743–8.
20. Startek M, Szafranski P, Gambin T, Campbell IM, Hixson P, Shaw CA, et al. Genome-wide analyses of LINE-LINE-mediated nonallelic homologous recombination. Nucleic Acids Res. 2015;43(4):2188–98.
21. Batzer MA, Deininger PL. Alu repeats and human genomic diversity. Nat Rev Genet. 2002;3(5):370–9.
22. Teixeira-Silva A, Silva RM, Carneiro J, Amorim A, Azevedo L. The role of recombination in the origin and evolution of Alu subfamilies. PloS one. 2013;8(6):e64884.
23. Borun P, De Rosa M, Nedoszytko B, Walkowiak J, Plawski A. Specific Alu elements involved in a significant percentage of copy number variations of the STK11 gene in patients with Peutz-Jeghers syndrome. Fam Cancer. 2015;14(3):455–61.
24. Gu S, Yuan B, Campbell IM, Beck CR, Carvalho CM, Nagamani SC, et al. Alu-mediated diverse and complex pathogenic copy-number variants within human chromosome 17 at p13.3. Hum Mol Genet. 2015;24(14):4061–77.
25. Boone PM, Yuan B, Campbell IM, Scull JC, Withers MA, Baggett BC, et al. The Alu-rich genomic architecture of SPAST predisposes to diverse and functionally distinct disease-associated CNV alleles. Am J Hum Genet. 2014;95(2):143–61.
26. Giorgio E, Rolyan H, Kropp L, Chakka AB, Yatsenko S, Di Gregorio E, et al. Analysis of LMNB1 duplications in autosomal dominant leukodystrophy provides insights into duplication mechanisms and allele-specific expression. Hum Mutat. 2013;34(8):1160–71.
27. Quental R, Azevedo L, Rubio V, Diogo L, Amorim A. Molecular mechanisms underlying large genomic deletions in ornithine transcarbamylase (OTC) gene. Clin Genet. 2009;75(5):457–64.
28. Azevedo L, Stolnaja L, Tietzeova E, Hrebicek M, Hruba E, Vilarinho L, et al. New polymorphic sites within ornithine transcarbamylase gene: population genetics studies and implications for diagnosis. Mol Genet Metab. 2003; 78(2):152–7.
29. Ewald IP, Ribeiro PL, Palmero EI, Cossio SL, Giugliani R, Ashton-Prolla P. Genomic rearrangements in BRCA1 and BRCA2: a literature review. Genet Mol Biol. 2009;32(3):437–46.
30. Toft M, Ross OA. Copy number variation in Parkinson's disease. Genome Med. 2010;2(9):62.
31. Hedrich K, Eskelson C, Wilmot B, Marder K, Harris J, Garrels J, et al. Distribution, type, and origin of Parkin mutations: review and case studies. Mov Disord. 2004;19(10):1146–57.
32. Ross OA, Braithwaite AT, Skipper LM, Kachergus J, Hulihan MM, Middleton FA, et al. Genomic investigation of alpha-synuclein multiplication and parkinsonism. Ann Neurol. 2008;63(6):743–50.
33. Campbell IM, Gambin T, Dittwald P, Beck CR, Shuvarikov A, Hixson P, et al. Human endogenous retroviral elements promote genome instability via non-allelic homologous recombination. BMC Biol. 2014;12:74.
34. Bosch E, Jobling MA. Duplications of the AZFa region of the human Y chromosome are mediated by homologous recombination between HERVs and are compatible with male fertility. Hum Mol Genet. 2003;12(3):341–7.
35. Bergmann C, Zerres K, Senderek J, Rudnik-Schoneborn S, Eggermann T, Hausler M, et al. Oligophrenin 1 (OPHN1) gene mutation causes syndromic X-linked mental retardation with epilepsy, rostral ventricular enlargement and cerebellar hypoplasia. Brain. 2003;126(Pt 7):1537–44.
36. Antonell A, de Luis O, Domingo-Roura X, Perez-Jurado LA. Evolutionary mechanisms shaping the genomic structure of the Williams-Beuren syndrome chromosomal region at human 7q11.23. Genome Res. 2005;15(9):1179–88.
37. Pentao L, Wise CA, Chinault AC, Patel PI, Lupski JR. Charcot-Marie-Tooth type 1A duplication appears to arise from recombination at repeat sequences flanking the 1.5 Mb monomer unit. Nat Genet. 1992;2(4):292–300.
38. Weterman MA, van Ruissen F, de Wissel M, Bordewijk L, Samijn JP, van der Pol WL, et al. Copy number variation upstream of PMP22 in Charcot-Marie-Tooth disease. Eur J Hum Genet. 2010;18(4):421–8.
39. Zhang F, Seeman P, Liu P, Weterman MA, Gonzaga-Jauregui C, Towne CF, et al. Mechanisms for nonrecurrent genomic rearrangements associated with CMT1A or HNPP: rare CNVs as a cause for missing heritability. Am J Hum Genet. 2010;86(6):892–903.
40. Uddin RK, Zhang Y, Siu VM, Fan YS, O'Reilly RL, Rao J, et al. Breakpoint Associated with a novel 2.3 Mb deletion in the VCFS region of 22q11 and the role of Alu (SINE) in recurring microdeletions. BMC Med Genet. 2006;7:18.
41. Shishido E, Aleksic B, Ozaki N. Copy-number variation in the pathogenesis of autism spectrum disorder. Psychiatry Clin Neurosci. 2014;68(2):85–95.
42. Ferreira F, Esteves S, Almeida LS, Gaspar A, da Costa CD, Janeiro P, et al. Trimethylaminuria (fish odor syndrome): genotype characterization among Portuguese patients. Gene. 2013;527(1):366–70.
43. Quelhas D, Quental R, Vilarinho L, Amorim A, Azevedo L. Congenital disorder of glycosylation type Ia: searching for the origin of common mutations in PMM2. Ann Hum Genet. 2007;71(Pt 3):348–53.
44. Van Esch H. MECP2 duplication syndrome. Mol Syndromol. 2012;2(3-5):128–36.
45. Bauters M, Van Esch H, Friez MJ, Boespflug-Tanguy O, Zenker M, Vianna-Morgante AM, et al. Nonrecurrent MECP2 duplications mediated by genomic architecture-driven DNA breaks and break-induced replication repair. Genome Res. 2008;18(6):847–58.
46. Carvalho CM, Zhang F, Liu P, Patel A, Sahoo T, Bacino CA, et al. Complex rearrangements in patients with duplications of MECP2 can occur by fork stalling and template switching. Hum Mol Genet. 2009;18(12):2188–203.
47. Saunier S, Calado J, Benessy F, Silbermann F, Heilig R, Weissenbach J, et al. Characterization of the NPHP1 locus: mutational mechanism involved in deletions in familial juvenile nephronophthisis. Am J Hum Genet. 2000; 66(3):778–89.
48. Yuan B, Liu P, Gupta A, Beck CR, Tejomurtula A, Campbell IM, et al. Comparative genomic analyses of the human NPHP1 locus reveal complex genomic architecture and its regional evolution in primates. PLoS Genet. 2015;11(12):e1005686.
49. Konrad M, Saunier S, Heidet L, Silbermann F, Benessy F, Calado J, et al. Large homozygous deletions of the 2q13 region are a major cause of juvenile nephronophthisis. Hum Mol Genet. 1996;5(3):367–71.
50. Amos-Landgraf JM, Ji Y, Gottlieb W, Depinet T, Wandstrat AE, Cassidy SB, et al. Chromosome breakage in the Prader-Willi and Angelman syndromes involves recombination between large, transcribed repeats at proximal and distal breakpoints. Am J Hum Genet. 1999;65(2):370–86.
51. Bayes M, Magano LF, Rivera N, Flores R, Perez Jurado LA. Mutational mechanisms of Williams-Beuren syndrome deletions. Am J Hum Genet. 2003;73(1):131–51.
52. Willatt L, Cox J, Barber J, Cabanas ED, Collins A, Donnai D, et al. 3q29 microdeletion syndrome: clinical and molecular characterization of a new syndrome. Am J Hum Genet. 2005;77(1):154–60.
53. Ballif BC, Theisen A, Coppinger J, Gowans GC, Hersh JH, Madan-Khetarpal S, et al. Expanding the clinical phenotype of the 3q29 microdeletion syndrome and characterization of the reciprocal microduplication. Mol Cytogenet. 2008;1:8.
54. Soler-Alfonso C, Carvalho CM, Ge J, Roney EK, Bader PI, Kolodziejska KE, et al. CHRNA7 triplication associated with cognitive impairment and neuropsychiatric phenotypes in a three-generation pedigree. Eur J Hum Genet. 2014;22(9):1071–6.
55. Sharp AJ, Mefford HC, Li K, Baker C, Skinner C, Stevenson RE, et al. A recurrent 15q13.3 microdeletion syndrome associated with mental retardation and seizures. Nat Genet. 2008;40(3):322–8.
56. Shchelochkov OA, Li FY, Geraghty MT, Gallagher RC, Van Hove JL, Lichter-Konecki U, et al. High-frequency detection of deletions and variable rearrangements at the ornithine transcarbamylase (OTC) locus by oligonucleotide array CGH. Mol Genet Metab. 2009;96(3):97–105.
57. Mazoyer S. Genomic rearrangements in the BRCA1 and BRCA2 genes. Hum Mutat. 2005;25(5):415–22.
58. Sun C, Skaletsky H, Rozen S, Gromoll J, Nieschlag E, Oates R, et al. Deletion of azoospermia factor a (AZFa) region of human Y chromosome caused by recombination between HERV15 proviruses. Hum Mol Genet. 2000;9(15):2291–6.
59. Inoue K, Osaka H, Thurston VC, Clarke JT, Yoneyama A, Rosenbarker L, et al. Genomic rearrangements resulting in PLP1 deletion occur by nonhomologous end joining and cause different dysmyelinating phenotypes in males and females. Am J Hum Genet. 2002;71(4):838–53.

14

Whole transcriptome analysis of human erythropoietic cells during ontogenesis suggests a role of *VEGFA* gene as modulator of fetal hemoglobin and pharmacogenomic biomarker of treatment response to hydroxyurea in β-type hemoglobinopathy patients

Vasiliki Chondrou[1], Petros Kolovos[2], Argyro Sgourou[3], Alexandra Kourakli[4], Alexia Pavlidaki[1,8], Vlasia Kastrinou[1], Anne John[5], Argiris Symeonidis[4], Bassam R. Ali[5,6], Adamantia Papachatzopoulou[7], Theodora Katsila[1] and George P. Patrinos[1,5,6*]

Abstract

Background: Human erythropoiesis is characterized by distinct gene expression profiles at various developmental stages. Previous studies suggest that fetal-to-adult hemoglobin switch is regulated by a complex mechanism, in which many key players still remain unknown. Here, we report our findings from whole transcriptome analysis of erythroid cells, isolated from erythroid tissues at various developmental stages in an effort to identify distinct molecular signatures of each erythroid tissue.

Results: From our in-depth data analysis, pathway analysis, and text mining, we opted to focus on the *VEGFA* gene, given its gene expression characteristics. Selected *VEGFA* genomic variants, identified through linkage disequilibrium analysis, were explored further for their association with elevated fetal hemoglobin levels in β-type hemoglobinopathy patients. Our downstream analysis of non-transfusion-dependent β-thalassemia patients, β-thalassemia major patients, compound heterozygous sickle cell disease/β-thalassemia patients receiving hydroxyurea as fetal hemoglobin augmentation treatment, and non-thalassemic individuals indicated that *VEGFA* genomic variants were associated with disease severity in β-thalassemia patients and hydroxyurea treatment efficacy in SCD/β-thalassemia compound heterozygous patients.

Conclusions: Our findings suggest that *VEGFA* may act as a modifier gene of human globin gene expression and, at the same time, serve as a genomic biomarker in β-type hemoglobinopathy disease severity and hydroxyurea treatment efficacy.

Keywords: *VEGFA*, Beta-thalassemia, Transcriptomics, Ontogenesis, Sickle cell disease, Erythroid cell differentiation, Pharmacogenomics, Biomarkers

* Correspondence: gpatrinos@upatras.gr
[1]Department of Pharmacy, School of Health Sciences, University of Patras, University Campus, Rion, GR-265 04 Patras, Greece
[5]Department of Pathology, College of Medicine & Health Sciences, United Arab Emirates University, Al-Ain, United Arab Emirates
Full list of author information is available at the end of the article

Introduction

Hemoglobin is the key tetramer oxygen transport protein of red blood cells, composed of two pairs of identical globin chains (namely, the α-like and β-like chains). Different types of hemoglobin molecules are produced during embryonic, fetal, and adult erythropoiesis at different hematopoietic sites (yolk sac, fetal liver, and bone marrow, respectively) [34]. The differentiation of erythroid progenitors into mature erythrocytes as well as human globin expression needs to be strictly regulated aiming to maintain sufficient oxygen levels in all tissues [11, 20]. There are two developmental switches that occur upon the switch from primitive to definitive hematopoiesis and during the perinatal period. In the latter case, human fetal globin genes (*HBG1* and *HBG2*) that are expressed at high levels during the fetal stage are gradually downregulated, whereas human adult (*HBB* and *HBD*) globin genes are reciprocally upregulated. As a result, fetal hemoglobin (HbF) is expressed at high levels during fetal development and gradually declines to reach less than 2–3% of total hemoglobin levels shortly after birth.

Hemoglobinopathies are the most common single gene disorders and at the same time, one of the most devastating health problems worldwide, as their clinical phenotypes vary from mostly asymptomatic to severe anemia. Hemoglobinopathies are caused by quantitative (α- or β-thalassemia) or qualitative (hemoglobin variants and sickle cell disease, SCD) defects in hemoglobin production [5, 12]. Today, the most common therapeutic interventions for β-type hemoglobinopathies include regular blood transfusions, bone marrow transplantation, and transient pharmacological reactivation of HbF to compensate for the absent or deficient expression of adult hemoglobin. Hydroxyurea or hydroxycarbamide (HU) is the only FDA-approved drug for the treatment of SCD and β-thalassemia patients that transiently increases/reactivates HbF production and hence, ameliorates disease severity. However, HU is less effective in β-thalassemia than in SCD patients, while there is extreme inter-individual variability among β-type hemoglobinopathy patients in response to HU treatment [3, 23].

HbF production as well as the developmental switch from fetal to adult hemoglobin are regulated by various transcription factors and have been the focus of intensive investigations, since our understanding of the molecular mechanisms involved in fetal-to-adult globin gene switching would provide useful insights for β-type hemoglobinopathy therapeutics [19]. It has been proposed that there is a complex interplay between cis-acting elements within the human β-globin gene cluster and transcription factors, such as *MYB*, *BCL11A*, *KLF1* [39, 41], and others, that affect the rate of β-like globin gene transcription. Also, previous studies suggest that genomic loci residing outside the human β-globin gene cluster act as modifier genes to HbF production and are associated with elevated HbF levels and, as such, variable disease severity in β-type hemoglobinopathy patients and HU treatment response rate in SCD/β-thalassemia compound heterozygous patients [18, 25].

We have previously shown that genomic variants in the *MAP3K5*, *KLF10*, *SIN3A*, *NOS1*, *ARG1*, and *ARG2* genes are associated with elevated HbF levels and, hence, milder disease severity in β-type hemoglobinopathy patients and HU treatment response rate in SCD/β-thalassemia compound heterozygous patients [4, 7, 17, 40]. Herein, we adopted a whole transcriptome analysis of erythroid cells derived from human hematopoietic tissues of various developmental stages to identify candidate genes that are differentially expressed at various developmental stages. Following our data analysis coupled to pathway and linkage disequilibrium analyses, we show that selected *VEGFA* genomic variants are associated with β-thalassemia disease severity and HU treatment efficacy in SCD/β-thalassemia compound heterozygous patients, suggesting that *VEGFA* may be considered as a modifier gene for HbF production.

Material and methods

Subjects

For the purpose of microarray-based whole transcriptome analysis, we isolated and cultured erythroid progenitor cells from human fetal liver ($n = 4$), umbilical cord blood ($n = 5$), and adult peripheral blood ($n = 4$) samples, all from unrelated individuals of Caucasian origin. Human umbilical cord blood and fetal liver samples were collected and processed as described previously [24, 43, 44].

For tagSNP genotyping, we exploited a separate set of individuals, namely β-thalassemia major patients, non-transfusion-dependent thalassemia (NTDT) patients, SCD/β-thalassemia compound heterozygous patients, and ethnically matched healthy (non-thalassemic) individuals. β-thalassemia major patients differ from their NTDT counterparts in terms of their clinical phenotype and disease severity. In particular, β-thalassemia major patients require lifelong regular transfusions to survive and avoid disease complications, while NTDT patients present mild anemia (hemoglobin levels ranging from 7.7 to 11.2 g/dl) and need less frequent or no blood transfusions. The clinical phenotype of the NTDT patients included in this study cannot be attributed to α-globin gene variants (α-thalassemia) or hereditary persistence of fetal hemoglobin (HPFH syndrome). SCD/β-thalassemia compound heterozygous patients were systematically administered HU and characterized as "HU-responders" (plateau HbF levels above 20%) or "HU non-responders" (plateau HbF levels below 20%), based on their HbF expression levels following drug administration. All molecular, hematological, and clinical data of patient cohorts have been described in our previously published work [7, 15, 17, 32, 33, 40]. All tagSNP genotyping samples are of Hellenic origin, collected at the Patras University Hospital (Patras, Greece), AHEPA University Hospital (Thessaloniki, Greece), and Ippokrateio General Hospital of Thessaloniki (Thessaloniki, Greece).

Whole transcriptome analysis

Microarray-based whole transcriptome analysis was performed as described previously [4]. In brief, erythroid progenitor cells from fetal liver, umbilical cord blood, and adult peripheral blood samples were isolated and cultured ex vivo. Total RNA was extracted, labeled, and hybridized to the Affymetrix Human Genome Array v2.0 according to manufacturer's instructions (Affymetrix Inc., Santa Carla, CA, USA). Differential expression specifics were set by AltAnalyse. Probe sets were characterized and selected as significant, when their p value was < 0.05. Cluster 3.0 was used for data clustering of the short-listed probe sets [9] and JavaTree View Version 1.1.6r2 for data visualization [35]. A fold-change > 2 (FC > 2) is indicative of gene upregulation, whereas a fold-change < 2 (FC <2) corresponds to gene downregulation.

TagSNP selection and linkage disequilibrium analysis

TagSNP selection across the *VEGFA* gene was carried out by the tagSNP picker program via the International HapMap Project (HapMap data release 27, phase II + III, February 2009, on NCBI36 assembly) and the LD TAG SNP Selection (tagSNP) (National Institute of Environmental Health Sciences) web-based tool. A tagged pairwise method was used with an R-square cutoff value of 0.8 and minor allele frequency (MAF) cutoff value of 0.2 [42, 45]. Pairwise linkage disequilibrium (LD) calculations were based on phase genotyped data (SNAP v2.2) [22], utilizing the HapMap Phase II+III (release 28) [2] and the 1000 Genomes Project (http://www.1000genomes.org) dataset for Caucasians (CEU). Findings were visualized on HaploView 4.2 and by using the LDmatrix module on LDlink web tool [26].

Genotype analysis

Genomic DNA was extracted from whole blood leukocytes collected from healthy individuals and patients using the QIAamp Blood Kit (Qiagen GmbH, Hilden, Germany). Polymerase chain reaction (PCR) was carried out according to the KAPA2G Fast Hot Start protocol (KAPA Biosystems, MA, USA). A detailed description per tagSNP amplification conditions is available upon request. PCR products were purified with NucleoSpin Gel and PCR clean-up kit (Macherey-Nagel, GmbH, Düren, Germany) and subjected to direct DNA sequence analysis on an ABI Prim 3130xl DNA Analyser (Applied Biosystems) using the Big Dye® Terminator v3.1 Cycle Sequencing Kit (Applied Biosystems, CA, USA), according to the manufacturer's instructions.

In silico analyses

Pathway analysis was performed with STRING software v9.1 (http://string-db.org). An emphasis was given to text mining and predicted interactions, both direct (physical) and indirect (functional). Venn diagrams were drawn with VENNY v2.1 (http://bioinfogp.cnb.csic.es/tools/venny/index.html). Gene ontology (GO) term analysis was performed with PANTHER classification system. Molecular function and biological process subcategories were subsequently identified [27]. For our downstream analysis, and to further investigate the role of the *VEGFA* tagSNPs in HU-mediated HbF production, we explored their effect on splicing motifs (including the "accept" and "donor" splice sites), the branch point and auxiliary sequences that enhance (exonic splicing enhancers, ESE) or repress (exonic splicing silencers, ESS) splicing. For this, in silico prediction took place, using Human Splicing Finder (http://www.umd.be/HSF3). This is a system that has quickly become an international reference, as it combines 12 algorithms [10].

Statistical analysis

Hardy-Weinberg equilibrium was explored by Pearson's goodness-of-fit chi-square (degree of freedom = 1), log-likelihood ratio chi-square (degree of freedom = 1), and exact test. De Finetti diagrams were also constructed [37]. Genotype and allele frequencies were evaluated using Fisher's exact test. A two-tailed p value of < 0.05 was considered statistically significant. The *R* project for statistical computing (R i386 3.2.1) was used.

Results

Transcription profiling of human hematopoietic tissues during ontogenesis

Whole transcriptome analysis was performed to explore the transcription profiles of human hematopoietic tissues at different stages of ontogenesis. A unique molecular signature was obtained, consisting of genes that were differentially expressed among tissues that express (fetal liver, umbilical cord blood) HbF, do not express HbF, or marginally express (adult peripheral blood) HbF. Our comparative analysis includes three different datasets: (i) adult peripheral blood (low HbF) versus umbilical cord blood (high HbF), (ii) adult peripheral blood (low HbF) versus fetal liver (high HbF), and (iii) adult peripheral blood (low HbF) versus umbilical cord blood and fetal liver (high HbF).

When the first comparison was considered, a total of 165 probe sets representing 133 unique genes were differentially expressed (Additional file 1: Figure S1), while the second comparison revealed 1239 probe sets corresponding to 898 unique genes being differentially expressed (Additional file 1: Figure S2). When comparing all tissues (fetal liver and umbilical cord blood) that express high HbF levels versus peripheral blood that does not produce HbF, our analysis revealed 348 probe sets, corresponding to 264 unique genes that were differentially expressed among those tissues (Fig. 1). Data analysis revealed a candidate gene signature of erythropoiesis during human ontogenesis. Next, we focused on the comparison of the gene signature profile of those hematopoietic tissues, being most ontogenically distant, and thus, adult peripheral blood was compared to fetal liver (dataset ii) and/or adult peripheral blood was compared to umbilical cord blood and fetal liver (dataset iii). As indicated in Fig. 2 and Additional file 1: Tables S1 and S2, 103 genes were upregulated and 50 genes were downregulated, when datasets (ii) and (iii) were considered. Data were filtered on the basis of current publicly available literature and experimental evidence regarding gene-to-phenotype associations with β-hemoglobinopathies. We have subsequently performed GO term analysis. Pathway analysis and text mining were carried out for the genes included in the most dominant classifications of the GO term analysis. *VEGFA* was most prevalent in "Binding" (GO: 0005488), "Cellular process" (GO: 0009987), "Developmental process" (GO: 0002376) and "Response to stimulus" (GO: 0050896).

VEGFA was found to be upregulated (FC > 2) in adult peripheral blood (low HbF levels), when compared to umbilical cord blood and fetal liver (high HbF levels). *VEGFA* upregulation was even more profound, when adult peripheral blood was solely compared to fetal liver.

TagSNPs across the *VEGFA* gene are associated with high HbF levels

Three tagSNPs (rs3024997, rs2146323, and rs10434) across the *VEGFA* gene were selected with MAF > 0.2% (CEU population) and explored further for their association with disease severity, attributed to high HbF levels. rs3024997 (G>A) and rs2146323 (C>A) are localized within intron 2, while rs10434 (A>G) within the 3′-untranslated region (3′-UTR) of the *VEGFA* gene. Genotyping data of β-type hemoglobinopathy patients and healthy (non-thalassemic) individuals of Hellenic origin are summarized in Table 1 and Additional file 1: Tables S3 and S4. A strong association for rs3024997 (G > A) with disease severity became evident, when NTDT patients (mild disease phenotype) and β-thalassemia major patients (severe disease phenotype) were compared (p = 0.003), and the same was true when NTDT patients versus non-thalassemic individuals (p = 0.005) were considered. Since

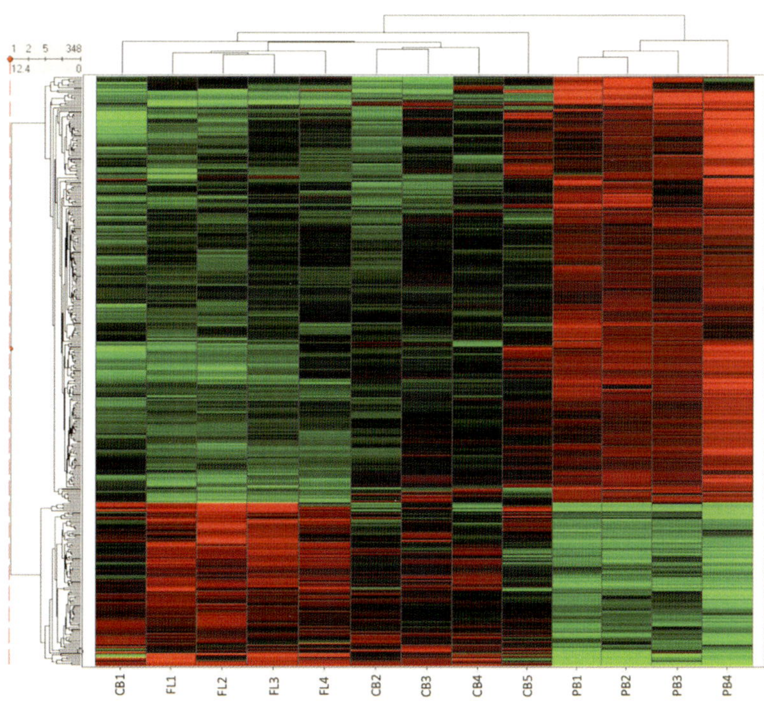

Fig. 1 Differential gene expression when adult peripheral blood is compared to cord blood and fetal liver. A total of 264 genes were up- (FC > 2) or downregulated (FC < 2), when tissues with low HbF expression levels were compared to their counterparts with high HbF expression levels. Columns represent samples; rows are genes. Genes that were upregulated are depicted in red and genes that were downregulated are depicted in green

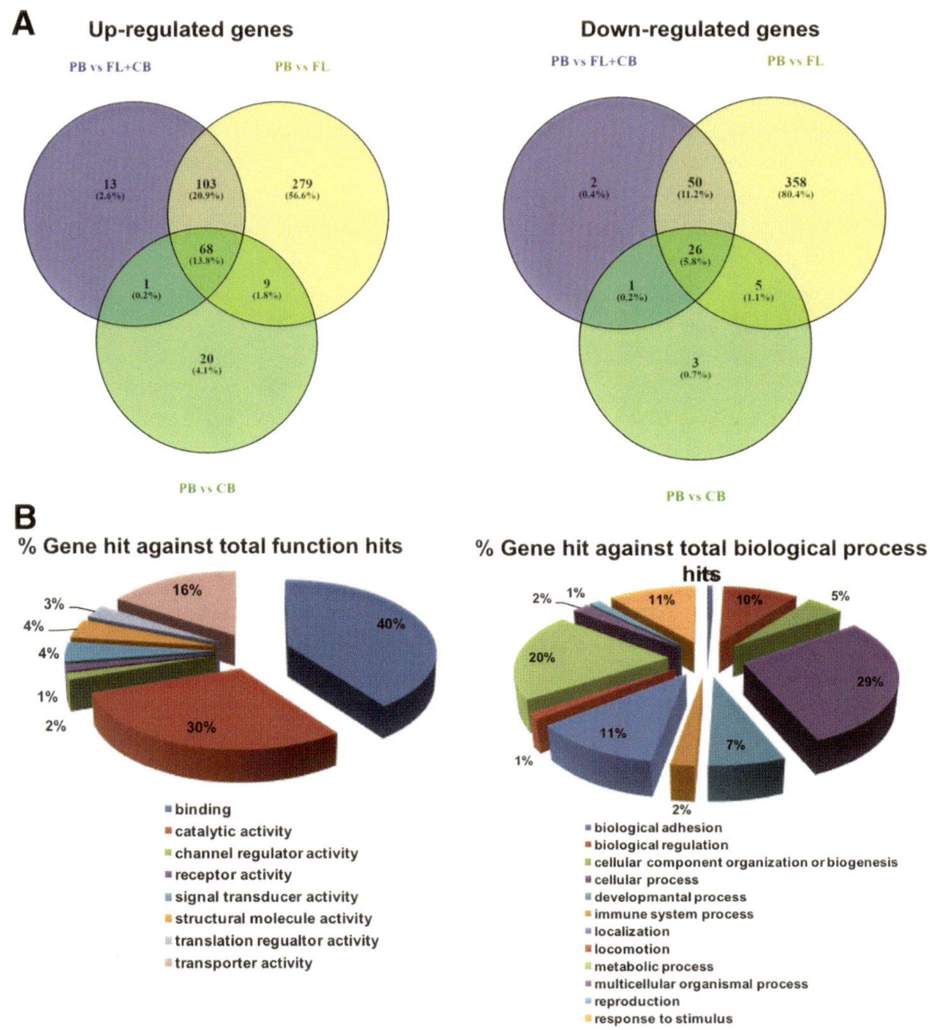

Fig. 2 Common and unique up- and downregulated genes during ontogenesis. **a** The number in each circle represents the number of differentially expressed genes among the groups in question. Common and unique genes are shown. **b** PANTHER analysis outcomes (GO; molecular function and biological process)

Table 1 Summary of our genotype analysis of β-type hemoglobinopathy patients of Hellenic origin and healthy (non-thalassemic) individuals

Study population	Genotype frequency (%)								
	rs3024997 (G>A)			rs2146323 (C>A)			rs10434 (A>G)		
	G/G	A/A	G/A	C/C	A/A	C/A	A/A	G/G	A/G
Healthy individuals	34	21	45	60	9	31	18	31	51
β-thalassemia major patients	26	16	58	51	3	46	21	33	46
NTDT patients	47	6	47	33	11	56	21	29	50
HU responders	26	16	58	43	10	48	26	26	48
HU non-responders	35	12	53	63	17	20	25	29	46

The number of individuals per group (n) is indicated in parentheses per tagSNP: rs3024997 healthy individuals (n = 112), NTDT patients (n = 17), β-thalassemia major patients (n = 112), HU responders (n = 19), HU non-responders (n = 26); rs2146323 healthy individuals (n = 115), NTDT patients (n = 18), β-thalassemia major patients (n = 114), HU responders (n = 21), HU non-responders (n = 30); rs10434 healthy individuals (n = 72), NTDT patients (n = 14), β-thalassemia major patients (n = 105), HU responders (n = 19), HU non-responders (n = 28)
HU hydroxyurea, *NTDT* non-transfusion-dependent thalassemia

the homozygous genotype for the rare allele (A) is less frequently found in NTDT patients, the presence of the A allele could be correlated with low HbF levels (Fig. 3a). rs2146323 (C > A) correlates well with disease severity and HbF levels, when (i) NTDT patients versus β-thalassemia major patients (p = 0.009), (ii) NTDT patients versus non-thalassemic individuals (p = 0.0005), and (iii) β-thalassemia major patients (p = 0.03) versus non-thalassemic individuals were considered. Our findings for the rare allele (A) suggest its association with high HbF levels (Fig. 3b). rs10434 (A > G) did not reach statistical significance, when genotype frequencies among patients and healthy individuals were compared.

TagSNPs across the *VEGFA* gene are associated with HU treatment efficacy in SCD/beta-thalassemia compound heterozygous patients

To explore if the selected tagSNPs across the *VEGFA* gene could serve as pharmacogenomic biomarkers, HU-responder and non-responder SCD/β-thalassemia patients were genotyped. A strong association for rs2146323 (C>A) with HU treatment efficacy (elevation of HbF levels) became evident (p = 0.0002), while neither of the rs3024997 (G>A) and rs10434 (A>G) tagSNPs reached statistical significance. As shown in Fig. 4 and Additional file 1: Table S4, pairwise LD calculations revealed that rs3024997 (G>A) and rs2146323 (C>A) are in complete LD (D′ = 1; $R^2 < 1$).

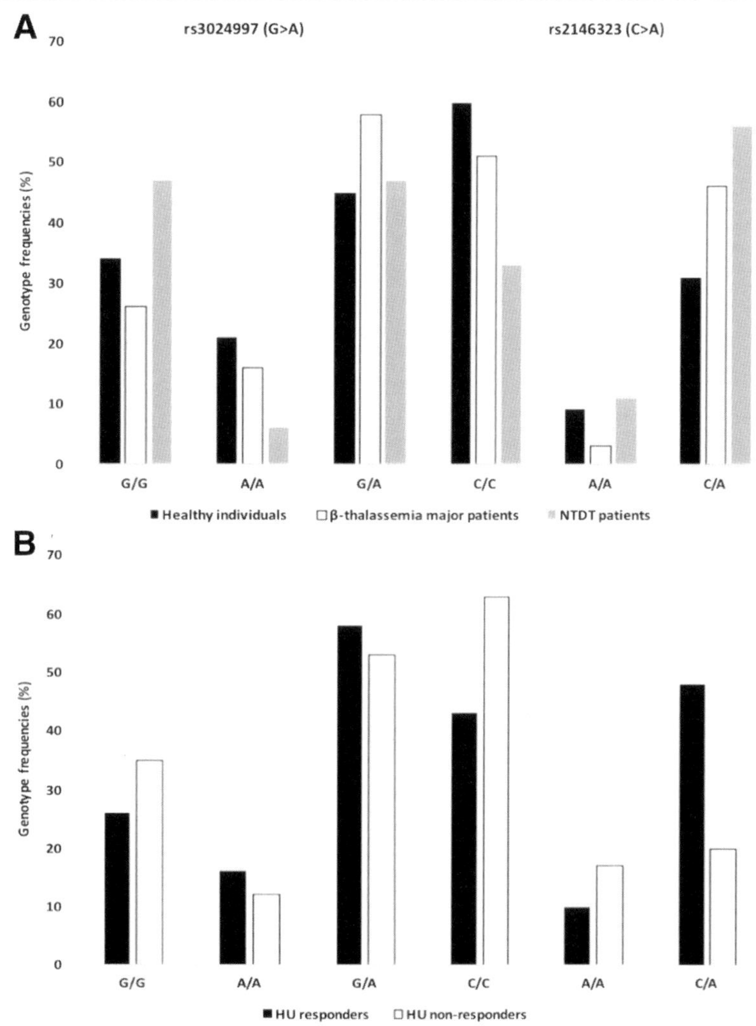

Fig. 3 TagSNPs across the *VEGFA* gene are associated with disease phenotype (**a**) and HU treatment efficacy (**b**). **a** disease phenotype, rs3024997 (G>A; healthy individuals vs. NTDT patients p = 0.005; β-thalassemia major patients vs. NTDT patients p = 0.003) and rs2146323 (C>A; healthy individuals vs. β-thalassemia major patients p = 0.03; healthy individuals vs. NTDT patients p = 0.0005; β-thalassemia major patients vs. NTDT patients p = 0.009). **b** HU treatment efficacy, rs2146323 (C>A; HU responders vs. HU non-responders p = 0.0002). HU: hydroxyurea

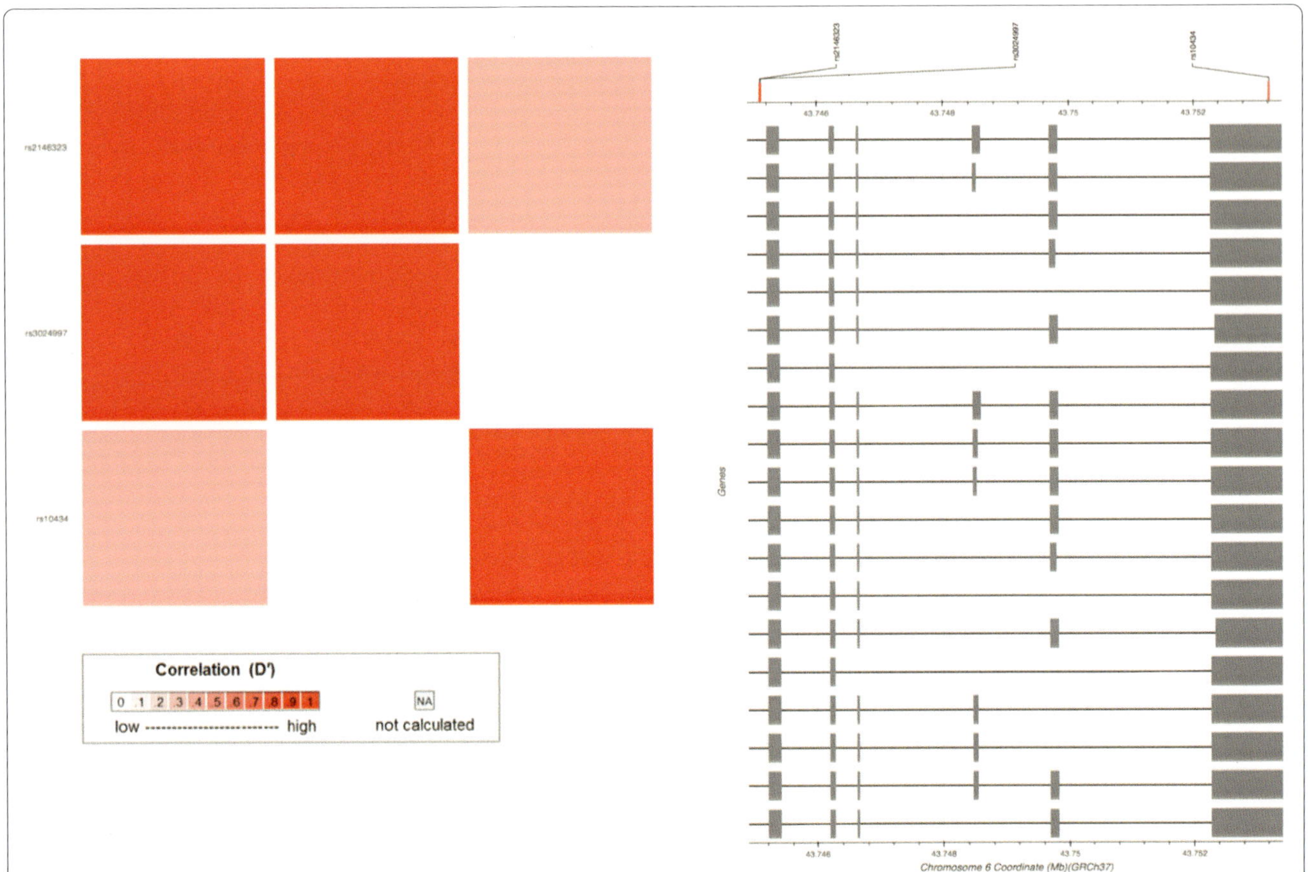

Fig. 4 Pairwise linkage disequilibrium (LD) calculations for the tagSNPs of interest across the *VEGFA* gene (CEU). LD is measured as D′ and R^2 (see also Additional file 1: Table S2)

In silico analyses

According to the Human Splicing Finder prediction algorithm, rs3024997 (G>A) was found to occur in a deep intronic position, resulting on the activation of an intronic cryptic acceptor site and thus, potential alteration of splicing. Yet, the RESCUE ESE, EIEs, PESE Octamers, ESE Finder-SRp40, and ESR Sequences prediction algorithms suggest the creation of an exonic splicing enhancer, probably, with no impact on splicing (Fig. 5). rs2146323 (C>A) causes no significant splicing motif alteration, suggesting that the other co-inherited variants are possibly the key in its association with high HbF levels.

Discussion

In humans, erythropoiesis as well as globin gene expression occurs at different sites during the various developmental

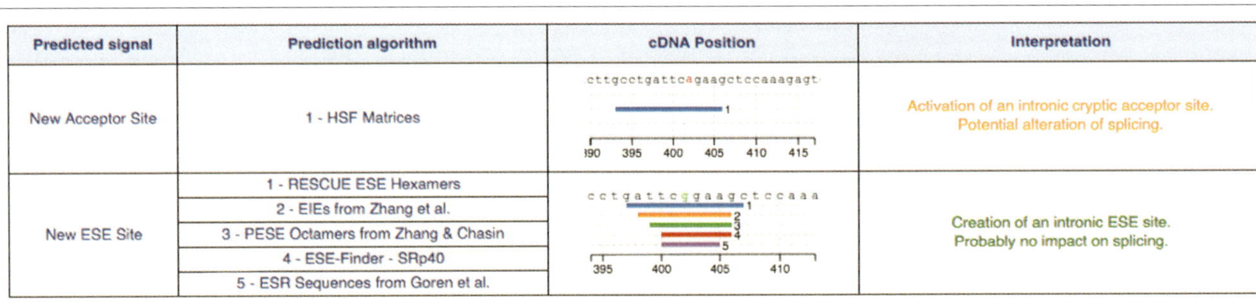

Fig. 5 In silico analysis of the role of rs3024997 on splicing. For rs3024997 (G > A), the Human Splicing Finder prediction algorithm supports the activation of an intronic cryptic acceptor site and thus, potential alteration of splicing. Yet, the RESCUE ESE, EIEs, PESE Octamers, ESE Finder-SRp40, and ESR Sequences prediction algorithms suggest the creation of an exonic splicing enhancer, probably, with no impact on splicing. The graphic representation of the region confirms individual outcomes per algorithm considered, each one corresponding at a different color and length. For more information on the data, please visit http://www.umd.be/HSF3/technicaltips.html

stages in a time-specific manner (tissue- and development-specific expression). Hemoglobin switch consists of two separate events; the first event occurs early in endometrial life (embryonic to fetal hemoglobin switch), whereas the second one begins a few weeks before birth and ends ~ 6 months after delivery (fetal-to-adult hemoglobin switch). The understanding of the molecular mechanisms that govern hemoglobin switch holds a great promise for curing β-type hemoglobinopathies [34].

We have previously demonstrated that several genes, residing outside the human β-globin gene cluster, can be held responsible as genes modifying HbF levels in β-type hemoglobinopathy patients, reflecting on the disease severity and HU treatment response [4, 7, 18, 40]. Herein, we adopted a whole transcriptome analysis on tissues that express high and low HbF levels in an effort to identify a unique molecular signature corresponding to high HbF levels.

Following whole transcriptome and pathway analysis, coupled to text mining, we focused on the *VEGFA* gene since it shows a consistent gene expression pattern in most comparisons. We employed linkage disequilibrium analysis to select *VEGFA* genomic variants to further explore their association with elevated HbF levels in β-type hemoglobinopathy patients. In humans, *VEGFA* (belongs to the family of vascular endothelial growth factors, VEGFs) is localized on chromosome 6p21.1 (14 kb), consisting of 8 exons and 7 introns [21]. Studies in knockout mice indicate the role of *VEGFA* in the development of the vascular and hematopoietic tissues. Casella et al. [6] found that *VEGFA* production is crucial for the survival and differentiation of adult hematopoietic stem cells (HSCs), while *VEGFA* has been also shown to participate in hematopoiesis by an internal autocrine loop mechanism and be associated with adult *HBB* gene expression [13, 14]. Nakayama et al. [31] have shown that *VEGFA* synergizes with BMP-4 on the development of hematopoietic cells [31]. The same authors reported that murine embryonic stem cells were white, when grown only in the presence of BMP-4, becoming red, after the addition of *VEGFA* (and stem cell factor (SCF)). A few years later, Adelman et al. [1] showed that the BMP/BMPR/Smad pathway induces the expression of KLF1 and GATA-1 transcription factors during the differentiation of embryonic bodies in mice, yet β-globin expression is only detected, when SCF and *VEGFA* were present [1].

Consistent with this work, our previous findings indicate that at the late stages of human ontogenesis, where HbF levels are low, *VEGFA* mRNA levels are high. In particular, *VEGFA* is upregulated in cultured erythroid progenitor cells derived from adult peripheral blood (low HbF expression levels), when compared to progenitors derived from fetal liver or umbilical cord blood and fetal liver. Furthermore, *VEGFA* is downregulated in erythroblasts, when compared to early (BFU-Es) or late (CFU-Es) erythroid progenitors in hematopoietic tissues expressing high levels of HbF (umbilical cord blood and fetal liver, Kolovos P, unpublished). Such findings support further the inverse correlation between *VEGFA* and HbF levels that we observed during ontogenesis.

High HbF levels may improve disease severity in β-thalassemia and SCD, as β-globin deficiency is balanced by γ-globin synthesis and HbF prevents the polymerization of hemoglobin S, respectively [36]. Following the completion of the Human Genome Project, family and genome-wide association studies reported several SNPs that are associated with high HbF levels or a high proportion of F cells in β-type hemoglobinopathy patients, revealing a relatively large number of genetic modifiers of HbF expression [18, 19].

Today, although several compounds that transiently induce HbF levels (5-azacitidine, dexitabine) have been studied, HU is the only FDA-approved sickle cell disease and β-thalassemia treatment. HU is a cytotoxic antineoplastic agent that was initially administered to patients with myelodysplastic diseases and immune deficiencies as it is an inhibitor of ribonucleotide reductase, an enzyme necessary for DNA synthesis and repair. The drug mechanism towards the induction of HbF is not fully known. In β-thalassemia patients, HU administration leads to a 2- to a ~9-fold increase in γ-globin mRNA levels [30]. Inter-individual variability remains an issue and several studies concur that genomic variants residing in genes not only within, but also outside the human β-globin gene cluster, correlate with disease severity and HU treatment efficacy [18, 25].

Interestingly, our whole transcriptome analysis revealed that among those genes with a similar, to *VEGFA*, expression profile, there are genes previously described to be correlated with differentially produced HbF levels and with response to HU treatment in β-type hemoglobinopathy patients [7, 16, 25].

Following our whole transcriptome analysis, we focused on *VEGFA* gene variants and genotyped non--transfusion-dependent β-thalassemia patients, β-thalassemia major patients, and healthy (non-thalassemic) individuals as well as a cohort of compound heterozygous SCD/β-thalassemia patients receiving HU as HbF augmenting therapy. rs3024997 (G>A) was found to be strongly associated with low HbF levels and the severe phenotype of β-thalassemia major. A strong association was also observed between rs2146323 (C>A) and high HbF levels in NTDT patients and hence, a milder clinical phenotype of the disease. rs2146323 (C>A) may also serve as a pharmacogenomic biomarker for HU treatment efficacy. rs10434 (A>G) did not reach statistical significance. Small sample size remains a major limitation in all studies focusing on HU treatment individualization, including ours, especially for NTDT patients, due to the scarcity of such patients. Herein, Fisher's exact test was chosen as the most appropriate test to guarantee type I error control, taking into account small sample sizes (Fisher's exact test is considered more accurate than the chi-square test or G-test of independence in such cases). Yet, the lack of association for rs10434 due to small sample sizes cannot be excluded. *VEFGA* genomic variants have also been found in asymptomatic individuals with high HbF levels (unpublished), suggesting a possible role of *VEGFA* in increasing HbF levels.

According to the outcome of our in silico analyses, rs3024997 (G>A) was found to occur in a deep intronic position, resulting on the activation of an intronic cryptic acceptor site and thus, potential alteration of splicing. Yet, the RESCUE ESE, EIEs, PESE Octamers, ESE Finder-SRp40, and ESR Sequences prediction algorithms suggested the creation of an exonic splicing enhancer, which has probably no impact on splicing. rs2146323 (C>A) causes no significant splicing motif alteration, suggesting that the other co-inherited variants are possibly the key in its association with high HbF levels. No doubt, coupled to the bioinformatics predictions described, functional analysis needs to be performed, such as functional minigene analysis and exon-tiling microarrays to confirm the role of these variants as predicted in silico [8, 28, 29, 38].

Our study has a number of limitations. First of all, we have not managed to isolate fetal tissues from enough number of individuals to replicate our findings and this is subject to future work that is currently ongoing. Secondly, the sample size of the subsequent follow-up study was equally small, due to the lack of sufficient number of well-characterized β-thalassemia/SCD as well as NTDT patients, which are scarce and truly unique to find. Our results are, nevertheless, indicative for future replication work to validate the suggested role of *VEGFA* as possible modifier of HbF levels in adult life.

Conclusion and future perspectives

Human hemoglobin switching still remains a great challenge, when β-type hemoglobinopathy management is considered. In a similar context, HbF production has attracted great interest over the last 50 years towards the amelioration of disease symptoms of β-type hemoglobinopathy patients. Taking into account that HU treatment efficacy exhibits great inter-individual variability, identification, and subsequently validation and clinical implementation of pharmacogenomic biomarkers hold promise for optimum patient stratification and disease management. Herein, our transcriptomics approach provided insights into the differential expression profiles of different erythroid tissues during human ontogenesis and suggested that *VEGFA* genomic variants serve both as genomic biomarkers for β-thalassemia disease severity and pharmacogenomic biomarkers for HU treatment efficacy in β-type hemoglobinopathy patients. In other words, a dual role is implied for *VEGFA* in erythropoiesis and HbF induction, which needs to be further investigated, if the molecular mechanism that delineate human hemoglobin switching is to be better defined and genome-based stratification of β-type hemoglobinopathy patients for HU treatment is to become reality. Notably, not all genomic loci that have been reported to increase HbF levels could be considered as pharmacogenomic biomarkers of HU treatment efficacy, as the clinical features in question, albeit related, are likely controlled by different molecular mechanisms. These findings, in conjunction to previous work conducted by our group and others, hold promise for the identification of pharmacogenomic biomarker for HbF-augmenting therapy, requiring carefully designed prospective clinical studies conducted by large multicenter consortia that include experienced clinicians and researchers from major clinical and academic centers.

Abbreviations

CEU: Caucasian; HbF: Fetal hemoglobin; HPFH: Hereditary persistence of fetal hemoglobin; HU: Hydroxyurea; NTDT: Non-transfusion-dependent thalassemia; SCD: Sickle cell disease

Acknowledgements

The authors are grateful to Dr. Stamatia Theodoridou (Ippokrateio General Hospital Thessaloniki, Thessaloniki, Greece) and Dr. Panagiota Chalkia (AHEPA University Hospital, Thessaloniki, Greece) for their valuable assistance with sample collection.

Funding

This work was partly funded by research grants from the Cypriot Research Promotion Foundation (HU_PHARMGK; RFP_046) and the European Commission (RD-Connect; FP7-305444; U-PGx; H2020-668353) to GPP. BRA is funded by the United Arab Emirates University Center-based grants through Zayed Center for Health Sciences.

Authors' contributions

GPP conceived the study. VC, TK, and GPP designed the study. AK and AS provided the samples. VC, PK, AS, VK, AP, and AJ performed the experiments. VC, PK, and TK analyzed the data. BRA and GPP provided funding for this work. VC, PK, BRA, TK, and GPP wrote the manuscript. All authors read and approved the manuscript.

Competing interests

The authors declare that they have no competing interests.

Author details

[1]Department of Pharmacy, School of Health Sciences, University of Patras, University Campus, Rion, GR-265 04 Patras, Greece. [2]Biotech Research and Innovation Centre (BRIC), University of Copenhagen, Copenhagen, Denmark. [3]Hellenic Open University, Patras, Greece. [4]Hematology Division, Department of Internal Medicine, Faculty of Medicine, University of Patras, Patras, Greece. [5]Department of Pathology, College of Medicine & Health Sciences, United Arab Emirates University, Al-Ain, United Arab Emirates. [6]Zayed Bin Sultan Center for Health Sciences, United Arab Emirates University, Al-Ain, United Arab Emirates. [7]Laboratory of General Biology, Faculty of Medicine, University of Patras, Patras, Greece. [8]Present address: Institut de Génétique et de Biologie Moléculaire et Cellulaire IGBMC/CNRS/INSERM/UDS, 67404 ILLKIRCH, BP 10142 CU de Strasbourg, France.

References

1. Adelman CA, Chattopadhyay S, Bieker JJ. The BMP/BMPR/Smad pathway directs expression of the erythroid-specific EKLF and GATA1 transcription factors during embryoid body differentiation in serum-free media. Development. 2002;129:539–49.
2. Barrett JC, Fry B, Maller J, Daly MJ. Haploview: analysis and visualization of LD and haplotype maps. Bioinformatics. 2004;21:263–5.
3. Bordbar MR, Silavizadeh S, Haghpanah S, Kamfiroozi R, Bardestani M, Karimi M. Hydroxyurea treatment in transfusion-dependent β-thalassemia patients. Iran Red Crescent Med J. 2014;16:e18028.
4. Borg J, Phylactides M, Bartsakoulia M, Tafrali C, Lederer C, Felice AE, Papachatzopoulou A, Kourakli A, Stavrou EF, Christou S. KLF10 gene expression is associated with high fetal hemoglobin levels and with response to hydroxyurea treatment in β-hemoglobinopathy patients. Pharmacogenomics. 2012;13:1487–500.
5. Cao A, Galanello R. Beta-thalassemia. Genet Med. 2010;12:61–76.
6. Casella I, Feccia T, Chelucci C, Samoggia P, Castelli G, Guerriero R, Parolini I, Petrucci E, Pelosi E, Morsilli O. Autocrine-paracrine VEGF loops potentiate the maturation of megakaryocytic precursors through Flt1 receptor. Blood. 2003;101:1316–23.
7. Chalikiopoulou C, Tavianatou A-G, Sgourou A, Kourakli A, Kelepouri D, Chrysanthakopoulou M, Kanelaki V-K, Mourdoukoutas E, Siamoglou S, John A. Genomic variants in the ASS1 gene, involved in the nitric oxide biosynthesis and signaling pathway, predict hydroxyurea treatment efficacy in compound sickle cell disease/β-thalassemia patients. Pharmacogenomics. 2016;17:393–403.
8. Cooper DN. Functional intronic polymorphisms: buried treasure awaiting discovery within our genes. Human Genom. 2010;4:284.
9. de Hoon MJ, Imoto S, Nolan J, Miyano S. Open source clustering software. Bioinformatics. 2004;20:1453–4.
10. Desmet F-O, Hamroun D, Lalande M, Collod-Béroud G, Claustres M, Béroud C. Human Splicing Finder: an online bioinformatics tool to predict splicing signals. Nucleic Acids Res. 2009;37:e67.
11. Dzierzak E, Philipsen S. Erythropoiesis: development and differentiation. Cold Spring Harbor Perspect Med. 2013;3:a011601.
12. Galanello R, Origa R. Beta-thalassemia. Orphanet J Rare Dis. 2010;5:11.
13. Gerber H-P, Ferrara N. The role of VEGF in normal and neoplastic hematopoiesis. J Mol Med. 2003;81:20–31.
14. Gerber H-P, Malik AK, Solar GP, Sherman D. VEGF regulates haematopoietic stem cell survival by an internal autocrine loop mechanism. Nature. 2002;417:954.
15. Giannopoulou E, Bartsakoulia M, Tafrali C, Kourakli A, Poulas K, Stavrou EF, Papachatzopoulou A, Georgitsi M, Patrinos GP. A single nucleotide polymorphism in the HBBP1 gene in the human β-globin locus is associated with a mild β-thalassemia disease phenotype. Hemoglobin. 2012;36:433–45.
16. Giardine B, Borg J, Higgs DR, Peterson KR, Philipsen S, Maglott D, Singleton BK, Anstee DJ, Basak AN, Clark B. Systematic documentation and analysis of human genetic variation in hemoglobinopathies using the microattribution approach. Nat Genet. 2011;43:295–301.
17. Gravia A, Chondrou V, Kolliopoulou A, Kourakli A, John A, Symeonidis A, Ali BR, Sgourou A, Papachatzopoulou A, Katsila T. Correlation of SIN3A genomic variants with β-hemoglobinopathies disease severity and hydroxyurea treatment efficacy. Pharmacogenomics. 2016;17:1785–93.
18. Gravia A, Chondrou V, Sgourou A, Papantoni I, Borg J, Katsila T, Papachatzopoulou A, Patrinos GP. Individualizing fetal hemoglobin augmenting therapy for β-type hemoglobinopathies patients. Pharmacogenomics. 2014;15:1355–64.
19. Hagh MF, Fard AD, Saki N, Shahjahani M, Kaviani S. Molecular mechanisms of hemoglobin F induction. Int J Hematol-Oncol Stem Cell Res. 2011;5:5–9.
20. Hattangadi SM, Wong P, Zhang L, Flygare J, Lodish HF. From stem cell to red cell: regulation of erythropoiesis at multiple levels by multiple proteins, RNAs, and chromatin modifications. Blood. 2011;118:6258–68.
21. Holmes DI, Zachary I. The vascular endothelial growth factor (VEGF) family: angiogenic factors in health and disease. Genome Biol. 2005;6:209.
22. Johnson, AD, Handsaker, RE, Pulit, SL, Nizzari, MM, O'donnell, CJ and De Bakker, PI. (2008). SNAP: a web-based tool for identification and annotation of proxy SNPs using HapMap. Bioinformatics 24, 2938-2939.
23. Koren A, Levin C, Dgany O, Kransnov T, Elhasid R, Zalman L, Palmor H, Tamary H. Response to hydroxyurea therapy in β-thalassemia. Am J Hematol. 2008;83:366–70.
24. Leberbauer C, Boulmé F, Unfried G, Huber J, Beug H, Müllner EW. Different steroids co-regulate long-term expansion versus terminal differentiation in primary human erythroid progenitors. Blood. 2005;105:85–94.
25. Ma Q, Wyszynski D, Farrell J, Kutlar A, Farrer L, Baldwin C, Steinberg M. Fetal hemoglobin in sickle cell anemia: genetic determinants of response to hydroxyurea. Pharmacogenom J. 2007;7:386.
26. Machiela MJ, Chanock SJ. LDlink: a web-based application for exploring population-specific haplotype structure and linking correlated alleles of possible functional variants. Bioinformatics. 2015;31:3555–7.
27. Mi H, Muruganujan A, Casagrande JT, Thomas PD. Large-scale gene function analysis with the PANTHER classification system. Nat Protocols. 2013;8:1551–66.
28. Millar DS, Horan M, Chuzhanova NA, Cooper DN. Characterisation of a functional intronic polymorphism in the human growth hormone (GHI) gene. Human Genom. 2010;4:289.
29. Moyer RA, Wang D, Papp AC, Smith RM, Duque L, Mash DC, Sadee W. Intronic polymorphisms affecting alternative splicing of human dopamine D2 receptor are associated with cocaine abuse. Neuropsychopharmacology. 2011;36:753–62.
30. Musallam KM, Taher AT, Cappellini MD, Sankaran VG. Clinical experience with fetal hemoglobin induction therapy in patients with β-thalassemia. Blood. 2013;121:2199–212.
31. Nakayama N, Lee J, Chiu L. Vascular endothelial growth factor synergistically enhances bone morphogenetic protein-4-dependent lymphohematopoietic cell generation from embryonic stem cells in vitro. Blood. 2000;95:2275–83.
32. Papachatzopoulou A, Kaimakis P, Pourfarzad F, Menounos PG, Evangelakou P, Kollia P, Grosveld FG, Patrinos GP. Increased γ-globin gene expression in β-thalassemia intermedia patients correlates with a mutation in 3′ HS1. Am J Hematol. 2007;82:1005–9.
33. Papachatzopoulou A, Kourakli A, Makropoulou P, Kakagianne T, Sgourou A, Papadakis M, Athanassiadou A. Genotypic heterogeneity and correlation to intergenic haplotype within high HbF β-thalassemia intermedia. Eur J Haematol. 2006;76:322–30.
34. Patrinos GP, Antonarakis SE. Human hemoglobin. In: Vogel and Motulsky's human genetics. Vergal Berlin Heidelberg: Springer; 2010. p. 365–401.
35. Saldanha AJ. Java Treeview—extensible visualization of microarray data. Bioinformatics. 2004;20:3246–8.
36. Sankaran VG. Targeted therapeutic strategies for fetal hemoglobin induction. ASH Educ Program Book. 2011;2011:459–65.
37. Sasieni PD. From genotypes to genes: doubling the sample size. Biometrics. 1997:1253–61.
38. Seo S, Takayama K, Uno K, Ohi K, Hashimoto R, Nishizawa D, Ikeda K, Ozaki N, Nabeshima T, Miyamoto Y. Functional analysis of deep intronic SNP rs13438494 in intron 24 of PCLO gene. PLoS One. 2013;8:e76960.
39. Suzuki M, Yamamoto M, Engel JD. Fetal globin gene repressors as drug targets for molecular therapies to treat the β-globinopathies. Mol Cell Biol. 2014;34:3560–9.
40. Tafrali C, Paizi A, Borg J, Radmilovic M, Bartsakoulia M, Giannopoulou E, Giannakopoulou O, Stojiljkovic-Petrovic M, Zukic B, Poulas K. Genomic variation in the MAP3K5 gene is associated with β-thalassemia disease severity and hydroxyurea treatment efficacy. Pharmacogenomics. 2013;14:469–83.
41. Tallack MR, Perkins AC. Three fingers on the switch: Krüppel-like factor 1 regulation of γ-globin to β-globin gene switching. Curr Opin Hematol. 2013;20:193–200.
42. Thorisson GA, Smith AV, Krishnan L, Stein LD. The international HapMap project web site. Genome Res. 2005;15:1592–3.
43. Van Handel, B, Prashad, SL, Hassanzadeh-Kiabi, N, Huang, A, Magnusson, M, Atanassova, B, Chen, A, Hamalainen, EI and Mikkola, HK. (2010). The first trimester human placenta is a site for terminal maturation of primitive erythroid cells. Blood 116, 3321-3330.
44. Xu, J, Shao, Z, Glass, K, Bauer, DE, Pinello, L, Van Handel, B, Hou, S, Stamatoyannopoulos, JA, Mikkola, HK and Yuan, G-C. (2012). Combinatorial assembly of developmental stage-specific enhancers controls gene expression programs during human erythropoiesis. Dev Cell 23, 796-811.
45. Xu Z, Taylor JA. SNPinfo: integrating GWAS and candidate gene information into functional SNP selection for genetic association studies. Nucleic Acids Res. 2009;37:W600–5.

15

Novel genetic risk variants for pediatric celiac disease

Angeliki Balasopoulou[1†], Biljana Stanković[2†], Angeliki Panagiotara[1], Gordana Nikčevic[2], Brock A. Peters[3,4], Anne John[5], Effrosyni Mendrinou[1], Apostolos Stratopoulos[1], Aigli Ioanna Legaki[1], Vasiliki Stathakopoulou[1], Aristoniki Tsolia[1], Nikolaos Govaris[1], Sofia Govari[1], Zoi Zagoriti[1], Konstantinos Poulas[1], Maria Kanariou[6], Nikki Constantinidou[6], Maro Krini[7], Kleopatra Spanou[6], Nedeljko Radlovic[8], Bassam R. Ali[5], Joseph Borg[9], Radoje Drmanac[3,4], George Chrousos[7], Sonja Pavlovic[2], Eleftheria Roma[7], Branka Zukic[2], George P. Patrinos[1,5] and Theodora Katsila[1*]

Abstract

Background: Celiac disease is a complex chronic immune-mediated disorder of the small intestine. Today, the pathobiology of the disease is unclear, perplexing differential diagnosis, patient stratification, and decision-making in the clinic.

Methods: Herein, we adopted a next-generation sequencing approach in a celiac disease trio of Greek descent to identify all genomic variants with the potential of celiac disease predisposition.

Results: Analysis revealed six genomic variants of prime interest: *SLC9A4* c.1919G>A, *KIAA1109* c.2933T>C and c. 4268_4269delCCinsTA, *HoxB6* c.668C>A, *HoxD12* c.418G>A, and *NCK2* c.745_746delAAinsG, from which *NCK2* c. 745_746delAAinsG is novel. Data validation in pediatric celiac disease patients of Greek ($n = 109$) and Serbian ($n = 73$) descent and their healthy counterparts ($n = 111$ and $n = 32$, respectively) indicated that *HoxD12* c. 418G>A is more prevalent in celiac disease patients in the Serbian population ($P < 0.01$), while *NCK2* c.745_ 746delAAinsG is less prevalent in celiac disease patients rather than healthy individuals of Greek descent ($P = 0.03$). *SLC9A4* c.1919G>A and *KIAA1109* c.2933T>C and c.4268_4269delCCinsTA were more abundant in patients; nevertheless, they failed to show statistical significance.

Conclusions: The next-generation sequencing-based family genomics approach described herein may serve as a paradigm towards the identification of novel functional variants with the aim of understanding complex disease pathobiology.

Keywords: Celiac disease, Genomic variants, Family genomics, Next-generation sequencing, Disease predisposition

Background

Celiac disease is a complex chronic immune-mediated disorder of the small intestine. Today, the pathobiology of the disease is unclear, perplexing differential diagnosis, patient stratification, and decision-making in the clinic. Genetics has been reported to play a key role. The *HLA-DQ2* gene is identified in up to 95 % of celiac disease patients, while most of the remaining patients have the *HLA-DQ8* gene. Notwithstanding, the Chinese and Japanese populations (devoid of *HLA-DQ2*) are not expected to develop the disease, yet this is not true for the individuals with the *HLA-DQ8* gene. Celiac disease is also associated with an extended ancestral haplotype that is defined by class I and II *HLA*s (*A*, *B*, *DR*, *DQ*). Notably, *HLA-DQ2* and/or *HLA-DQ8* expression is necessary but not sufficient for disease development. Thus, other genes are anticipated to be involved. Indeed, genome-wide association studies (GWAS) have revealed 26 non-*HLA* genetic loci-associated celiac disease and other autoimmune or chronic immune

* Correspondence: thkatsila@upatras.gr
†Equal contributors
[1]Department of Pharmacy, School of Health Sciences, University of Patras, University Campus, Rion, 265 04 Patras, Greece
Full list of author information is available at the end of the article

disorders (diabetes mellitus type I, rheumatoid arthritis) [1, 2]. In 2008 to 2011, several new celiac disease risk loci have been identified [3–5], bringing the number of known loci (including the *HLA* one) to 40 and indicating genes and gene regulatory elements of paramount importance. In 2015, five new genetic loci were identified, being independent of *HLA-DQA1* and *HLA-DQB1* and associated with celiac disease predisposition [6].

Although a genetic component has been described, disease occurrence has been also associated with environmental factors and gut microbiome. In all cases, gluten has been identified as the environmental trigger of the disease, leading to the stimulation of gluten-specific T cells. Differential diagnosis is still a major issue. Although a gold standard diagnostic approach has been defined (endoscopy with biopsy of the small intestine coupled to positive disease serology), several pathological conditions have been reported sharing similar mucosal transformations with celiac disease as well as other autoimmune disorders (thyroid disease, Addison disease, autoimmune liver disease, Sjögren syndrome) that occur ten times more frequently in celiac disease patients often masking celiac disease symptoms. Disease management options are restricted to a gluten-free lifestyle, which ultimately fails to protect patients from disease symptoms due to its chronic nature. Can we delineate individual variability towards differential diagnosis? Can we highlight the disease mechanisms in question to assist disease management?

So far, findings account for 49 % of the genetic basis of the disease. As in other immune-mediated diseases, genetic predisposition to celiac disease remains unresolved as we still need to explain the remaining major fraction of heritability, including rare as well as additional common risk variants. Causal variants and genes still need to be identified and/or more finely localized. In this context, the Immunochip Consortium was developed to explore comprehensive datasets containing common, low-frequency, and rare variants in related diseases (autoimmune thyroid disease, ankylosing spondylitis, Crohn disease, celiac disease, IgA deficiency, multiple sclerosis, primary biliary cirrhosis, psoriasis, rheumatoid arthritis, systemic lupus erythematosus, type 1 diabetes mellitus, and ulcerative colitis) [7].

As expected, the advent of technology and, in particular, next-generation sequencing has provided unprecedented opportunities to delineate disease pathobiology as well as inter-individual differences [8, 9]. Herein, we propose a multi-step next-generation sequencing-based family genomics approach, piloted in a celiac disease trio of Greek descent to identify novel genomic variants of functional significance with the aim of understanding disease pathobiology.

Methods

Case selection, DNA isolation, and whole-genome sequencing

A seven-member Greek family has been recruited (informed consents have been obtained), and a trio analysis (III-1, III-2, IV-3) has been performed using the celiac disease model (Additional file 1: Figure S1). A family-based design was employed rather than a population-based design, as the former is generally considered to be robust against population admixture and stratification and may yield both within- and between-family information [10]. Genomic DNA isolation was performed from saliva using the Oragene collection kit (DNA Genotek, Ontario, Canada) (Serbian cohort) and peripheral blood using an automated system (MagNA Pure Compact, Roche, Basel, Switzerland) (Greek cohort). Whole-genome sequencing was performed using Complete Genomics' (CA, USA) DNA nanoarray platform [11]. DNA sequencing coverage was 110×. Only high-quality call variants were included in the analysis (>93 %). Genomes were aligned with the hg19 reference genome.

Bioinformatics and in silico analyses

Next-generation sequencing data (Complete Genomics Inc., CA) were analyzed using Ingenuity Variant Analysis version 3.1.2 (Ingenuity® Systems, www.ingenuity.com). This is a well-established software that identifies associations between phenotypes, defined by the user by classification of the tested individuals, and variants in the sequenced genome. Upon classification of the family members by phenotype (celiac vs. normal), a number of variants were listed; the output was filtered into a smaller variant list upon classification of the family members by those being celiac patients vs. those who were healthy and known not to be celiac disease subjects. The genetic model used for this comparison was of an autosomal dominant model, since it traces the genetic inheritance from mother (III-2) to daughter (IV-3) in a highly penetrant form. A total of 263 genes followed an autosomal dominant pattern, and 227 variants were identified in the genetic model. Out of these, 6 genes and 7 variants were identified in the biological/phenotype pattern of celiac disease, due to either the past association of the genes considered or via the biological significance as determined by the IVA software.

Due to the large amount of variants which are normally present in the genome, even when excluding intronic sequences, several filtering steps are used in data analysis to include only the genes which are likely to be causative in the final output connected with just the disease of interest, in this case—celiac disease. All variants were filtered according to the analysis required, using custom scripts and Complete Genomics Analysis Tools

(CGA™ Tools). The filtering cascade utilized in the present data analysis is as follows:

1. Confidence: Only variants with call quality at least 20.0 in cases or at least 20.0 in controls (i.e., 99 % call accuracy) were included.
2. Common variants: All variants observed to have an allele frequency ≥3.0 % of the genomes in the 1000 genomes project OR ≥3.0 % of the public Complete Genomics genomes OR ≥3.0 % of the NHLBI ESP exomes were excluded.
3. Predicted deleterious: Only variants that are experimentally observed to be associated with a phenotype (Pathogenic, Possibly Pathogenic, Unknown Significance OR established gain of function in the literature OR gene fusions OR inferred activating mutations by Ingenuity OR predicted gain of function by BSIFT OR in a microRNA binding site OR Frameshift, in-frame indel, or stop codon change OR Missense and not predicted to be innocuous by SIFT OR disrupt splice site up to 2.0 bases into intron OR deleterious to a microRNA OR structural variant) were kept.
4. Genetic analysis: Only variants with the following genotype characteristics were kept: associated with gain of function OR heterozygous_alt OR haploinsufficient OR heterozygous OR homozygous OR heterozygous_amb OR compound_heterozygous OR hemizygous AND occur in at least 2 of the case samples at the gene level in the Case samples AND not which are associated with gain of function OR heterozygous_alt OR haploinsufficient OR heterozygous OR homozygous OR heterozygous_amb OR compound_heterozygous OR hemizygous AND occur in at least 1 of the control samples at the variant level in the control samples.
5. Biological context: Only variants that are within 1 hop (direct targets) of upstream regulators or downstream regulatory targets of such genes and that are known or predicted to affect celiac disease.

Variants of interest were annotated with Annovar in Galaxy [12] and compared with NCBI dbSNP build 137 (http://www.ncbi.nlm.nih.gov/projects/SNP/snp_summary.cgi), 69 reference genomes from Complete Genomes (http://www.completegenomics.com/publicdata/69Genomes/), and GWAS (http://www.genome.gov/gwastudies) to determine their novelty or otherwise. To obtain a list of variants of potential functional significance, we employed protein variation effect analyzer (PROVEAN) v1.1.3 (PROVEAN human genome variants tool) that provides both scale-invariant feature transform (SIFT) [13] and PROVEAN [14] predictions for a given list of human genome variants as well as accessory information (dbSNP rs IDs, gene description, PFAM domain, GO terms, etc.). PROVEAN is able to make predictions for any type of protein sequence alteration, including single or multiple amino acid substitutions, deletions, and insertions [15]. Additionally, Variant Effect Predictor [16] and RegulomeDB [8] were employed to allow further data interrogation.

Downstream molecular analysis

Selected variants were subsequently validated in pediatric celiac disease patients of Greek ($n = 109$) [17] and Serbian ($n = 73$) [18] descent and their healthy counterparts ($n = 111$ and $n = 32$, respectively). The diagnosis of celiac disease was based on the criteria of the European Society for Paediatric Gastroenterology, Hepatology and Nutrition (ESPGHAN) [19]. For children diagnosed prior to 1990, the "Interlaken criteria" were applied. The Ethics Committee of University Children's Hospital, University of Belgrade, and the Review Board of "Aghia Sophia" Children's Hospital have approved the study.

Amplification was carried out according to the KAPA2G Fast HotStart protocol (KAPABIOSYSTEMS, MA, USA); detailed information per SNP amplification conditions is available upon request. For *SLC9A4* c.1919G>A, an allele-specific polymerase chain reaction (PCR) assay was developed (two alternative reverse primers hybridizing exclusively either to the wild-type or the mutant allele). For *NCK2* c.745_746delAAinsG, PCR products were subjected to *XcmI* (New England Biolabs, MA, USA) restriction endonuclease analysis at 37 °C for 1.15 h and subsequent enzyme deactivation (65 °C, 20 min). Restriction fragments were visualized by 3 % agarose gel electrophoresis following ethidium bromide or Midori Green staining. For *HoxD12* c.418G>A, *HoxB6* c.668C>A, and *KIAA1109* c.2933T>C and c.4268_4269delCCinsTA, a PCR-based conventional Sanger resequencing approach was employed. Capillary electrophoresis was performed on the ABI Prism 3130xl DNA Analyzer (Applied Biosystems). Sanger sequencing was also employed to ensure PCR-RFLP and allele-specific PCR method verification.

Statistical analysis

Herein, a thorough statistical review and analysis has been attempted, having always in mind that we used the celiac disease model (trio analysis) as a reason to conduct a more refined approach in searching/genotyping the resulted variants in a selective population of celiac disease of Greek and Serbian descent. We tested for deviations from HWE using the chi-square goodness of fit test and principal component analysis. Considering that the χ^2 approximation can be poor when there are low genotype counts, a Fisher exact test (R genetics package) was also used, as it does not rely on the χ^2 approximation [20]. Tests were

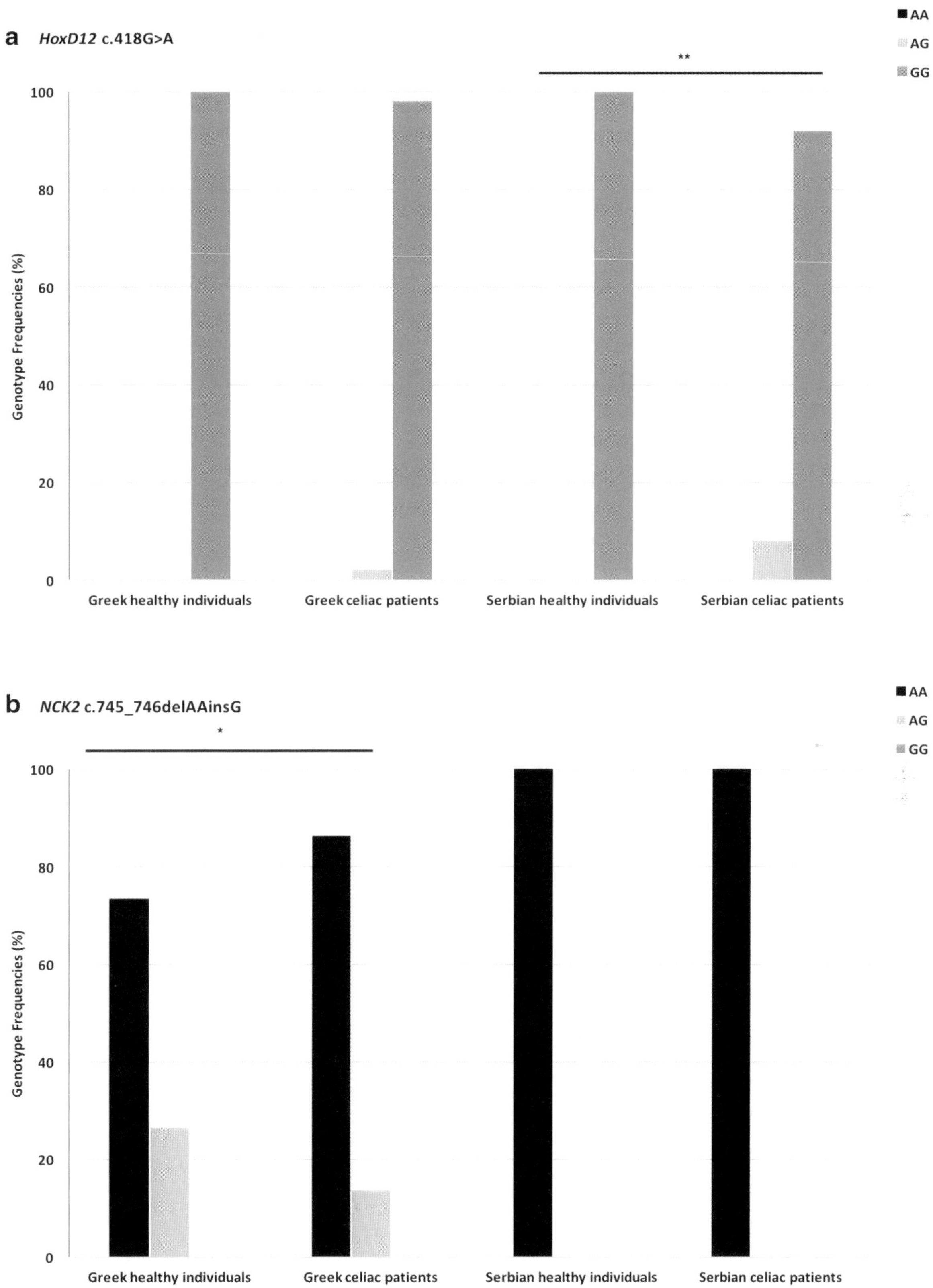

Fig. 1 Distribution of newly identified risk variants in Greek and Serbian populations. **a** *HoxD12* c.418G>A is more abundant in pediatric celiac disease patients of Greek and Serbian descent, reaching statistical significance (**$P < 0.01$) in the Serbian population. **b** *NCK2* c.745_746delAAinsG is more abundant in healthy individuals of Greek and Serbian descent, reaching statistical significance (*$P = 0.03$) in the Greek population

performed as two-tailed, and differences were considered statistically significant when $P < 0.05$. Focusing on case-control phenotypes, we tested the null hypothesis of no association between rows and columns of the 2×3 matrix that contains the counts of the three genotypes (the two homozygotes and the heterozygote) among cases and controls. Again, a Fisher exact test was preferred (to evaluate genotype and allele frequencies), as it is computationally more demanding, but it is easily implemented in R. We also performed the Armitage test (Monte Carlo method; it obtains results that are closer to an exact test, since the classical Cochran-Armitage trend test is based on approximation) [20].

Results and discussion

Whole-genome sequencing analysis of trio reveals newly identified genetic risk variants for pediatric celiac disease

Our multi-step next-generation sequencing-based family genomics approach revealed six genomic variants of prime interest: *SLC9A4* c.1919G>A, *HoxD12* c.418G>A, *KIAA1109* c.2933T>C and c.4268_4269delCCinsTA, *HoxB6* c.668C>A, and *NCK2* c.745_746delAAinsG. Susceptibility to celiac disease (CELIAC6) and to autoimmunity (AIS5) has been previously mapped to the 4q27 region, within a linkage disequilibrium block encompassing *KIAA1109*, *TENR*, *IL2*, and *IL21* genes [21]. So far, the most significant linkage outside the *HLA* region refers to rs13119723 ($P = 2.0 \times 10^{-7}$ in the *KIAA1109* gene on chromosome 4q27). Zhernakova and coworkers [2] hypothesized that the *KIAA1109/TENR/IL2/IL21* susceptibility region reported by van Heel and coworkers [21] might represent a general risk locus for multiple autoimmune diseases. Even though several CELIAC6 genomic variants have been reported [1, 2, 4, 21], this is the first time such a disease association is revealed for *KIAA1109* c.2933T>C and c.4268_4269delCCinsTA. *SLC9A4* c.1919G>A, *HoxD12* c.418G>A, *HoxB6* c.668C>A, and *NCK2* c.745_746delAAinsG are also reported for the first time as celiac disease risk variants (Fig. 1).

NCK2 c.745_746delAAinsG has not been annotated in either dbSNP or the 1000 Genomes Project/exome variant server data, and hence, it may be considered to be novel. *NCK2* codes for Human Nck2 (hNck2), a 380-residue adapter protein consisting of three SH3 domains and one SH2 domain. Nck2 plays a pivotal role in connecting and integrating signaling networks constituted by transmembrane receptors, such as ephrinB and effectors critical for cytoskeletal dynamics and remodeling [22–25]. A transient Nck2/PINCH-1 association process has been also reported that may trigger rapid focal adhesion turnover during integrin signaling, mediating cell shape change and migration [26, 27]. We showed that the novel variant identified herein results in a single amino acid change (p.K249E), being this exact amino acid that is reported of fundamental importance during the abovementioned Nck2 SH3 domain protein-protein interactions (Fig. 2a) [22, 26, 27]. p.K249E could severely alter this network of polar interactions and affect the interaction between the two proteins (Fig. 2b). In 2014, Nadalutti et al. [28] observed that celiac patient IgA antibodies disturb the extracellular protein cross-linking function of transglutaminase 2, thus altering cell-extracellular matrix interactions and thereby affecting endothelial cell adhesion, polarization, and motility.

In silico analyses

To ascertain whether the variants of interest have functional significance, in silico analysis was performed using

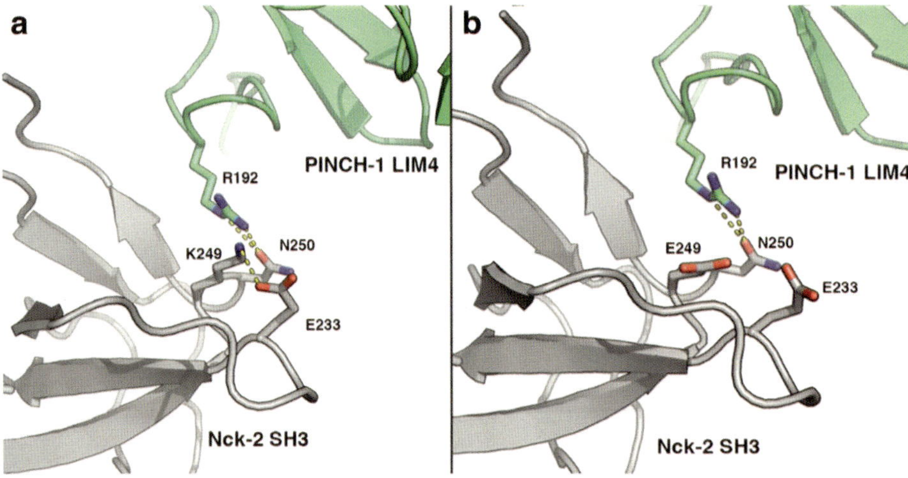

Fig. 2 **a** View of the SH3-3/LIM4 binding interface as previously shown by NMR spectroscopy [26]. The Nck2 DH3 domain interface is shown in *gray* and the PINCH-1 LIM4 domain in *green*. K249 interacts with E233 and is part of a network connecting R192 of LIM4 and N250 of SH3. **b** Structural model of the mutant p.K249E and the potential effect in the interactions between SH3 and LIM4

Table 1 In silico analyses outcome of the six variants of prime interest identified in the family trio

HUGO gene symbol	HGVS description of variant	AA position	Reference residue	Alternative residue	PROVEAN prediction			SIFT prediction		Variant effect predictor			
					Variation type	Score	Prediction	Score	Prediction	Consequence	Impact	PolyPhen	LoFtool
SLC9A4	c.1919G>A	640	R	K	Single AA change	−0.67	Neutral	0.140	Tolerated	Frameshift variant	High	–	0.911
NCK2	c.745_746delAAinsG	249	K	E	Single AA change	−1.97	Neutral	0.010	Damaging	Frameshift variant	High	–	0.223
HOXD12	c.418G>A	140	A	T	Single AA change	−0.01	Neutral	0.201	Tolerated	Frameshift variant	High	–	0.432
KIAA1109	c.2933T>C	978	I	T	Single AA change	−0.25	Neutral	0.187	Tolerated	Frameshift variant	High	–	0.845
	c.4268_4269delCCinsTA	1423	T	I	Single AA change	−1.22	Neutral	0.108	Tolerated	Missense variant	Moderate	Benign (0.031)	0.845
HOXB6	c.668C>A	223	A	D	Single AA change	−.029	Neutral	0.230	Tolerated	Frameshift variant	High	–	–

Source: PROVEAN v1.1.3 (PROVEAN human genome variants tool, http://provean.jcvi.org/genome_submit_2.php?species=human) and Variant Effect Predictor (http://grch37.ensembl.org/Homo_sapiens/Tools/VEP). Assembly: GRCh37. PROVEAN introduces a delta alignment score based on the reference and variant versions of a protein query sequence with respect to sequence homologs (NCBI NR protein database through BLAST, http://www.ncbi.nlm.nih.gov/). The default score threshold was set at −2.5 for binary classification (deleterious <−2.5 vs. neutral > −2.5). Similarly, (through PSI-BLAST, http://blast.ncbi.nlm.nih.gov/Blast.cgi?CMD=Web&PAGE=Proteins&PROGRAM=blastp&RUN_PSIBLAST=on), SIFT (http://sift.jcvi.org/) may be applied to naturally occurring non-synonymous variants. SIFT score ranges from 0 to 1. A SIFT score of ≤0.05 corresponds to a "damaging" prediction, whereas a SIFT score >0.05 predicts that the variant is likely to be "tolerated." VEP; Consequence—consequence type of this variation, Impact—a subjective classification of the severity of the variant consequence (high: the variant is assumed to have disruptive impact in the protein, probably causing protein truncation or loss of function or triggering nonsense mediated decay, moderate: a non-disruptive variant that might change protein effectiveness, low: assumed to be mostly harmless or unlikely to change protein behavior, modifier: usually non-coding variants affecting non-coding genes, where predictions are difficult or there is no evidence of impact), PolyPhen—the PolyPhen prediction and/or score, LoFtool—provides a per-gene rank of genic intolerance and consequent susceptibility to disease based on the ratio of loss of function (LoF) to synonymous mutations in ExAC data

Table 2 Genotyping data of celiac disease pediatric patients of Greek and Serbian descent and healthy individuals

Population groups	Genotype frequency (%)											
	HoxB6 c.668C>A			*SLC9A4* c.1919G>A			*KIAA1109* c.2933T>C			*KIAA1109* c.4268_4269delCCinsTA		
	TT	GG	GT	AA	GG	AG	TT	CC	CT	CC/CC	TA/TA	CC/TA
Healthy individuals of Greek descent	0	100	0	0	96	4	86	1	13	100	0	0
Patients of Greek descent	0	100	0	0	93	7	81	2	16	98	0	2
Healthy individuals of Serbian descent	0	100	0	0	97	3	80	0	20	100	0	0
Patients of Serbian descent	0	100	0	0	93	7	81	0	19	100	0	0

In both Greek and Serbian patients, *SLC9A4* c.1919G>A and *KIAA1109* c.2933T>C and c.4268_4269delCCinsTA were more abundant in patients; nevertheless, they failed to show statistical significance, possibly due to a small sample size

the SIFT and PROVEAN algorithms [13, 14], as well as Variant Effect Predictor [16] and Regulome DB [8]. As summarized in Table 1, analyses yielded that all variants share an effect to protein structure, which in the case of *NCK2* c.745_746delAAinsG is considered to be damaging. Regulome DB questioned a possible role of the variants of interest in terms of transcription factor binding sites, chromatin states, eQTLs, differentially methylated regions, validated functional SNPs and DNase sensitivity. All variants had minimum or no impact (Additional file 2: Table S1).

Replication analyses

Replication analyses were carried out in two cohorts to account for population differences. We found that *NCK2* c.745_746delAAinsG is a novel variant that is more abundant in healthy individuals, reaching statistical significance ($P = 0.03$) in the Greek population. Moreover, *HoxD12* c.418G>A, a frameshift variant, was more abundant in pediatric celiac disease patients, reaching statistical significance ($P < 0.01$) in the Serbian population. When celiac disease risk assessment is considered, it is important to note that apart from genotype data, records related to family history along with gender and country of residence should not be disregarded [29]. In both Greek and Serbian patients, *SLC9A4* c.1919G>A and *KIAA1109* c.2933T>C and c.4268_4269delCCinsTA were more abundant in patients; nevertheless, they failed to show statistical significance, possibly due to small sample sizes. All the studied variants satisfied the Hardy-Weinberg equilibrium. All variants were verified as non-frequent ones in agreement with PROVEAN's scoring scheme, separating disease-associated variants from common ones [14]. Genotype frequencies (%) are summarized in Fig. 1 and Table 2.

Conclusions

In relation to disease diagnosis and prognosis, data interpretation requires an understanding of the variation in risk-associated variants. In celiac disease, in particular, this knowledge is still largely lacking. As whole-genome and/or whole-exome sequencing approaches begin to be employed in clinical care, the understanding of detected sequence variations on diagnosis (and prognosis) is still not a trivial undertaking. We envisage that the clinical implementation of next-generation sequencing will play a crucial role in delineating inter-individual variability and identification of novel variants towards improved therapeutic modalities. Herein, we propose a multi-step next-generation sequencing-based family genomics approach, similar to our previous conducted cancer genomics study [30], but piloted towards a complex genetic disease, such as celiac disease, to analyze a family trio of Greek descent to identify novel genomic variants of functional significance with the aim of understanding complex disease pathobiology. Recently, we have outlined the paradigm of pharmacometabolomics-aided pharmacogenomics in autoimmune diseases to address the interplay of genomic and environmental influences with information technologies to facilitate data analysis as well as sense- and decision-making on the basis of synergy between artificial and human intelligence. We propose that better-informed, rapid, and cost-effective "omics" studies need the implementation of holistic and multidisciplinary approaches [31].

Acknowledgements
Not applicable

Funding
This study was funded by the European Commission (RD-CONNECT; FP7-304555) research grant to GPP.

Authors' contributions
TK and GPP conceived and designed the study. AB, AP, BS, GN, AJ, EM, AS, AIL, VS, AT, NG, SG, ZZ, MK, MK, KS, and TK carried out the PCR-based conventional Sanger resequencing approach. BAP and RD supervised the next-generation sequencing analyses. TK carried out the in silico analyses. BRA, NC, ER, JB, KP, GC, BZ, NR, RD, SP, TK, and GPP drafted the manuscript. All authors read and approved the final manuscript.

Competing interests
The authors declare the following competing interests: BAP and RD are employees of the Complete Genomics Inc. (Mountain View, CA, USA).

Author details
[1]Department of Pharmacy, School of Health Sciences, University of Patras, University Campus, Rion, 265 04 Patras, Greece. [2]Institute of Molecular Genetics and Genetic Engineering, University of Belgrade, Belgrade, Serbia. [3]Complete Genomics Inc., Mountain View, CA, USA. [4]BGI Shenzhen, Shenzhen 51803, People's Republic of China. [5]Department of Pathology,

College of Medicine and Health Sciences, United Arab Emirates University, Al Ain, United Arab Emirates. [6]Department of Immunology and Histocompatibility, "Aghia Sophia" Children's Hospital, Athens, Greece. [7]First Department of Pediatrics, National and Kapodistrian University of Athens Medical School, Athens, Greece. [8]Department of Gastroenterology and Nutrition, University Children's Hospital, Medical Faculty, University of Belgrade, Belgrade, Serbia. [9]Department of Applied Biomedical Science, Faculty of Health Sciences, University of Malta, Msida, Malta.

References

1. Burton PR, et al. Genome-wide association study of 14,000 cases of seven common diseases and 3,000 shared controls. Nature. 2007;447(7145):661–78.
2. Zhernakova A, et al. Meta-analysis of genome-wide association studies in celiac disease and rheumatoid arthritis identifies fourteen non-HLA shared loci. PLoS Genet. 2011;7(2):e1002004.
3. Hunt KA, et al. Novel celiac disease genetic determinants related to the immune response. Nat Genet. 2008;40(4):395–402.
4. Romanos J, et al. Six new coeliac disease loci replicated in an Italian population confirm association with coeliac disease. J Med Genet. 2009; 46(1):60–3.
5. Trynka G, et al. Dense genotyping identifies and localizes multiple common and rare variant association signals in celiac disease. Nat Genet. 2011;43(12): 1193–201.
6. Gutierrez-Achury J, et al. Fine-mapping in the MHC region accounts for 18 % additional genetic risk for celiac disease. Nat Genet. 2015;47(6):577–8.
7. Cortes A, Brown MA. Promise and pitfalls of the Immunochip. Arthritis Res Ther. 2011;13(1):1.
8. Boyle AP, et al. Annotation of functional variation in personal genomes using RegulomeDB. Genome Res. 2012;22(9):1790–7.
9. Mizzi C, et al. Personalized pharmacogenomics profiling using whole-genome sequencing. Pharmacogenomics. 2014;15(9):1223–34.
10. Laird NM, Lange C. Family-based designs in the age of large-scale gene-association studies. Nat Rev Genet. 2006;7(5):385–94.
11. Drmanac R, et al. Human genome sequencing using unchained base reads on self-assembling DNA nanoarrays. Science. 2010;327(5961):78–81.
12. Hiltemann S, et al. CGtag: complete genomics toolkit and annotation in a cloud-based Galaxy. GigaScience. 2014;3:1.
13. Kumar P, Henikoff S, Ng PC. Predicting the effects of coding non-synonymous variants on protein function using the SIFT algorithm. Nat Protoc. 2009;4(8):1073–81.
14. Choi Y, et al. Predicting the functional effect of amino acid substitutions and indels. PLoS One. 2012;7(10):e46688.
15. Boycott KM, et al. Rare-disease genetics in the era of next-generation sequencing: discovery to translation. Nat Rev Genet. 2013;14(10):681–91.
16. McLaren W, et al. Deriving the consequences of genomic variants with the Ensembl API and SNP Effect Predictor. Bioinformatics. 2010;26(16):2069–70.
17. Krini M, et al. HLA class II high-resolution genotyping in Greek children with celiac disease and impact on disease susceptibility. Pediatr Res. 2012;72(6):625–30.
18. Stanković B, et al. HLA genotyping in pediatric celiac disease patients. Bosn J Basic Med Sci. 2014;14(3):171.
19. Walker-Smith J, et al. Revised criteria for diagnosis of coeliac disease. Report of working group of ESPGAN. Arch Dis Child. 1990;65:909–11.
20. Balding DJ. A tutorial on statistical methods for population association studies. Nat Rev Genet. 2006;7(10):781–91.
21. van Heel DA, et al. A genome-wide association study for celiac disease identifies risk variants in the region harboring IL2 and IL21. Nat Genet. 2007;39(7):827–9.
22. Liu J, et al. Structural insight into the binding diversity between the human Nck2 SH3 domains and proline-rich proteins. Biochemistry. 2006;45(23):7171–84.
23. Mayer BJ. SH3 domains: complexity in moderation. J Cell Sci. 2001;114(7):1253–63.
24. Koytiger G, et al. Phosphotyrosine signaling proteins that drive oncogenesis tend to be highly interconnected. Mol Cell Proteomics. 2013;12(5):1204–13.
25. Ran X, Song J. Structural insight into the binding diversity between the Tyr-phosphorylated human ephrinBs and Nck2 SH2 domain. J Biol Chem. 2005; 280(19):19205–12.
26. Vaynberg J, et al. Structure of an ultraweak protein-protein complex and its crucial role in regulation of cell morphology and motility. Mol Cell. 2005; 17(4):513–23.
27. Velyvis A, et al. Structural and functional insights into PINCH LIM4 domain-mediated integrin signaling. Nat Struct Mol Biol. 2003;10(7):558–64.
28. Nadalutti CA, et al. Celiac disease patient IgA antibodies induce endothelial adhesion and cell polarization defects via extracellular transglutaminase 2. Cell Mol Life Sci. 2014;71(7):1315–26.
29. Liu E, et al. Risk of pediatric celiac disease according to HLA haplotype and country. N Engl J Med. 2014;371(1):42–9.
30. Karageorgos I, et al. Identification of cancer predisposition variants in apparently healthy individuals using a next-generation sequencing-based family genomics approach. Hum Genomics. 2015;9(1):1.
31. Katsila T, et al. Pharmacometabolomics-aided pharmacogenomics in autoimmune disease. EBioMedicine. 2016;5:40–5.

16

Evaluation of a bone morphogenetic protein 6 variant as a cause of iron loading

Cameron J. McDonald[1†], Gautam Rishi[2†], Eriza S. Secondes[2], Lesa Ostini[1], Daniel F. Wallace[2], Darrell H. G. Crawford[3], Hanlon Sia[4], Paul Clark[5] and V. Nathan Subramaniam[2*]

Abstract

Background: Atypical iron overload without variation in the five clinically associated hereditary hemochromatosis genes is now recognized; however, their etiology remains unknown. Since the identification of iron overload in the bone morphogenetic protein 6 (*Bmp6*) knockout mouse, the search has been on for clinically pathogenic variants in the *BMP6* gene. A recent report proposes that variants in the pro-peptide region of *BMP6* are the underlying cause of several cases of iron overload. We performed targeted next-generation sequencing on three cases of atypical iron overload with Asian ethnicity and identified a p.Q118dup (aka p.E112indelEQ, p.Q115dup, p.Q118_L119insQ) variant in *BMP6*. The purpose of this study was to characterize the molecular function of the identified BMP6 variant. Molecular characterization by immunofluorescence microscopy and Western blotting of transfected cells, bioinformatics, and population analyses was performed.

Results: In contrast to reports for other BMP6 pro-peptide variants in this region, our data indicates that this variant does not affect the function of the mature BMP6 protein.

Conclusions: Our data suggest that assignment of disease causation in clinical cases of iron overload to pro-peptide variants in BMP6 should thus be treated with caution and requires biological characterization.

Keywords: Next-generation sequencing, Hemochromatosis, Causal variant, Iron overload, BMP6

Background

Hereditary hemochromatosis (HH) is relatively common in individuals of northern European descent, with the majority of cases caused by mutations in the *HFE* (hemochromatosis) gene [1, 2]. Conversely, mutations in *HFE* are rare in non-European populations, and mutations in other genes involved in the regulation of iron homeostasis are more common, such as hemojuvelin (*HFE2*), hepcidin (*HAMP*), transferrin receptor 2 (*TFR2*), and ferroportin (*SLC40A1*), collectively termed non-*HFE* HH [3]. Potentially, all regulators of iron homeostasis are functional gene candidates for non-*HFE* HH [4]. BMP6 (bone morphogenetic protein 6) is a key regulator of iron homeostasis [5]. *Bmp6* null mice have significant iron overload due to deficiency of the iron-regulatory hormone hepcidin [6, 7].

Under normal conditions, *Bmp6* expression is upregulated by increased iron and increases the expression of hepcidin which in turn limits iron absorption and recycling [8]. A recent report associated heterozygosity for three variants p.P95S, p.L96P, and p.Q113E in the BMP6 pro-peptide region with nine clinical cases of unexplained atypical iron overload [9]. The functional link between BMP6 and iron overload remains to be explained, however, and further validation is necessary to better assess causality of these variants [10]. In addition, p.E112Q and p.R257H have also been associated with more severe iron overload in patients with *HFE* mutations [11]. Here, we report on three clinical cases of unexplained atypical iron overload carrying an amino acid insertion within the same region of the BMP6 pro-peptide.

Results

Three cases are reported in this study; in each case, *HFE* genotyping was negative, and liver specialist assessment was undertaken. Case 1 was a 62-year-old male who over the past 7 years had raised serum ferritin (SF) ranging

* Correspondence: nathan.subramaniam@qut.edu.au
†Equal contributors
[2]Institute of Health and Biomedical Innovation and School of Biomedical Sciences, Queensland University of Technology (QUT), 60 Musk Avenue, Kelvin Grove, Brisbane, Queensland 4059, Australia
Full list of author information is available at the end of the article

between 1261 and 1675 μg/L (normal range 30–300 μg/L), with transferrin saturation (TS) 40 to 53% (normal range 20–55%). His alanine aminotransferase (ALT), aspartate aminotransferase (AST), and gamma-glutamyl transferase (GGT) levels all remained normal during this time. Liver biopsy revealed grade 4 stainable iron in hepatocytes, with accentuation of iron in the pericanalicular region (Fig. 1). No other pathology was noted. In case 2, a male aged 51 who did not consume any alcohol, presented with a SF of 1714 μg/L and TS of 34%. ALT, AST, and GGT were all normal although ultrasound revealed a diffusely echogenic liver suggesting fatty liver. Ferriscan identified a hepatic iron concentration of 44 μmol/g (normal range 3–33 μmol/g). In case 3, also male aged 62 presented with a SF of 1133 μg/L and TS of 90%. His ALT, AST, and GGT levels were mildly elevated. Liver biopsy demonstrated grade 1 iron with a hepatic iron content of 39 μmol/g and F1 fibrosis. Case 3's pathophysiology is complex with positivity for α-thalassemia trait and hepatitis C virus (genotype 2).

Targeted next-generation sequencing revealed that all three patients were negative for mutations in the five currently clinically associated HH genes. Further analysis identified a tri-nucleotide duplication in *BMP6*, c.353-355dupAGC (NM_001718.4), resulting in the in-frame duplication of glutamine p.Q118dup (NP_001709.1), which was confirmed by Sanger sequencing. The nomenclature for this variant is noted in three different forms across various datasets: dbSNP rs771616962 refers to this variant as p.Q118_L119insQ, wANNOVAR, and the NHLBI Exome Sequencing Project (http://evs.gs.washington.edu/EVS/) (ESP) dataset as p.E112delinsEQ and Exome Aggregation Consortium database (ExAC) [12] as p.Gln115dup. While all of these references result in the same outcome, extension of the poly-Q stretch, the various designations may cause underestimation of its population frequency. This variant, or its pseudonyms, is not present in the 1000 Genomes database; however, it is present in the ESP (MAF = 0.016) and ExAC (MAF = 0.041).

To investigate possible functional effects of the p.Q118dup variant on BMP6, immunofluorescence microscopy studies were conducted using BMP6 wildtype and p.Q118dup proteins with a pro-peptide N-terminus HA tag and a mature protein C-terminus V5 tag. We used both CHO cells and liver endothelial (SK-HEP-1) cells as a model for examining the molecular and functional effects of the p.Q118dup variant. CHO cells (Fig. 2a) and SK-HEP-1 cells (Fig. 3a) stably expressing these constructs showed some peri-nuclear Golgi localization of p.Q118dup pro-peptide; however, this was very mild and not consistent within all cells. No difference in localization was observed for the mature V5-tagged protein in either the CHO or endothelial cell models.

Discussion

BMP6 is an important signaling molecule required for iron homeostasis [6, 8]. In response to increase in body iron levels *BMP6* levels increase, this results in an increase in BMP-SMAD signaling. The increased BMP_SMAD signaling then leads to an increase in hepcidin production. Recently, Daher and colleagues reported on three BMP6 pro-domain variants associated with iron overload and attributed the cause to reduced export of BMP6 [9]. We compared levels of the full-length and mature wildtype and mutant BMP6 protein in cell lysate and conditioned media (Fig. 2b, c). This revealed no difference in the capacity of cells to export p.Q118dup BMP6 protein compared to wildtype. Recent studies have suggested that the endothelial cells may be responsible for BMP6 production in response to iron [13]. Using an endothelial cell model, we show that there is

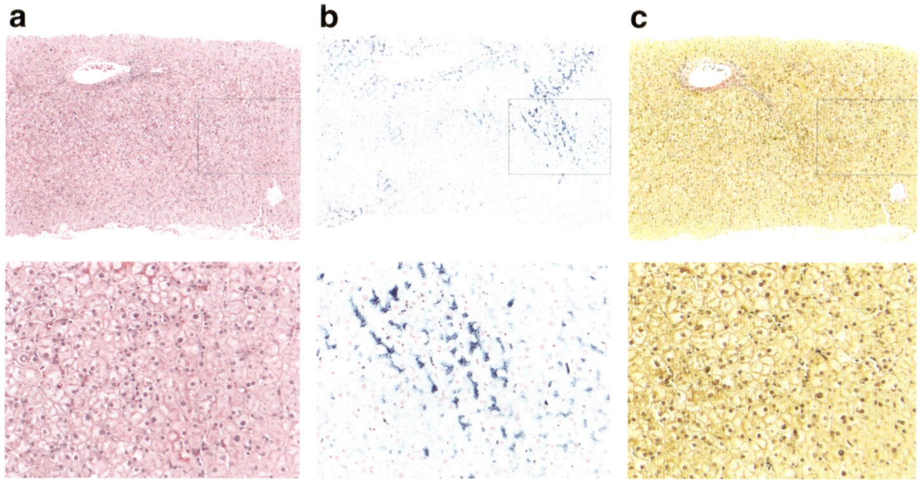

Fig. 1 Liver biopsy histology of case 1. Histological sections stained with **a** H&E, **b** Perls, and **c** Van Gieson's stain showing significant stainable iron, without pathology

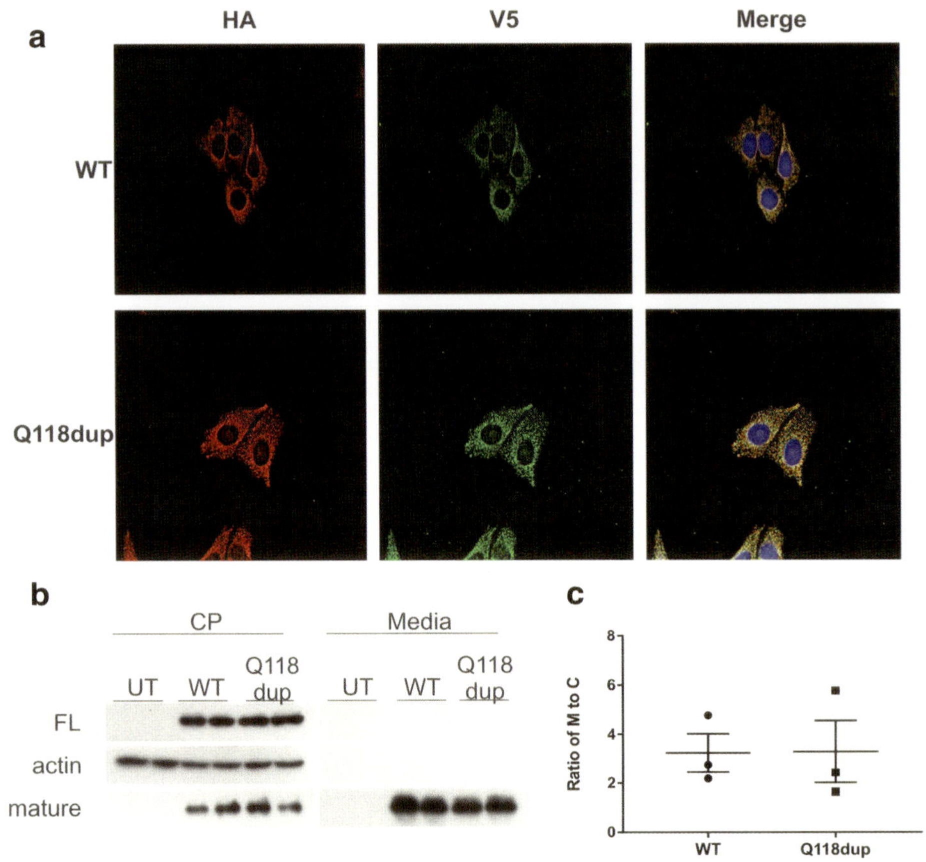

Fig. 2 Cellular characterization of p.Q118dup BMP6 protein in CHO cells. **a** Representative immunofluorescence image of stably transfected CHO cells. The HA tag on the N-terminus of the pro-peptide, and the V5 tag on the C-terminus of the mature protein co-localize, and no difference in localization of the wildtype (WT) and p.Q118dup variant of BMP6 was observed. **b** Western blot identifying the full-length (FL) and mature BMP6 proteins in cell lysate (CP) and conditioned media (M) from untransfected (UT), wildtype (WT), and p.Q118dup (Q118dup) BMP6 transfected CHO cells. **c** Quantification of Western blot shown in **b** ($n = 3$). The ratio of mature proteins in conditioned media (M) to cell lysate (CP) shows no difference in protein secretion between WT and p.Q118dup BMP6 transfected cells

no difference in the expression of the mature BMP6 protein for either the wildtype or p.Q118dup variant of BMP6 (Fig. 3b).

As population frequency can provide insight into the likelihood of a variant being benign, we investigated the frequency of p.Q118dup in the ExAC dataset (http://exac.broadinstitute.org/) which contains exome sequences from 60,706 unrelated individuals, and carrier rates were then calculated using the Hardy-Weinberg equation. This analysis reveals that in East Asians, p.Q118dup has a carrier rate of 1 in 3 (MAF = 0.191), with other ethnicities also showing lower though still significant carrier rates, confirming the experimental result that this variant is unlikely to affect gene function. Finally, we examined the classification of the p.Q118dup variant according to the "standards and guidelines for the interpretation of sequence variants" as set out by the American College of Medical Genetics and Genomics [14]. Based on the above data plus bioinformatic functional impact prediction using several tools available through ANNOVAR, it confirmed a categorization of the BMP6 pro-peptide p.Q118dup variant as benign.

Conclusions

The data from this study suggest no functional relationship between the p.Q118dup BMP6 pro-peptide variant and iron overload. Recognition of this variant as non-deleterious and not causative is notably important for this specific variant, as cursory literature and database analysis may easily lead to the alternate and incorrect assumption that this variant is likely causative of the disease.

Firstly, the alternative nomenclature of p.E112indelEQ (which while technically incorrect is the annotation returned by several common sequence alignment programs) places this variant at the same location as the p.Q113E variant recently reported by Daher et al. [9] to be deleterious and the cause of atypical iron overload in two members of a single family. Secondly, the absence of p.Q118dup from the two most commonly known variant data sets, dbSNP and 1000 Genomes, erroneously suggests

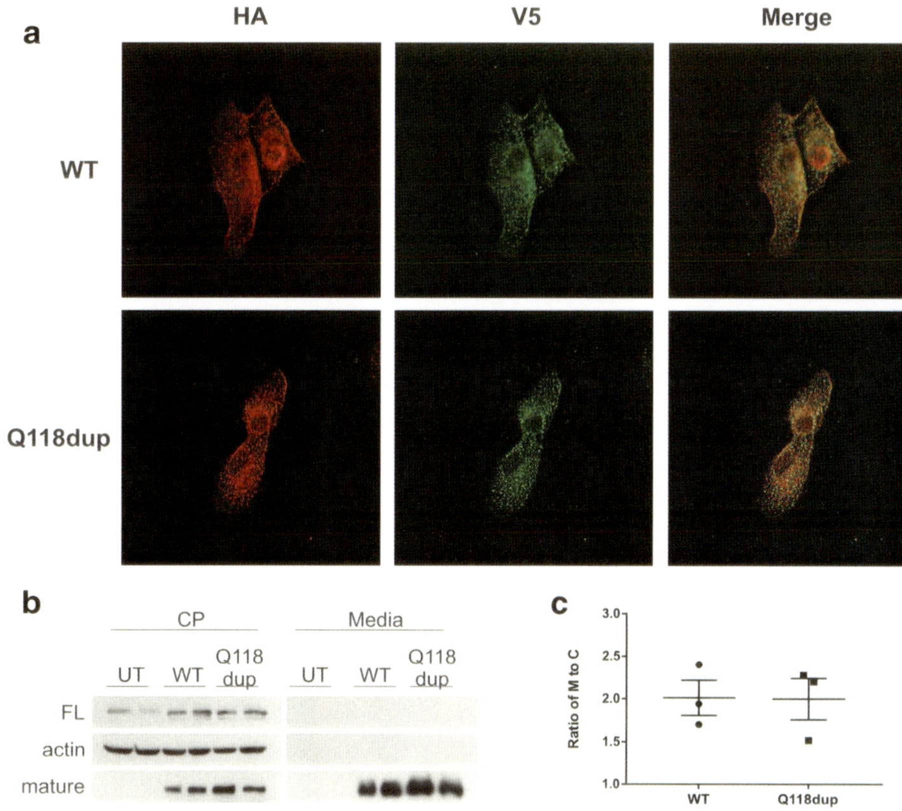

Fig. 3 Cellular characterization of p.Q118dup BMP6 protein in a hepatic endothelial cell model, SK-HEP-1. **a** Immunofluorescence of stably transfected SK-HEP-1 cells. No difference in localization of the wildtype and p.Q118dup variant of BMP6 was observed. HA tag, N-terminus of pro-peptide; V5 tag, C-terminus of mature protein. **b** Western blot identifying the full-length (FL) and mature BMP6 proteins in cell lysate (CP) and conditioned media from untransfected (UT), wildtype (WT), and p.Q118dup BMP6 transfected SK-HEP-1 cells. **c** Quantification of Western blot shown in **b** ($n = 3$). The ratio of mature proteins in conditioned media to cell lysate shows no difference in protein secretion between WT and p.Q118dup BMP6 transfected cells

that this variant is novel and thus is not carried in the healthy population. Finally, using CHO and hepatocyte endothelial cell models, we showed no difference in the localization or secretion between the wildtype and p. Q118dup BMP6 variant.

These data demonstrated no relationship between *BMP6* variants and atypical iron overload and provided no functional evidence of causality for the identified variant. Furthermore, the analysis raises uncertainty about the population prevalence of *BMP6* variants and their potential role in iron overload conditions. This has important clinical implications, for monitoring and treatment, and should lead to pause before suggesting genetic and family counseling based on *BMP6* variation. Atypical, non-HFE-related iron overload remains an important question; however, despite prior literature and the appeal of its underlying biological plausibility, the genetic causes of some forms of HH appear elusive. Further research will be required to uncover the potential genetic causes of these atypical iron overload disorders.

Methods

Patients and consent

This study was approved by and performed in accordance with the ethical standards of the QIMR Berghofer Human Research Ethics Committee and with the Helsinki Declaration of 1975, as revised in 1983. Informed and written consent was obtained for the studies described in this report.

Cases of clinically identified atypical iron overload of unknown cause were referred to our laboratory for sequencing by primary clinicians. Cases were required to demonstrate persistently (two or more occasions) abnormal iron indices (including significantly elevated serum ferritin >1000 μg/L for males and >700 for females) and to be negative for p. C282Y homozygosity. Referring clinicians were also requested to undertake a detailed iron metabolism-specific patient history for other possible attributing causes, such as high alcohol consumption. In total, 31 referred patients have been sequenced to date at our center [15].

Next-generation sequencing

Sequencing of genomic DNA using an iron-associated gene panel, covering 39 genes and 11 promoters associated with iron overload or anemia, was performed as previously described [15]. Samples were sequenced to an average of 400-fold coverage using an Ion Torrent PGM, with post run QC/QA filtering performed using Torrent Suite (v3.6; Life Technologies). Sequences were mapped to the Human Genome (HG19) and variants identified using the Torrent Variant Caller (version 3.6.59049 with Germ Line - Low Stringency configuration). Identified variants were annotated using the wANNOVAR tool [16], and candidate mutations confirmed by Sanger sequencing.

BMP6 expression constructs

Constructs containing double-tagged human *BMP6* coding sequence were synthesized and validated by BioMatik (Delaware, USA). Constructs were generated for both the wildtype and p.Q118dup sequence and contained a hemagglutinin (HA)—tag inserted between amino acids 23 and 24 (N-terminus of the pro-protein) and a V5-tag at the carboxyl-terminus of the mature protein.

Transfections

Chinese hamster ovary (CHO) cells and the hepatic endothelial cell line, SK-HEP-1 [17] (HTB-52, ATCC, Manassas, Virginia), were transiently transfected with the *BMP6* expression constructs by reverse transfection using Viafect (Promega, Alexandria, NSW, Australia) according to the manufacturer's instructions. Stably expressing cells were obtained by placing transfected cells under selection with puromycin at 10 μg/ml (CHO cells) or 1 μg/ml (SK-HEP-1 cell).

Immunofluorescence

Transfected cells were plated on glass coverslips to a confluency of 50–70% for 24 h. Cells were washed twice in PBSCM (phosphate buffered saline with 1 mM $CaCl_2$, 1 mM $MgCl_2$) and then fixed (in methanol at − 20 °C for 5 min for CHO cells then at room temperature (RT) for 10 min and in 3% paraformaldehyde for SK-HEP Hep-1 cells which were then permeabilized using 0.1% saponin in PBSCM for 15 min). Primary antibodies were then applied: anti-HA at 1:10 (12CA5, tissue culture supernatant) and anti-V5 at 1:3000 (Merck-Millipore). After three PBSCM washes, cells were incubated in Alexa Fluor donkey secondary antibodies: anti-mouse 488/594 and anti-rabbit 594/488 (Invitrogen). Following three final PBSCM washes, coverslips were mounted in Prolong Gold antifade mounting media (Invitrogen) and imaged by microscopy at × 63 magnification using a Zeiss Axioscope NLO-780 or a Leica TCS SP5. Z stacks were imaged for each focal point, and the final images were processed using the in-built deconvolution algorithms in the Zen software. The immunofluorescence studies were performed at least three times for each cell line.

Western blotting

Conditioned media from transfected cells were precipitated with 10% trichloroacetic acid overnight at 4 °C, and the precipitate was washed with cold acetone and resuspended in SDS sample buffer (SB) (50 mm Tris pH 6.8, 2% SDS, 10% glycerol, 0.1% bromophenol blue, 5% β-mercaptoethanol). Cell lysates were also resuspended in SDS SB, and all samples were loaded onto a 12% SDS-PAG and electrophoresed. Following transfer onto 0.2 μm nitrocellulose (Bio-Rad), blots were blocked for 3 h at RT in Western blocking buffer WBB (10% skim milk powder in 0.5% Tween-20 in TBS (TBST)). Primary anti-V5 (2.5 ng/ml) or anti-HA (1:100) diluted in WBB was applied overnight at 4 °C. Following three washes in TBST, blots were incubated with secondary anti-mouse horseradish peroxidase (1:10,000 in WBB) for 1 h at RT. Blots were washed extensively with TBST, Luminata Forte Western Chemiluminescent HRP Substrate (Merck-Millipore) was applied for 5 min, and blots were then exposed to film. Western blotting was repeated three times for each cell line and quantified. Band volume and density were quantitated using ImageJ software (National Institutes of Health, Maryland, USA).

Abbreviations

ALT: Alanine aminotransferase; AST: Aspartate aminotransferase; BMP: Bone morphogenetic protein; ESP: NHLBI Exome Sequencing Project 6500 database; ExAC: Exome Aggregation Consortium database; GGT: Gamma-glutamyl transferase; SF: Serum ferritin; TS: Transferrin saturation

Acknowledgements

The authors gratefully acknowledge the support of the patients in this study.

Funding

This work was supported in part by the project grants (APP1031325 and APP1048000) from the National Health and Medical Research Council (NHMRC) of Australia to VNS. VNS is the recipient of an NHMRC Senior Research Fellowship (APP1024672 and APP1118888).

Authors' contributions

CJM, DFW, GR, and VNS designed the studies. CJM, GR, ES, and LO performed the experiments. CJM, GR, LO, DFW, and VNS analyzed the data. DHGC, HS, and PC contributed to clinical aspects of the study. CJM, GR, and VNS wrote the manuscript. CJM, GR, DFW, DHGC, HS, and PC critically reviewed the manuscript. VNS provided the funding. All authors read and approved the final manuscript.

Competing interests

The authors declare that they have no competing interests.

Author details

[1]QIMR Berghofer Medical Research Institute, Brisbane, Australia. [2]Institute of Health and Biomedical Innovation and School of Biomedical Sciences, Queensland University of Technology (QUT), 60 Musk Avenue, Kelvin Grove, Brisbane, Queensland 4059, Australia. [3]Faculty of Medicine and Biomedical Sciences, The University of Queensland, Brisbane, Australia. [4]ICON Cancer Care, Southport, Australia. [5]Princess Alexandra and Mater Hospitals, Brisbane, Australia.

References

1. Allen KJ, Gurrin LC, Constantine CC, Osborne NJ, Delatycki MB, Nicoll AJ, McLaren CE, Bahlo M, Nisselle AE, Vulpe CD, et al. Iron-overload-related disease in HFE hereditary hemochromatosis. N Engl J Med. 2008;358(3):221–30.
2. Feder JN, Gnirke A, Thomas W, Tsuchihashi Z, Ruddy DA, Basava A, Dormishian F, Domingo R Jr, Ellis MC, Fullan A, et al. A novel MHC class I-like gene is mutated in patients with hereditary haemochromatosis. Nat Genet. 1996;13(4):399–408.
3. McDonald CJ, Wallace DF, Crawford DH, Subramaniam VN. Iron storage disease in Asia-Pacific populations: the importance of non-HFE mutations. J Gastroenterol Hepatol. 2013;28(7):1087–94.
4. Wallace DF, Subramaniam VN. Non-HFE haemochromatosis. World J Gastroenterol. 2007;13(35):4690–8.
5. Rishi G, Subramaniam VN. The liver in regulation of iron homeostasis. Am J Physiol Gastrointest Liver Physiol. 2017;313(3):G157–65.
6. Meynard D, Kautz L, Darnaud V, Canonne-Hergaux F, Coppin H, Roth MP. Lack of the bone morphogenetic protein BMP6 induces massive iron overload. Nat Genet. 2009;41(4):478–81.
7. Andriopoulos B Jr, Corradini E, Xia Y, Faasse SA, Chen S, Grgurevic L, Knutson MD, Pietrangelo A, Vukicevic S, Lin HY, et al. BMP6 is a key endogenous regulator of hepcidin expression and iron metabolism. Nat Genet. 2009;41(4):482–7.
8. Kautz L, Besson-Fournier C, Meynard D, Latour C, Roth MP, Coppin H. Iron overload induces BMP6 expression in the liver but not in the duodenum. Haematologica. 2011;96(2):199–203.
9. Daher R, Kannengiesser C, Houamel D, Lefebvre T, Bardou-Jacquet E, Ducrot N, de Kerguenec C, Jouanolle AM, Robreau AM, Oudin C, et al. Heterozygous mutations in BMP6 pro-peptide lead to inappropriate hepcidin synthesis and moderate iron overload in humans. Gastroenterology. 2016;150(3):672–683 e674.
10. McDonald CJ, Rishi G, Wallace DF, Subramaniam VN. Genetic variants in the BMP6 pro-peptide may not cause iron loading and should be interpreted with caution. Gastroenterology. 2016;151(4):770–1.
11. Piubelli C, Castagna A, Marchi G, Rizzi M, Busti F, Badar S, Marchetti M, De Gobbi M, Roetto A, Xumerle L, et al. Identification of new BMP6 pro-peptide mutations in patients with iron overload. Am J Hematol. 2017;92(6):562–8.
12. Lek M, Karczewski KJ, Minikel EV, Samocha KE, Banks E, Fennell T, O'Donnell-Luria AH, Ware JS, Hill AJ, Cummings BB, et al. Analysis of protein-coding genetic variation in 60,706 humans. Nature. 2016;536(7616):285–91.
13. Canali S, Zumbrennen-Bullough KB, Core AB, Wang CY, Nairz M, Bouley R, Swirski FK, Babitt JL. Endothelial cells produce bone morphogenetic protein 6 required for iron homeostasis in mice. Blood. 2017;129(4):405–14.
14. Richards S, Aziz N, Bale S, Bick D, Das S, Gastier-Foster J, Grody WW, Hegde M, Lyon E, Spector E, et al. Standards and guidelines for the interpretation of sequence variants: a joint consensus recommendation of the American College of Medical Genetics and Genomics and the Association for Molecular Pathology. Genet Med. 2015;17(5):405–24.
15. McDonald CJ, Ostini L, Wallace DF, Lyons A, Crawford DH, Subramaniam VN. Next-generation sequencing: application of a novel platform to the analysis of atypical iron disorders. J Hepatol. 2015;63(5):1288-93.
16. Kircher M, Witten DM, Jain P, O'Roak BJ, Cooper GM, Shendure J. A general framework for estimating the relative pathogenicity of human genetic variants. Nat Genet. 2014;46(3):310–5.
17. Heffelfinger SC, Hawkins HH, Barrish J, Taylor L, Darlington GJ. SK HEP-1: a human cell line of endothelial origin. In Vitro Cell Dev Biol. 1992; 28A(2):136–42.

17

Bayesian variable selection for parametric survival model with applications to cancer omics data

Weiwei Duan[1,2,3,4†], Ruyang Zhang[1,2,3,4†], Yang Zhao[1,2,3,4], Sipeng Shen[1,2,3,4], Yongyue Wei[1,2,3,4], Feng Chen[1,2,3,4*] and David C. Christiani[2,3,5,6]

Abstract

Background: Modeling thousands of markers simultaneously has been of great interest in testing association between genetic biomarkers and disease or disease-related quantitative traits. Recently, an expectation-maximization (EM) approach to Bayesian variable selection (EMVS) facilitating the Bayesian computation was developed for continuous or binary outcome using a fast EM algorithm. However, it is not suitable to the analyses of time-to-event outcome in many public databases such as The Cancer Genome Atlas (TCGA).

Results: We extended the EMVS to high-dimensional parametric survival regression framework (SurvEMVS). A variant of cyclic coordinate descent (CCD) algorithm was used for efficient iteration in M-step, and the extended Bayesian information criteria (EBIC) was employed to make choice on hyperparameter tuning. We evaluated the performance of SurvEMVS using numeric simulations and illustrated the effectiveness on two real datasets. The results of numerical simulations and two real data analyses show the well performance of SurvEMVS in aspects of accuracy and computation. Some potential markers associated with survival of lung or stomach cancer were identified.

Conclusions: These results suggest that our model is effective and can cope with high-dimensional omics data.

Keywords: Survival analysis, Bayesian variable selection, EM algorithm, Omics, Non-small cell lung cancer, Stomach adenocarcinoma

Introduction

With the development of high-throughput sequence technology, large-scale omics data are generated rapidly for discovering new biomarkers [1, 2]. The public databases such as The Cancer Genome Atlas (TCGA) and Gene Expression Omnibus (GEO) provide great opportunities to understand complex diseases comprehensively on a molecular level [3, 4] and subsequently facilitate growing demanding statistical approaches designed to cope with these large-scale data [5]. Analyzing biomarkers one at a time is the most common strategy to detect the underlying causal markers [6, 7]. However, this one-by-one method ignores the correlation between biomarkers and needs multiple corrections for controlling false positives. Furthermore, multiple regression is performed increasingly because it is powerful to identify causal markers after the strongest associations have been accounted for [8–10]. It can also avoid multiple correction and enable accurate effect estimation [11, 12]. Nevertheless, omics data generally have the property of high dimensionality, which makes the classical multiple regression yield unstable parameter estimations with high standard errors. Due to this limitation, least absolute shrinkage and selection operator (LASSO) regression and its variants shrink the effects of noise toward zero while adding a penalty term to the likelihood function. The approach can easily be conducted on a large-scale variable selection analysis [13, 14]. The LASSO can also be explained from Bayesian perspectives, namely Bayesian

* Correspondence: fengchen@njmu.edu.cn
†Weiwei Duan and Ruyang Zhang contributed equally to this work.
[1]Department of Biostatistics, School of Public Health, Nanjing Medical University, 101 Longmian Avenue, Nanjing 211166, Jiangsu, China
[2]China International Cooperation Center for Environment and Human Health, Nanjing Medical University, 101 Longmian Avenue, Nanjing 211166, Jiangsu, China
Full list of author information is available at the end of the article

LASSO (BL) [15]. That is, we can generate the LASSO estimators by imposing a Laplace prior on coefficients of explanatory variables. Compared with a frequentist penalty, Bayesian regression is more flexible to induce different shrinkage by specifying various priors.

George and McCulloch [16] proposed a two-component "spike-and-slab" mixture prior, consisting of the "spike" to be either a point mass at zero or a normal distribution with a very narrow variance while a "slab" be a normal distribution with a large variance. Indicator variables are utilized to denote which component each marker belongs to, which is known as Bayesian variable selection (BVS). BVS and its expansions are widely used in genomic studies, including marker detection and disease risk prediction [11, 12, 17]. But, most Bayesian studies have used a Markov Chain Monte Carlo (MCMC) algorithm to explore the posterior distribution of unknown parameters via numerical approximations in high-dimensional models, which is quite time consuming for getting a stable chain. For example, the BayesR model required ~ 18 h to complete an analysis of a bipolar disorder genome-wide association data with ~ 3800 individuals (80% of whole samples) and ~ 300,000 genotype markers [12]. In order to facilitate Bayesian computation, variational inference [18–20] and expectation-maximization (EM) algorithm are commonly used for Bayesian posterior inference [21]. Ročková and George [22] proposed EM variable selection (EMVS) for continuous outcomes to rapidly identify promising high posterior models and parameter estimates. The continuous conjugate spike-and-slab prior adopted by EMVS leads to fast closed form expression for the EM algorithm. Nevertheless, there has been considerable interest in discovering associations between biomarkers and prognosis.

Analyzing time-to-event data, namely survival analysis, plays a very important role in statistics, which arises in many fields, such as medicine, genetics, industrial engineering, sociology, and economics [23–25]. Modeling survival data using Cox proportional hazards regression is popular for its robust to the unknown baseline hazard [26]. Alternatively, being well known for parametric survival analysis, accelerated failure time (AFT) model tends to give more precise estimates of interest parameters if the distribution of survival time is chosen correctly, in addition, the parameter estimates from AFT are robust to omitted covariates [27]. Under the scenario of high-dimensional survival analysis, a lot of works have been done usually by adding a penalty term to likelihood. In a Bayesian framework, we usually need to assign a semi-parametric or nonparametric prior processes to the (cumulative) baseline hazard function in a Cox model [28, 29], which does not allow us to naturally choose a fully parametric survival model for the subsequent analyses. As a parametric model, the Weibull regression induces a very flexible model since it is a unique parametric model which has both AFT and the proportional hazards properties [30].

In this study, we extended EMVS to parametric survival model (SurvEMVS) with Weibull distribution assumption. A fast EM algorithm was used to obtain posterior modes of interested parameters, in which a variant of the fast cyclic coordinate descent (CCD) method is nested. We used simulation trials to explore performance in comparison with an alternative frequentist variable selection strategy, namely Cox LASSO regression. After that, we applied SurvEMVS to a lung cancer genotype data and a stomach cancer gene expression data. Further details of this work were given below.

Methods

Statistical framework

Survival times of n individuals in sample are designed by $T_i = \min(t_i, c_i)$, $i = 1, \ldots, n$, where t_i and c_i are lifetime and fixed censoring time for a specific individual i, respectively. The survival outcome from a follow-up study can be conveniently represented by pair of random variables (T_i, δ_i), where δ_i indicates whether the lifetime t_i corresponds to an event ($\delta_i = 1$) or is censored ($\delta_i = 0$). In this study, we consider right censoring scheme and non-informative censoring mechanism for each individual without note elsewhere. Under parametric framework, $f(T_i| \theta)$ and $S(T_i| \theta)$ are defined as probability density and survival function of survival time T_i, respectively, parametrized by θ. Let $L = \prod_{i=1}^{n} f(T_i|\theta)^{\delta_i} S(T_i|\theta)^{(1-\delta_i)}$ be the likelihood of the parametric model with an i.i.d assumption. Weibull distribution can be fully parametrized by the parameter pair $\theta = (\lambda, \alpha)$, where λ and α are scale and shape parameter, respectively. The density and survival function of Weibull distribution T are $f(T| \lambda, \alpha) = \alpha T^{\alpha-1} \lambda \exp(-\lambda T^{\alpha})$ and $S(T| \lambda, \alpha) = \exp(-\lambda T^{\alpha})$, respectively. Typically in a regression model, the scale parameter is defined as $\lambda = 1/\exp(Zu + X\beta)$, where $X_{n \times p}$ represents a column-scaled matrix of tumor biomarkers such as gene expression, genotype or DNA methylation, $\boldsymbol{\beta}$ is a $p \times 1$vector of marker effects, $Z_{n \times (1+q)}$is a covariates matrix of intercept and q clinical variables such as gender, age, and tumor histological grade, $\mathbf{u}$ is a $(q + 1)$-dimensional effect vector of $Z_{n \times (1+q)}$. With the condition of $p > n$(i.e., high dimension), a penalize term is necessary for inducing a sparse solution of $\boldsymbol{\beta}$. Under the Bayesian framework, we want to impose a well-known spike-and-slab prior on each β_j to facilitate Bayesian variable selection [16]. A vector of binary latent variables $\boldsymbol{\gamma} = (\gamma_1, \ldots, \gamma_p)^T$, $\gamma_j \in \{0, 1\}$ are introduced as indicator variables, where $\gamma_j = 1$ donates that jth explanatory variable is to be included in the model. Conditional on $\boldsymbol{\gamma}$, the continuous prior being assigned to $\boldsymbol{\beta}$ is,

$$\pi(\boldsymbol{\beta}|\sigma^2, \boldsymbol{\gamma}) = \mathbf{N}_p(\mathbf{0}, \mathbf{D}_{\sigma^2, \boldsymbol{\gamma}}), \tag{1}$$

where $\mathbf{D}_{\sigma^2,\boldsymbol{\gamma}} = \sigma^2\ diag(a_1, ..., a_p)$and $a_j = (1 - \gamma_j)v_0 + \gamma_j v_1$. As suggested by [22], we set these hyperparameters v_0 and v_1 to be small and large positive values, respectively. σ^2 is a common variance parameter with an inverse gamma prior $\pi(\sigma^2) = IG(v/2, v\eta/2)$. The binomial prior is chosen for the indicator variable $\boldsymbol{\gamma}$, i.e., $\pi(\boldsymbol{\gamma}|\theta) = \prod_{j=1}^{p} \theta^{\gamma_j}(1-\theta)^{1-\gamma_j}$, where θ is a hyperparameter and we impose a *Beta*(*a*, *b*) prior on it. The constant prior is chosen for α and $\mathbf{u}$, i.e., $\pi(\alpha) \propto 1$ and $\pi(\mathbf{u}) \propto 1$.

Generally speaking, MCMC is usually used for simulating the posterior distribution of unknown parameters $\boldsymbol{\beta}$, $\boldsymbol{\gamma}$, θ, σ^2, α, and $\mathbf{u}$. But here we employ an EM algorithm to seek the posterior mode of each parameter because this algorithm provides substantial computational advantage, especially for high-dimensional data analysis. Concerning about the unknown status $\boldsymbol{\gamma}$ for variables, we replace this "missing data" by its conditional expectation given the current estimates for other parameters and observed data (E-step) [31]. Then, an M-step is followed by maximizing the expected complete-data log-posterior with respect to $\boldsymbol{\beta}$, θ, σ^2, α, and $\mathbf{u}$. As a result of iterations between the E-step and M-step, each estimator will converge toward a local maximum of the posterior distribution. More specifically, the objective function can be expressed as:

$$\begin{aligned} Q(\beta, \theta, \sigma^2, \alpha, \mathbf{u}|T, \delta) &= E_{\gamma|\cdot}[\log \pi(\beta, \gamma, \theta, \sigma^2, \alpha, \mathbf{u}|T, \delta)] \\ &= C + \log L + E_{\gamma|\cdot}[\log \pi(\beta|\sigma^2, \gamma)] \\ &+ E_{\gamma|\cdot}[\log \pi(\gamma|\theta)], \\ +\log \pi(\theta) + \log \pi(\sigma^2) &+ \log \pi(\alpha) + \log \pi(\mathbf{u}) \end{aligned} \quad (2)$$

where $E_{\boldsymbol{\gamma}\,|\,\cdot}(\cdot)$ denotes the expectation with regard to $\boldsymbol{\gamma}$ given estimations in current iteration. Furthermore, $E_{\boldsymbol{\gamma}|\cdot}[\ \log\pi(\boldsymbol{\beta}|\sigma^2, \boldsymbol{\gamma})] = C_1 - \frac{p}{2}\ \log\sigma^2 - \frac{1}{2\sigma^2}\sum_{j=1}^{p}\beta_j^2 E_{\boldsymbol{\gamma}|\cdot}[(1-\gamma_j)v_0 + \gamma_j v_1]^{-1}$, and $E_{\boldsymbol{\gamma}|\cdot}[\ \log\pi(\boldsymbol{\gamma}|\theta)] = \sum_{j=1}^{p} E_{\boldsymbol{\gamma}|\cdot}[\gamma_j] \log(\frac{\theta}{1-\theta}) + p\ \log(1-\theta)$, both C and C_1 are constants. Next, our EM algorithm for Bayesian Weibull regression proceeds as follows.

(1) Initialize the unknown parameters: $\boldsymbol{\beta}^{(0)}$, $\theta^{(0)}$, $\sigma^{2(0)}$, $\alpha^{(0)}$, $\mathbf{u}^{(0)}$.

(2) E-step:

As can be seen from the formula (2) above, there are two parts that need further evaluation, namely $E_{\boldsymbol{\gamma}\,|\,\cdot}[\gamma_j]$ and $E_{\boldsymbol{\gamma}\,|\,\cdot}[(1 - \gamma_j)v_0 + \gamma_j v_1]^{-1}$. In particular, $E_{\boldsymbol{\gamma}\,|\,\cdot}[\gamma_j]$ is a conditional expectation of γ_j and depends on observed data (T, δ) only by means of current parameter estimates $\boldsymbol{\beta}^{(k)}$, $\theta^{(k)}$, $\sigma^{2(k)}$ because of the hierarchical structure of $\boldsymbol{\gamma}$; therefore, we have

$$E_{\boldsymbol{\gamma}|\cdot}\left[\gamma_j\right] = P\left(\gamma_j = 1|\boldsymbol{\beta}^{(k)}, \theta^{(k)}, \sigma^{2(k)}\right) = p_j^*, \quad (3)$$

where $p_j^* = \frac{\pi(\beta_j^{(k)}|\sigma^{2(k)}, \gamma_j=1)P(\gamma_j=1|\theta^{(k)})}{\pi(\beta_j^{(k)}|\sigma^{2(k)}, \gamma_j=1)P(\gamma_j=1|\theta^{(k)}) + \pi(\beta_j^{(k)}|\sigma^{2(k)}, \gamma_j=0)P(\gamma_j=0|\theta^{(k)})}$,

meanwhile, the second part will be easily derived as

$$E_{\boldsymbol{\gamma}|\cdot}\left[\left(1-\gamma_j\right)v_0 + \gamma_j v_1\right]^{-1} = \frac{1-p_j^*}{v_0} + \frac{p_j^*}{v_1} = d_j^*. \quad (4)$$

(3) M-step:

Next, we derive the M-step for the objective function $Q(\boldsymbol{\beta}, \theta, \sigma^2, \alpha, \mathbf{u}|\ T, \delta)$.

1) Differentiating $Q(\cdot|\ T, \delta)$ with regard to $\boldsymbol{\beta}$ needs to solve the following expression

$$\boldsymbol{\beta}^{(k+1)} = \arg\min_{\boldsymbol{\beta}}\left\{-\ \log L + \frac{1}{2\sigma^2}\left\|\mathbf{D}^{*1/2}\boldsymbol{\beta}\right\|^2\right\}, \quad (5)$$

where $\mathbf{D}^{*1/2}$ is the square root of the $p \times p$ diagonal matrix $\mathbf{D}^* = diag(d_1^*, ..., d_p^*)$. It can be shown that the formula (5) above for Weibull model is convex, and a wide variety of numerical optimization algorithms can be applicable. For generalizing our algorithm to high-dimensional data, the commonly used multidimensional Newton-Raphson method is not recommended because of large memory requirements and intensive computations. In this research, we employ the cyclic coordinate descent (CCD) algorithm due to its efficiency and ease of implementation, which makes one-dimensional optimization available [32]. Briefly, the CCD minimizes the objective function with regard to β_j, holding all other variables constant. Similar to the combined local and global (CLG) algorithm of [33, 34], we modify the update for β_j in two ways. First, in order to avoid big steps in Newton iteration, we specify a positive value Δ_j for the *j*th maker to restrict the maximum change of β_j between two adjacent iterations. Second, for one-dimensional optimization, we update β_j only once instead of multiple iterations till convergence before updating β_{j+1}. Moreover, considering that it is unnecessary to take much time to update the amount of possible neural markers (that is, their minuscule effects contribute less to outcome, with no need for accurate estimations) when p is large, we partially update those markers with "large" effect ($|\beta_j|$is greater than a threshold β', e.g., 1E−08) after a small number (k') of full iterations for all makers, which speeds up computation considerably.

2) Differentiating $Q(\cdot \mid T, \delta)$ with regard to u_j, $j = 1, \ldots, q + 1$one-by-one using one-dimensional optimization reveals the following form

$$u_j^{(k+1)}\Big|_{\boldsymbol{\beta}^{(k+1)},\alpha,\sigma^2,\theta,u_{j-}^{(k+1)},u_{j+}} = u_j - \frac{\partial \log L}{\partial u_j}\left(\frac{\partial^2 \log L}{\partial u_j^2}\right)^{-1}, \tag{6}$$

with all other parameters being fixed at current estimates.

3) Differentiating $Q(\cdot \mid T, \delta)$ with regard to α derives the following form

$$\alpha^{(k+1)}\Big|_{\boldsymbol{\beta}^{(k+1)},\mathbf{u}^{(k+1)},\sigma^2,\theta} = \alpha - \frac{\partial \log L}{\partial \alpha}\left(\frac{\partial^2 \log L}{\partial \alpha^2}\right)^{-1}. \tag{7}$$

4) For σ^2, we have

$$\sigma^{2(k+1)} = \frac{\sum_{j=1}^{p}\beta_j^{(k+1)2}d_j^* + \nu\eta}{p+\nu+2}. \tag{8}$$

5) For θ, we have

$$\theta^{(k+1)} = \frac{\sum_j^p p_j^* + a-1}{a+b+p-2}. \tag{9}$$

(4) Iterations between the E-step and M-step are in progress. SurvEMVS will be terminated if the convergence criterion is satisfied as follows: $\sum_{i=1}^{n}|\mathbf{X}_i^T(\boldsymbol{\beta}^{(k)}-\boldsymbol{\beta}^{(k-1)})|/(1+\sum_{i=1}^{n}|\mathbf{X}_i^T\boldsymbol{\beta}^{(k)}|) < \xi$, where $\mathbf{X}\boldsymbol{\beta}^{(k)}$ is predictive vector at kth iteration, and ξ is a small value (say 10^{-4}). Summarizing, Additional file 1: Figure S1 presents pseudocode for our implementation of SurvEMVS.

Simulation studies

In this section, we used simulations to validate the performance of proposed SurvEMVS. Cox LASSO model [35] was considered as a benchmark for comparison. The effect sizes and directions of Cox LASSO estimates were adjusted for consistency with our parametric model, which made the direct comparison between two methods. For each simulation scenario, we replicated the simulation 50 times and then summarized these results.

Marker values were simulated from a multivariate normal distribution $N_{50}(0, \Sigma)$, where Σ is a variance-covariance symmetric matrix with $\Sigma_{jj} = 1$ and $\Sigma_{ij} = 0.6^{|i-j|}$, $i \neq j$. For large p markers, we repeatedly sampled from the above distribution and then combined them by column. Thus, we obtained an $n \times p$ matrix with multiple independent blocks and 50 makers in each block were correlated. Assuming $\lambda_i = \exp(-\sum_j^p x_{ij}\beta_j)$, we simulated survival time t_i for each subject from an exponential distribution t_i~exponential(λ_i) , and random censoring time c_i from a uniform distribution $c_i \sim U(0, K)$, and chose K such that on average 40% subjects were right censored. The observed censored survival time T_i was generated by $\min(t_i, c_i)$. Furthermore, additional simulations where survival times are generated from Weibull distribution (with $\alpha = 2$) were used to show effectiveness of our method. As is well-known, the true distribution of survival time in a real data is unclear and does not coincide with the Weibull assumption exactly. Therefore, we simulated a vector of Gamma-distributed survival time on purpose, thus assigning weakness setting to SurvEMVS. The shape and rate parameters of gamma distribution were set to be 0.8 and $1/\lambda_i$, respectively. We randomly sampled six causal markers and set coefficients to be {0.2, −0.2, 0.3, −0.3, 0.4, −0.4}. Sample size (n) was set to be 500, and number of makers is set to be 1000 or 5000. Moreover, we generated 100 samples as a test dataset in each replication to appreciate the predictive performance of two approaches. The detailed simulation scenarios were summarized in Table 1.

Hyperparameters tuning and performance metric

The performance of SurvEMVS depended on the hyperparameters v_0 and v_1, which made us be interested in a running model based on more than one combination of v_0 and v_1. The speed of the EM algorithm made it feasible to consider a sequence of models as (v_0, v_1) varied over many candidates, from which we could select an optimal combination based on some criteria. According to [22], large v_1 and small v_0 could accommodate all plausible β_j. In order to acquire sparse solution in large p data, we set a sequence of candidates $\{1/10p, 1/5p, 1/2p, 1/p, 2/p, 5/p, 10/p, 0.05\}$ (0.05 was reserved if $p > 500$) to v_0 unless otherwise noted, which was dynamic with p. Three candidates from {10, 100, 500} were assigned to v_1. Therefore, there were 24 combinations for hyperparameter tuning. The procedure of fitting Cox LASSO by widely used R package *glmnet* gave the similar parameter tuning as we did here.

On account of making parameter selection from the 24 combinations of v_0 and v_1, we needed a metric to

Table 1 Parameters settings for simulation studies

Parameter	Scenario					
	1	2	3	4	5	6
Censoring rate	40%					
Causal effects	− 0.2, 0.2, − 0.3, 0.3, − 0.4, 0.4					
Replications	50					
Sample size of test dataset	100					
Distribution of survival time (shape)	Exponential		Weibull (2)		Gamma (0.8)	
Sample size (*n*) / No. of makers(*p*)	500/1000	500/5000	500/1000	500/5000	500/1000	500/5000

measure the performance of the fitted models. Cross-validation partial likelihood (CVPL) was generally used for parameter selection in Cox model [35, 36], while some employed cross-validation score in parametric survival model [36]. Subsequently, one candidate of hyperparameters was chosen to minimize one of these metrics. However, these metrics involving random cross-validation (CV) make the hyperparameter selection not stable as well as time demanding, and depend on the folds. Other criteria without CV like the Akaike information criterion (AIC), the Bayesian information criterion (BIC), and the generalized cross-validation (GCV) tend to select many spurious variables especially in high-dimensional problem [37, 38]. In this paper, we considered a metric, namely extended Bayesian Information Criteria (EBIC), which was utilized for model selection at first [39]. The constant prior behind the BIC assigns high probabilities to the models with a larger number of markers, which was apparently unreasonable and strongly against the principle of parsimony. The EBIC was proposed to take away this disadvantage of the BIC. The EBIC is defined as,

$$\mathrm{EBIC}_\gamma = -2\log L + p_m \log n + 2\tau \binom{p}{p_m}, 0 \le \tau \le 1, \tag{10}$$

where p_m is the number of selected variables in a fitted model. The EBIC with $\tau = 0$ reduces to the original BIC. Minimizing the EBIC with larger τ will get a much more parsimonious model. Thus, EBIC1, EBIC2, and EBIC3 were served as metrics for hyperparameter tuning with regard to $\tau = 0,\ 0.5,\ 1$, respectively.

In simulation studies, the optimal SurvEMVS model selected by the EBIC was compared with Cox LASSO in aspects with variable selection, effect estimation, and model prediction. We utilized false positive rate (FPR), true positive rate (TPR), and false discovery rate (FDR) as evaluation indicators for variable selection. Note that $P(\gamma_j = 1|\hat{\beta}_j, \hat{\theta}, \hat{\sigma}^2) \ge 0.5$ meant the *j*th maker was selected. Mean square error (MSE) denoted by $\sum_{j=1}^{p} (\hat{\beta}_j - \beta_j)^2 / p$ was used to appreciate effect estimations for makers. The predictive accuracy of the fitted model be applied to test dataset was evaluated by Harrell's *c* statistic [40], as known as the area under the ROC curve (AUC).

Implementation

We considered $a = b = 1$ in beta prior for θ which yielded a uniform distribution. As noted in [22], we had inverse gamma prior for σ^2 with $\nu = \eta = 1$ to make this prior relatively non-influential. We ran all analyses using R software (v3.41) on a machine with Intel® Xeon® X5690 3.46-GHz processors. Cox LASSO model was implemented with the *glmnet* package in R. Tenfold cross-validation was used to choose an optimal penalization parameter λ_{lasso} in *glmnet*, which determined an optimal Cox LASSO model. Two LASSO models selected by "minimum cvm" and "1 standard error" of λ_{lasso} were considered as LASSO.min and LASSO.se, respectively. We employed the PLINK tool for quality control of genotype data [41].

Results

Simulation studies

Iteration and tuning plot

By analogy with LASSO solution path plot that shows the estimates change with an increasing penalty parameter, here we want to investigate the impact of parameters tuning for v_0. Figure 1a displays a solution path of SurvEMVS under Scenario 1 with v_1=10. Large effects (red dots) will be firstly incorporated into the fitting model with v_0 increasing, and a remarkable separation between the positive and negative effects appears when v_0 is larger than 0.03. However, the estimated effects for zeros inflate because of less shrinkage at large v_0. We also present the iteration plot to detect the convergence property of our approach. From Fig. 1b, SurvEMVS makes a fast convergence to posterior estimates only in several steps. Moreover, neutral effects (black dot line) get close to zero in the fourth iteration, which means that we can concentrate iterations on large effects after a

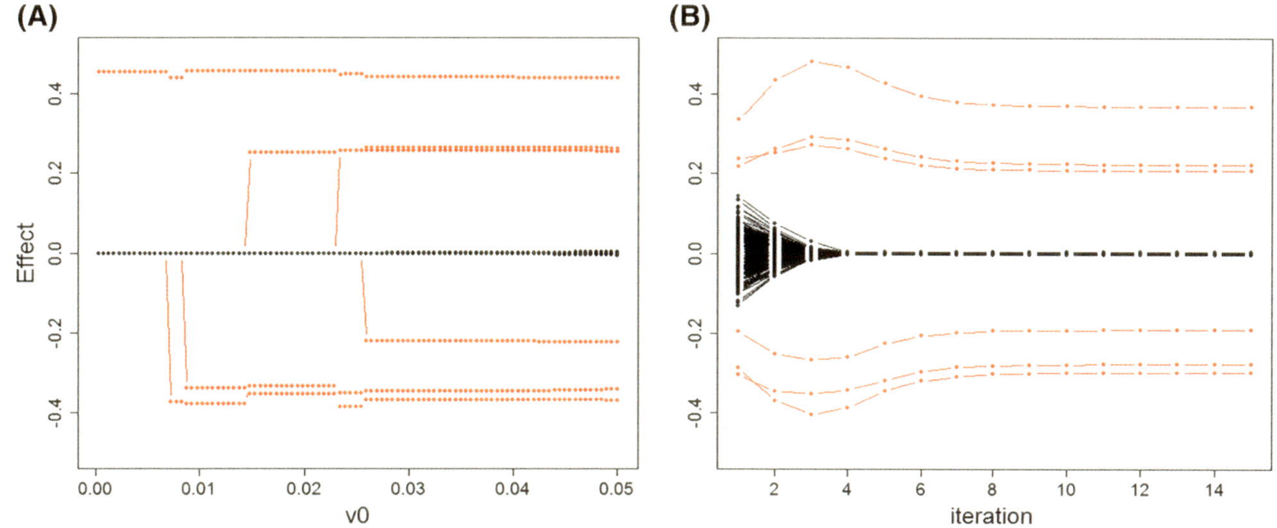

Fig. 1 Solution path and iteration path of the proposed SurvEMVS under Scenario 1. Red dots represent the changes of estimated effects for the true signals. **a** Solution path. **b** Iteration path ($\upsilon_0 = 0.05$)

number of full iterations for all makers and further accelerate the posterior computation.

Variable selection

In SurvEMVS, conditional posterior probabilities are used to guide variable selection. Table 2 shows comparison results between SurvEMVS and Cox LASSO in variable selection for Scenarios 1 and 2. For Scenario 1 with $p = 1{,}000$, all models except LASSO.min can reduce noise markers with low FDRs, and all of three models with regard to SurvEMVS acquire high TPRs. When simulated p increases to 5000 (Scenario 2), FPR and FDR of BIC (i.e., EBIC1) inflate seriously. These indicate that proper extra penalty on the BIC of SurvEMVS brings to a moderate result of variable selection. We summarize the results of Scenarios 3 and 4 with Weibull distribution in Additional file 1: Table S1, and the results of Scenarios 5 and 6 with gamma distribution in Additional file 1: Table S2. Each of them presents a similar trend with scenarios of exponential distribution.

Table 2 TPR, FPR, and FDR in variable selection with 50 replications (exponential distribution)

Method	Scenario 1 ($p = 1000$)			Scenario 2 ($p = 5000$)		
	TPR	FPR	FDR	TPR	FPR	FDR
LASSO.se	0.657	1.25E−03	0.239	0.327	1.36E−04	0.258
LASSO.min	0.920	2.11E−02	0.792	0.713	4.60E−03	0.843
EBIC ($\tau = 0$)	0.743	1.19E−03	0.209	0.703	5.78E−03	0.872
EBIC ($\tau = 0.5$)	0.730	7.85E−04	0.151	0.480	1.48E−04	0.204
EBIC ($\tau = 1.0$)	0.710	6.24E−04	0.127	0.377	2.00E−05	0.042

Abbreviations: TPR, true positive rate; FPR, false positive rate; FDR, false discovery rate

Parametric estimation

Figure 2 and Additional file 1: Figures S2-S6 show the parameter estimations of five models for all scenarios. Averaged estimated effects (*black vertical lines*) of estimated effects for all makers are calculated over 50 trials. Triangles in all figures label the locations and effect sizes of the pre-specified causal makers. In all scenarios, SurvEMVS gives a lower bias than Cox LASSO. Biases of all models increase with number of variants. Two models of SurvEMVS (i.e., EBIC2 and EBIC3) present a similar estimator, while the estimated effects in EBIC1 for zeros inflate under scenarios with $p = 5{,}000$ (rough X-axis in Additional file 1: Figures S2, S4 and S6). In order to make a comprehensive evaluation of bias and variance, we use the MSE metric and present the results in the left panels of Fig. 3 and Additional file 1: Figures S7 and S8. Both the EBIC2 and EBIC3 are well performed under all scenarios, whereas the EBIC1 model get a high MSE with $p = 5{,}000$. There is no apparent difference between the results of exponential, Weibull, and gamma distribution.

Prediction accuracy

In order to appreciate prediction accuracy of the fitted models, we summarize AUC results by box plot in the right panels of Fig. 3 and Additional file 1: Figures S7 and S8. Generally speaking, the EBIC2 model performs best under our simulation settings, while the LASSO.min presents similar prediction but with larger variance. In accordance with the conclusion of "Parametric estimation", prediction accuracy of the BIC model descends with p varying from 1000 to 5000. Moreover, SurvEMVS with exponential or Weibull settings gain slightly larger AUC than those with the gamma settings. Furthermore, the

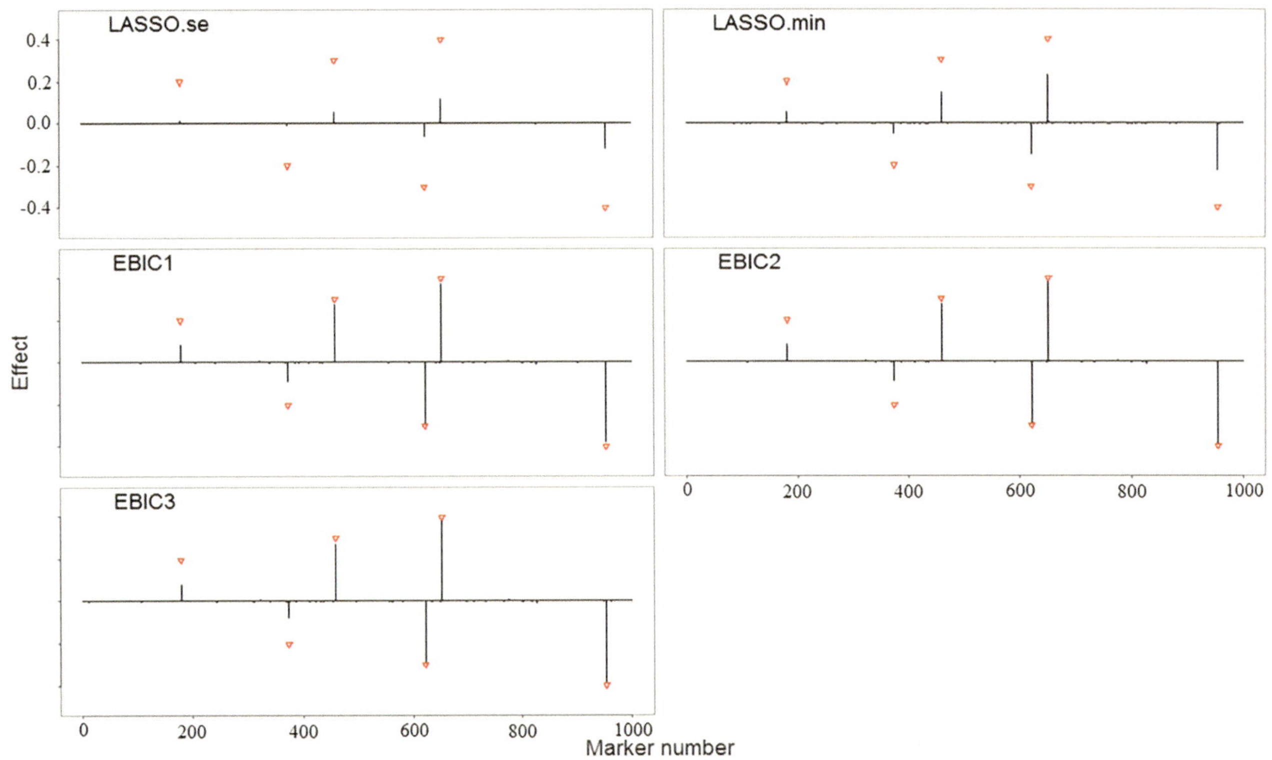

Fig. 2 Averaged estimated effect (*black vertical lines*) for each marker over 50 replications under Scenario 1. Red triangles label true effect sizes and locations of the causal markers

LASSO.se model almost provides the lowest AUC among simulation scenarios. All the above results indicate that the BIC is not suitable for large p scenario.

In summary, the EBIC2 model works best under almost all scenarios in terms of variable selection, parameter estimation, and prediction accuracy. Besides, Additional file 1: Table S3 shows the time consumption in different scenarios. In comparison with Cox LASSO, SurvEMVS takes more computational time but is still fast enough. Note that time used in Additional file 1: Table S3 is for reference only, as it varies depending on context, such as convergence criterion, programming language, computer performance, and algorithm optimization.

Real data analysis

Harvard lung cancer data

This dataset from The Harvard Lung Cancer Susceptibility Study GWAS includes 526 late-stage (III and IV) patients with non-small cell lung cancer (NSCLC) recruited from Massachusetts General Hospital (Boston, MA). More details about participants' recruitment have been described previously [42]. We note that it is appropriate to assess an association study restricted to late-stage cancer because some gene functions work primarily in the late stage and are not present in preinvasive stages of cancer [43]. DNA was genotyped using Illumina 610K Quad chip. After quality control protocol described by [44], there were 512,885 SNPs remaining. Those patients with more than 5 years of overall survival were considered as right censored, and finally, the censor rate was equal to 20.27%. We assumed an additive genetic model and imputed missing genotypes by mean of each SNP. We adjusted for age, sex, smoking status, cell type, stage, surgery (yes vs. no), and the top four principal components in the subsequent analysis. Considering that the number of SNPs related to NSCLC survival was not expected to be too large, we filtered the SNPs by a commonly used single locus Cox model. This filter yielded a de-noising of outcome so that the subsequent analyses became more efficient. By setting a threshold of P value less than 5E−3, 3911 SNPs were left for the subsequent analysis.

The EBIC2 was used to choose an optimal model from the candidates we noted above. Finally, 14 SNPs were detected by the proposed EBIC2 model with $\upsilon_1 = 100$ and υ_0=2.56E-03. We further analyzed and annotated these SNPs by TCGA (with an online tool UALCAN [45]), KEGG pathway, and PubMed database. Interestingly, seven of all listed in Table 3 may have potential functional influence on carcinogenesis or prognosis. For example, rs1506943 is located at ~33 kb downstream of RXRG (retinoid X receptor gamma) on Chromosome 1. This gene is expressed at significantly lower levels in TCGA-LUAD (lung adenocarcinoma)

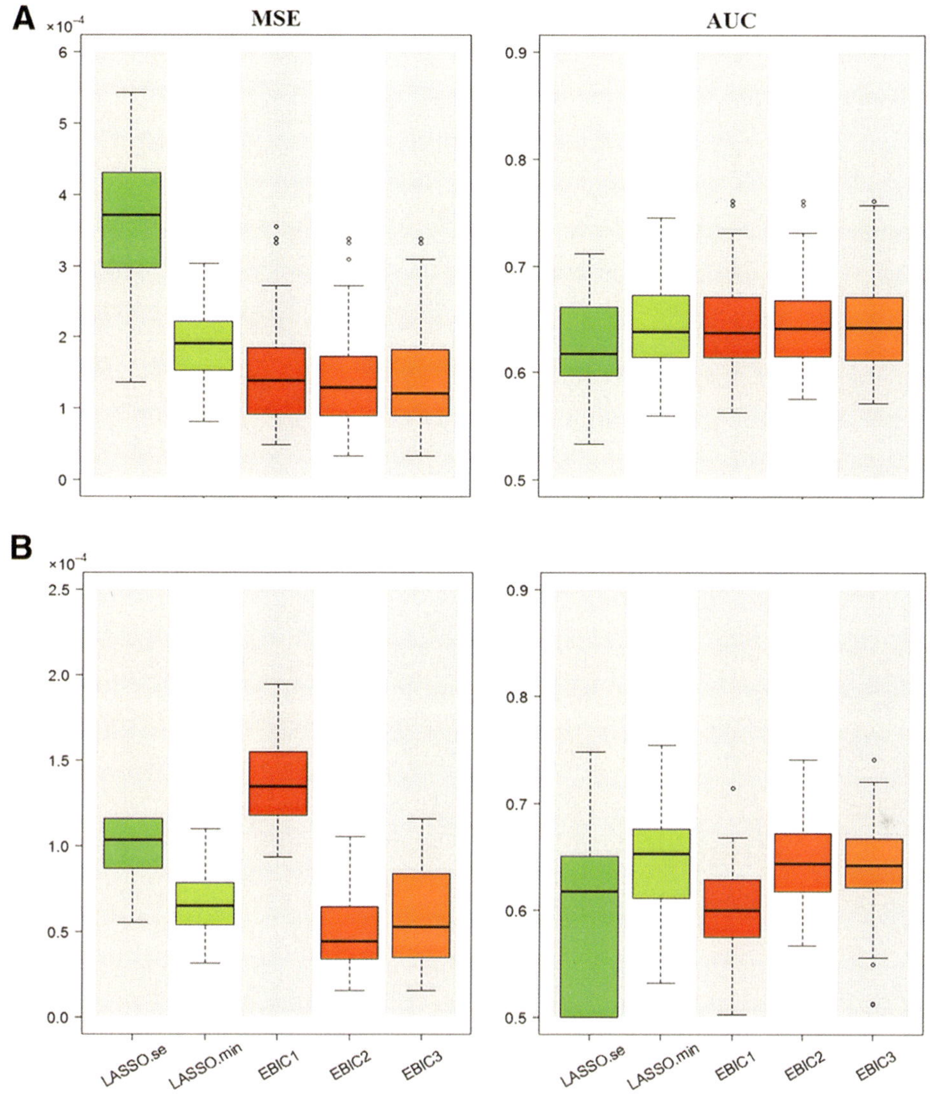

Fig. 3 MSE of parameter estimation and AUC of prognosis prediction for Scenarios 1 and 2. **a**, **b** The results of Scenarios 1 and 2, respectively

and TCGA-LUSC (lung squamous cell carcinoma) tumor samples and samples of other research [46]. Additionally, it also participates in non-small cell lung cancer pathways and other cancer-related pathways. rs2074986 is located at DNase I hypersensitive site (DHS) of GFRA1 on Chromosome 10. GFRA1 released by nerves enhances cancer cell perineural invasion [47], whose expression is reduced in tumor samples of TCGA-LUAD and TCGA-LUSC compared with normal samples. In addition, the high expression level in TCGA-LUAD tumor samples may contribute to good prognosis ($P = 0.0025$). We also provided the estimated effects of 14 SNPs by SurvEMVS in Additional file 1: Table S4 along with classical Weibull regression estimations for them (that is, only 14 SNPs and clinical variables are fitted by Weibull regression). In this way, SurvEMVS applied in high-dimensional data can also generate approximate estimates with Weibull regression. We plotted Kaplan-Meier (KM) survival curve of patients with high, moderate, and low risk defined by tertiles of risk scores $-\sum_j^p x_{ij}\beta_j$ (Additional file 1: Figure S9). The log-rank test was used to compare the survival estimates among the three groups, and the results show that higher prognostic risk score is significantly associated with shorter survival ($P < 1E{-}16$). However, Cox LASSO models did not identify any SNP.

TCGA stomach adenocarcinoma (TCGA-STAD) expression data

We accessed this RNA-seq transcriptomic data from TCGA database by R/Bioconductor package *TCGAbiolinks* [48], which was used to do subsequent quality control, normalization, differential expression analysis

Table 3 Validation analysis of the seven potential SNPs identified by SurvEMVS using external database

SNP (Cytoband)	Gene symbol (annotation)	TCGA	KEGG	PubMed
rs1506943_G (1q23.3)	LMX1A-RXRG (Intergenic)	RXRG: low expression in LUAD and LUSC tumor samples	RXRG participates in non-small cell lung cancer pathway and other cancer related pathways (hsa05200, 05222)	This gene is expressed at significantly lower levels in non-small cell lung cancer cells [46].
rs1921660_G (2q37.3)	GBX2-ASB18 (Intergenic)	GBX2: high expression is associated with bad prognosis ($P = 0.0052$)	–[a]	Enhanced GBX2 expression stimulates growth of human prostate cancer cells [64, 65].
rs981852_C (3p14.2)	FHIT (Intron)	Low expression in LUSC tumor samples	FHIT participates in non-small cell lung cancer pathway and Small cell lung cancer pathway (hsa05222, 05223)	–
rs2044831_G (7p14.1)	EPDR1 (Coding)	Low expression in LUSC tumor samples	–	EPDR1 is highly expressed in colorectal tumor cells [66].
rs263264_G, (8q24.2)	ADCY8 (Intron)	–	ADCY8 participates multiple signal pathways and pathways in cancer	–
rs2074986_G (10q25.3)	GFRA1 (DHS)	Low expression in LUAD and LUSC tumor samples; High expression in LUAD is associated with good prognosis ($P = 0.0025$)	–	GFRA1 released by nerves enhances cancer cell perineural invasion [47]; Methylation changes of GFRA1 may be a potential biomarker for prediction of gastric carcinoma metastasis [67].
rs4885110_A (13q22.1)	LINC00393-KLF12 (Intergenic)	KLF12: low expression in LUAD tumor samples	–	KLF12 is an important regulator of gene expression during carcinogenesis [68–70].

[a]Negative results of validation analysis

(DEA), and visualization. The clinical information is summarized in Additional file 1: Table S5. Similar to the first real data analysis, we built final models only using filtered expression markers by DEA rather than all markers. There were 2711 markers left passing a selection threshold defined at fold change (FC) > 2 and testing FDR < 0.01. Due to the relative high missing rate, we made use of multivariate imputation by chained equations (MICE) to deal with missing clinical covariates [49]. After removing the patients with missing or zero survival time, we apply SurvEMVS and Cox LASSO to a matrix with 390 rows and 2716 columns (including 5 clinical covariates listed in Additional file 1: Table S5).

We used the EBIC2 to select best model from the candidates above. Three markers were identified by the proposed model ($v_0 = 3.69E{-}03$ and $v_1 = 500$) including CTLA4, NACAD, and SERPINE1, mapped to 2q33.2, 7p13, and 7q22.1, respectively. Meanwhile, the LASSO.-min detected ALG11, GAMT, and PLCXD3 in addition to the overlap genes CTLA4 and SERPINE1. Estimated effects of the selected markers in both two models are provided (Additional file 1: Table S6) along with classical Weibull regression and Cox model estimations for them (like the first application). We can see that many effects estimated by Cox LASSO are small while SurvEMVS presents similar estimations with its counterpart in the low-dimensional Weibull regression. According to tertiles of risk scores, we equally divided the patients into high-, moderate-, and low-risk groups. Figure 4 presents the KM curves of SurvEMVS (left panel) and Cox LASSO (right panel), respectively, and both of them show a higher risk score which is significantly associated with shorter survival (Log-rank test $P = 3.87E{-}07$ for SurvEMVS and $P = 1.02E{-}04$ for Cox LASSO).

Furthermore, in order to validate the results, we used external data from GEO database. Five datasets (GSE14210, GSE15459, GES29272, GSE51105, and GSE62254) are included for their proper sample sizes. Table 4 presents the estimated hazard ratios along with 95% confidence intervals (CI) and P value extracted from an online tool (KM plotter, *Web resource*). We also show the combined results using meta-analysis. As a result, CTLA4 and NACAD were successfully validated and have the same direction of the effects on prognosis with those estimated by SurvEMVS in TCGA-STAD data. Interestingly, CTLA4 encodes CTLA-4 (cytotoxic T-lymphocyte-associated protein 4) which inhibits T cell activation and downregulates immune response. Antagonistic antibody against CTLA has become a targeted drug (Ipilimumab, approved by FDA for melanoma in

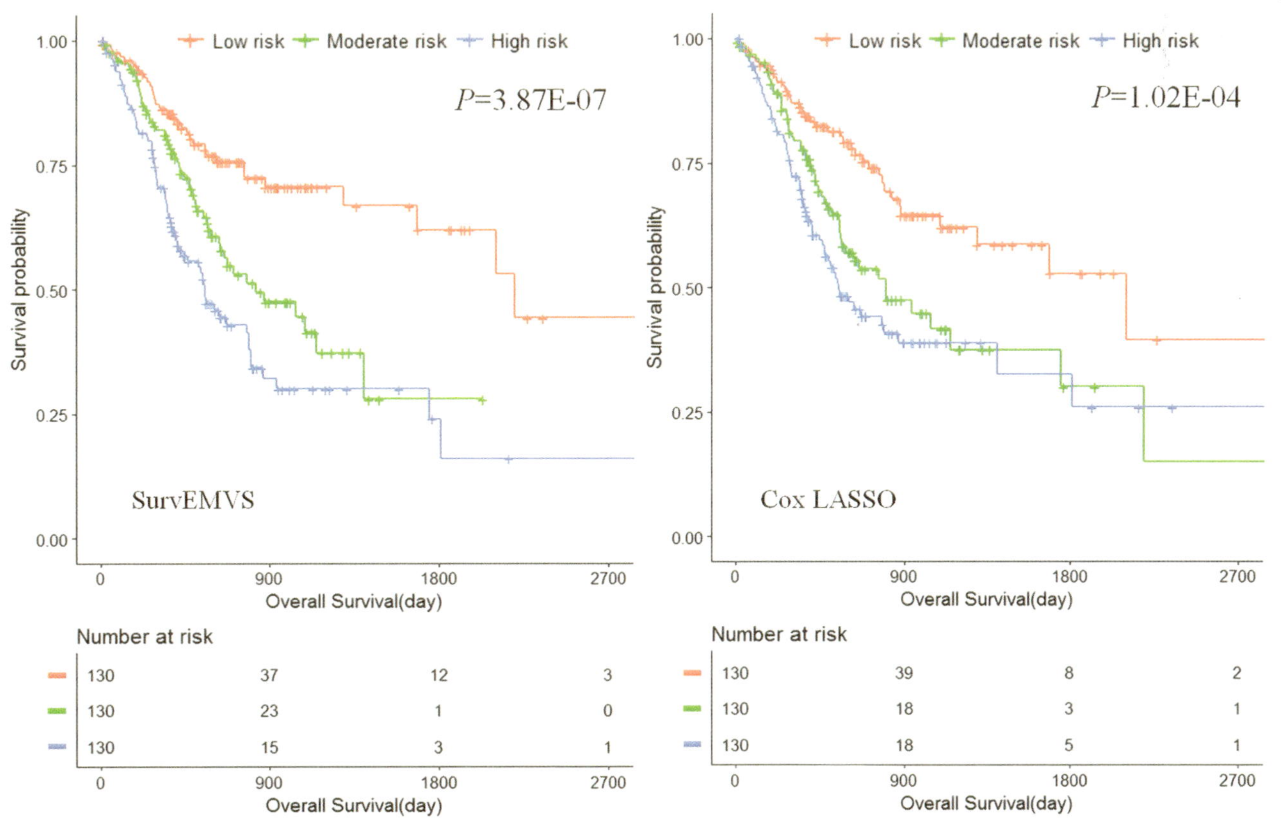

Fig. 4 Kaplan-Meier survival curve of patients with high, moderate, and low risk. P value is calculated using log-rank test

Table 4 Validation analysis of five genes using five GEO datasets

Gene symbol	GSE14210 (*N* = 119)	GSE15459 (*N* = 197)	GSE29272 (*N* = 126)	GSE51105 (*N* = 93)	GSE62254 (*N* = 283)	Heterogeneity-*P* (I^2)	Combined (random)
CTLA4 (2q33.2)	–[a]	0.77 (0.52~1.12) 1.7E−01	–	0.45 (0.25~0.82) 7.6E−03	0.59 (0.41~0.85) 4.1E−03	3.0E−01 16.9%	0.62 (0.48~0.82) 5.6E−04
PLCXD3 (5p13.1)	–	0.77 (0.51~1.15) 2.0E−01	–	1.60 (0.98~2.6) 5.8E−02	1.92 (1.32~2.79) 5.0E−04	4.0E−03 82.1%	1.33 (0.75~2.36) 3.3E−01
NACAD (7p13)	1.47 (0.97~2.24) 7.1E−02	1.47 (0.93~2.34) 9.8E−02	1.61 (1.04~ 2.49) 3.0E−02	1.76 (1.06~2.92) 2.7E−02	2.03 (1.41~2.92) 9.3E−05	7.7E−01 0.0%	1.68 (1.39~2.04) 1.2E−07
SERPINE1 (7q22.1)	1.46 (0.99~2.16) 5.6E−02	0.83 (0.56~1.24) 3.7E−01	0.73 (0.48~ 1.10) 1.3E−01	1.27 (0.76~2.12) 3.7E−01	1.57 (1.08~2.28) 1.6E−02	2.2E−02 65.0%	1.12 (0.82~1.53) 4.7E−01
GAMT (19p13.3)	1.17 (0.81~1.70) 4.0E−01	0.69 (0.46~1.03) 6.6E−02	1.81 (1.07~ 3.06) 2.6E−02	0.54 (0.32~0.92) 2.2E−02	1.75 (1.22~2.51) 2.2E−03	< 1.0E−03 81.8%	1.08 (0.69~1.68) 7.5E−01

The contents of each cell represent estimated hazard ratio (HR), 95%CI of HR, and hypothesis testing *P* value of HR, and in each dataset, the samples are categorized into two groups using a best cutoff of expression level. Combined results are derived by meta-analysis with random effect model

[a]Expression data of the gene is not available in the corresponding GEO database

2011), which is the first approved and popular immune checkpoint blockade therapy [50, 51]. Some research also indicates CTLA4 may have influence on gastric cancer germination and progression [52, 53]. GAMT and PLCXD3 detected by Cox LASSO display strong heterogeneity on effects (81.8% and 82.1%, respectively) with five datasets and no significant association in the combined analysis. Note that ALG11 is not identified in the five data. Although we acquire a negative consequence of SERPINE1 (also known as plasminogen activator inhibitor-1, PAI-1) in validation analysis; interestingly, it has been widely studied and is well known for participating p53 signaling pathway and playing a crucial role in tumor progression and angiogenesis [54, 55].

Discussion

High-throughput sequencing technology, which has become cheaper, promotes the development of precision medicine [56]. Picking up underlying markers affecting disease prognosis from thousands of candidates calls for high-dimensional survival model besides generally used one-by-one Cox proportional hazards model. In this paper, we propose a parametric survival counterpart of EMVS, namely SurvEMVS, which employs a fast EM algorithm to fit all candidate biomarkers simultaneously and to explore posterior distribution of the unknown parameters, consequently to identify important signals and make effect estimations.

Much work has concentrated on developing new Bayesian methods on high-dimensional parametric survival model in application to medical or genetic data. For example, Sha et al. built AFT models with less common distribution (i.e., log-normal and log-t) for microarray data using a discrete spike-and-slab prior, where a time-consuming MCMC procedure was employed to simulate posterior distribution [57]. Mittal et al. developed four parametric models, i.e., exponential, Weibull, log-logistic, and log-normal distribution, by assigning Gaussian and Laplace prior to effects, where maximum a posterior (MAP) was used to acquire posterior modes of effects; however, this work lacked numerical study to evaluate their models, as well as discussion on variables selected in real data analysis from medical reasonability [58]. Newcombe et al. imposed a discrete spike-and-slab prior on coefficients of Weibull regression, where reversible jump MCMC being used for the posterior computation is ineffective. Moreover, it is unrepresentative of their application to a low-dimensional breast cancer data [59].

SurvEMVS imposes a continuous spike-and-slab mixture prior on effects to facilitate the separation of different effect sizes. This two-component prior can provide an indicator vector to guide variable selection whereby using a local version of the median probability model [22, 60]. In contrast, the EM algorithm or variational approximation employing one-component prior such as Laplace or t distribution does not involve variable inclusion indicators, and consequently makes variable selection indirectly [20]. Due to the unavailable closed form of maximization about maker effects in M-step, a variant of CCD algorithm serves to be feasible for obtaining approximate solutions. Consequently, our EM steps incorporating this fast CCD make the fitting much effective. One focus of this study is how to choose an optimal model from the hyperparameter tuning process. The EBIC, an extension of the BIC, is adopted with reason as follows: in comparison with the EBIC, the normally used AIC, BIC, or GCV would generate more spurious signal when applied to high-dimensional data, while CV-based metrics demand more computation and are unstable since the folds in CV are selected randomly. This is, to our knowledge, the first application of EBIC to the high-dimensional parametric survival analysis.

Over a range of simulation scenarios, our method with EBIC2 generally performs better than Cox LASSO in variable selection, parameter estimation, and prediction. In contrast, owing to imposing a single penalty on all effects, Cox LASSO yields high biased estimators. Our simulations also show the EBIC is appropriate for model selection, while the BIC (i.e., EBIC1) perform worst in situation with very large number of markers. For $p > n$ problem in omics data, we recommend $\tau = 0.5$ for EBIC in multi-stage study because it offers a good trade-off between the well-controlled FDR and the TPR and provides more opportunity to new findings. However, if one is strict to control false discovery, $\tau = 1$, is recommended. Subsequently, we conducted two real data applications. In the first study with a lung cancer genotype data, 14 SNPs were detected by SurvEMVS, and further validation analyses using external data or function annotation resulted in 7 outstanding SNPs. In order to widen the application range of SurvEMVS considerably, we utilized a stomach cancer expression data in the second study. Expression levels of three genes are associated with cancer prognosis, and two of them are validated by extra GEO datasets along with one (namely SERPINE1) involved in tumor progression. The identification of well-known CTLA4 illustrates the availability of SurvEMVS. However, further functional experiments are needed for evidence of biologic plausibility of those identified markers.

Although we did not directly compare our EM algorithm with its MCMC counterpart, the speed advantage is apparent, according to the results of our EM algorithm under each optimal model converge needing 174 and 238 iterations in the two real data applications, which is much less than the chain length being set up for MCMC (usually > 10,000 for stable estimation). The model thus resembles a distinct iteration increase of real data application relative to a simulation study. We can explain that ideal conditions (e.g., sparse structure with independent markers) along with strong shrinkage of candidate hyperparameters (producing a parsimonious model) favor rapid convergence, but generally are not available under real data applications, which leads to more iterations demanding (but still fast enough) not only for SurvEMVS but also for other model [20].

However, we acknowledge that there are several limitations of the present study. First, SurvEMVS incorporating the EM, which seeks for a posterior mode rather than a whole posterior distribution of the parameter, cannot provide uncertain measure for estimators. We can directly disentangle this disadvantage by the bootstrap method, but have to bear expensive computations. Actually, another compromise may be adopted: the estimates of SurvEMVS can be considered as initial values of a following MCMC algorithm, which makes the MCMC procedure avoid the burn-in stage and finally yield fast and accurate estimators with uncertain measurement. Second, the most worrying thing of the parametric model is a situation of going against the parametric assumption for survival distribution. We show that SurvEMVS is robust for the status with moderately deviating from the Weibull premise. However, we believe that SurvEMVS will be less effective if the real survival time distinctly violates the Weibull distribution. We can bypass this limitation using a non-parametric AFT model like in [61], in which a Dirichlet process is used to make the model robust over a wider range of unknown baseline hazard. In addition, a lot of new directions for methodological work will arise from the current study. One obvious extension to our method will consider multivariate "*g*-priors" to reflect the effect correlations within the correlated markers [62]. Another interesting extension will involve introducing a newly developed spike-and-slab Laplace prior [63]. Going forward, the meaningful extension of SurvEMVS will integrate functional annotations or multi-omics data to powerfully mine association signals in future work.

Conclusions

We present a new implementation of the EM algorithm for Bayesian variable selection under a Weibull survival model. Both of our simulation studies and two real data analyses show that the proposed method is effective and can cope with high-dimensional omics data.

Additional file

Additional file 1: Table S1. TPR, FPR and FDR in variable selection with 50 replications (Weibull distribution). **Table S2.** TPR, FPR and FDR in variable selection with 50 replications (Gamma distribution). **Table S3.** Computational time (minutes) for application in simulation trials. **Table S4.** The estimated effects of 14 SNPs by SurvEMVS and classical Weibull regression. **Table S5.** Demographic and clinical characteristics of STAD patients. **Table S6.** The estimated effects of gene expression levels selected by SurvEMVS and Cox LASSO with their counterparts in low dimension scenario (i.e., Weibull regession and Cox model, respectively). **Figure S1.** Pseudocode for implementation of SurvEMVS. **Figure S2.** Averaged estimated effect (*black vertical lines*) for each marker over 50 replications under Scenario 2. **Figure S3.** Averaged estimated effect (*black vertical lines*) for each marker over 50 replications under Scenario 3. **Figure S4.** Averaged estimated effect (*black vertical lines*) for each marker over 50 replications under Scenario 4. **Figure S5.** Averaged estimated effect (*black vertical lines*) for each marker over 50 replications under Scenario 5. **Figure S6** Averaged estimated effect (*black vertical lines*) for each marker over 50 replications under Scenario 6. **Figure S7.** MSE of parameter estimation and AUC of prognosis prediction for Scenarios 3 and 4. **Figure S8.** MSE of parameter estimation and AUC of prognosis prediction for Scenarios 5 and 6. **Figure S9.** Kaplan-Meier survival curve of patients with high, moderate, and low risk.

Abbreviations

AFT: Accelerated failure time; CCD: Cyclic coordinate descent; EBIC: Extended Bayesian Information Criteria; EM: Expectation-maximization; GEO: Gene Expression Omnibus; LASSO: Least absolute shrinkage and selection operator; MCMC: Markov Chain Monte Carlo; TCGA: The Cancer Genome Atlas

Acknowledgements

We thank the participants and staff for their important contributions to this study.

Funding

This study was funded by National Natural Science Foundation of China (81530088 and 81473070 to F.C.), National Key Research and Development Program of China (2016YFE0204900 to F.C.), the National Institutes of Health (CA092824 and CA209414 to D.C.C.), Natural Science Foundation of the Jiangsu Higher Education Institutions of China (14KJA310002 to F.C.), Research and Innovation Project for College Graduates of Jiangsu Province of China (KYLX16_1123 to W.D.), Priority Academic Program Development of Jiangsu Higher Education Institutions (PAPD), and Top-notch Academic Programs Project of Jiangsu Higher Education Institutions (TAPP: PPZY2015A067). Y.W. and R.Z. were partially supported by the Outstanding Young Teachers Training Program of Nanjing Medical University.

Authors' contributions

WD, RZ, FC, and DCC contributed to the conception and design. WD contributed to the development of methodology. YZ and DCC contributed to the acquisition of data. WD, RZ, YZ, YW, and SS contributed to the analysis and interpretation of data. WD, RZ, and FC contributed to the writing, review, and revision of the manuscript. All authors read and approved the final manuscript.

Competing interests

The authors declare that they have no competing interests.

Author details

[1]Department of Biostatistics, School of Public Health, Nanjing Medical University, 101 Longmian Avenue, Nanjing 211166, Jiangsu, China. [2]China International Cooperation Center for Environment and Human Health, Nanjing Medical University, 101 Longmian Avenue, Nanjing 211166, Jiangsu, China. [3]Joint Laboratory of Health and Environmental Risk Assessment (HERA), Nanjing Medical University School of Public Health / Harvard School of Public Health, 101 Longmian Avenue, Nanjing 211166, Jiangsu, China. [4]Key Laboratory of Biomedical Big Data of Nanjing Medical University, 101 Longmian Avenue, Nanjing 211166, Jiangsu, China. [5]Department of Environmental Health, Harvard School of Public Health, Boston, MA, USA. [6]Pulmonary and Critical Care Division, Department of Medicine, Massachusetts General Hospital/Harvard Medical School, Boston, MA 02114, USA.

References

1. Metzker ML. Sequencing technologies - the next generation. Nat Rev Genet. 2010;11(1):31.
2. Veeramah KR, Hammer MF. The impact of whole-genome sequencing on the reconstruction of human population history. Nat Rev Genet. 2014;15(3):149.
3. Network TCGA. Comprehensive molecular characterization of gastric adenocarcinoma. Nature. 2014;513(7517):202–9.
4. Edgar R, Domrachev M, Lash AE. Gene expression omnibus: NCBI gene expression and hybridization array data repository. Nucleic Acids Res. 2002; 30(1):207–10.
5. Yang J, Lee SH, Goddard ME, Visscher PM. GCTA: a tool for genome-wide complex trait analysis. Am J Hum Genet. 2011;88(1):76–82.
6. Hu Z, Wu C, Shi Y, Guo H, Zhao X, Yin Z, Yang L, Dai J, Hu L, Tan W. A genome-wide association study identifies two new lung cancer susceptibility loci at 13q12.12 and 22q12.2 in Han Chinese. Nat Genet. 2011; 43(8):792–6.
7. Dong J, Hu Z, Wu C, Guo H, Zhou B, Lv J, Lu D, Chen K, Shi Y, Chu M. Association analyses identify multiple new lung cancer susceptibility loci and their interactions with smoking in the Chinese population. Nat Genet. 2012;44(8):895.
8. Zhou X, Stephens M. Genome-wide efficient mixed model analysis for association studies. Nat Genet. 2012;44(7):821.
9. Chen H, Wang C, Conomos MP, Stilp AM, Li Z, Sofer T, Szpiro AA, Chen W, Brehm JM, Celedón JC. Control for population structure and relatedness for binary traits in genetic association studies via logistic mixed models. Am J Hum Genet. 2016;98(4):653–66.
10. Yang J, Zaitlen NA, Goddard ME, Visscher PM, Price AL. Advantages and pitfalls in the application of mixed-model association methods. Nat Genet. 2014;46(2):100–6.
11. Guan Y, Stephens M. Bayesian variable selection regression for genome-wide association studies and other large-scale problems. Ann Appl Stat. 2011;5(3):1780–815.
12. Moser G, Sang HL, Hayes BJ, Goddard ME, Wray NR, Visscher PM. Simultaneous discovery, estimation and prediction analysis of complex traits using a Bayesian mixture model. PLoS Genet. 2015;11(4):e1004969.
13. Tibshirani R. Regression shrinkage and selection via the lasso: a retrospective. J R Stat Soc B. 2011;73:273–82.
14. Zou H. The adaptive lasso and its oracle properties. J Am Stat Assoc. 2006; 101(476):1418–29.
15. Casella TP, George. The Bayesian lasso. J Am Stat Assoc. 2008;103(482):681–6.
16. George EI, Mcculloch RE. Approaches for Bayesian variable selection. Stat Sin. 1997;7(2):339–73.
17. Zhou X, Carbonetto P, Stephens M. Polygenic modeling with Bayesian sparse linear mixed models. PLoS Genet. 2013;9(2):e1003264.
18. Carbonetto P, Stephens M. Scalable variational inference for Bayesian variable selection in regression, and its accuracy in genetic association studies. Bayesian Anal. 2012;7(1):73–107.
19. Logsdon BA, Carty CL, Reiner AP, Dai JY, Kooperberg C. A novel variational Bayes multiple locus Z-statistic for genome-wide association studies with Bayesian model averaging. Bioinformatics. 2012;28(13):1738.
20. Duan W, Zhao Y, Wei Y, Yang S, Bai J, Shen S, Du M, Huang L, Hu Z, Chen F. A fast algorithm for Bayesian multi-locus model in genome-wide association studies. Mol Gen Genet. 2017;292(4):923–34.
21. Hayashi T, Iwata H. EM algorithm for Bayesian estimation of genomic breeding values. BMC Genet. 2010;11(1):3.
22. Ročková V, George EI. EMVS: the EM approach to Bayesian variable selection. J Am Stat Assoc. 2014;109(506):828–46.
23. Oakes D. Biometrika centenary: survival analysis. Biometrika. 2001;88(1):99–142.
24. Ziegel ER. Modelling for survival data in medical research by D. Collett: Chapman & Hall; 1994. https://www.crcpress.com/Modelling-Survival-Data-in-Medical-Research-Third-Edition/Collett/p/book/9781439856789.
25. Hosmer DW, Lemeshow S. Applied survival analysis: regression modeling of time to event data: Wiley-Interscience; 1999. https://www.wiley.com/en-us/Applied+Survival+Analysis%3A+Regression+Modeling+of+Time+to+Event+Data%2C+2nd+Edition-p-9780471754992.
26. Cox DR. Regression models and life-tables: Springer New York; 1992. https://link.springer.com/chapter/10.1007%2F978-1-4612-4380-9_37.
27. Keiding N, Andersen PK, Klein JP. The role of frailty models and accelerated failure time models in describing heterogeneity due to omitted covariates. Stat Med. 1997;16(1 3):215.
28. Robins JM, Scheines R, Spirtes P, Wasserman L. A Bayesian justification of Cox's partial likelihood. Biometrika. 2003;90(3):629–41.
29. Zucknick M, Saadati M, Benner A. Nonidentical twins: comparison of frequentist and Bayesian lasso for Cox models. Biom J. 2015;57(6):959–81.
30. Klein JP, Moeschberger ML. Survival analysis: techniques for censored and truncated data. 2nd ed; 2003.
31. Dempster AP, Laird NM, Rubin DB. Maximum likelihood from incomplete data via the EM algorithm. J R Stat Soc. 1977;39(1):1–38.
32. Luenberger DG, Ye Y. Linear and nonlinear programming: Addison-Wesley; 1984. https://link.springer.com/book/10.1007%2F978-0-387-74503-9.
33. Tong Z, Oles FJ. Text categorization based on regularized linear classification methods. Inf Retr. 2001;4(1):5–31.
34. Genkin A, Lewis DD, Madigan D. Large-scale Bayesian logistic regression for text categorization. Technometrics. 2007;49(3):291–304.
35. Simon N, Friedman J, Hastie T, Tibshirani R. Regularization paths for Cox's proportional hazards model via coordinate descent. J Stat Softw. 2011;39(05):1–13.
36. Van Houwelingen HC, Bruinsma T, Hart AAM, Van'T Veer LJ, Wessels LFA. Cross-validated cox regression on microarray gene expression data. Stat Med. 2006;25(18):3201.
37. Bogdan M, Ghosh JK, Doerge RW. Modifying the Schwarz Bayesian information criterion to locate multiple interacting quantitative trait loci. Genetics. 2004;167(2):989–99.
38. Siegmund D. Model selection in irregular Problems: applications to mapping quantitative trait loci. Biometrika. 2004;91(4):785–800.
39. Chen J, Chen Z. Extended Bayesian information criteria for model selection with large model spaces. Biometrika. 2008;95(3):759–71.
40. Jr HF, Lee KL, Mark DB. Multivariable prognostic models: issues in developing models, evaluating assumptions and adequacy, and measuring and reducing errors. Stat Med. 1996;15(4):361–87.
41. Purcell S, Neale B, Todd-Brown K, Thomas L, Ferreira MAR, Bender D, Maller J, Sklar P, Bakker PIWD, Daly MJ. PLINK: a tool set for whole-genome association and population-based linkage analyses. Am J Hum Genet. 2007; 81(3):559–75.
42. Asomaning K, Miller DP, Liu G, Wain JC, Lynch TJ, Su L, Christiani DC. Second hand smoke, age of exposure and lung cancer risk. Lung Cancer. 2008;61(1):13.
43. Machida EO, Brock MV, Hooker CM, Nakayama J, Ishida A, Amano J, Picchi MA, Belinsky SA, Herman JG, Taniguchi S. Hypermethylation of ASC/TMS1 is a sputum marker for late-stage lung cancer. Cancer Res. 2006;66(12):6210.
44. Zhao Y, Wei Q, Hu L, Chen F, Hu Z, Heist RS, Su L, Amos CI, Shen H, Christiani DC. Polymorphisms in MicroRNAs are associated with survival in non-small cell lung cancer. Cancer Epidemiol Biomarkers Prev. 2014;23(11): 2503–11.
45. Chandrashekar DS, Bashel B, Sah B, Creighton CJ, Ponce-Rodriguez I, Bvsk C, Varambally S. UALCAN: a portal for facilitating tumor subgroup gene expression and survival analyses. Neoplasia. 2017;19(8):649.
46. Brabender J, Danenberg KD, Metzger R, Schneider PM, Lord RV, Groshen S, Tsao-Wei DD, Park J, Salonga D, Holscher AH, et al. The role of retinoid X receptor messenger RNA expression in curatively resected non-small cell lung cancer. Clin Cancer Res. 2002;8(2):438–43.
47. He S, Chen CH, Chernichenko N, He S, Bakst RL, Barajas F, Deborde S, Allen PJ, Vakiani E, Yu Z. GFRα1 released by nerves enhances cancer cell perineural invasion through GDNF-RET signaling. Proc Natl Acad Sci U S A. 2014;111(19):E2008.
48. Colaprico A, Silva TC, Olsen C, Garofano L, Cava C, Garolini D, Sabedot TS, Malta TM, Pagnotta SM, Castiglioni I. TCGAbiolinks: an R/ Bioconductor package for integrative analysis of TCGA data. Nucleic Acids Res. 2016;44(8):e71.
49. White IR, Royston P, Wood AM. Multiple imputation using chained equations: issues and guidance for practice. Stat Med. 2011;30(4):377–99.
50. Pardoll DM. The blockade of immune checkpoints in cancer immunotherapy. Nat Rev Cancer. 2012;12(4):252–64.
51. Wei SC, Levine JH, Cogdill AP, Zhao Y, Anang NAS, Andrews MC, Sharma P, Wang J, Wargo JA, Pe'er D, et al. Distinct cellular mechanisms underlie anti-CTLA-4 and anti-PD-1 checkpoint blockade. Cell. 2017;170(6):1120–1133.e1117.
52. Hou R, Cao B, Chen Z, Li Y, Ning T, Li C, Xu C, Chen Z. Association of cytotoxic T lymphocyte-associated antigen-4 gene haplotype with the susceptibility to gastric cancer. Mol Biol Rep. 2010;37(1):515–20.
53. Kim JW, Nam KH, Ahn SH, Park DJ, Kim HH, Kim SH, Chang H, Lee JO, Kim YJ, Lee HS, et al. Prognostic implications of immunosuppressive protein expression in tumors as well as immune cell infiltration within the tumor microenvironment in gastric cancer. Gastric Cancer. 2016;19(1):42–52.

54. Rakic JM, Maillard C, Jost M, Bajou K, Masson V, Devy L, Lambert V, Foidart JM, Noel A. Role of plasminogen activator-plasmin system in tumor angiogenesis. Cell Mol Life Sci. 2003;60(3):463–73.
55. Takayama Y, Hattori N, Hamada H, Masuda T, Omori K, Akita S, Iwamoto H, Fujitaka K, Kohno N. Inhibition of PAI-1 limits tumor angiogenesis regardless of angiogenic stimuli in malignant pleural mesothelioma. Cancer Res. 2016; 76(11):3285.
56. Collins FS, Varmus H. A new initiative on precision medicine. N Engl J Med. 2015;372(9):793.
57. Sha N, Tadesse MG, Vannucci M. Bayesian variable selection for the analysis of microarray data with censored outcomes. Bioinformatics. 2006;22(18): 2262–8.
58. Mittal S, Madigan D, Cheng JQ, Burd RS. Large-scale parametric survival analysis. Stat Med. 2013;32(23):3955–71.
59. Newcombe P, Raza AH, Blows F, Provenzano E, Pharoah P, Caldas C, Richardson S. Weibull regression with Bayesian variable selection to identify prognostic tumour markers of breast cancer survival. Stat Methods Med Res. 2014;26(1):414.
60. Barbieri M, Berger J. Optimal predictive model selection. Ann Stat. 2004; 32(3):870–97.
61. Zhang Z, Sinha S, Maiti T, Shipp E. Bayesian variable selection in the accelerated failure time model with an application to the surveillance, epidemiology, and end results breast cancer data. Stat Methods Med Res. 2016. https://doi.org/10.1177/0962280215626947.
62. Zellner A. On assessing prior distributions and Bayesian regression analysis with G-prior distributions. Bayesian Inference Decis Tech. 1986;6:233–43.
63. Ročková V, George EI. The Spike-and-Slab LASSO. J Am Stat Assoc. 2018; 113(521):431–44. https://doi.org/10.1080/01621459.2016.1260469.
64. Gao AC, Lou W, Isaacs JT. Enhanced GBX2 expression stimulates growth of human prostate cancer cells via transcriptional up-regulation of the interleukin 6 gene. Clin Cancer Res. 2000;6(2):493–7.
65. Gao AC, Lou W, Isaacs JT. Down-regulation of homeobox gene GBX2 expression inhibits human prostate cancer clonogenic ability and tumorigenicity. Cancer Res. 1998;58(7):1391.
66. Nimmrich I, Erdmann S, Melchers U, Chtarbova S, Finke U, Hentsch S, Hoffmann I, Oertel M, Hoffmann W, Müller O. The novel ependymin related gene UCC1 is highly expressed in colorectal tumor cells. Cancer Lett. 2001; 165(1):71–9.
67. Liu Z, Zhang J, Gao Y, Pei L, Zhou J, Gu L, Zhang L, Zhu B, Hattori N, Ji J. Large-scale characterization of DNA methylation changes in human gastric carcinomas with and without metastasis. Clin Cancer Res. 2014; 20(17):4598–612.
68. Godinheymann N, Brabetz S, Murillo MM, Saponaro M, Santos CR, Lobley A, East P, Chakravarty P, Matthews N, Kelly G. Tumour-suppression function of KLF12 through regulation of anoikis. Oncogene. 2015;35(25):3324.
69. Yu N, Migita T, Hosoda F, Okada N, Gotoh M, Arai Y, Fukushima M, Ohki M, Miyata S, Takeuchi K. Krüppel-like factor 12 plays a significant role in poorly differentiated gastric cancer progression. Int J Cancer. 2009;125(8):1859.
70. Rozenblum E, Vahteristo P, Sandberg T, Bergthorsson JT, Syrjakoski K, Weaver D, Haraldsson K, Johannsdottir HK, Vehmanen P, Nigam S, et al. A genomic map of a 6-Mb region at 13q21-q22 implicated in cancer development: identification and characterization of candidate genes. Hum Genet. 2002;110(2):111–21.

18

BRCA1 and *BRCA2* mutations and clinical interpretation in 398 ovarian cancer patients: comparison with breast cancer variants in a similar population

Florencia C. Cardoso[1], Susana Goncalves[3], Pablo G. Mele[2], Natalia C. Liria[1], Leonardo Sganga[3], Ignacio Diaz Perez[3], Ernesto J. Podesta[2] and Angela R. Solano[1,2*]

Abstract

Background: Ovarian cancer is the leading cause of death worldwide among gynecologic malignancies. The recent approval of inhibitors of poly (ADP-ribose) polymerase (iPARP) in the treatment of ovarian cancer in the presence of a *BRCA1/2* mutation has sparked the analysis of women with such diagnosis, which can further benefit from the detection of carriers in the family. Germline sequence and large rearrangements for *BRCA1/2* were tested in 398 consecutive epithelial ovarian cancer (EOC) patients.

The aim of this study was to identify the frequency and spectrum of germline *BRCA1/2* pathogenic alterations in a cohort of patients with ovarian serous carcinoma, with a view to adequately selecting patients for prevention through family counseling and correlating this frequency with platinum sensitivity as a guidance to identify patients eligible for iPARP in our population.

Results: A total of 96 patients carried a pathogenic germline mutation, accounting for an overall 24.1% mutation incidence. Among mutation carriers, *BRCA1 showed* 62.5% incidence, *BRCA2* rendered 36.5%, and one patient exhibited a mutation in both genes. Three pathogenic mutations were recurrent mutations detected five, three, and four times and represented 12.5% of the mutated samples. Worth highlighting, a 50% mutation incidence was detected when breast and ovarian cancer coexisted in the same patient. Novel mutations amounted to 9.4% of the total mutations, as compared to 4.7% in breast cancer. Forty out of 60 *BRCA1* mutations were beyond the ovarian cancer cluster region (OCCR), in stark contrast with 22 out of 36 *BRCA2* mutations being inside the OCCR. Taken together, germline *BRCA1/2* mutations in EOC patients showed a distinct mutational spectrum compared to our previously published data on breast cancer patients.

Conclusions: In sum, our study provides novel data on ovarian *BRCA1/2* mutation prevalence worldwide, enhances adequate patient selection for family counseling and prevention, and sheds light on the benefits of iPARP treatment.

Keywords: Ovarian cancer, *BRCA1/2* and ovarian cancer, iPARP treatment

* Correspondence: asolano@cemic.edu.ar
[1]Genotipificación y Cáncer Hereditario, Centro de Educación Médica e Investigaciones Clínicas "Norberto Quirno" (CEMIC), Galván 4102, C1431FWO Ciudad Autonoma de Buenos Aires, Argentina
[2]Instituto de Investigaciones Biomédicas (INBIOMED), Facultad de Medicina, Universidad de Buenos Aires-CONICET, Paraguay 2155 - Piso 5, C1121ABG Ciudad Autonoma de Buenos Aires, Argentina
Full list of author information is available at the end of the article

Background

Ovarian cancer is the leading cause of death worldwide among gynecologic malignancies. Argentina exhibits mid-high rates, and, in 2016, the National Cancer Institute, Ministry of Health (Instituto Nacional del Cáncer, INC, Ministerio de Salud de la Nación), reported a total of 2274 ovarian cancer cases out of a total of 60,209 women cancer cases, which represents 3.8% (Argentina, 2016, SIVER-Ca, INC, Ministerio de Salud de la Nación).

Genetic testing for *BRCA1/2* mutation carriers proves critical to clinical decisions, as more than 90% of the cases of epithelial ovarian cancer (EOC) are diagnosed with bulky intra-abdominal disease or distant metastases [1]. The importance of *BRCA1/2* mutation screening in ovarian cancer patients has been further underscored by recent findings showing that mutation carriers have increased sensitivity to inhibitors of poly (ADP-ribose) polymerase (PARP) [2, 3]. In fact, PARP inhibitors (iPARP) have recently been approved for the treatment of advanced ovarian cancer patients carrying either germline or somatic mutations in *BRCA1/2* genes [4]. Moreover, *BRCA1/2* mutation status has been shown to predict response to iPARP. Individuals with germline *BRCA1/2* alterations treated with iPARP have a significant increase in progression-free survival compared with patients with wild-type *BRCA1/2* [3, 5].

The reported prevalence of *BRCA1/2* mutations in patients with ovarian cancer varies across different studies and ethnic populations. A report interpreting the results of 14 studies from eight Western countries, summarized in a meta-analysis, has shown the overall incidence of germline mutations to be 18.0% for *BRCA1* and 6.9% for *BRCA2*, although this incidence ranges between 3.4 and 47% for *BRCA1* and between 1 and 12% for *BRCA2* [6] when considering specific populations. Reports from Asia have revealed the following figures: in South Korea [7], only one pathogenic mutation was found in the *BRCA1* gene among 37 EOC patients; a Japanese study [8] found 5.3% cases with germline mutations in *BRCA1* and 7.4% in *BRCA2*; in Hong Kong [9], the publication of a series of 60 ovarian cancer patients analyzed for the whole coding region of *BRCA1* but only the exon 11 of *BRCA2* rendered 11.3% and 2.1% patients carrying a mutation, respectively, including the c.1081delG in *BRCA1*, which seemed to be a founder mutation from Southern Chinese populations, and two recurrent mutations, i.e., c.2371-2372delTG in *BRCA1* and c.3337C>T in *BRCA2*; finally, in the Chinese population [10], the rate of mutation carriers among patients was reported to be 16.7%, with the description of a presumably very frequent non-founder mutation, i.e. c.5470_5477del8 in *BRCA1*, and the conclusion that the spectrum of *BRCA1/2* mutations greatly differs from that described in Western studies.

Relatively few studies have been reported on South American populations, and the most readily available results are based on small-size cohorts. A Colombian study has reported 100 patients with ovarian cancer diagnosis and 15% of mutation detection—13% in *BRCA1* and 2% in *BRCA2*—including an 11% accounting for a founder mutation [11]. A review of Latin American and Caribbean studies summarizes breast/ovarian cancer cases from a few countries. However, only a limited number of studies used full sequencing analysis and ovarian cancer was not clearly disclosed, which prevented the review from reaching conclusions [12].

To gain a more complete insight into the prevalence of *BRCA1/2* mutations in EOC patients from Argentina, we performed a cohort study of 398 unselected consecutive EOC patients for *BRCA1/2* mutation screening using the next-generation sequencing (NGS) approach and multiplex ligation-dependent probe amplification (MLPA) for large rearrangements.

The aim of this study was to identify the frequency and spectrum of germline *BRCA1/2* pathogenic alterations in a cohort of patients with ovarian serous carcinoma, with a view to adequately selecting patients for prevention through family counseling and correlating this frequency with platinum sensitivity as a guidance to identify patients eligible for iPARP in our population. In addition, and considering similarities in the population analyzed, this study presents a comparison with results previously published by our group [13] on *BRCA1/2* mutations in breast cancer patients.

Methods

Study subjects

Subjects were selected among women diagnosed with epithelial ovarian cancer and referred to Centro de Educación Médica e Investigaciones Clínicas (CEMIC) for genetic testing from January 2014 to June 2017. A total of 398 patients were included in the study, 299 of whom were selected by the inclusion criteria required for treatment with iPARP (high-grade ovarian serous carcinoma, relapsed, second-line platinum-sensitive). Routine procedure included signing a written informed consent to genetic testing (including anonymized disclosure of the data) from each patient, approved by the Ethics Committee from CEMIC, and a Pretest Counseling for Susceptibility Testing (purpose of testing), as described in the American Society of Clinical Oncology Policy Statement Update [14].

Subjects enrolled in this study showed a mean age at diagnosis of 53.5 ± 12 years, within a range of 18 to 84 years of age. Eligible patients included women with newly diagnosed, histologically confirmed, or chemotherapy-treated serous ovarian cancer, regardless of chemotherapy line. Although data on family history (FH) were collected as part of the study, recruitment was independent of FH conditions.

BRCA testing

Genomic DNA of the 398 blood samples was isolated by MagNA Pure® LC instrument with total DNA isolation kit I (Roche Diagnostics). Analysis of *BRCA1/2* genes included complete sequencing and study of large rearrangements.

The Ion AmpliSeq*BRCA1/2* community panel was used for the targeted NGS, as it allows to amplify the entire coding sequences of *BRCA1* and *BRCA2*, including 20–50 bases of adjacent intronic sequence of each exon. Sequencing of the amplified regions was performed with the next-generation platform Personal Genome Machine® System. As a control, the STR variants of every sample were previously traced and intra NGS [15] was used to ensure the identification of the sample and avoid possible processing. The few codifying sequences with low readings were analyzed by Sanger reaction in order to reach 100% coverage.

The raw signal data and the sequence reads were processed with Ion Torrent Suite software (Thermo Fisher Scientific) on a Torrent server. The pipeline included signaling processing, base calling, quality score assignment, adapter trimming, PCR duplicate removal, read alignment to the reference human genome 19, quality control of mapping quality, coverage analysis, and variant calling. Coverage analysis used plug-in software in the Torrent server. The variant caller parameter setting was germline PGM (Life Technologies).

After data analysis, single-nucleotide variants, insertions, deletions, and splice site alternations were registered, and all variants detected were reported. Sanger DNA sequencing was used to confirm all clinically relevant variants detected (classes 3, 4, and 5) using the specific gene primers. Clinical significance was determined according to the report in the reference databases (ClinVar [16], LOVD 3.0 [17], UMD [18]—last access December 29, 2017). For missense mutations not reported or reported with uncertain clinical significance (VUS), in silico programs were used to predict the change in protein function using software Align-GVGD, SIFT, and Mutations Taster.

Large rearrangements were measured by MLPA using SALSA MLPA Probemix P002-D1 and P045-B3 provided by MRC-Holland, and Coffalyser.net software was used for data analysis.

In a preliminary analysis for a panel of genes, 30 samples were exome sequenced and then filtered for the following: *ATM, BRCA1, BRCA2, BRIP1, CDH1, CHEK2, MSH2, MLH1, MSH6, PMS2, EPCAM, NBN, NF1, PALB2, PTEN, RAD51C, RAD51D, STK11*, and *TP53*. Full exonic ± 20 bases of adjacent intronic sequence for each gene were assured. These genes were selected according to the genes listed in the NCCN guidelines (Genetic/Familial High-Risk Assessment: Breast and Ovarian—Version 2.2017), for which there are risk and management recommendations of patients with a pathogenic mutation. In other words, these actionable genes allow clinical measures such as monitoring, treatment, counseling, and prevention for both the probands and their families.

We routinely share our genetic variants and collected at Leiden Open Variation Database (Chapter for Argentina) [19]. In the case of the novel variants, the registration numbers of each of the variants in the LOVD database [17] are shown in Table 2.

Genetic variant classification

The novel variants were classified according to the recommendation guidelines of the American College of Medical and Genomics (ACMG) [20]. As they correspond to variants not reported in the population and disease database all comply with the PM2 criteria of the ACMG Guidelines, this is a criterion of moderate pathogenicity. According to this:

Probably pathogenic mutations were defined as follows:

1. Nonsense and frameshift variants that generate a premature stop codon, except for the variants that generate a premature stop codon after codon 3326 in the BRCA2 gene (criterion PVS1 of the ACMG guidelines)
2. Splice site variants that are found in intronic or exonic variant in the exon-intron border (criterion PVS1 of the ACMG guidelines)

Variants of uncertain clinical significance (VUS) were defined as follows:

1. Missense variants where multiple lines of computational evidence support to deleterious effect on the gene or gene product or no impact on gene or gene product (criteria PP3 and BP4 respectively of ACMG guidelines)
2. Synonymous (silent) variant for which splicing prediction algorithms predict no impact to the splice consensus sequence nor the creation of a new splice site and the nucleotide is not highly conserved (criterion BP7 ACMG guidelines)
3. Intronic variants distant from the intron-exon boundary

Results

The sequencing of *BRCA1/2* in 398 consecutive EOC patients, including 299 patients selected for iPARP treatment, rendered a total of 96 patients carrying a pathogenic germline mutation. These cases are listed in Additional file 1, which indicates patients selected for iPARP treatment in italics and patients with novel mutations in bold. Overall mutation incidence amounted to 24.1% ($n = 398$), while mutation incidence among patients selected for iPARP treatment was 20.7% ($n = 299$) and mutation incidence among non-iPARP-selected patients was 34.3% ($n = 99$).

The mutations found were as follows: 60 in *BRCA1* (62.5%), 35 in *BRCA2* (36.5%), and 1 in both genes (1%) (Table 1). The mean age of diagnosis for the patients carrying a mutation was 53.7 years, which was non-statistically different from 54.3 years in the non-detected-mutation group. The low end of the age range among patients with a non-detected mutation, as well as among patients with both breast and ovary cancer diagnosis was 31 years of age, much higher than that of the mutation-carrying group at 18 years (Table 1). Remarkably, the patients diagnosed with both cancers showed a 50% rate of mutation detection (Table 1), again with similar distribution in both genes: 69% detected in *BRCA1*, 27.6% in *BRCA2*, and 3.4% in both genes.

Key to validating our population detection methods and interpretation, only 3.38% variants were found of unknown significance (VUS). Out of the total number of mutations detected, nine were found to be novel deleterious mutations (9.4%), three of them in *BRCA1* and six in *BRCA2*, as listed in Table 2. Of note, *BRCA1* mutation c.3578_3759delCT has been previously described by our group in an unrelated patient [21], although this patient had breast cancer diagnosed at 31 years; *BRCA2* mutation c.7805+2_7805+3delTA has also been already described [13] but is included now as belonging to an ovary cancer patient. Novel intronic variants detected to be yet classified were c.670+31A>C, c.4357+22C>T, c.80 +52T>A, and c.516+3A>T.

Regarding recurrent pathogenic mutations, present in 3 or more patients each, 2 were detected in *BRCA1* and 1 in *BRCA2*, including 12 patients among mutation carriers (12.5%) (Table 3). These recurrent mutations were c.4964_4982del19 and c.5266dupC in *BRCA1* and c.5351dupA in *BRCA2*, with five, three, and four detections, respectively.

The FH group—understood as having at least 1 relative developing breast and/or ovarian cancer among first- or second-degree relatives—accounted for 158 cases, among which 55 rendered mutations (34.8%), including the patient with a mutation in both genes. In turn, the non-FH group included 105 patients, 10 of whom were mutation carriers (9.5%). No FH records were available for the remaining 135 patients, 31 of whom revealed a mutation (23.0%) (Table 4).

Regarding the spectrum of mutations along the genes (Fig. 1), 40 out of 60 mutations detected in *BRCA1* were located outside the ovarian cancer cluster region (OCCR), in contrast with the findings for *BRCA2*, in which 22 out of 36 were located inside the OCCR. In the case of the patient carrying a mutation in the two genes, both mutations were outside the OCCR. These mutations were c.-19-?_80+?del and c.1909+1G>A for *BRCA1* and *BRCA2*, respectively (Additional file 1).

Discussion

In the current study, we have assessed the *BRCA1/2* mutation status in 398 EOC patients with two main goals: the benefits of detecting hereditary breast/ovarian cancer syndrome for prevention and the possibility of selecting patients for treatment with iPARP. Results showed most mutations to be found in the *BRCA1* gene, reinforcing once again the well-established association of ovary cancer and a mutation in *BRCA1*. In our series, however, most of the mutations were outside the region of OCCR of *BRCA1*, even as the most recent and detailed publication [22] reinforcing the necessity of reporting regional genetic variants [19] and depositing genetic variants in open access databases. The apparent differences with the reported data [22] may very likely due to that no data was included from South America (or may be very little hidden in one of the categories); it is important to remark that the Hispanic demographic group in this very wide population analysis refers to a migration denomination in the USA and does not reflect South America and specifically, our country [13].

Our assay is a comprehensive analysis, and our group has vast experience in the regionality of the mutation spectra in our patients [13, 23], which is reflected in the low rate of 3.38% of VUS found in this series. The frequency of mutations detected reached 24.1% (Table 1), a value closer to the highest described in the literature [24, 25], lower than other published results [8, 11, 26–31]. The 99 patients not selected for iPARP treatment showed a striking proportion of 34.3% mutation carriers, which may stem from

Table 1 *BRCA1/2* sequence: summary of patients analyzed

Diagnosis	*n*	Age (range)[a]	BRCA mutated (%)	*BRCA1* mutation carriers (*n*)	*BRCA2* mutation carriers (*n*)	Non mutated (%)
EOC (total)	398	53.5 (18–84)	96 (24.1)	61[b]	36[b]	302 (75.9)
EOC and BC	58	56.5 (31–78)	29 (50.0)	21[b]	9[b]	29 (50.0)

The total number of patients analyzed was diagnosed with epithelial ovarian cancer (398). Among these, 58 patients also had a diagnosis of breast cancer (EOC and BC)

EOC epithelial ovarian cancer, *BC* breast cancer, *n* number of cases

[a]Age at ovary cancer diagnosis

[b]One of the patients with high-grade ovarian serous carcinoma and breast cancer had a mutation in both genes

Table 2 Novel variants in *BRCA1* (NM_007294.3) and *BRCA2* (NM_000059.3) genes detected in 398 probands with diagnosis of epithelial ovarian cancer

Sample ID	Gene	Exon/intron	Mutation[a]	Predicted effect[b]	MT	CS[c]	LOVD (genomic variant #)
BR1229	1B	11	c.2005dupA	p.(Met669Asnfs*4)	F	LP	198881
BR2066	1B	11	c.3758_3759delCT	p.(Ser1253*)	F	LP	196851
BR1037	1B	11	c.876_879delCACT	p.(Thr293Lysfs*4)	F	LP	198751
BR1410	2B	11	c.2133C>A	p.(Cys711*)	N	LP	202233
BR0986	2B	11	c.2860G>T	p.(Glu954*)	N	LP	197664
BR0832	2B	11	c.4419delC	p.(Asn1473Lysfs*6)	F	LP	201398
BR2072	2B	11	c.5253C>A	p.(Tyr1751*)	N	LP	203562
BR1464	2B	14	c.7308delC	p.(Asn2436Lysfs*31)	F	LP	206927
BR0495	2B	16i	c.7805+2_7805+3delTA		S	LP	199222
BR1104	1B	11	c.2357T>C	p.(Leu786Pro)	M	VUS	200898
BR0889	1B	11	c.3168C>T	p.(Ser1056=)	Syn	VUS	200773
BR1061	1B	10i	c.670+31A>C		S	VUS	196392
BR2063	1B	13i	c.4357+22C>T		S	VUS	209404
BR1078	1B	2i	c.80+52T>A		S	VUS	196406
BR0913	2B	6i	c.516+3A>T		S	VUS	199956

MT mutation type, *F* frameshift, *N* nonsense, *S* splicing, *M* missense, *Syn* synonym, *LP* likely pathogenic, *VUS* variant of uncertain significance
[a]HGVS nomenclature at cDNA level
[b]HGVS nomenclature at protein level
[c]CS: interpretation and classification of the variants was carried out according to the recommendations of the ACMG guidelines

the fact that CEMIC is a reference center for hereditary breast-ovary cancer patient analysis.

The worldwide age range of patients diagnosed with EOC included in *BRCA1/2* analyses [8, 11, 24–32] starts around 30 years, with the exception of Colombia [11] (16 years) and Argentina [13] (18 years). The lower-end value of the range does not reflect the most frequent age of diagnosis, as cases diagnosed in the patient's sixties are common, frequently with a mutation detected. This is reflected in the similar mean age among all the results published.

The high 50% rate of *BRCA1/2* mutations detected in 58 patients with both cancers diagnosis (Table 1) is in line with other studies on similar patients, although in smaller numbers, such as the Japanese study with 3 cases [8], all with a mutation detected. This is also in agreement with our previous publication [13], in which we analyzed 14 patients with breast and ovary cancer, 11 of whom (78.6%) bore a pathogenic mutation. Interestingly, seven mutations were found in common with the current series of patients, as follows: c.211A>G, c.1687C>T, c.1892dupT, c.5266dupC, c.5468-1G>A, c.2808_2811delACAA, and c.5351dupA (Additional file 1).

Table 3 Recurrent mutations in *BRCA1/2* detected in 398 probands with epithelial ovarian cancer

Mutation/times detected	Unrelated probands (% of the total probands)
BRCA1	
c.4964_4982del19 - p.(Ser1655Tyrfs*16)/5	5 (1.3)
c.5266dupC - p.(Gln1756Profs*74)/3	3 (0.8)
BRCA2	
c.5351dupA - p.(Asn1784Lysfs*3)/4	4 (1.0)
Total recurrent	12 (3.1)
Total recurrent (12)/total mutated (96) = 12.5%	–

Worth pointing out, the gene spectrum (Fig. 1), including data on the OCCR and the recurrent mutations described (Table 3), does not visualize a panel or hot spot of mutations to abbreviate the analysis of *BRCA1/2* in our ovarian cancer population.

As an additional comment regarding FH (not included in the criteria for the selection of patients), complementary data in the analysis of the results reveals large differences obtained in mutation detection between the FH and non-FH groups (34.8% vs 9.5%, p value = 0.000003, significant at $p < 0.05$), which is in contrast with results previously published [8]. This discrepancy may be explained by the larger number of patients studied in our report (398 vs 95), and our higher rate of mutations detected (24.1% vs 12.6%).

In turn, the following observations when comparing the findings described for ovarian cancer patients with our previous publication including a vast majority of breast cancer patients [13] are as follows: (a) the rate of

Table 4 Family history in patients with epithelial ovarian cancer

Family history	Number of probands (% of total)	Patients with a mutation detected (%)
Yes[a]	158 (39.7)	55 (34.8)
No	105 (26.4)	10 (9.5)
Not known	135 (33.9)	31 (23.0)

[a]Yes: family history with at least 1 relative developing breast and/or ovarian cancer among first- or second-degree relatives

mutation detection was higher in ovarian cancer patients with 24.1% vs breast cancer with 19.04% (p value = 0.035611, significant at $p < 0.05$); (b) the rate of novel mutations showed a tendency: 9.4% for ovarian cancer vs 4.7% for breast cancer. The population analyzed was 398 subjects for ovary cancer and 940 subjects for breast cancer with a detection rate of 2.26% (9 out 398) and 0.85% (8 out 940) novel variants, respectively (p value = 0.035249, significant at $p < 0.05$); (c) the rate of recurrent mutations was similar for both groups. Interestingly, the spectrum of recurrent mutations for both genes was spread along both genes.

A promising turn in the treatment of ovarian cancer has been the attempt at repairing double-strand DNA damage by homologous recombination repair pathway (HRR) mechanisms. *BRCA1* and *BRCA2* are genes centrally involved in this process, and mutations resulting in damaged *BRCA1* or *BRCA2* proteins can lead to various types of cancer such as breast, ovarian, or prostate cancer among the most closely associated. Even in the presence of a pathogenic mutation in *BRCA*, single-strand break repair by non-homologous end joining is an alternative pathway to repair double-strand breaks, avoiding cell death pathways like apoptosis. iPARP cause HRR leading gene-deficient (including *BRCA1/2*) cancer cells to die by apoptosis. This is known as "synthetic lethality," a concept developed upon evidence on sensitivity of *BRCA1/2* defective cells to platinum salts [33, 34].

Preliminary results from exome analysis of a panel of genes (see the "Methods" section) in 30 patients showed the following non-*BRCA1/2* mutations: in *EPCAM*, c.412C>T p.(Arg138*), and coexisting mutations as follows: in *MUTYH*, c.1105delC - p.(Ala371Profs*23) and in heterozygosis and *RAD51D*, c.1A>G p.(Met1Val). The application of these results is still under consideration, although the involvement of the *RAD51D* gene in the HRR mechanism should be highlighted.

Conclusion

In sum, the strength of our study lies in the inclusion of 299 patients exclusively selected for treatment with iPARP, plus an extra of 99 cases which could also benefit from treatment, the use of thorough methodology and

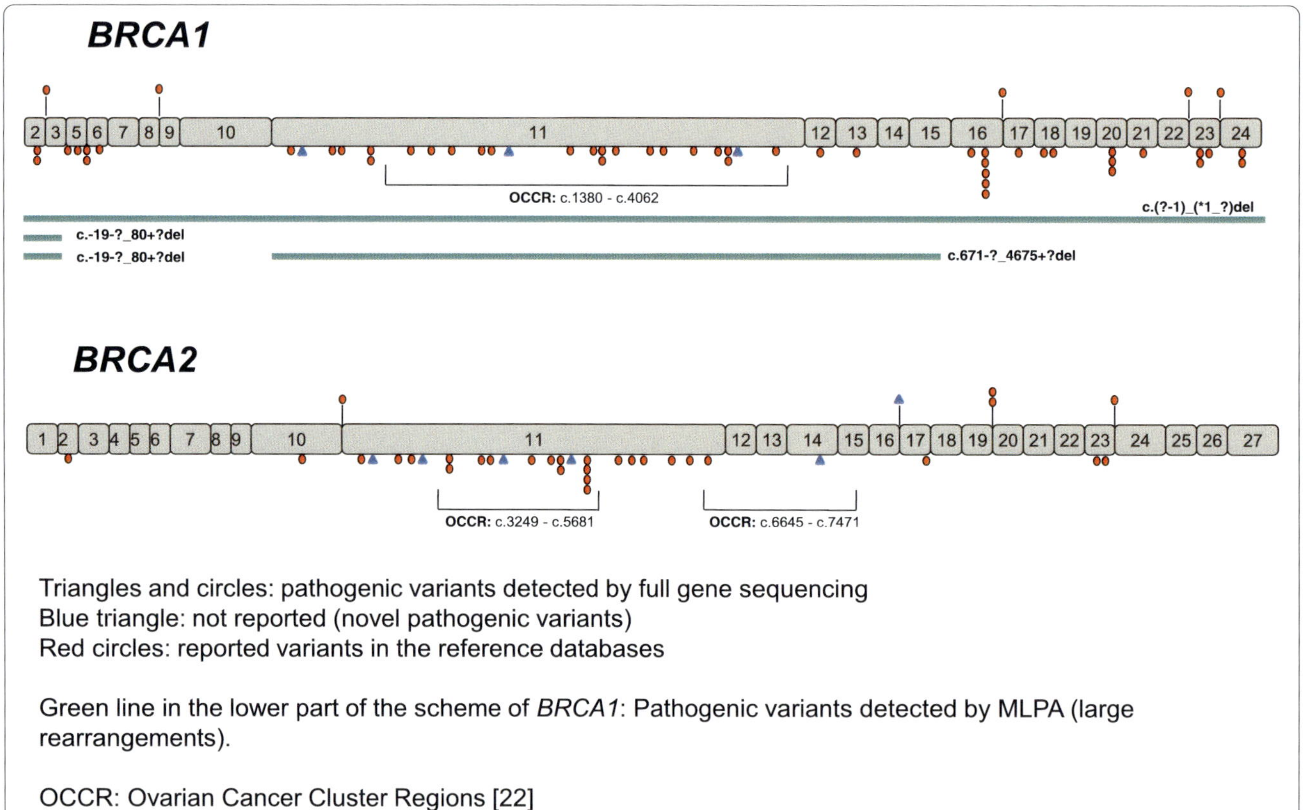

Fig. 1 Schematic representation of the 96 BRCA1/2 pathogenic mutations detected in 398 patients with diagnosis of epithelial ovarian cancer

knowledge of our population regional variants [13, 23], as supported by the 3.38% of VUS found. The findings reported here thus offer *BRCA* mutation carriers the benefit of treatment possibilities and allow precise identification of hereditary breast-ovary disease and the preventive measures associated.

Abbreviations
EOC: Epithelial ovarian cancer; NGS: Next-generation sequencing; OCCR: Ovarian cancer cluster region; PARP inhibitors: Poly (ADP-ribose) polymerase inhibitors

Acknowledgements
The authors are grateful to all the women who participated in this study. We also want to thank the clinic team for the careful selection and dedication to the patient attention, specially to Angel Martin, Arroyo Gerardo, Bas Carlos, Bruno Luisina, Caceres Valeria, Crimi Gabriel, Caminos Facundo, Colica Maria, Damiano Mario, De La Vega Maximo, Diaz Canton Enrique, Dodyk Patricia, Escudero Miguel, Fernandez Leyes Marcelo, Garrido Rosa, Gomez Abuin Gonzalo, Greco Martin, Ivulich Carlos, Kalfayan Pablo, Lacava Juan, Levit Patricio, Llugdar Jose, Mainella Andrea, Mampel Alejandra, Marmissolle Fabiana, Masllorens Francisca, Perazzo Florencia, Petracci Fernando, Real Nilda, Recondo Gonzalo, Richardet Martin, Riggi Maria, Santillan Francisco, Trigo Valeria, Yanzi Alvaro, and Zeff Natalia. We thank María M. Rancez for providing language help and writing assistance.

Funding
This study is partially funded by grant from the Instituto Nacional del Cáncer, Ministerio de Salud de la República Argentina, Res. 0515.

Authors' contributions
AS, FC, and EP had full access to all the data in the study and take responsibility for the integrity of the data and the accuracy of the data analysis. AS, FC, SG, and EP provided the study concept and design. FC, NL, and LS are responsible for the patients sample organization and collection. PM, IDP, and LS contributed to the literature analysis and statistical evaluation. AS, FC, SG, and EP did the acquisition, analysis, and interpretation of the data. All authors critically revised the manuscript for important intellectual content. All authors read and approved the final manuscript.

Competing interests
SG is the medical director in AstraZeneca Argentina and Uruguay MC. LS is the diagnosis manager in AstraZeneca Argentina MC. IDP is the oncology medical manager in AstraZeneca Argentina and Uruguay MC. The other authors declare that they have no competing interest.

Author details
[1]Genotipificación y Cáncer Hereditario, Centro de Educación Médica e Investigaciones Clínicas "Norberto Quirno" (CEMIC), Galván 4102, C1431FWO Ciudad Autonoma de Buenos Aires, Argentina. [2]Instituto de Investigaciones Biomédicas (INBIOMED), Facultad de Medicina, Universidad de Buenos Aires-CONICET, Paraguay 2155 - Piso 5, C1121ABG Ciudad Autonoma de Buenos Aires, Argentina. [3]AstraZeneca Argentina MC, Vedia 3616, C1430DAH Ciudad Autonoma de Buenos Aires, Argentina.

References

1. Hoskins WJ. Prospective on ovarian cancer: why prevent? J Cell Biochem Suppl. 1995;23:189–99.
2. Audeh MW, Carmichael J, Penson RT, Friedlander M, Powell B, Bell-McGuinn KM, Scott C, Weitzel JN, Oaknin A, Loman N, et al. Oral poly(ADP-ribose) polymerase inhibitor olaparib in patients with BRCA1 or BRCA2 mutations and recurrent ovarian cancer: a proof-of-concept trial. Lancet. 2010; 376(9737):245–51.
3. Ledermann J, Harter P, Gourley C, Friedlander M, Vergote I, Rustin G, Scott C, Meier W, Shapira-Frommer R, Safra T, et al. Olaparib maintenance therapy in platinum-sensitive relapsed ovarian cancer. N Engl J Med. 2012;366(15): 1382–92.
4. Kim G, Ison G, McKee AE, Zhang H, Tang S, Gwise T, Sridhara R, Lee E, Tzou A, Philip R, et al. FDA approval summary: olaparib monotherapy in patients with deleterious germline BRCA-mutated advanced ovarian cancer treated with three or more lines of chemotherapy. Clin Cancer Res. 2015;21(19): 4257–61.
5. Ledermann JA, Drew Y, Kristeleit RS. Homologous recombination deficiency and ovarian cancer. Eur J Cancer. 2016;60:49–58.
6. Zhong Q, Peng HL, Zhao X, Zhang L, Hwang WT. Effects of BRCA1- and BRCA2-related mutations on ovarian and breast cancer survival: a meta-analysis. Clin Cancer Res. 2015;21(1):211–20.
7. Kim YT, Nam EJ, Yoon BS, Kim SW, Kim SH, Kim JH, Kim HK, Koo JS, Kim JW. Germline mutations of BRCA1 and BRCA2 in Korean sporadic ovarian carcinoma. Gynecol Oncol. 2005;99(3):585–90.
8. Sakamoto I, Hirotsu Y, Nakagomi H, Ouchi H, Ikegami A, Teramoto K, Amemiya K, Mochizuki H, Omata M. BRCA1 and BRCA2 mutations in Japanese patients with ovarian, fallopian tube, and primary peritoneal cancer. Cancer. 2016;122(1):84–90.
9. Khoo US, Ngan HY, Cheung AN, Chan KY, Lu J, Chan VW, Lau S, Andrulis IL, Ozcelik H. Mutational analysis of BRCA1 and BRCA2 genes in Chinese ovarian cancer identifies 6 novel germline mutations. Hum Mutat. 2000; 16(1):88–9.
10. Khoo US, Chan KY, Cheung AN, Xue WC, Shen DH, Fung KY, Ngan HY, Choy KW, Pang CP, Poon CS, et al. Recurrent BRCA1 and BRCA2 germline mutations in ovarian cancer: a founder mutation of BRCA1 identified in the Chinese population. Hum Mutat. 2002;19(3):307–8.
11. Rodriguez AO, Llacuachaqui M, Pardo GG, Royer R, Larson G, Weitzel JN, Narod SA. BRCA1 and BRCA2 mutations among ovarian cancer patients from Colombia. Gynecol Oncol. 2012;124(2):236–43.
12. Dutil J, Golubeva VA, Pacheco-Torres AL, Diaz-Zabala HJ, Matta JL, Monteiro AN. The spectrum of BRCA1 and BRCA2 alleles in Latin America and the Caribbean: a clinical perspective. Breast Cancer Res Treat. 2015;154(3):441–53.
13. Solano AR, Cardoso FC, Romano V, Perazzo F, Bas C, Recondo G, Santillan FB, Gonzalez E, Abalo E, Viniegra M, et al. Spectrum of BRCA1/2 variants in 940 patients from Argentina including novel, deleterious and recurrent germline mutations: impact on healthcare and clinical practice. Oncotarget. 2017;8(36):60487–95.
14. Robson ME, Bradbury AR, Arun B, Domchek SM, Ford JM, Hampel HL, Lipkin SM, Syngal S, Wollins DS, Lindor NM. American Society of Clinical Oncology policy statement update: genetic and genomic testing for cancer susceptibility. J Clin Oncol. 2015;33(31):3660–7.
15. Marqués JM, Repetto L, Guggeri V, Russo E, García A, Agorio A, Torres A, Azambuja CJ. Sample ID quality control and methodological improvements for NGS gene panels. In: 65th Annual Meeting of The American Society of Human Genetics. (Abst.1959F); 2015.
16. ClinVar, National Center for Biotechnology http://www.ncbi.nlm.nih.gov/clinvar/. Accesed 29 Dec 2017.
17. Leiden Open Variation Database 3.0. https://databases.lovd.nl/shared/genes. Accesed 29 Dec 2017.
18. Universal Mutation Database http://www.umd.be/. Accesed 29 Dec 2017.
19. Leiden Open Variation Database (Chapter for Argentina). http://ar.lovd.org. Accesed 29 Dec 2017.
20. Richards S, Aziz N, Bale S, Bick D, Das S, Gastier-Foster J, Grody WW, Hegde M, Lyon E, Spector E, et al. Standards and guidelines for the interpretation of sequence variants: a joint consensus recommendation of the American College of Medical Genetics and Genomics and the Association for Molecular Pathology. Genet Med. 2015;17(5):405–24.
21. Solano AR, Aceto GM, Delettieres D, Veschi S, Neuman MI, Alonso E, Chialina S, Chacon RD, Renato MC, Podesta EJ. BRCA1 and BRCA2 analysis of Argentinean breast/ovarian cancer patients selected for age and family history highlights a role for novel mutations of putative south-American origin. SpringerPlus. 2012;1:20.
22. Rebbeck TR, Mitra N, Wan F, Sinilnikova OM, Healey S, McGuffog L, Mazoyer S, Chenevix-Trench G, Easton DF, Antoniou AC, et al. Association of type and location of BRCA1 and BRCA2 mutations with risk of breast and ovarian cancer. JAMA. 2015;313(13):1347–61.

23. Aceto GM, Solano AR, Neuman MI, Veschi S, Morgano A, Malatesta S, Chacon RD, Pupareli C, Lombardi M, Battista P, et al. High-risk human papilloma virus infection, tumor pathophenotypes, and BRCA1/2 and TP53 status in juvenile breast cancer. Breast Cancer Res Treat. 2010;122(3):671–83.
24. Gallagher DJ, Konner JA, Bell-McGuinn KM, Bhatia J, Sabbatini P, Aghajanian CA, Offit K, Barakat RR, Spriggs DR, Kauff ND. Survival in epithelial ovarian cancer: a multivariate analysis incorporating BRCA mutation status and platinum sensitivity. Ann Oncol. 2011;22(5):1127–32.
25. Vencken PM, Kriege M, Hoogwerf D, Beugelink S, van der Burg ME, Hooning MJ, Berns EM, Jager A, Collee M, Burger CW, et al. Chemosensitivity and outcome of BRCA1- and BRCA2-associated ovarian cancer patients after first-line chemotherapy compared with sporadic ovarian cancer patients. Ann Oncol. 2011;22(6):1346–52.
26. Yang D, Khan S, Sun Y, Hess K, Shmulevich I, Sood AK, Zhang W. Association of BRCA1 and BRCA2 mutations with survival, chemotherapy sensitivity, and gene mutator phenotype in patients with ovarian cancer. JAMA. 2011; 306(14):1557–65.
27. Alsop K, Fereday S, Meldrum C, deFazio A, Emmanuel C, George J, Dobrovic A, Birrer MJ, Webb PM, Stewart C, et al. BRCA mutation frequency and patterns of treatment response in BRCA mutation-positive women with ovarian cancer: a report from the Australian Ovarian Cancer Study Group. J Clin Oncol. 2012;30(21):2654–63.
28. Dann RB, DeLoia JA, Timms KM, Zorn KK, Potter J, Flake DD 2nd, Lanchbury JS, Krivak TC. BRCA1/2 mutations and expression: response to platinum chemotherapy in patients with advanced stage epithelial ovarian cancer. Gynecol Oncol. 2012;125(3):677–82.
29. McLaughlin JR, Rosen B, Moody J, Pal T, Fan I, Shaw PA, Risch HA, Sellers TA, Sun P, Narod SA. Long-term ovarian cancer survival associated with mutation in BRCA1 or BRCA2. J Natl Cancer Inst. 2013;105(2):141–8.
30. Shi T, Wang P, Xie C, Yin S, Shi D, Wei C, Tang W, Jiang R, Cheng X, Wei Q, et al. BRCA1 and BRCA2 mutations in ovarian cancer patients from China: ethnic-related mutations in BRCA1 associated with an increased risk of ovarian cancer. Int J Cancer. 2017;140(9):2051–9.
31. Hyman DM, Long KC, Tanner EJ, Grisham RN, Arnold AG, Bhatia J, Phillips MF, Spriggs DR, Soslow RA, Kauff ND, et al. Outcomes of primary surgical cytoreduction in patients with BRCA-associated high-grade serous ovarian carcinoma. Gynecol Oncol. 2012;126(2):224–8.
32. Pennington KP, Walsh T, Harrell MI, Lee MK, Pennil CC, Rendi MH, Thornton A, Norquist BM, Casadei S, Nord AS, et al. Germline and somatic mutations in homologous recombination genes predict platinum response and survival in ovarian, fallopian tube, and peritoneal carcinomas. Clin Cancer Res. 2014;20(3):764–75.
33. Fedier A, Steiner RA, Schwarz VA, Lenherr L, Haller U, Fink D. The effect of loss of Brca1 on the sensitivity to anticancer agents in p53-deficient cells. Int J Oncol. 2003;22(5):1169–73.
34. Evers B, Drost R, Schut E, de Bruin M, van der Burg E, Derksen PW, Holstege H, Liu X, van Drunen E, Beverloo HB, et al. Selective inhibition of BRCA2-deficient mammary tumor cell growth by AZD2281 and cisplatin. Clin Cancer Res. 2008;14(12):3916–25.

19

Linking a role of lncRNAs (long non-coding RNAs) with insulin resistance, accelerated senescence, and inflammation in patients with type 2 diabetes

Chandrakumar Sathishkumar, Paramasivam Prabu, Viswanathan Mohan and Muthuswamy Balasubramanyam*

Abstract

Background: Studying epigenetics is expected to provide precious information on how environmental factors contribute to type 2 diabetes mellitus (T2DM) at the genomic level. With the progress of the whole-genome resequencing efforts, it is now known that 75–90% of the human genome was transcribed to generate a series of long non-coding RNAs (lncRNAs). While lncRNAs are gaining widespread attention as potential and robust biomarkers in the genesis as well as progression of several disease states, their clinical relevance and regulatory mechanisms are yet to be explored in the field of metabolic disorders including diabetes. Despite the fact that Asian Indians are highly insulin resistant and more prone to develop T2DM and associated vascular complications, there is virtually lack of data on the role of lncRNAs in the clinical diabetes setting. Therefore, we sought to evaluate a panel of lncRNAs and senescence-inflammation signatures in peripheral blood mononuclear cells (PBMCs) from patients with type 2 diabetes (T2DM; $n = 30$) compared to individuals with normal glucose tolerance (NGT; $n = 32$).

Results: Compared to control subjects, expression levels of lncRNAs in PBMCs from type 2 diabetes patients showed significantly ($p < 0.05$) increased levels of HOTAIR, MEG3, LET, MALAT1, MIAT, CDKN2BAS1/ANRIL, XIST, PANDA, GAS5, Linc-p21, ENST00000550337.1, PLUTO, and NBR2. In contrast, lncRNA expression patterns of THRIL and SALRNA1 were significantly ($p < 0.05$) decreased in patients with T2DM compared to control subjects. At the transcriptional level, senescence markers (p53, p21, p16, and β-galactosidase), proinflammatory markers (TNF-α, IL6, MCP1, and IL1-β), and epigenetic signature of histone deacetylase-3 (HDAC3) were significantly ($p < 0.05$) elevated in patients with type 2 diabetes compared to control subjects. Interestingly, mRNA expression of Sirt1 and telomere length were significantly ($p < 0.05$) decreased in patients with type 2 diabetes compared to control subjects. Majority of the altered lncRNAs were positively correlated with poor glycemic control, insulin resistance, transcriptional markers of senescence, inflammation, and HDAC3 and negatively correlated with telomere length. Logistic regression analysis revealed a significant association of altered lncRNA signatures with T2DM, but this association was lost after adjusting for insulin resistance (HOMA-IR) and senescence markers.

Conclusion: Our study provides a clinically relevant evidence for the association of altered lncRNAs with poor glycemic control, insulin resistance, accelerated cellular senescence, and inflammation.

Keywords: lncRNA, SASP, HDAC3, Type 2 diabetes, Insulin resistance, Inflammation

* Correspondence: balusignal@gmail.com
Department of Cell and Molecular Biology and Dr. Rema Mohan High-Throughput Screening (HTS) Lab, Madras Diabetes Research Foundation and Dr. Mohan's Diabetes Specialties Centre, Gopalapuram, Chennai 600 086, India

Introduction

According to the latest edition of International Diabetes Federation Atlas [1], around 425 million people worldwide have diabetes and India alone harbors more than 73 millions of people with diabetes. While more than 90% of the diabetic population is affected majorly by type 2 diabetes mellitus (T2DM), it is a complex multi-factorial disease involving genetic, epigenetic, and environmental components. Several studies imply that accelerated aging, cellular senescence, and proinflammation are closely linked to the etiology of type 2 diabetes and insulin resistance [2, 3]. Although the association between the proinflammation and senescence in the development of insulin resistance and type 2 diabetes is well known, the underlying molecular mechanisms and upstream regulatory networks are only poorly understood. Epigenetics appears to play a major role in the regulation of inflammation and cellular senescence—the dual pathological features commonly associated with type 2 diabetes [4]. Aberrant epigenetic modifications such as DNA methylation, histone modification, and non-coding RNA alterations are well-recognized drivers for the cancer phenotype, but the accumulating evidence also implies their role in the etiology of diabetes and cardiovascular diseases.

Of the total genome that is transcribed, only 2% codes for proteins, whereas the vast majority of it is transcribed as non-coding RNAs which include long non-coding RNAs (lncRNAs), microRNAs, and others [5]. Of late, lncRNAs have gradually come into the spotlight for the increased appreciation of their functional importance both in health and disease [6]. lncRNAs were also found next to protein-coding genes that are under tight transcriptional control, and often, their expression pattern correlates with tissue differentiation, development, and disease [7]. The widespread dysregulation of lncRNA expression in several disease states and the finding that many lncRNAs are enriched for SNPs that associate with human traits/diseases have highlighted their role as master regulators [8, 9]. Challenging the concept that protein-coding genes are the sole contributors to the development of human disease, recent studies emphasize that lncRNAs mediate disease pathogenesis and hence should be studied and targeted for therapeutic benefits [10]. Accumulating literature on genetic, experimental, and epidemiological studies also highlights a growing list of lncRNAs that control glucose homeostasis and contribute to the pathogenesis of diabetes and its complications. Despite the fact that Asian Indians are highly insulin resistant [11] and more prone to develop T2DM and associated vascular complications [12], there is lack of data on the role of lncRNAs in the clinical diabetes setting and this is the rationale behind our study. Therefore, we planned to study the potential interactions among insulin resistance, cellular senescence, and proinflammation with a central focus on lncRNAs so as to better understand the clinical significance of these molecular perturbations in type 2 diabetes.

Research design and methods

Recruitment of the study subjects

Study participants with normal glucose tolerance (NGT; $n = 32$) and patients with type 2 diabetes (T2DM; $n = 30$) were recruited from Dr. Mohan's Diabetes Specialties Centre, Chennai, India, and from the ongoing epidemiological cohorts. The study was approved by the institutional ethics committee of the Madras Diabetes Research Foundation and conducted according to the principles of Declaration of Helsinki. Written informed consent was obtained from all the study participants prior to the start of the study. All the study participants were clinically well characterized into respective groups according to the World Health Organization (WHO) classification criteria. While all the diabetic patients were on oral hypoglycemic agent (OHA) treatment, < 10% were also on insulin, in addition to OHA.

Anthropometric measurements

Anthropometric measurements including weight, height, and waist circumference were obtained using standardized techniques. Height was noted down with a tape measured to the nearest centimeter. Weight was measured with traditional spring balance that was kept on a firm horizontal surface. Body mass index (BMI) was calculated using the formula: weight (kg)/height (m^2). Waist circumference was measured using a non-stretchable fiber measuring tape. Blood pressure was recorded from the right arm in a sitting position to the nearest 2 mmHg with a mercury sphygmomanometer (Diamond Deluxe BP apparatus, Pune, India). Two readings were taken 5 min apart, and the mean of the two readings was represented as the blood pressure.

Biochemical and clinical investigations

Fasting plasma glucose (glucose oxidase–peroxidase method), serum cholesterol (cholesterol oxidase–peroxidase–amidopyrine method), serum triglycerides (glycerol phosphate oxidase–peroxidase–amidopyrine method), and HDL cholesterol (direct method–polyethylene glycol-pretreated enzymes) were measured using Hitachi-912 Autoanalyser (Hitachi, Mannheim, Germany). The intra and inter assay co-efficient of variation for the biochemical assays was < 5%. Low-density lipoprotein (LDL) cholesterol was calculated using the Friedewald formula [13]. Glycated hemoglobin (HbAlc) was estimated by high-pressure liquid chromatography using the variant analyzer (Bio-Rad, Hercules, Calif., USA). Serum insulin was estimated using enzyme-linked immunosorbent assay (Calbiotech, CA). Insulin resistance was calculated using the homeostasis assessment model (HOMA-IR) using the formula: fasting insulin (μIU/mL) × fasting glucose (mmol/L)/22.5.

Blood collection and isolation of peripheral blood mononuclear cells (PBMCs)

Fasting blood (5–8 mL) was collected into the vacutainer tube and processed immediately for cell isolation within 2 h from the time of collection. Blood was processed for peripheral blood mononuclear cell (PBMC) isolation using Histopaque-1077 (Sigma-Aldrich) according to the standard protocol by overlaying the blood on density gradient solution and centrifugation at 1500–1800 rpm for 30 min. The buffy coat layer containing the PBMCs was aspirated, washed thrice with phosphate-buffered saline (PBS; pH 7.2–7.4), and aliquoted for various experiments.

RNA extraction and cDNA synthesis

Total RNA was extracted using TRIzol reagent (Invitrogen) according to the manufacturer's protocol. RNA quantity and quality were assessed by NanoDrop 2000 (Thermo Scientific) instrument. For the first-strand cDNA synthesis reaction, total RNA (1 μg) was adjusted with nuclease-free water and mixed with the cDNA synthesis master mix containing 100 units of RevertAid M-MuLV reverse transcriptase enzyme and 2× buffer, random hexamer primers (1×), 20 units of RNase inhibitor, and 10 mM dNTP solution mix. The resultant samples were incubated at 42 °C for 60 min for the first-strand cDNA synthesis followed by a 5-min incubation at 95 °C for enzyme deactivation. cDNA reaction negative control without reverse transcriptase enzyme (−RT) was also performed.

lncRNA/mRNA expression by Q-PCR

A panel of lncRNAs was chosen for this study based on their involvement in metabolic disorders as well as their emerging roles in senescence [14, 15]. The relative expression of the lncRNA/mRNA signatures were analyzed by preparing reaction mixer with FastStart Universal SYBR Green Master (Roche) and the corresponding gene-specific primers (Sigma) with diluted cDNA and final volume made up to 20 μL using nuclease-free water. Quantification and analysis were carried out in LightCycler® 96 real-time PCR System (Roche). The target gene expression was normalized to the house-keeping gene 18SrRNA (lncRNA) and β-actin (mRNA), and relative expression was determined using $2^{-\Delta\Delta CT}$ method. Non-template control (NTC) was also performed for each reaction assay plate.

DNA isolation and measurement of telomere length

For the measurement of telomere length, DNA was isolated from the whole blood by phenol–chloroform extraction and ethanol precipitation [16]. Relative telomere length was determined by real-time PCR approach as previously described by Cawthon [17] with a minor modification in the PCR temperature conditions. This method measures the factor by which the ratio of telomere repeat copy number to single-gene copy number differs between a sample and that of a reference DNA sample. PCR amplification was achieved using telomere (T) and single copy gene, 36B4 (encodes acidic ribosomal phosphoprotein) primers (S), which serves as a quantitative control. The mean telomere repeat gene sequence (T) to a reference single copy gene (S) was represented as T/S ratio—a reflection of relative telomere length [3].

Statistical analysis

All data are represented as mean ± standard error mean (SEM) unless otherwise mentioned as standard deviation (SD). Based on our pilot study on the expression levels of lncRNAs and using the SPSS software, the minimum sample size required for the study was calculated as 28 in each group considering the level of significance set at 0.05 and the statistical power at 0.90. Comparison between groups was performed using the independent sample Student *t* test with $p < 0.05$ as the criterion for statistical significance. Pearson correlation analysis was done between variables and the risk factors. Binary logistic regression analysis was performed to show the association between lncRNAs (independent variable) and diabetes (dependent variable). All analyses were done using SPSS Statistics (version 20.0) and GraphPad Prism (version 6).

Results

Clinical and biochemical characteristics of the study groups

Clinical and biochemical characteristics of the study subjects are depicted in Table 1. BMI and waist circumference were slightly and significantly higher in patients with type 2 diabetes compared to control subjects. Patients with type 2 diabetes exhibited significantly ($p < 0.001$) increased fasting plasma glucose and HbA1c compared to the control subjects. T2DM patients were also hyperinsulinemic and insulin resistant as characterized by significantly elevated fasting insulin levels and HOMA-IR values, respectively. Blood pressure and lipid parameters did not differ significantly between the groups.

Altered lncRNA signatures in T2DM

Compared to control subjects, expression profiling of lncRNAs in PBMCs from type 2 diabetes patients showed significantly ($p < 0.05$) increased levels of HOTAIR, MEG3, LET, MALAT1, MIAT, CDKN2BAS1/ANRIL, XIST, PANDA, GAS5, Linc-p21, ENST00000550337.1, PLUTO, and NBR2 (Fig. 1). In contrast, lncRNA expression patterns of THRIL and SALRNA1 were significantly ($p < 0.05$) decreased in patients with T2DM compared to control subjects (Fig. 1).

Table 1 Clinical and biochemical characterization of the study subjects

Parameter	Normal glucose tolerance [NGT] ($n = 32$)	Type 2 diabetes mellitus [T2DM] ($n = 30$)	p value
Age (years)	44 ± 8	46 ± 8	0.218
Gender—male (female)	18 (14)	18 (12)	–
Body mass index (kg/m^2)	25 ± 3.1	27 ± 4	*0.015*
Waist circumference (cm)	85 ± 8	94 ± 9	*< 0.001*
Fasting plasma glucose (mg/dL)	87 ± 9	136 ± 24	*< 0.001*
Glycated hemoglobin—HbA1c (%)	5.6 ± 0.34	8.1 ± 1.9	*< 0.001*
HOMA-IR	1.8 ± 0.8	6.9 ± 3	*< 0.001*
Fasting insulin (μIU/mL)	8.6 ± 3.5	22 ± 7.2	*< 0.001*
Systolic blood pressure (mmHg)	120 ± 25	131 ± 21	0.079
Diastolic blood pressure (mmHg)	79 ± 13	80 ± 8	0.795
Total cholesterol (mg/dL)	174 ± 28	169 ± 37	0.545
Serum triglycerides (mg/dL)	132 ± 71	138 ± 49	0.737
HDL cholesterol (mg/dL)	41 ± 10	39 ± 7	0.352
LDL cholesterol (mg/dL)	107 ± 21	102 ± 34	0.568
VLDL	27 ± 14	28 ± 10	0.732

Data represented as mean ± SD. Italicized value represents statistically significant compared to NGT

Augmentation of HDAC3 and impaired Sirt1 expression in T2DM

Transcriptional profiling revealed that mRNA expression of HDAC3 was significantly ($p < 0.05$) increased while the Sirt1 level was significantly ($p < 0.05$) decreased in patients with type 2 diabetes compared to control subjects (Fig. 2).

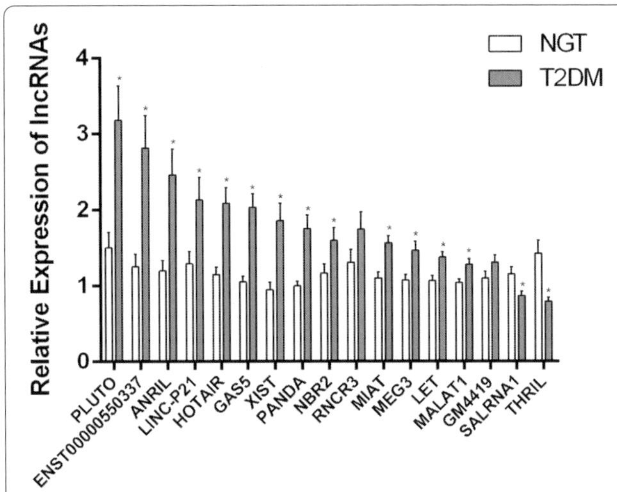

Fig. 1 Quantitative real-time PCR analysis of a panel of lncRNA expression levels in PBMCs from the study groups (NGT vs T2DM). Bars represent the mean ± SEM; *p value < 0.05 compared to control subjects

Altered senescence, inflammation, and telomere length in T2DM

At the transcriptional level, senescence markers, viz., p53, p21, p16, and β-galactosidase 1 (GLB1), were significantly ($p < 0.05$) elevated in patients with type 2 diabetes compared to control subjects (Fig. 3a). As a final read-out of augmented cellular senescence, patients with T2DM were also characterized by significantly ($p < 0.05$) shortened telomeres compared to control subjects (Fig. 3b). Interestingly, mRNA expression levels of proinflammatory gene mediators, viz. TNF-α, IL6, MCP1 and IL1-β, were also significantly upregulated ($p < 0.05$) in PBMCs from patients with type 2 diabetes, implying an acquisition state of senescence-associated secretory phenotype (Fig. 4).

Correlation analysis

A detailed correlation analysis of lncRNAs with various clinical and biochemical parameters (Additional file 1: Table S1) and molecular parameters (Additional file 2: Table S2) of the study subjects were summarized in the supplement tables. Majority of the altered lncRNAs were positively correlated with poor glycemic control, insulin resistance, transcriptional markers of senescence, inflammation, and HDAC3 and negatively correlated with telomere length. In contrast, expression levels of lncRNAs, viz., SALRNA1 and THRIL, were negatively correlated to glycemic control, insulin resistance, markers of senescence, inflammation, and HDAC3 and positively correlated to telomere length.

Logistic regression analysis

Logistic regression analysis using type 2 diabetes as dependent variable revealed that altered expression levels of lncRNAs, viz., PLUTO, ENST00000550337.1, CDKN2BAS1, LincRNA-P21, HOTAIR, GAS5, XIST, PANDA, NBR2, MIAT, MEG3, LET, MALAT1, SALRNA1, and THRIL, were associated significantly with T2DM, and this statistical significance was persisted even after adjusting for confounding factors like age and BMI. Interestingly, this statistical association was lost when adjusted for HOMA-IR and senescence markers. This implies that the association between lncRNAs and T2DM could be closely linked to insulin resistance and accelerated senescence with downstream inflammatory signaling (Table 2).

Discussion

Recent literature implies that the dysregulation of lncRNA expression and functionality contributes to several pathophysiological states as several lncRNAs get

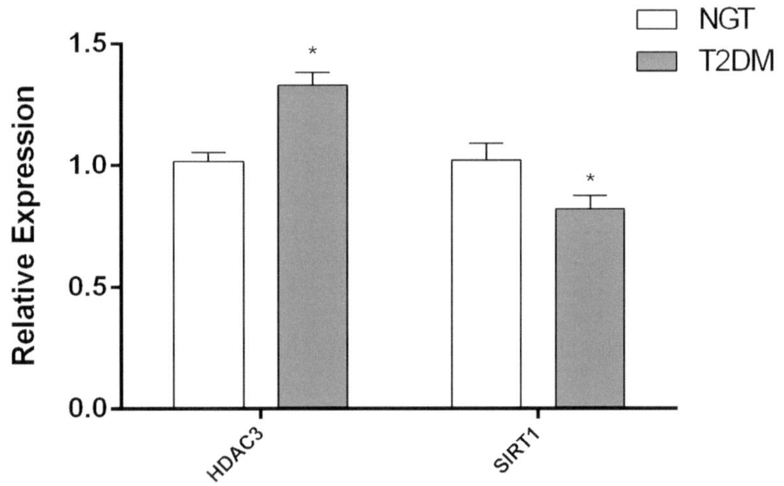

Fig. 2 Quantitative real-time PCR analysis of HDAC3 and SIRT1 in PBMCs from the study groups (NGT vs T2DM). Bars represent the mean ± SEM; *p value < 0.05 compared to control subjects

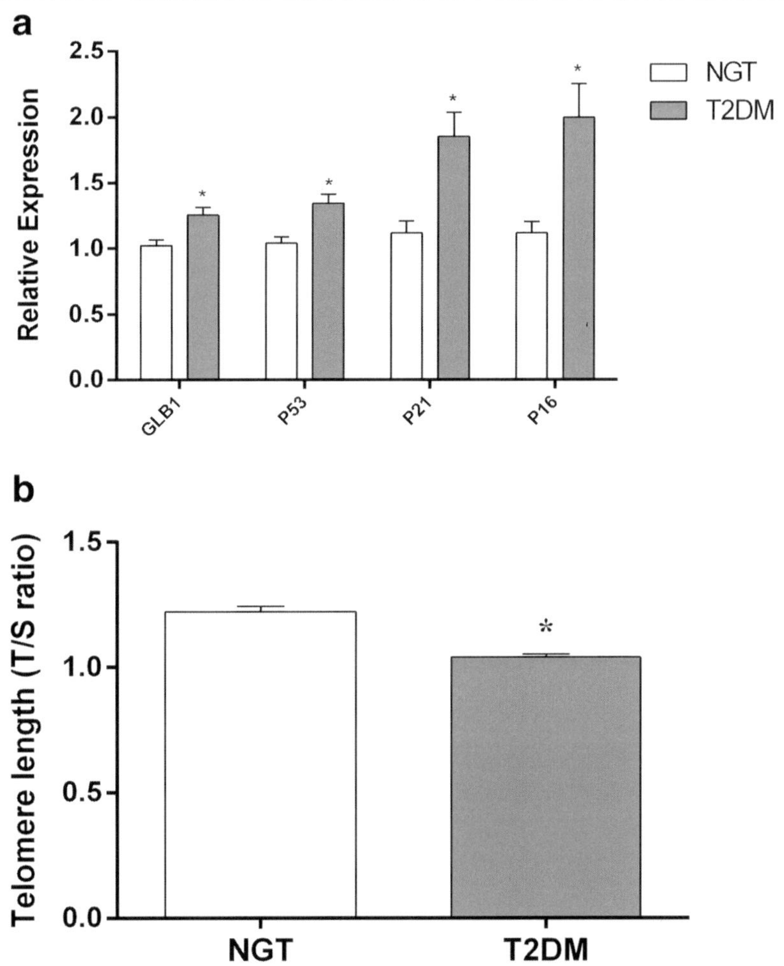

Fig. 3 Quantitative real-time PCR analysis of senescence marker gene expression levels, viz., GLB1, P53, P21, and P16 (**a**), and telomere length (**b**) in PBMCs from the study groups (NGT vs T2DM). Bars represent the mean ± SEM; *p value < 0.05 compared to control subjects

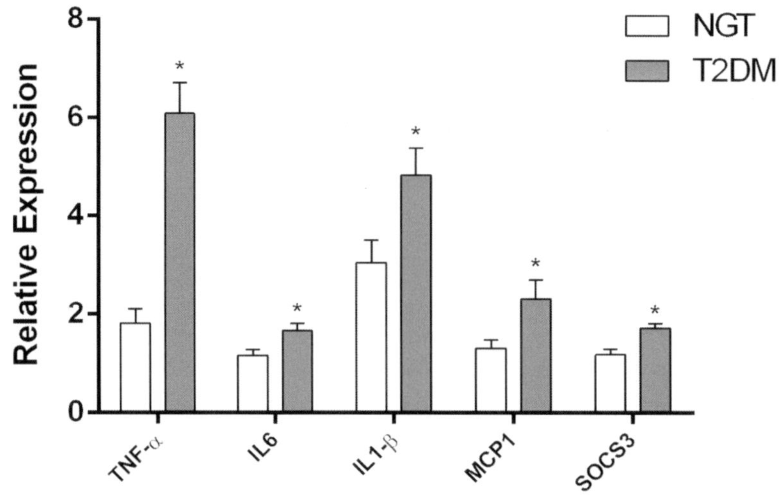

Fig. 4 Quantitative real-time PCR analysis of inflammatory signature gene expression levels, viz., TNFα, IL6, MCP1, IL1β, and SOCS3 in PBMCs from the study groups (NGT vs T2DM). Bars represent the mean ± SEM; *p value < 0.05 compared to control subjects

validated as bona fide prognostic/diagnostic markers and drug targets [9, 18, 19]. The role of lncRNAs in the pathogenesis of type 2 diabetes mellitus and related complications has only recently been recognized, but there is already some evidence for their involvement in many of the pathophysiological mechanisms that are linked to the genesis and progression of disease [20, 21]. Despite the fact that Asian Indians are highly insulin resistant [10], more prone to develop type 2 diabetes mellitus (T2DM) and associated vascular complications [11], and exhibit increased susceptibility to early β-cell dysfunction [22], there is virtually lack of data on the role of lncRNAs in the clinical diabetes setting. Our study is the first report from India to show an association of altered signatures of lncRNAs in T2DM with pathological connectivity reflected by poor glycemic control, insulin resistance, accelerated cellular senescence, and meta-inflammation.

Table 2 Binary logistic regression analysis using type 2 diabetes as dependent variable

	Unadjusted		Adjusted for age and BMI		Adjusted for HOMA-IR		Adjusted for senescence markers (GLB, P53, P21, P16, and TL)		Adjusted for inflammatory markers (TNF-α, IL6, MCP1, IL1-β, and SOCS3)	
	β	*p*	*β*	*p*	*β*	*p*	*β*	*p*	*β*	*p*
PLUTO	1.721	*0.005*	1.827	*0.003*	23.673	0.063	1.848	0.210	2.204	*0.025*
ENST00000550337.1	2.023	*0.004*	1.925	*0.013*	2.984	0.132	33.73	0.184	4.026	*0.038*
CDKN2BAS1	3.173	*0.006*	4.925	*0.002*	4.188	0.068	2.741	0.100	2.995	*0.044*
lincRNA-p21	1.867	*0.021*	1.970	*0.033*	3.492	0.096	2.283	0.311	6.395	*0.013*
HOTAIR	4.348	*0.001*	5.256	*0.001*	2.556	0.342	1.651	0.524	8.125	*0.015*
GAS5	10.642	*0.001*	14.054	*0.001*	20.820	0.226	22.512	0.128	12.214	0.069
XIST	0.388	*0.003*	3.824	*0.004*	3.677	0.145	2.318	0.386	3.166	*0.024*
PANDA	7.960	*0.003*	15.737	*0.002*	30.052	*0.041*	27.726	0.151	3.548	0.253
NBR2	2.045	*0.041*	1.728	0.159	1.496	0.522	1.869	0.443	2.675	0.141
RNCR3	1.464	0.144	1.650	0.065	1.795	0.394	1.582	0.410	1.740	0.225
MIAT	6.591	*0.002*	5.293	*0.012*	8.383	0.235	8.753	0.181	5.388	0.118
MEG3	5.669	*0.013*	6.444	*0.017*	17.060	0.141	12.830	0.063	57.903	*0.023*
LET	7.116	*0.014*	5.806	*0.036*	6.736	0.068	4.399	0.534	2.079	0.584
MALAT1	9.945	*0.008*	5.156	*0.046*	4.712	0.193	12.858	0.343	33.033	0.086
GM4419	2.468	0.104	2.142	0.242	3.254	0.232	4.832	0.293	1.937	0.433
SALRNA1	0.161	*0.013*	0.114	*0.009*	0.029	0.127	0.072	0.057	0.092	0.100
THRIL	0.047	*0.001*	0.529	*0.001*	0.013	0.084	0.063	0.139	0.333	0.271

Our study is in consistent with the recent literature of several lncRNAs upregulated in diabetes state. In support of our findings, increased expression of GAS5 [23] and lncRNA ENST00000550337.1 [24] was reported in type 2 diabetes even with high diagnostic claim and biomarker value. A role for lncRNAs XIST [25] and GM4419 [26] was implicated in diabetic nephropathy while alterations in PANDA [27] and NBR2 [28] P21 [29] were linked to cellular senescence, AMPK regulation, and liver fibrosis, respectively. Expression levels of lncRNA-LET was shown to be decreased in a certain type of cancers [30], but we observed it to be upregulated in patients with type 2 diabetes. MIAT is identified to be involved in various diseases, particularly myocardial infarction, diabetic retinopathy, and various other microvascular complications [31]. Similarly, lncRNA RNCR3 was shown to be increased in retinal vasculature of an animal model as well as in vitro cell model [32]. While lncRNA PLUTO has been shown to be downregulated in islets from donors who are patients with type 2 diabetes and pre-diabetes subjects [33], our study observed a highly significant upregulation of PLUTO in patients with type 2 diabetes. Previous studies also reported that upregulated expression of lncRNA MALAT1 was linked to hyperglycemia-induced inflammation and endothelial dysfunction [34], diabetic nephropathy [35], and gestational diabetes mellitus [36]. In vitro studies demonstrated that HOTAIR interacts with the various chromatin-modifying enzymes and thereby participates in the regulation of gene expression [37]. A functional role for HOTAIR in the diabetes pathogenesis is yet to be established; however, its role has been hinted to be associated with regional adiposity [38]. lncRNA MEG3 has an important regulatory role in beta cell function [39], and the knock-down of MEG3 has been shown contributing to the pathology of diabetic microvascular complication [40]. In contrast, MEG3 gene expression was shown upregulated in the hepatocytes from mice fed with high-fat diet as well as in ob/ob mice and this has been linked to increased hepatic gluconeogenesis [41].

Our study provides the first preliminary evidence that expression of the long non-coding RNAs, THRIL, and SALRNA1 were decreased in patients with type 2 diabetes and negatively correlated with hyperglycemia, senescence, and inflammation. THRIL was shown to regulate TNF-α expression through an epigenetic mechanism, and TNF-α can also reduce THRIL expression via a negative feedback action [42]. Similarly, SAL-RNA1 was earlier identified as putative age-delaying lncRNA, since its reduction with small inhibitory RNAs (siRNA) induced rapid aging changes of the fibroblasts, such as large cell morphology, positive β-galactosidase activity, and upregulation of p53 [43]. Notably, lncRNA ANRIL shown upregulated in our study was also linked to CDKN2A/B, a strong type 2 diabetes risk gene variant [44, 45].

It is interesting to note that the majority of differentially expressed lncRNAs in patients with type 2 diabetes observed in our study are involved in cell cycle regulation and senescence and their expression levels correlated to poor glycemic control, insulin resistance, accelerated senescence, and inflammation. Several lncRNAs were reported to influence the molecular processes that underlie age-associated phenotypes and play an important role in accelerated aging [4, 46]. Type 2 diabetes has been linked to cellular senescence, senescence-associated secretory phenotype (SASP), and accelerated aging [47, 48], and our lab was the first one in the world literature to report an association of increased telomere shortening in patients with type 2 diabetes [2, 3]. Earlier, we have also shown increased HDAC3 epigenetic signature in patients with type 2 diabetes [49], and in the present study, there was a positive correlation of HDAC3 mRNA expression with majority of the lncRNAs and this endorses the concerted and coordinated interactions between lncRNAs and histone modifications [50].

Our work offers an avenue for several translational applications including a role of lncRNAs in lifestyle changes. Recent findings suggest a putative role of non-coding RNAs in physical activity and several miRNAs have been identified as modulators of exercise-induced adaption at both systemic and tissue levels [51]. Contrast to miRNAs, little is known about the role of long non-coding RNAs (lncRNAs) in exercise. Identification of the role of lncRNAs in exercise will improve our understanding of exercise physiology and has the potential to enhance the application of current therapeutic approaches. In fact, a micropeptide encoded by a putative lncRNA has been shown to regulate muscle performance [52]. Although very little is known about the relationship between lncRNAs and dietary factors, it appears that dietary manipulation could also beneficially alter the expression of lncRNAs and thereby ensure health [53].

One of the limitations of our study is of its cross-sectional nature as well as small sample size, and hence, the findings of the study and its conclusions should be interpreted with caution. From this pilot study, we could not extrapolate causal link of alterations in lncRNAs with type 2 diabetes, and it needs replication and prospective follow-up studies. Secondly, considering the tissue-specific and heterogeneous actions of lncRNAs, the alterations seen in PBMCs might only mirror disease-pathology directionality. However, the altered expression profile of lncRNAs in PBMCs has been shown to reflect the pathophysiology in different disease states including multiple sclerosis [54], myocardial infarction [55], and rheumatoid arthritis [56]. In fact, a recent study of deep RNA sequencing uncovered a repertoire of human macrophage lncRNAs modulated by macrophage activation and closely linked it to the pathophysiology of cardiometabolic diseases [57].

Conclusion

To conclude, our study is of its first kind in India to report altered lncRNA profiles linked to poor glycemic control, insulin resistance, senescence, and proinflammation in patients with type 2 diabetes. A better understanding of the mechanisms underlying the functions of lncRNAs will help us to understand the ever-expanding pathophysiology of diabetes and its complications and thereby adapt to prevention strategies as well as to develop novel therapeutic agents.

Abbreviations

BMI: Body mass index; GLB1: β-Galactosidase 1; HbA1C: Glycated hemoglobin; HDAC: Histone deacetylase; HOMA-IR: Homeostatic model assessment-insulin resistance; IL-1β: Interleukin-1 beta; IL-6: Interleukin-6; lncRNAs: Long non-coding RNAs; MCP-1: Monocyte chemoattractant protein 1; NFκB: Nuclear factor kappa-light-chain-enhancer of activated B cells; NGT: Normal glucose tolerance; P16: Cyclin-dependent kinase inhibitor 2A; P21: Cyclin-dependent kinase inhibitor 1A; P53: Tumor protein/tumor suppressor 53; PBMCs: Peripheral blood mononuclear cells; SASP: Senescence-associated secretory phenotype; Sirt1: Sirtuin (silent mating-type information regulation 2 homolog) 1; SOCS-3: Suppressor of cytokine signaling 3; T2DM: Type 2 diabetes mellitus; TNF-α: Tumor necrosis factor-α

Funding

The authors acknowledge research grant support from the Department of Biotechnology (DBT), New Delhi, and the Indian Council of Medical Research (ICMR), Govt. of India and senior research fellowship assistance from the Council of Scientific and Industrial Research (CSIR), New Delhi, India.

Authors' contributions

MB conceived, designed, supervised, and commented on all drafts of this paper. CS and PP coordinated the clinical sample collection, conducted the overall experiments, and participated in the data collection and analysis and molecular investigations and helped in the drafts. VM and MB contributed to the data interpretation and manuscript completion. All authors read and approved the final manuscript.

Competing interests

The authors declare that they have no competing interests.

References

1. International Diabetes Federation. IDF diabetes atlas. 8th ed. Brussels: International Diabetes Federation; 2017.
2. Adaikalakoteswari A, Balasubramanyam M, Mohan V. Telomere shortening occurs in Asian Indian type 2 diabetic patients. Diabet Med. 2005;22:1151–6.
3. Monickaraj F, Aravind S, Gokulakrishnan K, Sathishkumar C, Prabu P, Prabu D, Mohan V, Balasubramanyam M. Accelerated aging as evidenced by increased telomere shortening and mitochondrial DNA depletion in patients with type 2 diabetes. Mol Cell Biochem. 2012;365:343–50.
4. Grammatikakis I, Panda AC, Abdelmohsen K, Gorospe M. Long noncoding RNAs (lncRNAs) and the molecular hallmarks of aging. Aging. 2014;6: 992–1009.
5. Hangauer MJ, Vaughn IW, McManus MT. Pervasive transcription of the human genome produces thousands of previously unidentified long intergenic noncoding RNAs. PLoS Genet. 2013;9:e1003569.
6. Morris KV, Mattick JS. The rise of regulatory RNA. Nat Rev Genet. 2014;15: 423–37.
7. Batista PJ, Chang HY. Long noncoding RNAs: cellular address codes in development and disease. Cell. 2013;152:1298–307.
8. Du Z, Fei T, Verhaak RGW, Su Z, Zhang Y, Brown M, Chen Y, Liu SX. Integrative genomic analyses reveal clinically relevant long noncoding RNAs in human cancer. Nat Struct Mol Biol. 2013;20:908–13.
9. Jain S, Thakkar N, Chhatai J, Bhadra M, Bhadra U. Long non-coding RNA: functional agent for disease traits. RNA Biol. 2016;14:1–14.
10. DiStefano JK. The emerging role of long noncoding RNAs in human disease. Methods Mol Biol. 2018;1706:91–110.
11. Sharp PS, Mohan V, Levy JC, Mather HM, Kohner EM. Insulin resistance in patients of Asian Indian and European origin with non-insulin dependent diabetes. Horm Metab Res. 1987;19:84–5.
12. Unnikrishnan R, Pradeepa R, Joshi SR, Mohan V. Type 2 diabetes: demystifying the global epidemic. Diabetes. 2017;66:1432–42.
13. Friedewald WT, Levy RI, Fredrickson DS. Estimation of the concentration of low-density lipoprotein cholesterol in plasma, without use of the preparative ultracentrifuge. Clin Chem. 1972;18:499–502.
14. Montes M, Lund AH. Emerging roles of lncRNAs in senescence. FEBS J. 2016; 283:2414–26.
15. Kim C, Kang D, Lee EK, Lee JS. Long noncoding RNAs and RNA-binding proteins in oxidative stress, cellular senescence, and age-related diseases. Oxidative Med Cell Longev. 2017;2017:2062384.
16. Köchl S, Niederstätter H, Parson W. DNA extraction and quantitation of forensic samples using the phenol-chloroform method and real-time PCR. Methods Mol Biol. 2005;297:13–30.
17. Cawthon RM. Telomere measurement by quantitative PCR. Nucleic Acids Res. 2002;30:e4730.
18. Matsui M, Corey DR. Non-coding RNAs as drug targets. Nat Rev Drug Discov. 2017;16:167–79.
19. Ghanbari M, Peters MJ, de Vries PS, Boer CG, van Rooij JGJ, Lee YC, Kumar V, Uitterlinden AG, Ikram MA, Wijmenga C, et al. A systematic analysis highlights multiple long non-coding RNAs associated with cardiometabolic disorders. J Hum Genet. 2018;63:431–46.
20. Leti F, DiStefano JK. Long noncoding RNAs as diagnostic and therapeutic targets in type 2 diabetes and related complications. Genes (Basel). 2017;22:8.
21. Goyal N, Kesharwani D, Datta M. Lnc-ing non-coding RNAs with metabolism and diabetes: roles of lncRNAs. Cell Mol Life Sci. 2018;75:1827–37.
22. Mohan V, Amutha A, Ranjani H, Unnikrishnan R, Datta M, Anjana R, Staimez L, Ali MK, Narayan VKM. Associations of β-cell function and insulin resistance with youth-onset type 2 diabetes and prediabetes among Asian Indians. Diabetes Technol Ther. 2013;15:315–22.
23. Carter G, Miladinovic B, Patel AA, Deland L, Mastorides S, Patel NA. Circulating long noncoding RNA GAS5 levels are correlated to prevalence of type 2 diabetes mellitus. BBA Clinical. 2015;4:102–7.
24. Li X, Zhao Z, Gao C, Rao L, Hao P, Jian D, Li W, Tang H, Li M. The diagnostic value of whole blood lncRNA ENST00000550337.1 for pre-diabetes and type 2 diabetes mellitus. Exp Clin Endocrinol Diabetes. 2017;125:377–83.
25. Huang Y-S, Hsieh H-Y, Shih H-M, Sytwu H-K, Wu C-C. Urinary Xist is a potential biomarker for membranous nephropathy. Biochem Biophys Res Commun. 2014;452:415–21.
26. Yi H, Peng R, L-y Z, Sun Y, H-m P, H-d L, Yu L-j, A-l L, Y-j Z, W-h J, et al. LincRNA-Gm4419 knockdown ameliorates NF-κB/NLRP3 inflammasome-mediated inflammation in diabetic nephropathy. Cell Death Dis. 2017;8:e2583.
27. Puvvula P, Desetty R, Pineau P, Marchio A, Moon A, Dejean A, Bischof O. Long noncoding RNA PANDA and scaffold-attachment-factor SAFA control senescence entry and exit. Nat Commun. 2014;5:5323.
28. Liu X, Gan B. lncRNA NBR2 modulates cancer cell sensitivity to phenformin through GLUT1. Cell Cycle. 2016;15:3471–81.
29. Yu F, Lu Z, Chen B, Dong P, Zheng J. Identification of a novel lincRNA-p21-miR-181b-PTEN signaling cascade in liver fibrosis. Mediat Inflamm. 2016; 2016:9856538.
30. Sun Q, Liu H, Li L, Zhang S, Liu K, Liu Y, Yang C. Long noncoding RNA-LET, which is repressed by EZH2, inhibits cell proliferation and induces apoptosis of nasopharyngeal carcinoma cell. Med Oncol. 2015;32:226.
31. Liao J, He Q, Li M, Chen Y, Liu Y, Wang J. LncRNA MIAT: myocardial infarction associated and more. Gene. 2015;578:158–61.
32. Shan K, Jiang Q, Wang QX, Wang NY, Yang H, Yao DM, Liu C, Li MX, Yao J, Liu B, et al. Role of long non-coding RNA-RNCR3 in atherosclerosis-related vascular dysfunction. Cell Death Dis. 2016;7:e2248.

33. Akerman I, Tu Z, Beucher A, Rolando D, Sauty-Colace C, Benazra M, Nakic N, Yang J, Wang H, Pasquali L, et al. Human pancreatic β cell lncRNAs control cell-specific regulatory networks. Cell Metab. 2017;25:400–11.
34. Puthanveetil P, Chen S, Feng B, Gautam A, Chakrabarti S. Long non-coding RNA MALAT1 regulates hyperglycaemia induced inflammatory process in the endothelial cells. J Cell Mol Med. 2015;19:1418–25.
35. Li X, Zeng L, Cao C, Lu C, Lian W, Han J, Zhang X, Zhang J, Tang T, Li M. Long noncoding RNA MALAT1 regulates renal tubular epithelial pyroptosis by modulated miR-23c targeting of ELAVL1 in diabetic nephropathy. Exp Cell Res. 2017;350:327–35.
36. Zhang Y, Wu H, Wang F, Ye M, Zhu H, Bu S. Long non-coding RNA MALAT1 expression in patients with gestational diabetes mellitus. Int J Gynecol Obstet. 2018;140:164–9.
37. Gupta RA, Shah N, Wang KC, Kim J, Horlings HM, Wong DJ, Tsai M-C, Hung T, Argani P, Rinn JL, et al. Long non-coding RNA HOTAIR reprograms chromatin state to promote cancer metastasis. Nature. 2010;464:1071–6.
38. Divoux A, Karastergiou K, Xie H, Guo W, Perera RJ, Fried SK, Smith SR. Identification of a novel lncRNA in gluteal adipose tissue and evidence for its positive effect on preadipocyte differentiation. Obesity. 2014;22:1781–5.
39. You L, Wang N, Yin D, Wang L, Jin F, Zhu Y, Yuan Q, De W. Downregulation of long noncoding RNA Meg3 affects insulin synthesis and secretion in mouse pancreatic beta cells. J Cell Physiol. 2016;231:852–62.
40. Qiu G-Z, Tian W, Fu H-T, Li C-P, Liu B. Long noncoding RNA-MEG3 is involved in diabetes mellitus-related microvascular dysfunction. Biochem Biophys Res Commun. 2016;471:135–41.
41. Zhu X, Wu Y-B, Zhou J, Kang D-M. Upregulation of lncRNA MEG3 promotes hepatic insulin resistance via increasing FoxO1 expression. Biochem Biophys Res Commun. 2016;469:319–25.
42. Li Z, Chao T-C, Chang K-Y, Lin N, Patil VS, Shimizu C, Head SR, Burns JC, Rana TM. The long noncoding RNA THRIL regulates TNFα expression through its interaction with hnRNPL. Proc Natl Acad Sci. 2014;111:1002–7.
43. Abdelmohsen K, Panda A, Kang MJ, Xu J, Selimyan R, Yoon JH, Martindale JL, De S, Wood WH, Becker KG, et al. Senescence-associated lncRNAs: senescence-associated long noncoding RNAs. Aging Cell. 2013;12:890–900.
44. Kommoju U, Samy S, Maruda J, Irgam K, Kotla J, Velaga L, Reddy B. Association of CDKAL1, CDKN2A/B & HHEX gene polymorphisms with type 2 diabetes mellitus in the population of Hyderabad, India. Indian J Med Res. 2016;143:455–63.
45. Chidambaram M, Radha V, Mohan V. Replication of recently described type 2 diabetes gene variants in a South Indian population. Metabolism. 2010;59: 1760–6.
46. Degirmenci U, Lei S. Role of lncRNAs in cellular aging. Front Endocrinol. 2016;7:151.
47. Palmer AK, Tchkonia T, LeBrasseur NK, Chini EN, Xu M, Kirkland JL. Cellular senescence in type 2 diabetes: a therapeutic opportunity. Diabetes. 2015;64: 2289–98.
48. Prattichizzo F, Nigris V, Sala L, Procopio A, Olivieri F, Ceriello A. "Inflammaging" as a druggable target: a senescence-associated secretory phenotype—centered view of type 2 diabetes. Oxidative Med Cell Longev. 2016;2016:1810327.
49. Sathishkumar C, Prabu P, Balakumar M, Lenin R, Prabhu D, Anjana R, Mohan V, Balasubramanyam M. Augmentation of histone deacetylase 3 (HDAC3) epigenetic signature at the interface of proinflammation and insulin resistance in patients with type 2 diabetes. Clin Epigenetics. 2016;8:125.
50. Han P, Chang C-P. Long non-coding RNA and chromatin remodeling. RNA Biol. 2015;12:1094–8.
51. Wang H, Liang Y, Li Y. Non-coding RNAs in exercise. Non-coding RNA Investigation. 2017;1:10. https://doi.org/10.21037/ncri.2017.09.01.
52. Anderson DM, Anderson KM, Chang C-L, Makarewich CA, Nelson BR, McAnally JR, Kasaragod P, Shelton JM, Liou J, Bassel-Duby R, et al. A micropeptide encoded by a putative long noncoding RNA regulates muscle performance. Cell. 2015;160:595–606.
53. Beaver LM, Kuintzle R, Buchanan A, Wiley MW, Glasser ST, Wong CP, Johnson GS, Chang JH, Löhr CV, Williams DE, et al. Long noncoding RNAs and sulforaphane: a target for chemoprevention and suppression of prostate cancer. J Nutr Biochem. 2017;42:72–83.
54. Zhang F, Gao C, Ma XF, Peng XL, Zhang RX, Kong DX, Simard AR, Hao JW. Expression profile of long noncoding RNAs in peripheral blood mononuclear cells from multiple sclerosis patients. CNS Neurosci Ther. 2016; 22:298–305.
55. Vausort M, Wagner DR, Devaux Y. Long noncoding RNAs in patients with acute myocardial infarction. Circ Res. 2014;115:668–77.
56. Yuan M, Wang S, Yu L, Qu B, Xu L, Liu L, Sun H, Li C, Shi Y, Liu H. Long noncoding RNA profiling revealed differentially expressed lncRNAs associated with disease activity in PBMCs from patients with rheumatoid arthritis. PLoS One. 2017;12:e0186795.
57. Zhang H, Xue C, Wang Y, Shi J, Zhang X, Li W, Nunez S, Foulkes AS, Lin J, Hinkle CC, Yang W, Morrisey EE, Rader DJ, Li M, Reilly MP. Deep RNA sequencing uncovers a repertoire of human macrophage long intergenic noncoding RNAs modulated by macrophage activation and associated with cardiometabolic diseases. J Am Heart Assoc. 2017;6. https://doi.org/10.1161/JAHA.117.007431.

Identification of TBX2 and TBX3 variants in patients with conotruncal heart defects by target sequencing

Huilin Xie[1†], Erge Zhang[1†], Nanchao Hong[1], Qihua Fu[2], Fen Li[3], Sun Chen[1], Yu Yu[1*] and Kun Sun[1*]

Abstract

Background: Conotruncal heart defects (CTDs) are heterogeneous congenital heart malformations that result from outflow tract dysplasia; however, the genetic determinants underlying CTDs remain unclear. Increasing evidence demonstrates that dysfunctional TBX2 and TBX3 result in outflow tract malformations, implying that both of them are involved in CTD pathogenesis. We screened for TBX2 and TBX3 variants in a large cohort of CTD patients ($n = 588$) and population-matched healthy controls ($n = 300$) by target sequencing and genetically analyzed the expression and function of these variants.

Results: The probably damaging variants p.R608W, p.T249I, and p.R616Q of TBX2 and p.A192T, p.M65L, and p.A562V of TBX3 were identified in CTD patients, but none in controls. All altered amino acids were highly conserved evolutionarily. Moreover, our data suggested that mRNA and protein expressions of TBX2 and TBX3 variants were altered compared with those of the wild-type. We screened PEA3 and MEF2C as novel downstream genes of TBX2 and TBX3, respectively. Functional analysis revealed that TBX2R608W and TBX2R616Q variant proteins further activated HAS2 promoter but failed to activate PEA3 promoter and that TBX3A192T and TBX3A562V variant proteins showed a reduced transcriptional activity over MEF2C promoter.

Conclusions: Our results indicate that the R608W and R616Q variants of TBX2 as well as the A192T and A562V variants of TBX3 contribute to CTD etiology; this was the first association of variants of TBX2 and TBX3 to CTDs based on a large population.

Keywords: TBX2, TBX3, Variant, Conotruncal heart defects, Target sequencing

Background

Conotruncal heart defects (CTDs) are a group of complex congenital heart malformations with an estimated prevalence of 0.1% of live births and roughly 10–25% in congenital heart defects (CHD) [1] and are caused by abnormal development of the outflow tract (OFT) in embryo or abnormal configuration and arrangement of the ventricle, septal tissue, and large vessels; CTDs include the tetralogy of Fallot (TOF), persistent truncus arteriosus (PTA), double outlet of right ventricle (DORV), transposition of the great arteries (TGA), single atrium (SA), single ventricle (SV), and others. CTDs commonly occur in infants and children and are chief causes of infant death and childhood disability. Most CTD patients require catheter-based or surgical interventions early in life because without intervention, the diseases could lead to poor quality of life with mental and physical retardation, severe cardiac arrhythmias, heart failure, and even sudden death. Although therapeutic regimens have increased survival into adulthood in patients with CTDs, the morbidity and mortality rates remain high in survivors [2, 3]. In addition, CTDs induce heavy economic burdens on society, especially as the survival rates and the number of adults living with CTDs increase [4].

The development of the OFT in the embryonic stage is an elaborate regulatory process, which includes the formation and development of the secondary heart field (SHF) and cardiac neural crest (CNC), during which any abnormal factor of inheritance or environment can lead to abnormal proliferation, differentiation, or migration

* Correspondence: yuyu@xinhuamed.com.cn; sunkun@xinhuamed.com.cn
†Huilin Xie and Erge Zhang contributed equally to this work.
[1]Department of Pediatric Cardiovascular, Xin Hua Hospital, School of Medicine, Shanghai Jiao Tong University, Shanghai 200092, China
Full list of author information is available at the end of the article

of SHF and CNC cells, thereby causing CTDs [5–7]. Increasing studies demonstrated that genetic factors played primary roles in pathogenesis of CTDs, but the genetic determinants underlying CTDs remain unclear [8, 9].

In genetics, many transcription factors are recognized as major contributors to normal cardiac morphogenesis, including the T-box family of transcription factors [10]. TBX2 and TBX3 are members of the T-box family of transcription factors that are important for early cardiogenic lineage development as well as formation of chambers and the conduction system [11]. At embryonic day 8–10 mouse heart, Tbx2 was detected in the non-chamber myocardium, which included the atrioventricular canal (AVC), inner curvature, inflow tract, and OFT [12]. Tbx2 expression patterns during chick heart development are consistent with that of mouse [13]. Morphological defects of the heart were observed in Tbx2 knock-out mouse embryos, including abnormal atrioventricular morphology and outflow tract septation defects [14]. Mutations in TBX3 specifically cause ulnar-mammary syndrome [15]. TBX3 is most closely related to TBX2. Tbx3-null mouse embryos have atrioventricular alignment and OFT defects and various kinds of cardiac malformation, such as DORV and TGA. In addition, Tbx3 is involved in multiple signaling pathways that regulate OFT morphogenesis and SHF proliferation [16]. Both Tbx2 and Tbx3 express embryo mesoderm adjacent to CNC and the SHF [16–18]. Accordingly, overexpression/low expression or abnormal function of TBX2 and TBX3 causes heart defects and thus play an important role in heart development.

Current studies for TBX2 and TBX3 have typically focused on gene knock-out animal models to observe phenotype and explore mechanism; however, they have not investigated whether genetic variants were involved in pathogenesis in populations of CTD patients. Only Pang et al. reported variants (g.59477201C>T, g.59477347G>A, g.59477353delG, and g.59477371G>A) located at the TBX2 gene promoter in a cohort of 324 patients with ventricular septal defects, and the variants reduced the transcriptional activities of the TBX2 gene promoter [19]. Therefore, identifying rare variants of TBX2 and TBX3 in large CTD cohort is required urgently.

Here, we show several rare heterozygous variants of TBX2 and TBX3 by target sequencing in a cohort of 588 CTD patients without 22q11.2 deletion, but none in population-matched healthy controls. Our data shows that these variants alter mRNA and protein expression of TBX2 and TBX3. We screen PEA3 and MEF2C as novel downstream target genes of TBX2 and TBX3, respectively. Function analyses reveal that the variants of TBX2 or TBX3 may regulate PEA3, MEF2C, and HAS2 (the known downstream gene of TBX2) promoting CTD incidence, first defining the connection between TBX2/TBX3 variants and CTDs and further elucidating the genetic pathogenesis of CTDs.

Results

The variants of TBX2 and TBX3 identified in CTD patients

We found variants of TBX2 and TBX3 through target sequencing in 588 CTD patients and identified three variants of TBX2 in seven patients and three variants of TBX3 in six patients, including TOF, TGA, SA, and SV (Table 1). The variants of TBX2 were p.R608W, p.T249I, and p.R616Q (Fig. 1b, d, and f), and the variants of TBX3 were p.A192T, p.M65L, and p.A562V (Fig. 2b, d, and f). The p.R608W, p.T249I, and p.R616Q variants of TBX2 and p.A192T and p.M65L variants of TBX3 in both control and case groups were in HWE; the p.A562V variant of TBX3 in control group was in HWE, but in case group, it was not in HWE (Additional file 1: Table S1). However, these variants all led to amino acid substitutions and were predicted to be damaging as per SIFT, Polyphen-2, or Mutation Taster (Table 1).

Alignment of multiple TBX2 and TBX3 protein sequences and display of the structure of human TBX2 and TBX3 protein

All variation sites in this study were highly conserved in vertebrates, as shown in multiple TBX2 and TBX3 protein alignments (Fig. 3a, b), indicating that these variants were very important and might result in TBX2 and TBX3 gene function alterations. The human TBX2 spans 3396 bp, and has been mapped to chromosome 17q23, which is composed of seven exons and six introns (20). The T-box DNA-binding domain of TBX2 is located at amino acids 109–287 (Fig. 3c). The human TBX3 mapped to chromosome 12q24, spans 4814 bp and is composed of eight exons and seven introns. The T-box DNA-binding domain of TBX3 is located at amino acids 107–220 and 241–305 (Fig. 3d) (Uniprot: http://www.uniprot.org/).

Detection of TBX2 and TBX3 variant expression

To investigate whether the expression of the TBX2 and TBX3 variants were altered, we performed quantitative RT-PCR and Western blot. Quantitative RT-PCR analysis revealed that mRNA expression of R608W, T249I, and R616Q variants of TBX2 (Fig. 4a) and A192T and M65L variants of TBX3 (Fig. 4d) were greater than that of the group of the wild-type plasmid ($P < 0.05$). On Western blot, protein expression of R608W and R616Q variants (Fig. 4b, c) was distinctly greater than that of the wild-type TBX2 ($P < 0.05$), consistent with the mRNA expression of these two TBX2 variants; in contrast, protein expression of A192T and A562V variants (Fig. 4e, f) were notably lower than that of the wild-type TBX3 ($P < 0.05$), indicating that TBX3

Table 1 Clinical information and variant characteristics of TBX2 and TBX3 in patients with CTDs

Patient	Gender	Age	Cardiac phenotype	Gene	Location in gene	Function	Nucleotide change	Amino acid change	dbSNP ID	SIFT	Mutation taster	PolyPhen-2	ExAC allele frequency
1	F	4 months	TOF	TBX2	exon7	Missense	1822C>T	R608W	rs764896880	0.01	Disease causing	1.000	1.726e−05
2	F	8 months	TOF	TBX2	exon3	Missense	746C>T	T249I	rs778075071	0.02	Disease causing	0.967	6.633e−05
3	F	5 months	SV	TBX2	exon3	Missense	746C>T	T249I	rs778075071	0.02	Disease causing	0.967	6.633e−05
4	F	5 years	SV	TBX2	exon3	Missense	746C>T	T249I	rs778075071	0.02	Disease causing	0.967	6.633e−05
5	M	6 months	TOF	TBX2	exon7	Missense	1847G>A	R616Q	rs191930922	0.01	Disease causing	0.865	0.0008162
6	F	3 years	SA	TBX2	exon7	Missense	1847G>A	R616Q	rs191930922	0.01	Disease causing	0.865	0.0008162
7	M	1 year	TGA	TBX3	exon6	Missense	574G>A	A192T	rs768160499	0.11	Disease causing	1.000	2.471e−05
8	M	1 year	TOF	TBX3	exon1	Missense	193A>C	M65L	/	0.56	Disease causing	0.734	8.675e−06
9	M	5 months	TOF	TBX3	exon7	Missense	1685C>T	A562V	rs201325654	0.1	Disease causing	0.849	0.002761
10	M	6 months	TOF	TBX3	exon7	Missense	1685C>T	A562V	rs201325654	0.1	Disease causing	0.849	0.002761
11	F	5 months	TOF	TBX3	exon7	Missense	1685C>T	A562V	rs201325654	0.1	Disease causing	0.849	0.002761
12	F	6 months	TOF	TBX3	exon7	Missense	1685C>T	A562V	rs201325654	0.1	Disease causing	0.849	0.002761
13	M	4 years	TGA	TBX3	exon7	Missense	1685C>T	A562V	rs201325654	0.1	Disease causing	0.849	0.002761

F female, *M* male, *CTDs* conotruncal heart defects, *TOF* tetralogy of Fallot, *SA* single atrium, *SV* single ventricle, *TGA* transposition of the great arteries

variants might lead to protein degradation. Tbx3 is associated with SUMOylation (SUMO, small ubiquitin-related modifier) that may be a conserved mechanism controlling Tbx3 activity [21, 22]. Therefore, we observed the effect of ubiquitin-proteasome degradation and found that the reduction of A192T variant protein expression was rescued after adding the protease inhibitor, suggesting that the A192T variant decreased TBX3 protein stability by ubiquitin-proteasome degradation (Fig. 4g).

Nuclear localization of TBX2 and TBX3 variants

To detect the cellular distribution of TBX2 and TBX3 variant proteins, we carried out immunofluorescence assays that demonstrated that all the TBX2 and TBX3 variant proteins were expressed in the nucleus, as were wild-type TBX2 and TBX3 proteins (Fig. 4h, i). The result suggested that these variant proteins might affect TBX2 or TBX3 gene function through other mechanisms.

Screening of downstream target genes of TBX2 and TBX3

We selected several genes related to CTDs or OFT development from previous studies (BMP2 [13], BMP4 [13], FGF8 [23, 24], HAS2 [25], PEA3 [16]), and the MalaCards database (CRELD1, DKK1, FOG2, GATA4, GATA6, HAND2, MEF2C, PLXND1) and then screened the possible downstream genes of TBX2/TBX3 by observing mRNA expression alterations of these target genes after TBX2/TBX3 overexpression (Fig. 5a, b). The results showed that TBX2 activated HAS2 and PEA3, while TBX3 activated MEF2C ($P < 0.05$), indicating that these were downstream genes of TBX2/TBX3 in CTD incidence.

Transcriptional activity of TBX2 and TBX3 variant proteins

To evaluate the ability of the TBX2/TBX3 variants to regulate downstream genes, we constructed luciferase reporter genes for human HAS2, MEF2C, and PEA3 promoters selected from the mRNA expression screening and co-transfected them with wild-type or variants of TBX2/TBX3. Compared with wild-type TBX2, R608W and R616Q variant proteins were able to activate HAS2 promoter up to approximately 1.7 times ($P < 0.05$) and 2.6 times ($P < 0.01$), respectively (Fig. 6a), whereas the transcriptional activity of R608W and R616Q variant proteins to activate PEA3 promoter reduced by 45% ($P < 0.05$) and 55% ($P < 0.01$), respectively (Fig. 6b). Compared with

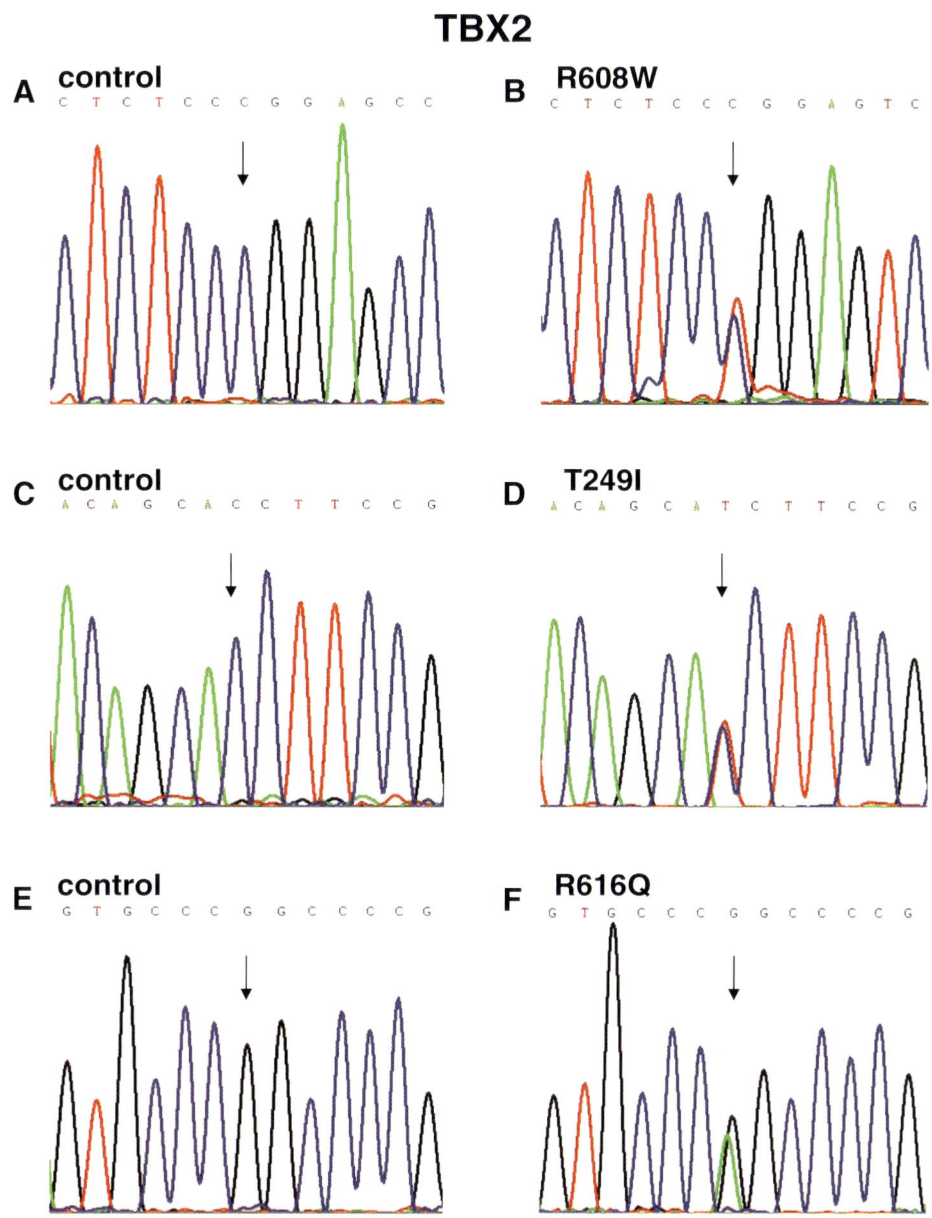

Fig. 1 Sequence chromatograms of TBX2 missense variants in patients and controls. **a**, **c**, and **e** Chromatograms of normal controls. **b**, **d**, and **f** Chromatograms of the three heterozygous variants. Arrows show heterozygous nucleotide changes

wild-type TBX3, A192T, and A562V variant proteins showed a reduced transcriptional activity over MEF2C promoter (Fig. 6c). Therefore, R608W and R616Q variants of TBX2 and A192T and A562V variants of TBX3 may affect TBX2/TBX3 regulation on downstream target genes through transcriptional activity alteration, thereby promoting CTD incidence.

Expression of TBX3 protein in the human embryo

TBX2 has been reported as being expressed at the AVC and OFT of the heart in animals and human embryos [12]. However, TBX3 expression has not been identified in the human embryo; therefore, we selected human embryos in Carnegie 13 stage, which is the crucial period of the OFT formation to carry out immunohistochemistry. The results showed that TBX3 was expressed in the nucleus in the OFT (Fig. 7c, d), indicating that TBX3 might have a function in the development of the OFT.

We show the illustration summarizing our results and claims (Fig. 8).

Discussion

Identifying rare variants of TBX2 and TBX3 in a large CTD cohort is required urgently; our study found six

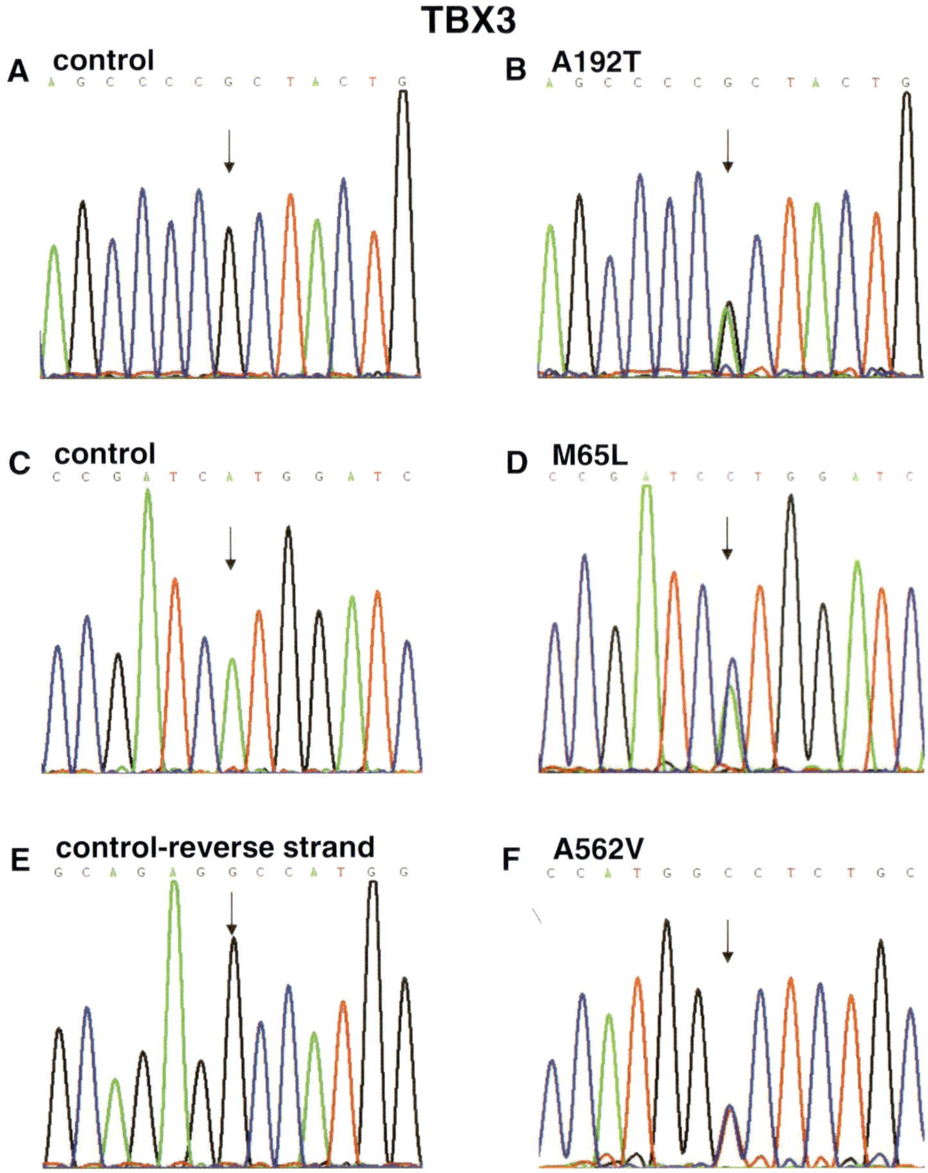

Fig. 2 Sequence chromatograms of TBX3 missense variants in patients and controls. **a**, **c**, and **e** Chromatograms of normal controls. **b**, **d**, and **f** Chromatograms of the three heterozygous variants. Arrows show heterozygous nucleotide changes

rare heterozygous variants of TBX2 and TBX3 in 13 patients from 588 sporadic patients with CTDs using target sequencing that included p.R608W, p.T249I, and p.R616Q variants of TBX2 and p.A192T, p.M65L, and p.A562V variants of TBX3, all of which were all highly conserved based on multiple sequence alignment, suggesting that these variants might have important biological functions. Among these variants, TBX3M65L was the novel variant first reported, and TBX2R608W had not been reported formerly in East Asians. The other four variants were reported in Ensemble (http://ensemblgenomes.org/); their functions had never been studied before. All these variants were predicted as damaging as per SIFT, Mutation Taster or Polyphen-2. Moreover, TBX2R608W, TBX2R616Q, TBX3A192T, and TBX3A562V showed altered expression and function compared with wild-type TBX2/TBX3. Nevertheless, none of the six variants affected the subcellular expression of TBX2 and TBX3 in nucleus, and it is possible that these variants were not located in the critical region that influenced the nuclear distribution of TBX2 and TBX3 [26].

Tbx2 and Tbx3 have common downstream target genes that have been identified as chamber myocardium-specific genes, including connexin 40 (Cx40), connexin 43 (Cx43), and natriuretic precursor peptide type A (Nppa) [27, 28].

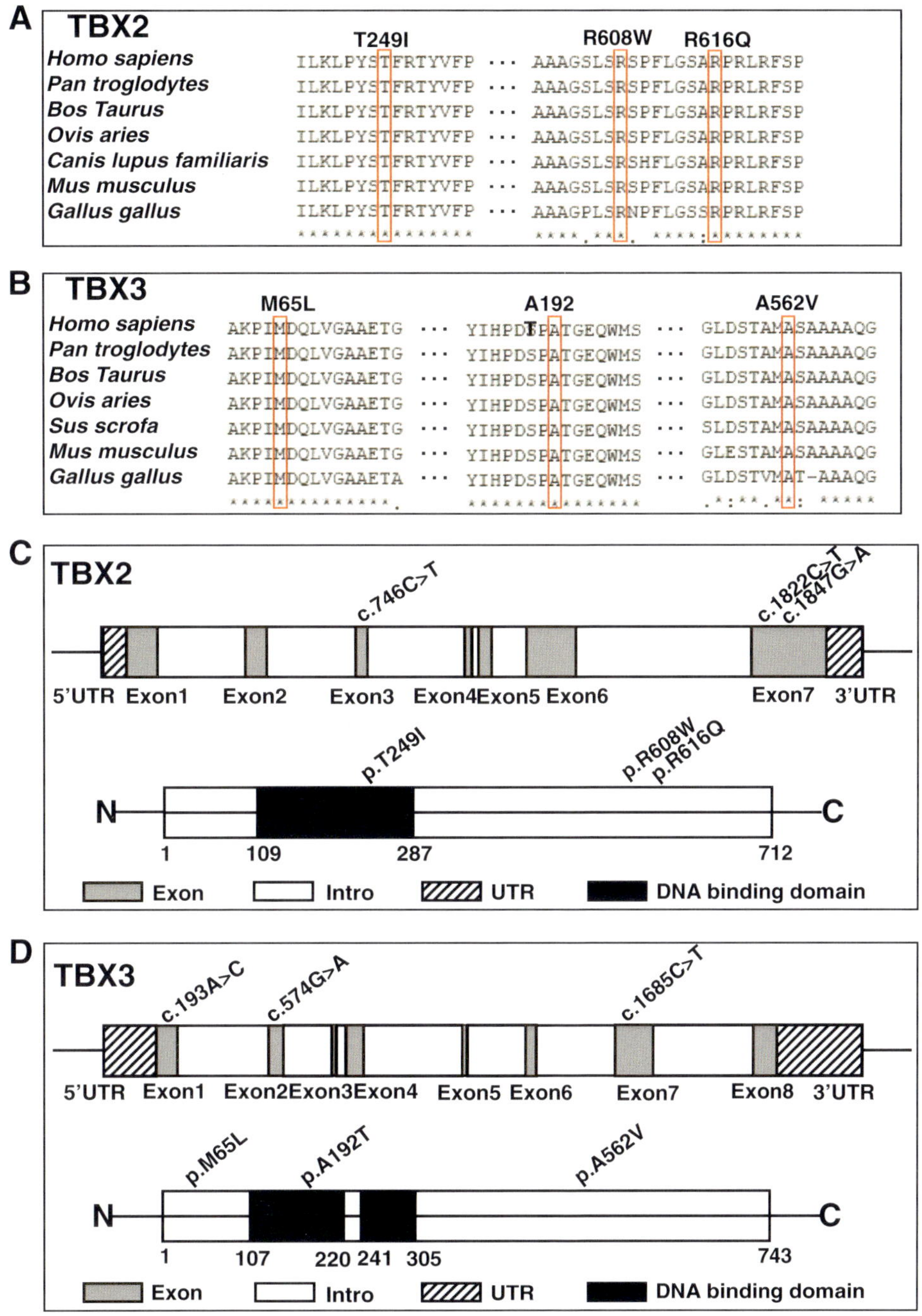

Fig. 3 Conservation and distribution of TBX2 and TBX3 variants. **a**, **b** Alignments of TBX2 and TBX3 protein among different species. All variants were highly conserved in vertebrates. **c**, **d** Diagram of the TBX2 and TBX3 gene exons and protein with location of variants identified in this study

Locally repressing these chamber specific genes is required for the formation of non-chamber myocardium and induction of the development of the AVC, inflow tract, and OFT [29, 30]. However, mRNA expression of Cx40, Cx43, and Nppa in HEK293 cells showed no difference after TBX2 or TBX3 overexpression (data not shown) probably due to the limitations of the cell line or the experimental model.

We screened 12 genes selected from previous studies and the MalaCards database (http://www.malacards.org/) as candidates for TBX2 or TBX3 downstream genes and found that mRNA expression of HAS2 and PEA3 in HEK293 cells were elevated substantially after TBX2 overexpression, while TBX3 transfection upregulated MEF2C abundance significantly. The activity of HAS2, MEF2C, and PEA3

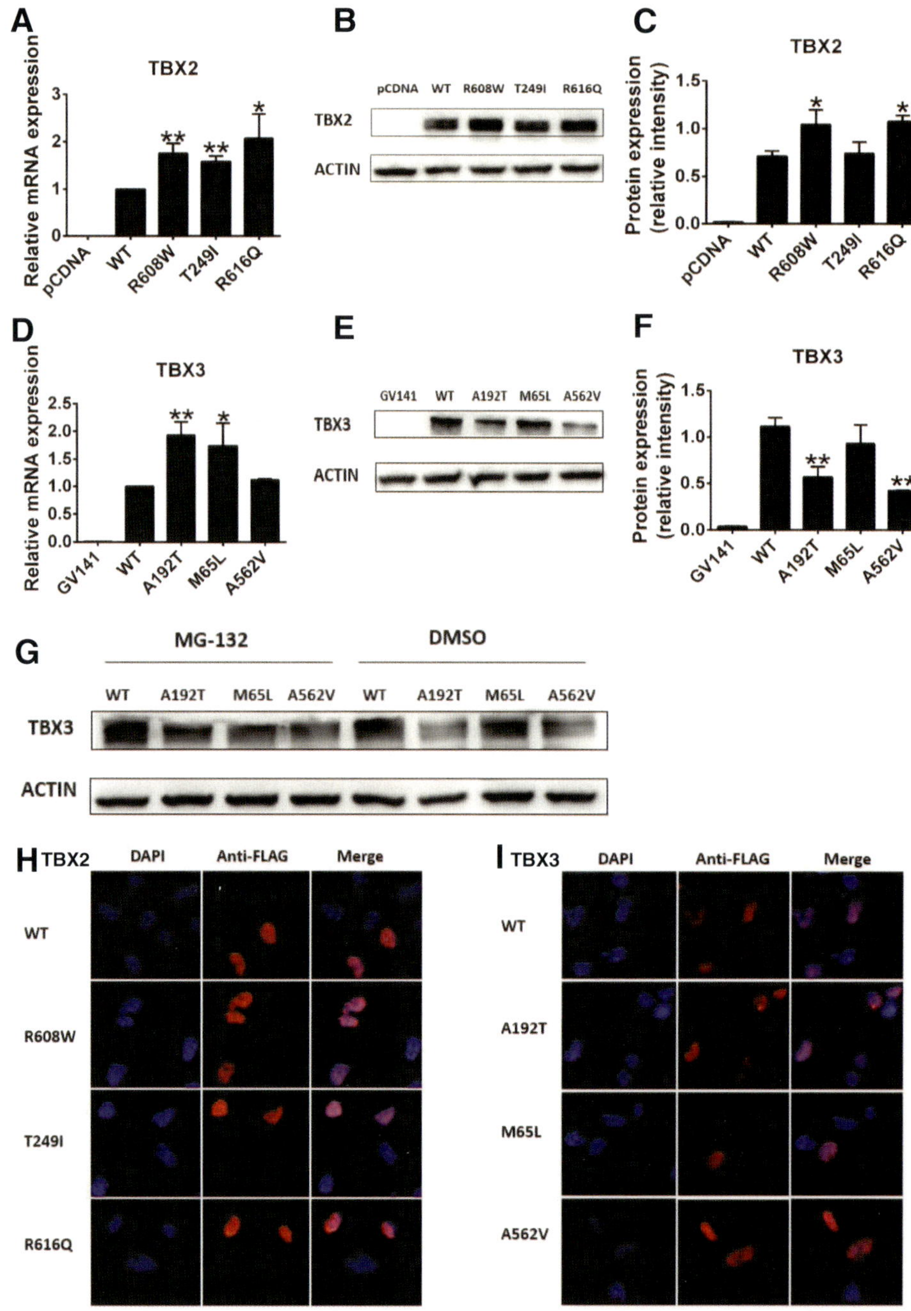

Fig. 4 mRNA abundance, protein expression level, and subcellular localization of TBX2 and TBX3. Plasmids were transfected into HEK 293T cells and harvested. **a**, **d** Relative mRNA expression of the blank vector, wild-type plasmid, and variants of TBX2 and TBX3 ($n = 3$). GAPDH was used as an internal control. **b**, **e** Western blot analysis of the blank vector, wild-type plasmid, and variants of TBX2 and TBX3. Actin was used as an internal control. **c**, **f** Density quantitation of TBX2 and TBX3 variant protein expression as shown in **b** and **e** ($n = 3$). **g** Western blot analysis of TBX3 variant protein degradation through the ubiquitin-proteasome pathway. MG-132 was the proteinase inhibitor and DMSO was used as control. **h**, **i** Representative images of immunofluorescence staining of TBX2 and TBX3 variants and wild-type proteins. $^*P < 0.05$, $^{**}P < 0.01$ versus WT; data represented here are obtained from three biological replicates

luciferase reporter genes was dramatically increased by wild-type TBX2/TBX3 compared with that of blank vectors, providing further evidence that the expression of HAS2, PEA3, and MEF2C was regulated by TBX2 or TBX3. HAS2 has conserved T-box binding sites among promoter regions and encodes hyaluronan synthases 2, the major enzyme responsible for hyaluronan (HA) production in the heart [31], and it is expressed in the OFT [20]. However, excess HA deposition may cause hemodynamic alterations

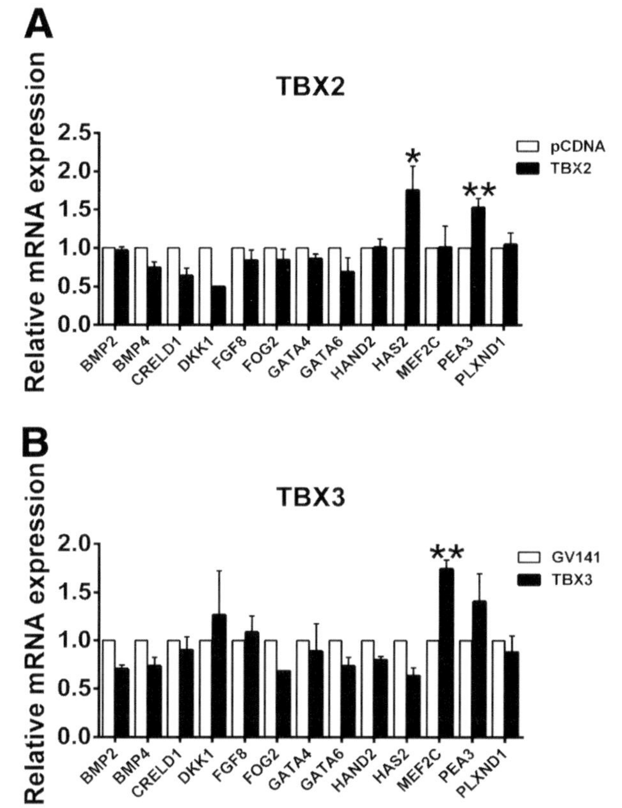

Fig. 5 Screening of downstream target genes related to CTDs of TBX2 or TBX3. **a**, **b** Relative mRNA expression of candidate downstream target genes affected by wild-type TBX2 or TBX3 transfection ($n = 3$). GAPDH was used as an internal control. $^{*}P < 0.05$, $^{**}P < 0.01$ versus pCDNA or GV141; data represented here are obtained from three biological replicates

and may block cardiomyocyte differentiation. Tbx2 contributes to the expansion of the extracellular matrix (ECM) and epithelial-mesenchymal transformation (EMT) by inducing Has2 myocardial expression and increasing HA deposition to drive endocardial cushion formation and altered cardiogenic lineage specification in embryonic hearts [25]. Overexpression of HAS2 leading to HA deposition may hinder cardiomyocyte differentiation. We found that TBX2 variants activated HAS2 and caused CTDs and were similar to this report. PEA3 (polyomavirus enhancer activator 3, currently called ETV4, ETS variant 4) is a transcription factor belonging to the PEA3 family and is involved in chromosomal translocation associated with Ewing tumors, whose overexpression promotes cell proliferation, motility, and invasion. The evidences suggest that PEA3 plays a role in cellular proliferation, differentiation, and migration [32, 33]. A previous study reported that Pea3 was associated with Tbx3 involved in regulating OFT morphogenesis [16]. However, in the present study, TBX3 did not affect mRNA expression of PEA3, whereas TBX2 markedly increased PEA3 mRNA abundance and promoter activity; meanwhile, the wild-type TBX2 protein was able to significantly activate its promoter and the TBX2 variant proteins failed to activate its promoter, indicating that PEA3 was a novel downstream gene of TBX2 causing CTDs. TBX2 contributes to oncogenesis and cell cycle regulation [34], analogous to the functions of PEA3 [32, 33]. Therefore, we inferred that TBX2 and PEA3 may engage in crosstalk during cell cycle regulation and that more studies are needed to determine whether they take part in cardiac development through the regulation that these pathways require. MEF2C (MEF2 polypeptide C) is a member of the MADS box transcription enhancer factor 2 (MEF2) family of proteins, which play roles in myogenesis. Previous studies demonstrated that MEF2C is required for proper OFT alignment [35]. Moreover, MEF2C has also been involved in congenital OFT defects in humans [36]. Our results showed that MEF2C was a novel downstream gene of TBX3 and that variants of TBX3 might regulate MEF2C to cause CTDs.

Previous studies reported Tbx2 and Tbx3 were transcriptional repressors [22, 23]. In contrast, TBX2 and TBX3 in our study were activators; we showed that wild-type TBX2 activated the HAS2 gene promoter and wild-type TBX3 activated the MEF2C gene promoter. On the one hand, TBX2 has the capacity to activate a promoter including multiple T-box elements by a weak activation domain located within the T-box [37]. We presumed that the regulating domain of TBX3 resembles that of TBX2. On the other hand, it can also be explained by the presumption that transcriptional repression of TBX2 and TBX3 may depend on the cell line and the primary cardiomyocyte; therefore, our results are limited by the single cell line we used.

Dysfunction of Tbx2 and Tbx3 leading to heart defects has been verified in animals, providing strong evidence that TBX2 and TBX3 are significant for human cardiac morphogenesis and the underlying etiology of CTDs. There were some limitations to our study; for example, the lack of parental samples limited our ability to study the genetic background of these variants. Nevertheless, this study provided the first genetic evidence of an association between malfunctioning TBX2 and TBX3 and CTDs based on a large population, contributing to prenatal diagnosis and prenatal consultation in favor of the early prophylaxis and allele-specific therapy of CTDs.

Conclusions

We found that the variants of TBX2 and TBX3 contributed to the occurrence of CTDs, and we explored the

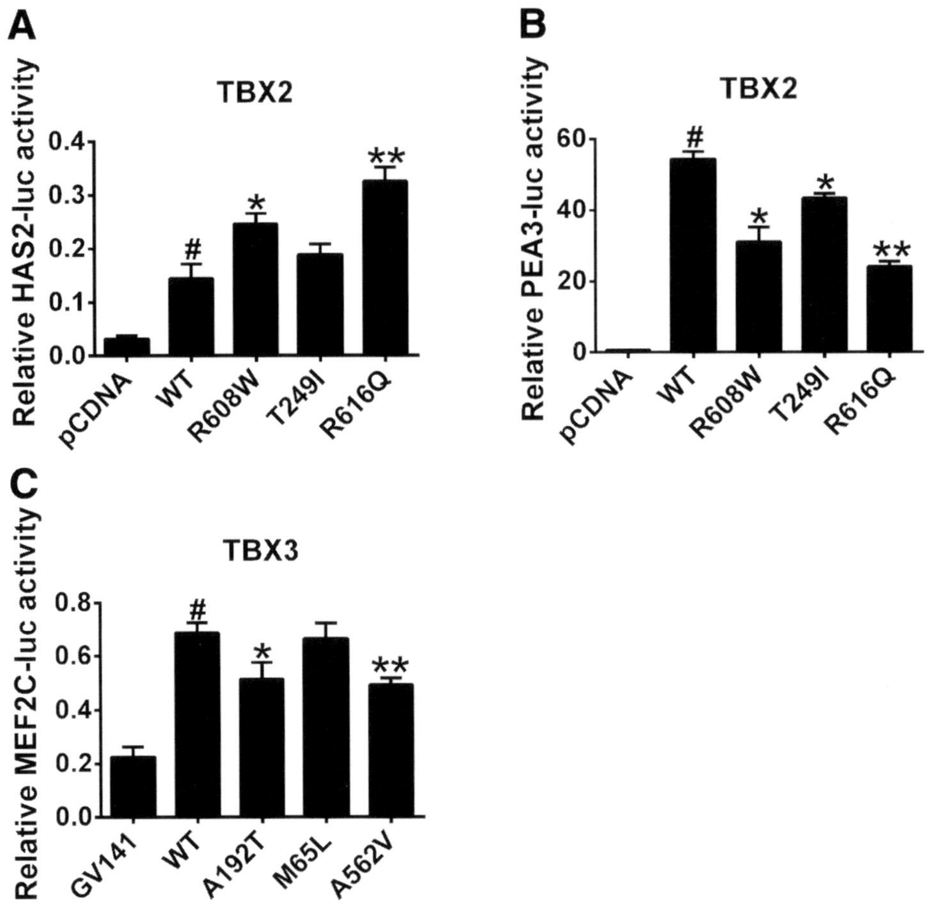

Fig. 6 The activity of HAS2, PEA3, and MEF2C luciferase reporter genes regulated by TBX2 or TBX3. HEK 293T cells that were co-transfected with vector or wild-type or variant plasmid and a luciferase reporter; transcriptional activity was measured by a luciferase reporter gene detection system. pRL-TK was used as an internal control. **a**, **b** Luciferase activity of HAS2, PEA3 promoter regulated by blank vector, and wild-type and variants of TBX2 ($n = 3$). **c** Luciferase activity of MEF2C promoter regulated by blank vector, wild-type, and variants of TBX3 ($n = 3$). $^{\#}P < 0.01$ versus pCDNA or GV141 and $^{*}P < 0.05$, $^{**}P < 0.01$ versus WT; data represented here are obtained from three biological replicates

interesting downstream genes of TBX2 and TBX3 to illuminate the mechanisms of CTD etiology. Meanwhile, our findings open new fields of investigation into CTD genetic pathogenesis.

Methods

Study population

Our study population included 588 sporadic nonsyndromic CTD patients diagnosed by echocardiogram, cardiac catheterization, or surgery from Shanghai Xin Hua Hospital. The participants are from the Chinese Han population and included 388 males and 200 females, with ages ranging from 0.1 to 17 years (Table 2). Patients with known syndromes or chromosomal abnormalities, such as 22q11.2 deletion, were excluded from our study. The controls were 300 healthy children without heart disease. Both patient and control groups gave informed consent for inclusion, and then, peripheral blood was collected for DNA extraction. The genomic DNA of participants was extracted by using the QIAamp DNA Blood Mini Kit (QIAGEN, Germany) following the manufacturer's instructions and was then stored at – 80 °C.

Target sequencing and variant analysis

Target sequencing was performed using the Illumina HiSeq 2000 platform for variants in TBX2 (GenBank accession number NC_000017.11, NM_005994.3) and TBX3 (GenBank accession number NC_000012.12, NM_016569.3). The candidate variants were validated by Sanger sequencing, and the primers were designed for PCR amplification of TBX2 and TBX3. To predict the effects of nonsynonymous variants, we used several bioinformatics criteria including SIFT (http://sift.jcvi.org/www/SIFT_enst_submit.html), Mutation Taster (http://www.mutationtaster.org/), and Polyphen-2 (http://genetics.bwh.havard.edu/pph2/). Amino acid substitutions were predicted as damaging when the score was ≤ 0.05 in SIFT or ≥ 0.85 in Polyphen-2. In our study, variants

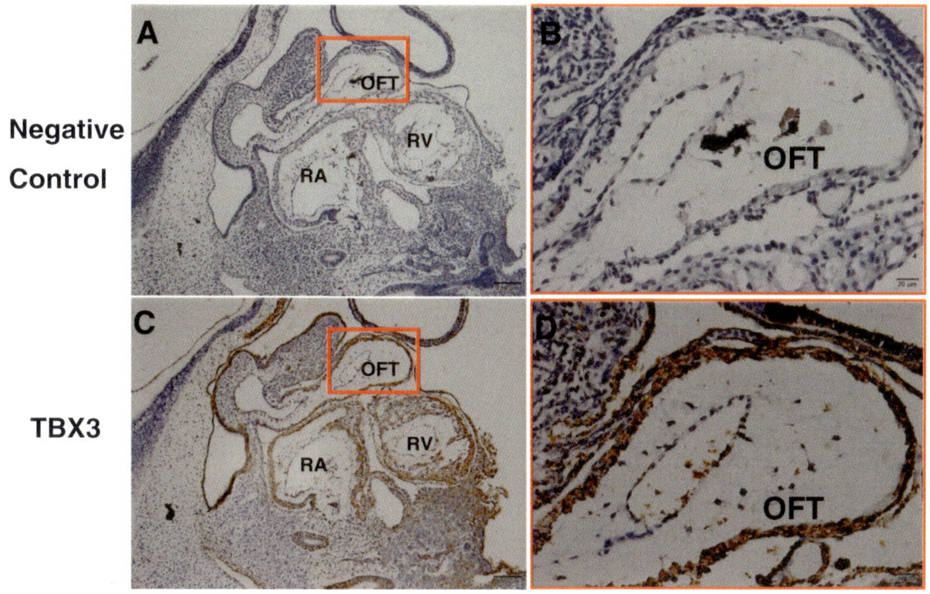

Fig. 7 Immunohistochemistry of TBX3 in human embryos in Carnegie 13 stage. **a**, **b** Negative control. **c**, **d** Wild-type TBX3. Scale bar 20 μm

with a minor allele frequency (MAF) < 0.5% were defined as rare [38].

Multiple TBX2 and TBX3 protein sequence alignment

TBX2 and TBX3 protein sequences from *Homo sapiens* (human), *Mus musculus* (house mouse), *Gallus gallus* (chicken), *Bos taurus* (cattle), *Canis lupus familiaris* (dog), *Pan troglodytes* (chimpanzee), and *Sus scrofa* (pig) were downloaded from NCBI (https://www.ncbi.nlm.nih.gov/protein/) and were aligned with ClustalX software to confirm the conservation of TBX2 and TBX3 sequences.

Plasmid construction and site-directed mutagenesis

The TBX2 and TBX3 cDNA plasmid was purchased from Genomeditech. Mutated primers were designed to amplify human TBX2 and TBX3 cDNA according to the protocol provided by the QuikChange SiteDirected Mutagenesis Kit (Stratagene, USA), and then, variant TBX2 cDNAs were cloned into a pCDNA3.1-3xFlag vectors while variant TBX3 cDNAs were cloned into GV141-3xFlag vectors. For recombining luciferase reporter plasmid, a 5′-flanking region of downstream gene promoter was subcloned into Kpn I and Bgl II sites of the pGL3 luciferase reporter-basic vector (Promega, USA).

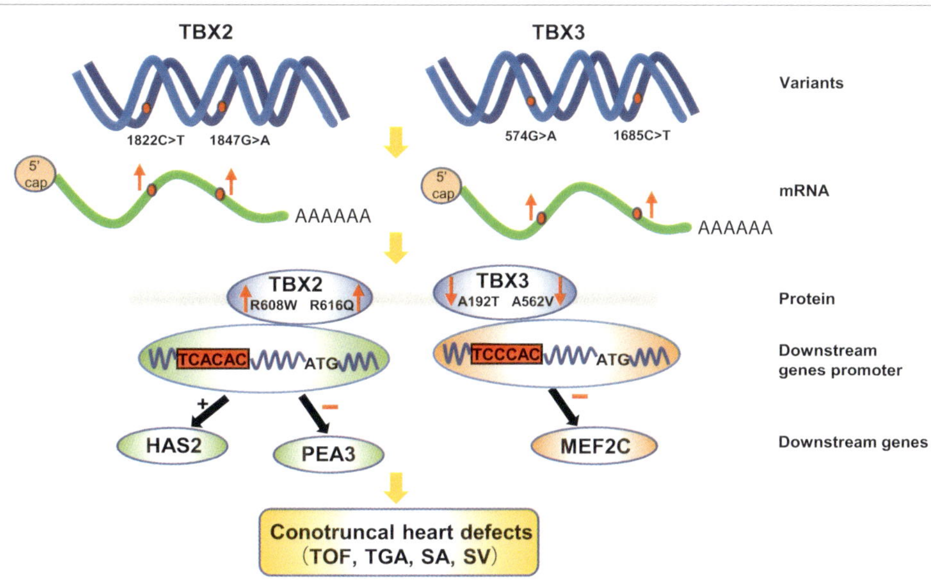

Fig. 8 The diagram of the regulation TBX2 and TBX3 variants involved in CTD pathogenesis

Table 2 Cardiac diagnoses for study population of patients with CTDs

Diagnoses	Number	Gender/number	Age
TGA	90	F18M72	1 day–16 years
TOF	234	F83M151	1 month–13 years
DORV	98	F32M66	1 month–17 years
PA/VSD	97	F36M61	3 months–12 years
IAA	13	F7M6	7 days–1 year
PTA	10	F5M5	3 days–2 years
SA/SV	46	F19M27	1 month–13 years
Total	588	F200M388	1 day–17 years

TGA transposition of the great arteries, *TOF* tetralogy of Fallot, *DORV* double outlet of right ventricle, *PA/VSD* pulmonary atresia with ventricular septal defect, *IAA* interruption of aortic arch, *PTA* persistent truncus arteriosus, *SA* single atrium, *SV* single ventricle, *F* female, *M* male

Cell cultures and transfection

HEK 293T cells (Human embryonic kidney cells) were maintained in Dulbecco's modified Eagle's medium (HyClone, USA) with 10% fetal bovine serum (MP Biomedicals, USA) and 1% penicillin-streptomycin (Gibco, USA). pcDNA3.1-3xFlag-TBX2 and GV141-3xFlag-TBX3 including wild-type and variants were transfected into 293T cells with FuGene HD (Promega, USA) according to the manufacturer's protocol after seeding 24 h.

Quantitative RT-PCR

Plasmids were transfected into HEK 293T cells that were seeded in 12-well plates. Cells were harvested 36 h after transfection. Total RNA was extracted with TRIzol reagent (Invitrogen, USA), and then, reverse transcription of cDNA was performed using Prime Script RT Master Mix (Takara, Japan) and was followed by quantitative RT-PCR using SYBR Premix Ex Taq (Takara, Japan) on an Applied Biosystems 7500 system (Applied Biosystems, USA). The relative quantification of expression was determined using the $2^{-\Delta\Delta Ct}$ method [39], and glyceraldehyde-3-phosphate dehydrogenase (GAPDH, human) was used as an internal control. Primer sequences of TBX2, TBX3, GAPDH, and candidate downstream genes are listed in Table 3.

Western blot

HEK 293T cells were transfected with 1 μg of wild-type and variant plasmid DNA. Cells were harvested 48 h after transfection. For protein degradation experiments, HEK 293T cells were cultured in the presence of 10 mM MG132 solution dissolved in DMSO for 8–10 h before harvest. Then, cells were lysed in RIPA lysis buffer (Beyotime, China) with PMSF (1:100). The proteins were subjected to 10% SDS-PAGE and were then transferred onto nitrocellulose membranes (Millipore, USA) and immunostained with rabbit anti-FLAG antibody (1:1000, Sigma-Aldrich, USA) and mouse anti-β-actin antibody (1:5000, Sigma-Aldrich, USA) at 4 °C overnight. The membranes were incubated with horseradish peroxidase-conjugated anti-rabbit secondary antibody (1:10000) and anti-mouse secondary antibody (1:10000). Immobilon Western Chemiluminescent HRP Substrate (Millipore, USA) was used for chemiluminescent immunodetection.

Table 3 Sequences of the primers used for real-time quantitative PCR

Gene	Forward (5′→3′)	Reverse (5′→3′)
GAPDH	GGAGCGAGATCCCTCCAAAAT	GGCTGTTGTCATACTTCTCATGG
TBX2	CACGGCTTCACCATCCTAAAC	TGCGGAAGGTGCTGTAAGG
TBX3	GAGGCTAAAGAACTTTGGGATCA	CATTTCGGGGTCGGCCTTA
BMP2	GAGGTCCTGAGCGAGTTCGA	ACCTGAGTGCCTGCGATACA
BMP4	ATGATTCCTGGTAACCGAATGC	CCCCGTCTCAGGTATCAAACT
CRELD1	GCTCCTATGAGTGCCGAGAC	CTACACTTCTTACAGCGACCTG
DKK1	ATAGCACCTTGGATGGGTATTCC	CTGATGACCGGAGACAAACAG
FGF8	GACCCCTTCGCAAAGCTCAT	CCGTTGCTCTTGGCGATCA
FOG2	GGCCTGAAAATCTGAGCTGC	CAGTCGTCTGTCTCAACTCCA
GATA4	CGACACCCCAATCTCGATATG	GTTGCACAGATAGTGACCCGT
GATA6	CTCAGTTCCTACGCTTCGCAT	GTCGAGGTCAGTGAACAGCA
HAND2	CGCCGACACCAAACTCTCC	TCGCCATTCTGGTCGTCCT
HAS2	CTCATCATCCAAAGCCTGTT	GCTGGGTCAAGCATAGTGTC
MEF2C	CCAACTTCGAGATGCCAGTCT	GTCGATGTGTTACACCAGGAG
PLXND1	AATGGGCGGAACATCGTCAAG	CGAGACTGGTTGGAAACACAG
PEA3	GAGAAACCTCTGCGACCATT	GCCCGTCCAGGCAATGAAAT

Luciferase assays

HEK 293T cells were transfected with 200 ng of wild-type or variant plasmid DNA, 200 ng of luciferase reporter plasmid, and 8 ng of an internal control reporter plasmid (pRL-TK) (Promega, USA) in a 48-well plate. The luciferase activity was measured on the Dual-Glo luciferase assay system (Promega, USA) following the manufacturer's protocol after 48 h.

Immunofluorescence assay

HEK 293T cells were seeded onto a 24-well plate covered with slips coated with poly-L-lysine (0.1 mg/mL) for 24 h and were then transfected with wild-type or variant plasmid DNA. Cells were harvested 24 h after transfection. Cells were incubated with rabbit anti-Flag antibody (1:100, Sigma-Aldrich, USA) diluted in PBS containing 5% BSA and 0.1% Triton X-100 at 4 °C overnight and followed by incubation with Cy3-conjugated goat anti-rabbit secondary antibody (1:250). Cell nuclei were stained by 4,6-diamidino-2-phenylindole (DAPI) (Vector Laboratories, USA). A Leica SP8 microscope was used for image analysis.

Tissue collection and immunohistochemistry

Human embryos of Carnegie 13 stage were acquired after medical termination of pregnancy at Shanghai Xin Hua Hospital. The medical ethics committee of Xin Hua Hospital approved the study. Embryos were fixed overnight in 4% paraformaldehyde in PBS, embedded in paraffin, and sectioned at a thickness of 7 μm. For immunolocalization of TBX3, paraffin sections were incubated with a primary rabbit anti-TBX3 antibody (1:50, Protein-tech), followed by horseradish peroxidase-conjugated secondary anti-rabbit antibody and DAB (Abcam, UK).

Statistical analysis

Each assay was performed for three independent biological replicates. The data are shown as the mean ± standard deviation (SD). Statistical differences were evaluated by one-way ANOVA and two-tailed unpaired *t* test. A P value < 0.05 was considered statistically significant.

Abbreviations

AVC: Atrioventricular canal; CNC: Cardiac neural crest; CTDs: Conotruncal heart defects; HA: Hyaluronan; OFT: Outflow tract; SHF: Secondary heart field; TBX2/3: T-box 2/3 [*Homo sapiens* (human)]; Tbx2/3: T-box 2/3 [*Mus musculus* (house mouse)]

Acknowledgements

We are grateful to all subjects who participated in this study.

Funding

This study received financial supports from the National Natural Science Foundation of China (81670285), the key international (regional) cooperation projects of the National Natural Science Foundation of China (81720108003), the multi-center clinical research project of Shanghai Jiao Tong University (DLY201609), and the public health system construction of Shanghai Municipal Commission of Health and Family Planning (GWIV-23), the Experts Recruitment Program of Xinhua Hospital (Re-013).

Authors' contributions

KS, YY, and HX conceived and designed the experiments; HX, EZ, and NH performed the experiments; HX, EZ, YY, and KS analyzed the data; QF, FL, and SC collected the blood samples from all subjects. HX wrote the first draft of the manuscript. YY and KS revised the manuscript. All authors contributed to writing this paper and approved the final manuscript.

Competing interests

The authors declare that they have no competing interests.

Author details

[1]Department of Pediatric Cardiovascular, Xin Hua Hospital, School of Medicine, Shanghai Jiao Tong University, Shanghai 200092, China. [2]Medical Laboratory, Shanghai Children's Medical Center, School of Medicine, Shanghai Jiao Tong University, Shanghai 200127, China. [3]Department of Pediatric Cardiology, Shanghai Children's Medical Center, School of Medicine, Shanghai Jiao Tong University, Shanghai 200127, China.

References

1. Hoffman JI, Kaplan S. The incidence of congenital heart disease. J Am Coll Cardiol. 2002;39(12):1890–900.
2. van der Bom T, Zomer AC, Zwinderman AH, Meijboom FJ, Bouma BJ, Mulder BJ. The changing epidemiology of congenital heart disease. Nat Rev Cardiol. 2011;8(1):50–60.
3. Tutarel O, Kempny A, Alonso-Gonzalez R, Jabbour R, Li W, Uebing A, Dimopoulos K, Swan L, Gatzoulis MA, Diller GP. Congenital heart disease beyond the age of 60: emergence of a new population with high resource utilization, high morbidity, and high mortality. Eur Heart J. 2014;35(11):725–32.
4. Verheugt CL, Uiterwaal CS, van der Velde ET, Meijboom FJ, Pieper PG, Sieswerda GT, Plokker HW, Grobbee DE, Mulder BJ. The emerging burden of hospital admissions of adults with congenital heart disease. Heart. 2010; 96(11):872–8.
5. Hutson MR, Kirby ML. Model systems for the study of heart development and disease. Cardiac neural crest and conotruncal malformations. Semin Cell Dev Biol. 2007;18(1):101–10.
6. Ward C, Stadt H, Hutson M, Kirby ML. Ablation of the secondary heart field leads to tetralogy of Fallot and pulmonary atresia. Dev Biol. 2005; 284(1):72–83.
7. Waldo KL, Hutson MR, Ward CC, Zdanowicz M, Stadt HA, Kumiski D, Abu-Issa R, Kirby ML. Secondary heart field contributes myocardium and smooth muscle to the arterial pole of the developing heart. Dev Biol. 2005;281(1): 78–90.
8. Jenkins KJ, Correa A, Feinstein JA, Botto L, Britt AE, Daniels SR, Elixson M, Warnes CA, Webb CL. Noninherited risk factors and congenital cardiovascular defects: current knowledge: a scientific statement from the American Heart Association Council on Cardiovascular Disease in the Yong: endorsed by the American Academy of Pediatrics. Circulation. 2007;115(23): 2995–3014.
9. Cooper WO, Hernandez-Diaz S, Arboast PG, Dudley JA, Deyer S, Giddeon PS, Hall K, Ray WA. Major congenital malformations after first-trimester exposure to ACE inhibitors. N Engl J Med. 2006;354(23):2443–51.
10. Meganathan K, Sotiriadou I, Natarajan K, Hescheler J, Sachinidis A. Signaling molecules, transcription growth factors and other regulators revealed from in-vivo and in-vitro models for the regulation of cardiac development. Int J Cardiol. 2015;183:117–28.
11. Plageman TF Jr, Yutzey KE. T-box genes and heart development: putting the "T" in heart. Dev Dyn. 2005;232(1):11–20.
12. Christoffels VM, Hoogaars WM, Tessari A, Clout DE, Moorman AF, Campione M. T-box transcription factor Tbx2 represses differentiation and formation of the cardiac chambers. Dev Dyn. 2004;229(4):763–70.

13. Yamada M, Revelli JP, Eichele G, Barron M, Schwartz RJ. Expression of chick Tbx-2, Tbx-3, and Tbx-5 genes during early heart development: evidence for BMP2 induction of Tbx2. Dev Biol. 2000;228(1):95–105.
14. Harrelson Z, Kelly RG, Goldin SN, Gibson-Brown JJ, Bollag RJ, Silver LM, Papaioannou VE. Tbx2 is essential for patterning the atrioventricular canal and for morphogenesis of the outflow tract during heart development. Development. 2004;131(20):5041–52.
15. Bamshad M, Lin RC, Law DJ, Watkins WC, Krakowiak PA, Moore ME, Franceschini P, Lala R, Holmes LB, Gebuhr TC, Bruneau BG, Schinzel A, Seidman JG, Seidman CE, Jorde LB. Mutations in human TBX3 alter limb, apocrine and genital development in ulnar-mammary syndrome. Nat Genet. 1997;16(3):311–5.
16. Mesbah K, Harrelson Z, Theveniau-Ruissy M, Papaioannou VE, Kelly RG. Tbx3 is required for outflow tract development. Circ Res. 2008;103(7):743–50.
17. Dupays L, Kotecha S, Angst B, Mohun TJ. Tbx2 misexpression impairs deployment of second heart field derived progenitor cells to the arterial pole of the embryonic heart. Dev Biol. 2009;333(1):121–31.
18. Mesbah K, Rana MS, Francou A, van Duijvenboden K, Papaioannou VE, Moorman AF, Kelly RG, Christoffels VM. Identification of a Tbx1/Tbx2/Tbx3 genetic pathway governing pharyngeal and arterial pole morphogenesis. Hum Mol Genet. 2012;21(6):1217–29.
19. Pang S, Liu Y, Zhao Z, Huang W, Chen D, Yan B. Novel and functional sequence variants within the TBX2 gene promoter in ventricular septal defects. Biochimie. 2013;95(9):1087–9.
20. Campbell C, Goodrich K, Casey G, Beatty B. Cloning and mapping of a human gene (TBX2) sharing a highly conserved protein motif with the Drosophila omb gene. Genomics. 1995;28(2):255–60.
21. Crum TL, Okkema PG. SUMOylation-dependent function of a T-box transcriptional repressor in Caenorhabditis elegans. Biochem Soc Trans. 2007; 35(6):1424–6.
22. Huber P, Crum T, Clary LM, Ronan T, Packard AV, Okkema PG. Function of the C. elegans T-box factor TBX-2 depends on SUMOylation. Cell Mol Life Sci. 2013;70(21):4157–68.
23. Firnberg N, Neubuser A. FGF signaling regulates expression of Tbx2, Erm, Pea3, and Pax3 in the early nasal region. Dev Biol. 2002;247(2):237–50.
24. Ilagan R, Abu-Issa R, Brown D, Yang YP, Jiao K, Schwartz RJ, Klingensmith J, Meyers EN. Fgf8 is required for anterior heart field development. Development. 2006;133(12):2435–45.
25. Shirai M, Imanaka-Yoshida K, Schneider MD, Schwartz RJ, Morisaki T. T-box 2, a mediator of Bmp-Smad signaling, induced hyaluronan synthase 2 and Tgfbeta2 expression and endocardial cushion formation. Proc Natl Acad Sci U S A. 2009;106(44):18604–9.
26. Yang YQ, Gharibeh L, Li RG, Xin YF, Wang J, Liu ZM, Qiu XB, Xu YJ, Xu L, Qu XK, Liu X, Fang WY, Huang RT, Xue S, Nemer G. GATA4 loss-of-function mutations underlie familial tetralogy of Fallot. Hum Mutat. 2013;34(12):1662–71.
27. Hoogaars WM, Tessari A, Moorman AF, de Boer PA, Hagoort J, Soufan AT, Campione M, Christoffels VM. The transcriptional repressor Tbx3 delineates the developing central conduction system of the heart. Cardiovasc Res. 2004;62(3):489–99.
28. Habets PE, Moorman AF, Clout DE, van Roon MA, Lingbeek M, van Lohuizen M, Campione M, Christoffels VM. Cooperative action of Tbx2 and Nkx2.5 inhibits ANF expression in the atrioventricular canal: implications for cardiac chamber formation. Genes Dev. 2002;16(10): 1234–46.
29. Ribeiro I, Kawakami Y, Büscher D, Raya A, Rodríguez-León J, Morita M, Rodríguez Esteban C, Izpisúa Belmonte JC. Tbx2 and Tbx3 regulate the dynamics of cell proliferation during heart remodeling. PLoS One. 2007;2(4):e398.
30. Singh R, Hoogaars WM, Barnett P, Grieskamp T, Rana MS, Buermans H, Farin HF, Petry M, Heallen T, Martin JF, Moorman AF, 't Hoen PA, Kispert A, Christoffels VM. Tbx2 and Tbx3 induce atrioventricular myocardial development and endocardial cushion formation. Cell Mol Life Sci. 2012; 69(8):1377–89.
31. Camenisch TD, Spicer AP, Brehm-Gibson T, Biesterfeldt J, Augustine ML, Calabro A Jr, Kubalak S, Klewer SE, McDonald JA. Disruption of hyaluronan synthase-2 abrogates normal cardiac morphogenesis and hyaluronan-mediated transformation of epithelium to mesenchyme. J Clin Invest. 2000; 106(3):349–60.
32. Akagi T, Kuure S, Uranishi K, Koide H, Costantini F, Yokota T. ETS-related transcription factors ETV4 and ETV5 are involved in proliferation and induction of differentiation-associated genes in embryonic stem (ES) cells. J Biol Chem. 2015;290(37):22460–73.
33. Oh S, Shin S, Janknecht R. ETV1, 4 and 5: an oncogenic subfamily of ETS transcription factors. Biochim Biophys Acta. 2012;1826(1):1–12.
34. Sinclair CS, Adem C, Naderi A, Soderberg CL, Johnson M, Wu K, Wadum L, Couch VL, Sellers TA, Schaid D, Slezak J, Fredericksen Z, Ingle JN, Hartmann L, Jenkins RB, Couch FJ. TBX2 is preferentially amplified in BRCA1- and BRCA2-related breast tumors. Cancer Res. 2002;62(13):3587–91.
35. Barnes RM, Harris IS, Jaehnig EJ, Sauls K, Sinha T, Rojas A, Schachterle W, McCulley DJ, Norris RA, Black BL. MEF2C regulates outflow tract alignment and transcriptional control of Tdgf1. Development. 2016;143(5):774–9.
36. Kodo K, Nishizawa T, Furutani M, Arai S, Ishihara K, Oda M, Makino S, Fukuda K, Takahashi T, Matsuoka R, Nakanishi T, Yamagishi H. Genetic analysis of essential cardiac transcription factors in 256 patients with non-syndromic congenital heart defects. Circ J. 2012;76(7):1703–11.
37. Paxton C, Zhao H, Chin Y, Langner K, Reecy J. Murine Tbx2 contains domains that activate and repress gene transcription. Gene. 2002;283(1–2):117–24.
38. Manolio TA, Collins FS, Cox NJ, Goldstein DB, Hindorff LA, Hunter DJ, McCarthy MI, Ramos EM, Cardon LR, Chakravarti A, et al. Finding the missing heritability of complex diseases. Nature. 2009;461(7265):747–53.
39. Livak KJ, Schmittgen TD. Analysis of relative gene expression data using real-time quantitative PCR and the 2(–Delta Delta C(T)) method. Methods. 2001;25(4):402–8.

Table 8 The expected accuracy results of the missense mutations of epidermal and hyperproliferative keratins in moderate psoriasis predicted as deleterious in PredictSNP and integrated tool

Gene	CDS mutation	AA mutation	Predict SNP		MAPP		PhD-SNP		PolyPhen-1		PolyPhen-2		SIFT		SNAP		PANTHER	
			Prediction	Accuracy	Prediction	Accuracy	Prediction	Accuracy	Prediction	Accuracy	Prediction	Accuracy	Prediction	Accuracy	Prediction	Accuracy	Prediction	Accuracy
K14	c.388C > G	p.L130V	DEL	0.76	DEL	0.72	DEL	0.86	DEL	0.74	DEL	0.65	DEL	0.79	NEU	0.58	DEL	0.77
	c.415G > C	p.A139P	DEL	0.87	DEL	0.59	DEL	0.82	DEL	0.74	DEL	0.65	DEL	0.53	DEL	0.56	DEL	0.74
	c.419A > T	p.N140I	DEL	0.87	DEL	0.84	DEL	0.86	DEL	0.74	DEL	0.81	DEL	0.79	DEL	0.62	DEL	0.87
	c.442C > T	p.R148C	DEL	0.76	DEL	0.59	DEL	0.88	DEL	0.74	DEL	0.68	DEL	0.79	NEU	0.55	DEL	0.87
	c.512A > T	p.D171V	DEL	0.76	DEL	0.59	DEL	0.82	DEL	0.74	DEL	0.56	DEL	0.79	NEU	0.50	DEL	0.74
	c.519G > T	p.R173S	DEL	0.76	DEL	0.59	DEL	0.61	DEL	0.59	DEL	0.43	DEL	0.79	NEU	0.50	DEL	0.74
	c.904G > C	p.A302P	DEL	0.61	DEL	0.75	DEL	0.82	DEL	0.59	NEU	0.64	DEL	0.79	NEU	0.50	DEL	0.84
	c.1057G > C	p.A353P	DEL	0.61	DEL	0.57	DEL	0.86	DEL	0.74	DEL	0.47	NEU	0.74	NEU	0.61	DEL	0.68
	c.1234A > T	P.I412F	DEL	0.87	DEL	0.63	DEL	0.77	DEL	0.74	DEL	0.81	DEL	0.79	DEL	0.56	–	0.00
K10	c.479A > C	p.Y160S	DEL	0.87	DEL	0.86	DEL	0.86	DEL	0.74	DEL	0.81	DEL	0.79	DEL	0.72	–	0.00
	c.520C > A	p.L174M	DEL	0.76	DEL	0.72	DEL	0.59	DEL	0.74	DEL	0.65	DEL	0.79	NEU	0.55	DEL	0.72
	c.674A > C	p.D225A	DEL	0.87	DEL	0.66	DEL	0.68	DEL	0.74	DEL	0.68	DEL	0.79	DEL	0.56	DEL	0.77
	c.704G > T	p.R235M	DEL	0.76	DEL	0.59	DEL	0.82	DEL	0.74	DEL	0.81	DEL	0.79	NEU	0.55	DEL	0.78
	c.711G > T	p.K237N	DEL	0.76	DEL	0.75	DEL	0.88	DEL	0.59	DEL	0.63	DEL	0.79	NEU	0.50	DEL	0.74
	c.785T > A	p.L262Q	DEL	0.76	DEL	0.41	DEL	0.61	DEL	0.74	DEL	0.81	DEL	0.79	NEU	0.50	DEL	0.78
K16	c.410C > T	p.A137V	NEU	0.63	NEU	0.70	NEU	0.45	DEL	0.59	NEU	0.61	DEL	0.79	NEU	0.71	DEL	0.68
	c.583G > T	p.A195S	NEU	0.65	NEU	0.66	NEU	0.51	NEU	0.67	DEL	0.47	DEL	0.45	NEU	0.71	DEL	0.72
	c.589C > A	p.L197M	NEU	0.60	NEU	0.79	DEL	0.59	NEU	0.67	DEL	0.59	DEL	0.45	NEU	0.83	DEL	0.67
	c.634C > G	p.L212V	NEU	0.60	DEL	0.51	NEU	0.51	NEU	0.67	DEL	0.45	DEL	0.53	NEU	0.77	DEL	0.71
	c.667C > G	p.L223V	DEL	0.76	DEL	0.75	DEL	0.77	DEL	0.74	DEL	0.65	DEL	0.79	NEU	0.55	DEL	0.71
K17	c.503A > T	p.D168V	DEL	0.87	DEL	0.63	DEL	0.82	DEL	0.59	DEL	0.68	DEL	0.79	DEL	0.56	DEL	0.87
	c.662A > T	p.N221I	DEL	0.72	NEU	0.77	DEL	0.59	DEL	0.74	DEL	0.81	DEL	0.79	DEL	0.56	DEL	0.74
	c.682G > C	p.A228P	DEL	0.72	DEL	0.48	DEL	0.88	DEL	0.74	DEL	0.50	DEL	0.46	NEU	0.61	DEL	0.73
	c.907C > T	p.L303F	DEL	0.51	NEU	0.75	NEU	0.51	DEL	0.74	DEL	0.65	DEL	0.79	NEU	0.50	DEL	0.78
	c.986C > T	p.A329V	DEL	0.55	DEL	0.48	DEL	0.77	NEU	0.67	DEL	0.40	DEL	0.46	NEU	0.61	DEL	0.72
	c.1070G > T	p.R357L	DEL	0.72	DEL	0.77	DEL	0.68	DEL	0.59	NEU	0.68	DEL	0.79	DEL	0.56	DEL	0.76
	c.1144G > T	p.A382S	NEU	0.83	NEU	0.64	NEU	0.51	NEU	0.67	NEU	0.70	NEU	0.71	NEU	0.71	DEL	0.57
	c.1210A > C	p.T404P	NEU	0.63	DEL	0.51	DEL	0.68	NEU	0.67	NEU	0.71	NEU	0.65	NEU	0.50	NEU	0.48

DEL deleterious, *NEU* neutral

Luciferase assays

HEK 293T cells were transfected with 200 ng of wild-type or variant plasmid DNA, 200 ng of luciferase reporter plasmid, and 8 ng of an internal control reporter plasmid (pRL-TK) (Promega, USA) in a 48-well plate. The luciferase activity was measured on the Dual-Glo luciferase assay system (Promega, USA) following the manufacturer's protocol after 48 h.

Immunofluorescence assay

HEK 293T cells were seeded onto a 24-well plate covered with slips coated with poly-L-lysine (0.1 mg/mL) for 24 h and were then transfected with wild-type or variant plasmid DNA. Cells were harvested 24 h after transfection. Cells were incubated with rabbit anti-Flag antibody (1:100, Sigma-Aldrich, USA) diluted in PBS containing 5% BSA and 0.1% Triton X-100 at 4 °C overnight and followed by incubation with Cy3-conjugated goat anti-rabbit secondary antibody (1:250). Cell nuclei were stained by 4,6-diamidino-2-phenylindole (DAPI) (Vector Laboratories, USA). A Leica SP8 microscope was used for image analysis.

Tissue collection and immunohistochemistry

Human embryos of Carnegie 13 stage were acquired after medical termination of pregnancy at Shanghai Xin Hua Hospital. The medical ethics committee of Xin Hua Hospital approved the study. Embryos were fixed overnight in 4% paraformaldehyde in PBS, embedded in paraffin, and sectioned at a thickness of 7 μm. For immunolocalization of TBX3, paraffin sections were incubated with a primary rabbit anti-TBX3 antibody (1:50, Protein-tech), followed by horseradish peroxidase-conjugated secondary anti-rabbit antibody and DAB (Abcam, UK).

Statistical analysis

Each assay was performed for three independent biological replicates. The data are shown as the mean ± standard deviation (SD). Statistical differences were evaluated by one-way ANOVA and two-tailed unpaired t test. A P value < 0.05 was considered statistically significant.

Abbreviations

AVC: Atrioventricular canal; CNC: Cardiac neural crest; CTDs: Conotruncal heart defects; HA: Hyaluronan; OFT: Outflow tract; SHF: Secondary heart field; TBX2/3: T-box 2/3 [*Homo sapiens* (human)]; Tbx2/3: T-box 2/3 [*Mus musculus* (house mouse)]

Acknowledgements

We are grateful to all subjects who participated in this study.

Funding

This study received financial supports from the National Natural Science Foundation of China (81670285), the key international (regional) cooperation projects of the National Natural Science Foundation of China (81720108003), the multi-center clinical research project of Shanghai Jiao Tong University (DLY201609), and the public health system construction of Shanghai Municipal Commission of Health and Family Planning (GWIV-23), the Experts Recruitment Program of Xinhua Hospital (Re-013).

Authors' contributions

KS, YY, and HX conceived and designed the experiments; HX, EZ, and NH performed the experiments; HX, EZ, YY, and KS analyzed the data; QF, FL, and SC collected the blood samples from all subjects. HX wrote the first draft of the manuscript. YY and KS revised the manuscript. All authors contributed to writing this paper and approved the final manuscript.

Competing interests

The authors declare that they have no competing interests.

Author details

[1]Department of Pediatric Cardiovascular, Xin Hua Hospital, School of Medicine, Shanghai Jiao Tong University, Shanghai 200092, China. [2]Medical Laboratory, Shanghai Children's Medical Center, School of Medicine, Shanghai Jiao Tong University, Shanghai 200127, China. [3]Department of Pediatric Cardiology, Shanghai Children's Medical Center, School of Medicine, Shanghai Jiao Tong University, Shanghai 200127, China.

References

1. Hoffman JI, Kaplan S. The incidence of congenital heart disease. J Am Coll Cardiol. 2002;39(12):1890–900.
2. van der Bom T, Zomer AC, Zwinderman AH, Meijboom FJ, Bouma BJ, Mulder BJ. The changing epidemiology of congenital heart disease. Nat Rev Cardiol. 2011;8(1):50–60.
3. Tutarel O, Kempny A, Alonso-Gonzalez R, Jabbour R, Li W, Uebing A, Dimopoulos K, Swan L, Gatzoulis MA, Diller GP. Congenital heart disease beyond the age of 60: emergence of a new population with high resource utilization, high morbidity, and high mortality. Eur Heart J. 2014;35(11):725–32.
4. Verheugt CL, Uiterwaal CS, van der Velde ET, Meijboom FJ, Pieper PG, Sieswerda GT, Plokker HW, Grobbee DE, Mulder BJ. The emerging burden of hospital admissions of adults with congenital heart disease. Heart. 2010; 96(11):872–8.
5. Hutson MR, Kirby ML. Model systems for the study of heart development and disease. Cardiac neural crest and conotruncal malformations. Semin Cell Dev Biol. 2007;18(1):101–10.
6. Ward C, Stadt H, Hutson M, Kirby ML. Ablation of the secondary heart field leads to tetralogy of Fallot and pulmonary atresia. Dev Biol. 2005; 284(1):72–83.
7. Waldo KL, Hutson MR, Ward CC, Zdanowicz M, Stadt HA, Kumiski D, Abu-Issa R, Kirby ML. Secondary heart field contributes myocardium and smooth muscle to the arterial pole of the developing heart. Dev Biol. 2005;281(1): 78–90.
8. Jenkins KJ, Correa A, Feinstein JA, Botto L, Britt AE, Daniels SR, Elixson M, Warnes CA, Webb CL. Noninherited risk factors and congenital cardiovascular defects: current knowledge: a scientific statement from the American Heart Association Council on Cardiovascular Disease in the Yong: endorsed by the American Academy of Pediatrics. Circulation. 2007;115(23): 2995–3014.
9. Cooper WO, Hernandez-Diaz S, Arboast PG, Dudley JA, Deyer S, Giddeon PS, Hall K, Ray WA. Major congenital malformations after first-trimester exposure to ACE inhibitors. N Engl J Med. 2006;354(23):2443–51.
10. Meganathan K, Sotiriadou I, Natarajan K, Hescheler J, Sachinidis A. Signaling molecules, transcription growth factors and other regulators revealed from in-vivo and in-vitro models for the regulation of cardiac development. Int J Cardiol. 2015;183:117–28.
11. Plageman TF Jr, Yutzey KE. T-box genes and heart development: putting the "T" in heart. Dev Dyn. 2005;232(1):11–20.
12. Christoffels VM, Hoogaars WM, Tessari A, Clout DE, Moorman AF, Campione M. T-box transcription factor Tbx2 represses differentiation and formation of the cardiac chambers. Dev Dyn. 2004;229(4):763–70.

13. Yamada M, Revelli JP, Eichele G, Barron M, Schwartz RJ. Expression of chick Tbx-2, Tbx-3, and Tbx-5 genes during early heart development: evidence for BMP2 induction of Tbx2. Dev Biol. 2000;228(1):95–105.
14. Harrelson Z, Kelly RG, Goldin SN, Gibson-Brown JJ, Bollag RJ, Silver LM, Papaioannou VE. Tbx2 is essential for patterning the atrioventricular canal and for morphogenesis of the outflow tract during heart development. Development. 2004;131(20):5041–52.
15. Bamshad M, Lin RC, Law DJ, Watkins WC, Krakowiak PA, Moore ME, Franceschini P, Lala R, Holmes LB, Gebuhr TC, Bruneau BG, Schinzel A, Seidman JG, Seidman CE, Jorde LB. Mutations in human TBX3 alter limb, apocrine and genital development in ulnar-mammary syndrome. Nat Genet. 1997;16(3):311–5.
16. Mesbah K, Harrelson Z, Theveniau-Ruissy M, Papaioannou VE, Kelly RG. Tbx3 is required for outflow tract development. Circ Res. 2008;103(7):743–50.
17. Dupays L, Kotecha S, Angst B, Mohun TJ. Tbx2 misexpression impairs deployment of second heart field derived progenitor cells to the arterial pole of the embryonic heart. Dev Biol. 2009;333(1):121–31.
18. Mesbah K, Rana MS, Francou A, van Duijvenboden K, Papaioannou VE, Moorman AF, Kelly RG, Christoffels VM. Identification of a Tbx1/Tbx2/Tbx3 genetic pathway governing pharyngeal and arterial pole morphogenesis. Hum Mol Genet. 2012;21(6):1217–29.
19. Pang S, Liu Y, Zhao Z, Huang W, Chen D, Yan B. Novel and functional sequence variants within the TBX2 gene promoter in ventricular septal defects. Biochimie. 2013;95(9):1087–9.
20. Campbell C, Goodrich K, Casey G, Beatty B. Cloning and mapping of a human gene (TBX2) sharing a highly conserved protein motif with the Drosophila omb gene. Genomics. 1995;28(2):255–60.
21. Crum TL, Okkema PG. SUMOylation-dependent function of a T-box transcriptional repressor in Caenorhabditis elegans. Biochem Soc Trans. 2007; 35(6):1424–6.
22. Huber P, Crum T, Clary LM, Ronan T, Packard AV, Okkema PG. Function of the C. elegans T-box factor TBX-2 depends on SUMOylation. Cell Mol Life Sci. 2013;70(21):4157–68.
23. Firnberg N, Neubuser A. FGF signaling regulates expression of Tbx2, Erm, Pea3, and Pax3 in the early nasal region. Dev Biol. 2002;247(2):237–50.
24. Ilagan R, Abu-Issa R, Brown D, Yang YP, Jiao K, Schwartz RJ, Klingensmith J, Meyers EN. Fgf8 is required for anterior heart field development. Development. 2006;133(12):2435–45.
25. Shirai M, Imanaka-Yoshida K, Schneider MD, Schwartz RJ, Morisaki T. T-box 2, a mediator of Bmp-Smad signaling, induced hyaluronan synthase 2 and Tgfbeta2 expression and endocardial cushion formation. Proc Natl Acad Sci U S A. 2009;106(44):18604–9.
26. Yang YQ, Gharibeh L, Li RG, Xin YF, Wang J, Liu ZM, Qiu XB, Xu YJ, Xu L, Qu XK, Liu X, Fang WY, Huang RT, Xue S, Nemer G. GATA4 loss-of-function mutations underlie familial tetralogy of Fallot. Hum Mutat. 2013;34(12):1662–71.
27. Hoogaars WM, Tessari A, Moorman AF, de Boer PA, Hagoort J, Soufan AT, Campione M, Christoffels VM. The transcriptional repressor Tbx3 delineates the developing central conduction system of the heart. Cardiovasc Res. 2004;62(3):489–99.
28. Habets PE, Moorman AF, Clout DE, van Roon MA, Lingbeek M, van Lohuizen M, Campione M, Christoffels VM. Cooperative action of Tbx2 and Nkx2.5 inhibits ANF expression in the atrioventricular canal: implications for cardiac chamber formation. Genes Dev. 2002;16(10): 1234–46.
29. Ribeiro I, Kawakami Y, Büscher D, Raya A, Rodríguez-León J, Morita M, Rodríguez Esteban C, Izpisúa Belmonte JC. Tbx2 and Tbx3 regulate the dynamics of cell proliferation during heart remodeling. PLoS One. 2007;2(4):e398.
30. Singh R, Hoogaars WM, Barnett P, Grieskamp T, Rana MS, Buermans H, Farin HF, Petry M, Heallen T, Martin JF, Moorman AF, 't Hoen PA, Kispert A, Christoffels VM. Tbx2 and Tbx3 induce atrioventricular myocardial development and endocardial cushion formation. Cell Mol Life Sci. 2012; 69(8):1377–89.
31. Camenisch TD, Spicer AP, Brehm-Gibson T, Biesterfeldt J, Augustine ML, Calabro A Jr, Kubalak S, Klewer SE, McDonald JA. Disruption of hyaluronan synthase-2 abrogates normal cardiac morphogenesis and hyaluronan-mediated transformation of epithelium to mesenchyme. J Clin Invest. 2000; 106(3):349–60.
32. Akagi T, Kuure S, Uranishi K, Koide H, Costantini F, Yokota T. ETS-related transcription factors ETV4 and ETV5 are involved in proliferation and induction of differentiation-associated genes in embryonic stem (ES) cells. J Biol Chem. 2015;290(37):22460–73.
33. Oh S, Shin S, Janknecht R. ETV1, 4 and 5: an oncogenic subfamily of ETS transcription factors. Biochim Biophys Acta. 2012;1826(1):1–12.
34. Sinclair CS, Adem C, Naderi A, Soderberg CL, Johnson M, Wu K, Wadum L, Couch VL, Sellers TA, Schaid D, Slezak J, Fredericksen Z, Ingle JN, Hartmann L, Jenkins RB, Couch FJ. TBX2 is preferentially amplified in BRCA1- and BRCA2-related breast tumors. Cancer Res. 2002;62(13):3587–91.
35. Barnes RM, Harris IS, Jaehnig EJ, Sauls K, Sinha T, Rojas A, Schachterle W, McCulley DJ, Norris RA, Black BL. MEF2C regulates outflow tract alignment and transcriptional control of Tdgf1. Development. 2016;143(5):774–9.
36. Kodo K, Nishizawa T, Furutani M, Arai S, Ishihara K, Oda M, Makino S, Fukuda K, Takahashi T, Matsuoka R, Nakanishi T, Yamagishi H. Genetic analysis of essential cardiac transcription factors in 256 patients with non-syndromic congenital heart defects. Circ J. 2012;76(7):1703–11.
37. Paxton C, Zhao H, Chin Y, Langner K, Reecy J. Murine Tbx2 contains domains that activate and repress gene transcription. Gene. 2002;283(1–2):117–24.
38. Manolio TA, Collins FS, Cox NJ, Goldstein DB, Hindorff LA, Hunter DJ, McCarthy MI, Ramos EM, Cardon LR, Chakravarti A, et al. Finding the missing heritability of complex diseases. Nature. 2009;461(7265):747–53.
39. Livak KJ, Schmittgen TD. Analysis of relative gene expression data using real-time quantitative PCR and the 2(−Delta Delta C(T)) method. Methods. 2001;25(4):402–8.

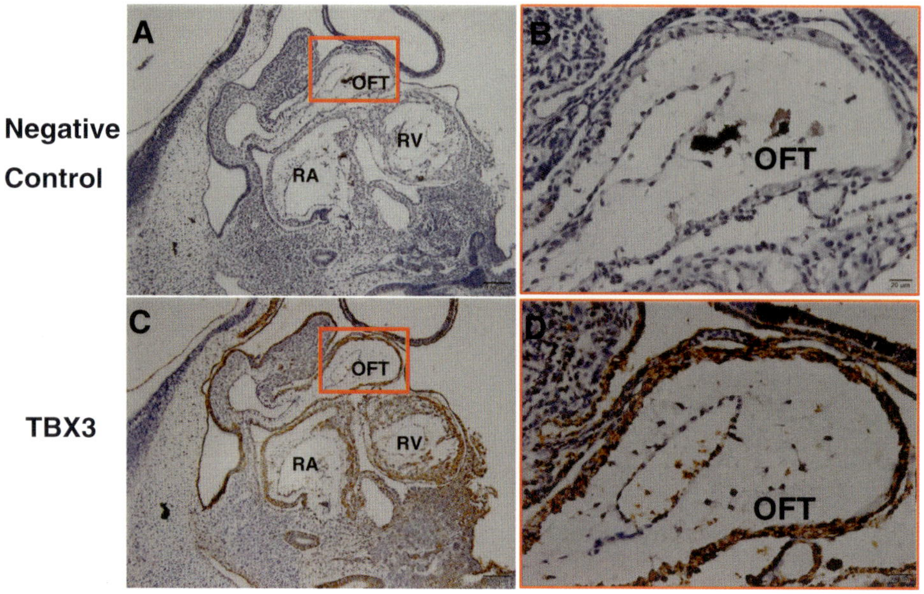

Fig. 7 Immunohistochemistry of TBX3 in human embryos in Carnegie 13 stage. **a**, **b** Negative control. **c**, **d** Wild-type TBX3. Scale bar 20 μm

with a minor allele frequency (MAF) < 0.5% were defined as rare [38].

Multiple TBX2 and TBX3 protein sequence alignment

TBX2 and TBX3 protein sequences from *Homo sapiens* (human), *Mus musculus* (house mouse), *Gallus gallus* (chicken), *Bos taurus* (cattle), *Canis lupus familiaris* (dog), *Pan troglodytes* (chimpanzee), and *Sus scrofa* (pig) were downloaded from NCBI (https://www.ncbi.nlm.nih.gov/protein/) and were aligned with ClustalX software to confirm the conservation of TBX2 and TBX3 sequences.

Plasmid construction and site-directed mutagenesis

The TBX2 and TBX3 cDNA plasmid was purchased from Genomeditech. Mutated primers were designed to amplify human TBX2 and TBX3 cDNA according to the protocol provided by the QuikChange SiteDirected Mutagenesis Kit (Stratagene, USA), and then, variant TBX2 cDNAs were cloned into a pCDNA3.1-3xFlag vectors while variant TBX3 cDNAs were cloned into GV141-3xFlag vectors. For recombining luciferase reporter plasmid, a 5′-flanking region of downstream gene promoter was subcloned into Kpn I and Bgl II sites of the pGL3 luciferase reporter-basic vector (Promega, USA).

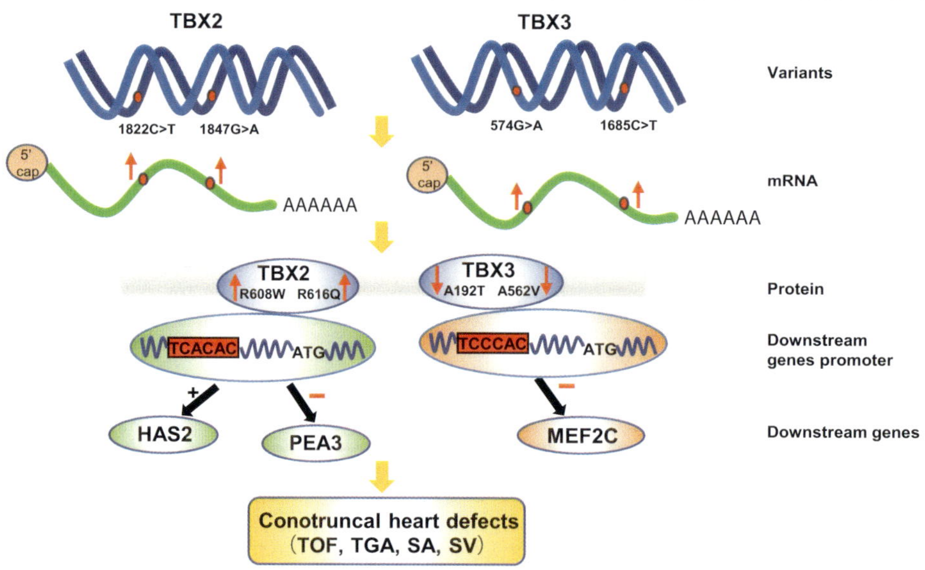

Fig. 8 The diagram of the regulation TBX2 and TBX3 variants involved in CTD pathogenesis

Table 2 Cardiac diagnoses for study population of patients with CTDs

Diagnoses	Number	Gender/number	Age
TGA	90	F18M72	1 day–16 years
TOF	234	F83M151	1 month–13 years
DORV	98	F32M66	1 month–17 years
PA/VSD	97	F36M61	3 months–12 years
IAA	13	F7M6	7 days–1 year
PTA	10	F5M5	3 days–2 years
SA/SV	46	F19M27	1 month–13 years
Total	588	F200M388	1 day–17 years

TGA transposition of the great arteries, *TOF* tetralogy of Fallot, *DORV* double outlet of right ventricle, *PA/VSD* pulmonary atresia with ventricular septal defect, *IAA* interruption of aortic arch, *PTA* persistent truncus arteriosus, *SA* single atrium, *SV* single ventricle, *F* female, *M* male

Cell cultures and transfection

HEK 293T cells (Human embryonic kidney cells) were maintained in Dulbecco's modified Eagle's medium (HyClone, USA) with 10% fetal bovine serum (MP Biomedicals, USA) and 1% penicillin-streptomycin (Gibco, USA). pcDNA3.1-3xFlag-TBX2 and GV141-3xFlag-TBX3 including wild-type and variants were transfected into 293T cells with FuGene HD (Promega, USA) according to the manufacturer's protocol after seeding 24 h.

Quantitative RT-PCR

Plasmids were transfected into HEK 293T cells that were seeded in 12-well plates. Cells were harvested 36 h after transfection. Total RNA was extracted with TRIzol reagent (Invitrogen, USA), and then, reverse transcription of cDNA was performed using Prime Script RT Master Mix (Takara, Japan) and was followed by quantitative RT-PCR using SYBR Premix Ex Taq (Takara, Japan) on an Applied Biosystems 7500 system (Applied Biosystems, USA). The relative quantification of expression was determined using the $2^{-\Delta\Delta Ct}$ method [39], and glyceraldehyde-3-phosphate dehydrogenase (GAPDH, human) was used as an internal control. Primer sequences of TBX2, TBX3, GAPDH, and candidate downstream genes are listed in Table 3.

Western blot

HEK 293T cells were transfected with 1 μg of wild-type and variant plasmid DNA. Cells were harvested 48 h after transfection. For protein degradation experiments, HEK 293T cells were cultured in the presence of 10 mM MG132 solution dissolved in DMSO for 8–10 h before harvest. Then, cells were lysed in RIPA lysis buffer (Beyotime, China) with PMSF (1:100). The proteins were subjected to 10% SDS-PAGE and were then transferred onto nitrocellulose membranes (Millipore, USA) and immunostained with rabbit anti-FLAG antibody (1:1000, Sigma-Aldrich, USA) and mouse anti-β-actin antibody (1:5000, Sigma-Aldrich, USA) at 4 °C overnight. The membranes were incubated with horseradish peroxidase-conjugated anti-rabbit secondary antibody (1:10000) and anti-mouse secondary antibody (1:10000). Immobilon Western Chemiluminescent HRP Substrate (Millipore, USA) was used for chemiluminescent immunodetection.

Table 3 Sequences of the primers used for real-time quantitative PCR

Gene	Forward (5′→3′)	Reverse (5′→3′)
GAPDH	GGAGCGAGATCCCTCCAAAAT	GGCTGTTGTCATACTTCTCATGG
TBX2	CACGGCTTCACCATCCTAAAC	TGCGGAAGGTGCTGTAAGG
TBX3	GAGGCTAAAGAACTTTGGGATCA	CATTTCGGGGTCGGCCTTA
BMP2	GAGGTCCTGAGCGAGTTCGA	ACCTGAGTGCCTGCGATACA
BMP4	ATGATTCCTGGTAACCGAATGC	CCCCGTCTCAGGTATCAAACT
CRELD1	GCTCCTATGAGTGCCGAGAC	CTACACTTCTTACAGCGACCTG
DKK1	ATAGCACCTTGGATGGGTATTCC	CTGATGACCGGAGACAAACAG
FGF8	GACCCCTTCGCAAAGCTCAT	CCGTTGCTCTTGGCGATCA
FOG2	GGCCTGAAAATCTGAGCTGC	CAGTCGTCTGTCTCAACTCCA
GATA4	CGACACCCCAATCTCGATATG	GTTGCACAGATAGTGACCCGT
GATA6	CTCAGTTCCTACGCTTCGCAT	GTCGAGGTCAGTGAACAGCA
HAND2	CGCCGACACCAAACTCTCC	TCGCCATTCTGGTCGTCCT
HAS2	CTCATCATCCAAAGCCTGTT	GCTGGGTCAAGCATAGTGTC
MEF2C	CCAACTTCGAGATGCCAGTCT	GTCGATGTGTTACACCAGGAG
PLXND1	AATGGGCGGAACATCGTCAAG	CGAGACTGGTTGGAAACACAG
PEA3	GAGAAACCTCTGCGACCATT	GCCCGTCCAGGCAATGAAAT

21

Mutational analysis of epidermal and hyperproliferative type I keratins in mild and moderate psoriasis vulgaris patients: a possible role in the pathogenesis of psoriasis along with disease severity

Tamilselvi Elango[1,5*†], Jingying Sun[1], Caihong Zhu[1], Fusheng Zhou[1], Yaohua Zhang[4], Liangdan Sun[1,2,3], Sen Yang[1,2,3] and Xuejun Zhang[1,2,3,4,5*†]

Abstract

Background: Mutations in keratin proteins have been vastly associated with a wide array of genodermatoses; however, mutations of keratins in psoriasis have not been fully investigated. The main aim of the current research was to identify the mutation in K14, K10, K16, and K17 genes in two stages of psoriasis patients.

Methods: Ninety-six psoriatic skin biopsies were collected. mRNA transcript of K14, K10, K16, and K17 was prepared, amplified, and sequenced. Sanger sequences of all keratins were further validated for mutational analysis using Mutation Surveyor and Alamut Visual. Then, in silico analysis of protein stability and protein and gene expression of all keratins was performed and validated.

Results: Out of 44 mutations, about 75% of keratins are highly pathogenic and deleterious. Remaining 25% mutations are less pathogenic and tolerated in nature. In these 33 deleterious mutations were immensely found to decrease keratin protein stability. We also found a correlation between keratin and Psoriasis Area and Severity Index score which added that alteration in keratin gene in skin causes severity of psoriasis.

Conclusions: We strongly concluded that acanthosis and abnormal terminal differentiation was mainly due to the mutation in epidermal keratins. In turn, disease severity and relapsing of psoriasis are mainly due to the mutation of hyperproliferative keratins. These novel keratin mutations in psoriatic epidermis might be one of the causative factors for psoriasis.

Keywords: Epidermal keratins, Hyperproliferative keratins, Psoriasis, Mutation, Sanger sequence, Immunofluorescence

Background

Keratinocytes play a special role in sensing epidermal barrier and regulating immune homeostasis [1]. Its functions mainly depend on structural proteins including keratins [2, 3]. Keratins are the main intermediate filament cytoskeleton in all epithelia [4]. In normal skin, basal cells express two keratins, K5 and K14, whereas suprabasal cells express differentiation-related keratins K1 and K10. These pairs act as a flexible scaffold enabling cells to resist physical stress and also play different cellular functions including protection from apoptosis and regulation of epithelial organization [5, 6]. Consequently, defects in intermediate filaments (Ifs) can lead to cell fragility and are linked to a wide array of genodermatoses and cancers [7, 8].

Psoriasis is a genetically determined chronic inflammatory skin disease characterized by acanthosis, abnormal keratinization, and inflammatory cell infiltrates [9]. In psoriatic lesions, terminal differentiation of keratinocytes is incomplete, which leads to preferential activation and

* Correspondence: tami24684@gmail.com; ayzxj@vip.sina.com
†Equal contributors
[1]Institute and Department of Dermatology, The First Affiliated Hospital, Anhui Medical University, Hefei, China
Full list of author information is available at the end of the article

proliferation of cells that do not mature properly. These changes are mainly associated with altered expression of keratin in psoriasis [10]. In psoriasis, the changes in keratin expression include a reduction in K1 and K10 and the induction of hyperproliferation-associated keratins K6, K16, and K17 [11–13]. Furthermore, the expression levels of K5 and K14 in the basal cell layer are also altered in the psoriatic epidermis. The hyperproliferation in psoriasis seemed to result from an increase in the number of transit amplifying cells, following depletion of the stem cell compartment [14, 15]. As a whole, these changes suggest that each keratin pair provides specific functional requirements to epidermal keratinocytes.

Over 90% of pathogenic mutations in keratinopathies are missense mutations with a small number of small in-frame insertions vs. deletion mutations and a few intronic splice site defects leading to larger in-frame deletions. Various cutaneous disorders are identified with mutated keratin proteins namely epidermolysis bullosa simplex (EBS) (K5, K14), ichthyosis (Kl, K2, and K10), palmoplantar keratoderma (K9), type I pachyonychia congenita (PC) (K6a and K16), seven type II pachyonychia congenita (K6b and K17), and monilethrix (K81, K83, and K86). [16–18]. In most of these conditions, the associated pathology results from fragile keratinocytes expressing the mutated keratin protein.

Since genome-wide association studies (GWAS), connecting the psoriasis to the late cornified envelope gene cluster has specified that epidermal abnormalities along with hyperproliferative keratin pattern play a major role in the pathogenesis of psoriasis [19, 20]. The main aim of this study is to identify the mutation of keratin in two stages of psoriasis, which mainly causes hyperproliferation along with defects in the cornification process. We speculated that mutation in K14 and K10 might serve as an important mechanism that affects keratinocyte proliferation in all stages of psoriasis, and also, mutation in hyperproliferative keratin K16 and K17 might be the foremost cause for the incurability and exacerbation of this disease. To verify our hypotheses, we examined Sanger sequence of the CDS region of all these keratins in both stages. For mutational analysis, we performed a computational analysis of all these keratins in both stages of psoriasis by using Mutation Surveyor and Alamut Visual software. In addition, effects of these mutations on protein stability were predicted by using in silico prediction tools. According to our result, the predicted deleterious mutations were mainly clustered in the rod domain on the keratin protein, which is crucial for keratin function. Most of the deleterious mutations were predicted to decrease protein stability which might cause the changes in protein expression of these keratins. All these changes might trigger or exacerbate psoriasis.

Materials and methods

Patients' details

Patients with psoriasis vulgaris ($n = 96$) who visited the Institute of Dermatology, Anhui Medical University (AHMU), between 2015 and 2017 were recruited in this study. The age of all patients ranged from 16 to 71 years (mean ± SD, 37.97 ± 14.03 years). In this study, based on body surface area involvement, we have categorized patients into two, (i) mild psoriasis patients ($n = 48$) and (ii) moderate psoriasis patients ($n = 48$). Severity of plaque psoriasis was graded into mild and moderate to severe disease. Mild disease was defined as body surface area (BSA) ≤ 10, Psoriasis Area and Severity Index (PASI) ≤ 10, and dermatology life quality index (DLQI) ≤ 10 and moderate to severe psoriasis as BSA > 10 or PASI > 10 and DLQI > 10 [21]. Patients were included in the study based on the following criteria: (i) at least one well-demarcated, erythematous, scaly lesion verified by at least two dermatologists; (ii) each lesion tissue was confirmed by clinical histopathology; (iii) no systematic anti-psoriatic treatment 2 weeks before skin biopsy; and (iv) no topical anti-psoriatic treatments for 1 week prior to biopsy. Informed consent was obtained from all individuals, under an AHMU-approved protocol. The study was approved by the institutional ethical committee and conducted according to the Declaration of Helsinki principles.

Collection of tissue samples

In all patients, 10 mm of lesional and nonlesional skin biopsies were taken after local anesthesia, lidocaine hydrochloride, and adrenaline bitartrate IP were given intradermally. Nonlesional skin biopsy served as control. Biopsies of psoriatic lesional skin were taken within a lesion, 1 cm from the edge of the plaque border. Biopsies of nonlesional skin were taken 2 cm beyond the plaque border. Skin biopsies were immediately frozen in liquid nitrogen.

Histology analysis

Formalin-fixed skin biopsy was embedded in paraffin and processed routinely. Hematoxylin-eosin staining was used to examine the histological changes in mild and moderate psoriatic skin.

RNA isolation and qRT-PCR

RNA from both skin tissues were isolated by TRIZOL Method, and RT-PCR was conducted using the High-Capacity cDNA Reverse Transcription Kits (Applied Biosystems, USA) according to the manufacturer's protocol. Taqman Master Mix (Applied Biosystems, Bedford, MA) was used with Taqman probes. Real-time quantitative PCR was performed with the ABI PRISM7700 Sequence Detection System. All expression values were normalized against

GAPDH. Relative mRNA expression levels of all examined genes were measured using the comparative $2^{-\Delta\Delta CT}$ [22]. All amplifications were done three times in triplicate.

PCR amplification, sequencing, and mutation screening

cDNA prepared from mild and moderate psoriatic RNA samples were amplified using a polymerase chain reaction (PCR). The primers were designed from the CDS region of all these keratins (Table 1). PCR reaction was performed using Biorad Thermal Cycler. The PCR conditions were as given in Table 1. Amplified PCR products were electrophoresed through a 1.5% agarose gel, to control the quality of fragments. Sanger sequencing reactions were performed on the purified PCR fragments using a BigDye® Terminator v3.1 Cycle Sequencing Kit (Applied Biosystems, USA) with the same primers as for the PCRs, forward and reverse primers in separate experiments. All genes were sequenced from both directions. Reactions were processed on the ABI3730xl instrument. Sequence reads were analyzed using Applied Biosystems. Sequence reads were aligned to human genome by using Bioedit software.

Mutation Surveyor is a useful in silico tool developed by SoftGenetics that assists the detection of sequence variations within Sanger sequencing traces. This tool can process up to 400 lanes of data at a time with high accuracy and sensitivity. It can effectively detect SNPs and mutation in their homozygous or heterozygous states as well as mosaicism [23]. In this study, we did sequence analysis and pathogenic variant identification by using Mutation Surveyor DNA variant analysis software (SoftGenetics, USA). For prediction of the mutation's pathogenicity, Alamut Visual software (Interactive Biosoftware, France) was used [24]. Studies have shown that Alamut Visual is the original decision-support software application, used by leading genetic clinicians and researchers around the world. This software was used for alignment, conservation, SIFT/PolyPhen dbSNP, and Exome Sequencing Project data collection to evaluate the variant in its surrounding genomic context [25, 26]. All variants were further annotated with the Exome Aggregation Consortium (ExAC) [27].

Prediction of deleterious mutations

Six best performing tools were combined into a consensus classifier PredictSNP1.0, which gives significantly improved prediction performance and at the same time returned results for all mutations, confirming that consensus prediction represents an accurate and robust alternative to the predictions delivered by individual tools. Also, this is a user-friendly web interface for all researchers and clinician which enables an easy access to all eight prediction tools, the consensus classifier PredictSNP, and annotations from the Protein Mutant Database and the UniProt database. Based on the above details, we used PredictSNP1.0 (http://loschmidt.chemi.muni.cz/predictsnp1), classifier webserver, to predict the effects of mutations on protein function [28]. PredictSNP1.0 runs and integrates MAPP, nsSNPAnalyzer, PANTHER, PhD-SNP, Polyphen-1, Polyphen-2, SIFT, and SNAP to predict disease-related amino acid mutations. The four tools use machine-learning methods; nsSNPAnalyzer uses random forest, PhD-SNP uses support vector machines, PolyPhen-2 uses Naive Bayes, and SNAP uses neural network. SIFT, MAPP, and PANTHER consider alignment score information, and PolyPhen-1 uses an expert set of empirical rules to predict possible impact of amino acid substitutions. PredictSNP1.0 displays the confidence scores generated by each tool and a consensus prediction as percentages by using their observed accuracy values to ease comparisons [29].

Table 1 Primer sequences and reaction conditions used for PCR

S. no.	Primer	Sequences (5'-3')	Length (bp)	Reaction conditions
1	K14 F	GTGGGCAGTGAGAAGGTGAC	966	Denaturation, 30 s at 94 °C
	K14 R	AGAGGAGAACTGGGAGGAGG		Annealing, 45 s at 59 °C Extension, 60 s at 72 °C No. of cycles, 35
2	K10 F	GGCTCATCAGGTGGCTAT	812	Denaturation, 30 s at 94 °C
	K10 R	CAGGCTTCAGCATCTTTG		Annealing, 45 s at 58 °C Extension, 60 s at 72 °C No. of cycles, 35
3	K16 F	GTGAAGATCCGTGACTGG	856	Denaturation, 30 s at 94 °C
	K16 R	TGCTGGGAGGAAAGGTGG		Annealing, 45 s at 56 °C Extension,60 s at 72 °C No. of cycles, 35
4	K17 F	CTTCCGCACCAAGTTTGA	753	Denaturation, 30 s at 94 °C
	K17 R	TTGCCATCCTGGACCTCT		Annealing, 45 s at 55 °C Extension, 60 s at 72 °C No. of cycles, 35

The effects of predicted deleterious mutations on protein stability

The effect of deleterious missense amino acid substitutions on K14, K10, K16, and K17 protein stability was analyzed with MUpro (http://mupro.proteomics.ics.uci.edu) [30] and I-Mutant2.0 (http://folding.biofold.org/i-mutant/i-mutant2.0.html) [31]. MUpro uses support vector machine (SVM) and neural network to predict the effect of amino acid changes on protein stability and calculates a score between − 1 and 1 as the confidence of prediction. A confidence score < 0 indicates the mutation decreases the protein stability, while a confidence score > 0 means the mutation increases the protein stability. I-Mutant 2.0 uses SVM to predict protein stability alterations upon mutations and provides the predicted free energy change value (DDG) and the sign of the prediction as increase or decrease. DDG is calculated as unfolding Gibbs free energy value (mutated protein) – unfolding Gibbs free energy value (wild-type protein) in Kcal/mole. DDG > 0 means increased protein stability, and DDG < 0 means decreased protein stability.

Visualization of predicted deleterious mutations on 3D keratin structure

The location of predicted deleterious mutations was detected by STRUM (http://zhanglab.ccmb.med.umich.edu/STRUM/), which constructs 3D models according to the iterative threading assembly refinement (I-TASSER) simulation [32].

Western blot analysis

Western blot was performed as previously described [33] using primary antibodies as follows: K14, K10, K16, and K17 and β-actin (Thermo-scientific, USA). Band intensity was analyzed using ImageJ software (http://rsb.info.nih.gov/ij/).

Immunofluorescence and confocal microscopy

Immunofluorescence assay was performed as described previously [34]. Skin biopsies were obtained from the lesional and nonlesional skin of each patient (control samples). Tissues were sectioned (4 μm) and stained with rabbit monoclonal anti-cytokeratin 14 and mouse monoclonal anti-cytokeratin10, 16, and 17 (Thermo-scientific, USA). An appropriate Alexa Fluor 488-conjugated anti-rabbit IgG and anti-mouse IgG (Thermo-scientific, USA) and DAPI staining of nuclei were used. The images were examined by the pathologist using an Olympus–Ix Microscope and merged using Image J Software.

Statistical analysis

Results were expressed as mean ± SD. Data were analyzed using SPSS 16.0 software. Nonlesional and lesional skin biopsy samples were compared by Student's T test. Spearman's coefficient was used to identify correlations between keratins and PASI score. $P < 0.05$ was considered to be significant.

Results

Baseline analysis of psoriatic lesion

The histological examination of nonlesional skin tissue shows normal rete ridges with stratum corneum whereas that of mild and moderate lesional skin revealed elongated rete ridges with deregulated stratum corneum (Fig. 1a). Histological analysis was further supported by PASI score. Forty-eight patients with mild psoriasis have a PASI score of 4.06 ± 2.46, and the remaining 48 patients with moderate psoriasis have a PASI score of 17.34 ± 5.64 (Fig. 1b).

Mutated keratin sequences identified through Sanger sequencing

Almost in all the keratin mutation and sequence studies, NCBI database is widely used, NM_000526.4 (K14), NM_000421.3 (K10), NM_005557.3 (K16), and NM_000422.2 (K17), as publicly available sequence data for healthy population (control). According to the above keratins, nucleotide accession number of these sequences is also retrieved from the Chinese population [35–39]. So, in order to predict the mutation in two stages of psoriasis, we have taken the K14, K10, K16, and K17 coding sequences of healthy population available in NCBI database with accession numbers NM_000526.4 (K14), NM_000421.3 (K10), NM_005557.3 (K16), and NM_000422.2 (K17), which were further aligned respectively with the Sanger sequences of K14, K10, K16, and K17 obtained in our patients by using BioEdit software (Additional file 1: Figs. S1 and S2). In mild psoriasis patients, we have identified nine and seven missense mutations in K14 and K10, respectively, as well as no missense mutation was found in K16 and K17. However, in moderate psoriasis, we found nine, six, five, and eight mutations of K14, K10, K16, and K17, respectively.

Some of our mutated K14, K10, and K17 sequences were matched to previously reported sequences in other skin disease (Table 2). In order to compare the mutation identified in psoriasis patients with other skin disease patients, we have used the following Clinvar data in the NCBI website (https://www.ncbi.nlm.nih.gov/clinvar/) (Tables 3 and 4). According to the Clinvar data of NM_000526.4 (K14), 11 missense mutations of K14 were found in EBS disease; comparing these mutations with our K14 results, three mutations were found to be identical in both diseases. Likewise, NM_000421.3 (K10) compared with K10 of our patients showed only one identical mutation. Compared with our results, no identical mutation was

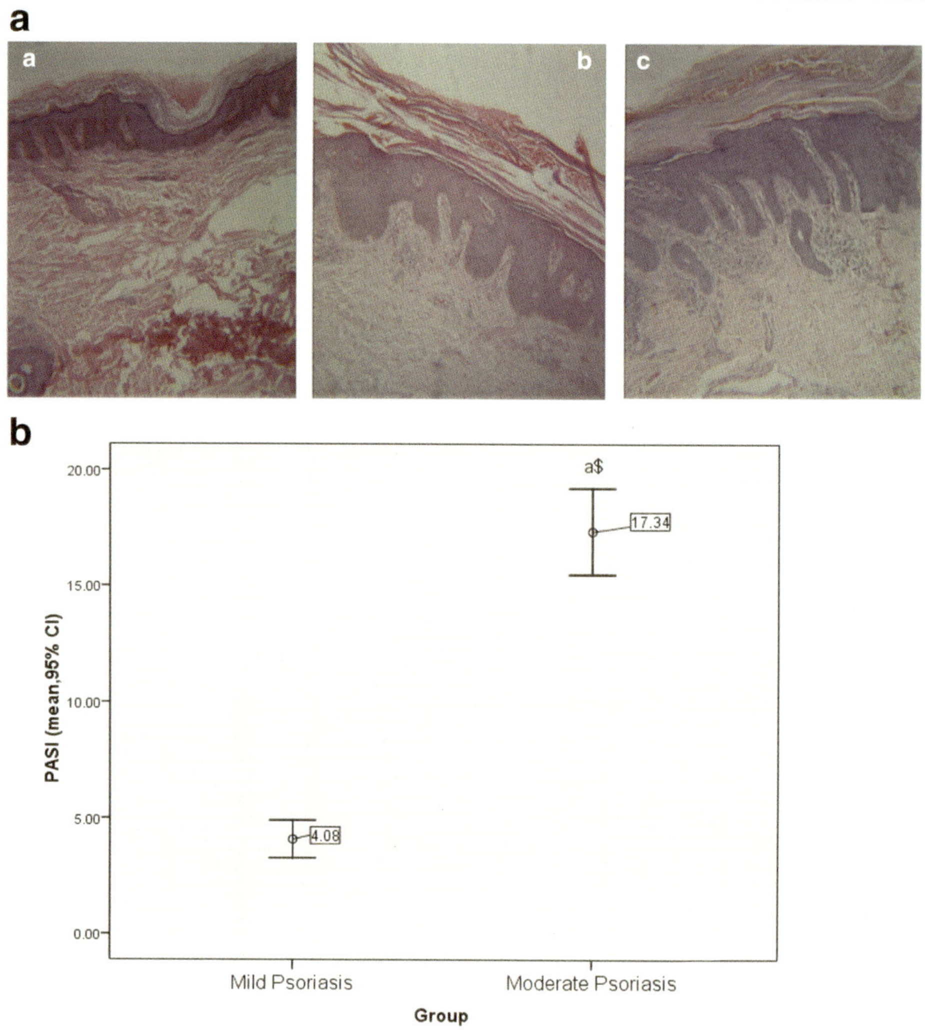

Fig. 1 Histological and clinical examinations of mild and moderate psoriatic skin. **a** Histological examination of skin biopsy. (A) Photomicrograph of nonlesional skin biopsy. (B), (C) Photomicrograph of mild and moderate psoriasis vulgaris showing Munro microabscess, acanthosis, rete ridge elongation, and acute infiltration of dermis. **b** Clinical evidence of mild and moderate psoriatic lesion by PASI score. All values were expressed as mean ± SD. "a" denotes comparison of PASI score of mild and moderate psoriasis. The dollar sign denotes $P < 0.001$

Table 2 Mutated epidermal and hyperproliferative keratin sequences identified in this study consistent with previous reports (clinvar and dbSNP in the NCBI website)

S. no.	Gene	Mutation region	Accession number	
			Clinvar	dbSNP
1	Keratin 14	C442 > T	RCV000056740.1	rs58378809
2		A1234 > T	RCV000056680.1	rs267607403
3		G1237 > A	RCV000056682.1	rs59780231
4		C1246 > T		rs777067461
5	Keratin 10	C520 > A	RCV000056502.1	
6	Keratin 17	C986 > T		rs780535087

found in both keratin 16 and 17. Based on per nucleotide sequence variation, percentage of background mutation rate was calculated. The high background mutation rates of K14 mutated nucleotide sequences in our patients were 33.3% G > C, followed by 22.2% A > T, 16.6% C > T, 11.1% G > T, and 5.5% of C > A, G > A, and C > G, whereas EBS disease condition obtained from the NCBI website showed high mutation rate of 36.3% G > A. Background mutation rates of psoriasis K10 were as follows: G > T, T > A, G > C, A > C, C > G, and C > A with percentages of 30.7, 15.3, and 7.6%. In EI disease, A > C nucleotide K10 mutation is found to be 23% followed with 15.3% of G > A and T > C. The most highest K16 mutated nucleotide found in our study is 40% of C > G whereas 25% of A > T, C > T, and G > T was found in K17.

Table 3 Comparison of publicly available mutated keratin 14 and keratin 10 sequence data of various skin disease patients with mutated sequence obtained in our study (psoriasis) from Clinvar NCBI database

S. no.	Name	Gene(s)	Condition(s)	Clinical significance (Last reviewed)	GRCh37		GRCh38		Variation ID	Allele ID(s)
					Chromosome	Location	Chromosome	Location		
1	NM_000526.4(KRT14): c.1264G > A (p.Glu422Lys)	KRT14	EBH-DM	Pathogenic (Apr 1, 2000)	17	39739497	17	41583245	14623	29662
2	NM_000526.4(KRT14): c.1256T > A (p.Leu419Gln)	KRT14	EBH-DM	Pathogenic (Apr 1, 2000)	17	39739505	17	41583253	14622	29661
3	NM_000526.4(KRT14): c.1243T > C (p.Tyr415His)	KRT14	EBH-DM	Pathogenic (Mar 27, 2015)	17	39739518	17	41583266	14621	29660
4	*NM_000526.4(KRT14): c.1237G > A (p.Ala413Thr)*	*KRT 14*	*Not provided*	*Pathogenic (Jul 31, 2012)*	*17*	*39739524*	*17*	*41583272*	*66319*	*77216*
5	*NM_000526.4(KRT14): c.1234A > T (p.Ile412Phe)*	*KRT14*	*Not provided*	*Pathogenic (Apr 2, 2018)*	*17*	*39739527*	*17*	*41583275*	*66317*	*77214*
6	NM_000526.4(KRT14): c.1228C > T (p.Gln410Ter)	KRT14	Not provided	Pathogenic (Sep 15, 2016)	17	39739533	17	41583281	66313	77210
7	NM_000526.4(KRT14): c.1162C > T (p.Arg388Cys)	KRT14	Not provided	Pathogenic (Oct 13, 2017)	17	39739599	17	41583347	66306	77203
8	NM_000526.4(KRT14): c.1151T > C (p.Leu384Pro)	KRT14	EBS, Koebner type	Pathogenic (Nov 22, 1991)	17	39739610	17	41583358	14611	29650
9	*NM_000526.4(KRT14): c.442C > T (p.Arg148Cys)*	*KRT14*	*EBS, Koebner type*	*Pathogenic (Apr 2, 2018)*	*17*	*39742645*	*17*	*41586393*	*66368*	*77265*
10	NM_000526.4(KRT14): c.374G > A (p.Arg125His)	KRT14	EBH-DM	Pathogenic (Oct 30, 2017)	17	39742713	17	41586461	14613	29652
11	NM_000526.4(KRT14): c.357G > A (p.Met119Ile)	KRT14	EBS, autosomal recessive	Pathogenic (Sep 1, 1997)	17	39742730	17	41586478	14620	29659
12	NM_000421.3(KRT10): c.1374-2A > C	KRT10	Not provided	Pathogenic (Nov 25, 2015)	17	38975415	17	40819163	449615	445767
13	NM_000421.3(KRT10): c.1374-2A > G	KRT10	EI, congenital reticular	Pathogenic (Oct 1, 2010)	17	38975415	17	40819163	14581	29620
14	NM_000421.3(KRT10): c.1373 + 2T > C	KRT10	Not provided	Pathogenic (May 9, 2017)	17	38975767	17	40819515	432261	426219
15	NM_000421.3(KRT10): c.1373 + 1G > A	KRT10	EI, congenital reticular	Pathogenic (Oct 1, 2010)	17	38975768	17	40819516	14582	29621
16	NM_000421.3(KRT10): c.1325T > A (p.Leu442Gln)	KRT10	BIE	Pathogenic (Feb 1, 1994)	17	38975817	17	40819565	14575	29614
17	NM_000421.3(KRT10): c.1300C > T (p.Gln434Ter)	KRT10	BIE	Pathogenic (Apr 1, 2006)	17	38975842	17	40819590	29764	38719
18	NM_000421.3(KRT10): c.1281C > A (p.Cys427Ter)	KRT10	BIE	Pathogenic (Jul 1, 2008)	17	38975861	17	40819609	29765	38720
19	NM_000421.3(KRT10): c.494G > C (p.Arg165Pro)	KRT10	Not provided	Likely pathogenic (Sep 1, 2016)	17	38978344	17	40822092	432167	426220
20	NM_000421.3(KRT10): c.482T > C (p.Leu161Ser)	KRT10	BIE	Pathogenic (Aug 21, 1992)	17	38978356	17	40822104	14569	29608
21	*NM_000421.3(KRT10): c.479A > C (p.Tyr160Ser)*	*KRT10*	*Not provided*	*Pathogenic (Apr 2, 2018)*	*17*	*38978359*	*17*	*40822107*	*66178*	*77075*
22	NM_000421.3(KRT10): c.478T > G (p.Tyr160Asp)	KRT10	BIE	Pathogenic (Feb 1, 1994)	17	38978360	17	40822108	14572	29611
23	NM_000421.3(KRT10): c.467G > A (p.Arg156His)	KRT10	BIE	Pathogenic (Sep 20, 2017)	17	38978371	17	40822119	14573	29612
24	NM_000421.3(KRT10): c.460A > C (p.Asn154His)	KRT10	BIE	Pathogenic (Feb 1, 1994)	17	38978378	17	40822126	14571	29610

EBH-DM epidermolysis bullosa herpetiformis-Dowling Meara, *EBS* epidermolysis bullosa simplex, *EI* erythroderma ichthyosiform, *BIE* Bullous ichthyosiform erythroderma
Italicized words indicate comparison of identical mutation obtained in our study (psoriasis) with other skin disease

Validation of mutation and their pathogenicity using Mutation Surveyor and Alamut Visual software

To validate and confirm the mutation, we did in silico analysis of all keratin sequences obtained in these patients by using Mutation Surveyor software. Similar to Sanger sequence results, in silico analysis also showed nine and seven missense mutations in K14 and K10, respectively, as well as no missense mutation was found in

Table 4 Comparison of publicly available mutated keratin 16 and keratin 17 sequence data of various skin disease patients with mutated sequence obtained in our study (psoriasis) from Clinvar NCBI database

S. no.	Name	Gene(s)	Condition(s)	Clinical significance (last reviewed)	GRCh37		GRCh38		Variation ID	Allele ID(s)
					Chromosome	Location	Chromosome	Location		
1	NM_005557.3(KRT16):c.395T > C (p.Leu132Pro)	KRT16	PC 1	Pathogenic (Jan 29, 2016)	17	39768546	17	41612294	14600	29639
2	NM_005557.3(KRT16):c.379C > G (p.Arg127Gly)	KRT16	Not provided	Pathogenic (May 11, 2015)	17	39768562	17	41612310	265217	260165
3	NM_000422.2(KRT17):c.1163T > C (p.Leu388Pro)	KRT17	Not provided	Not provided	17	39776929	17	41620677	66181	77078
4	NM_000422.2(KRT17):c.1112T > C (p.Leu371Pro)	KRT17	Not provided	Not provided	17	39776980	17	41620728	66180	77077
5	NM_000422.2(KRT17):c.325A > G (p.Asn109Asp)	KRT17	Not provided	Not provided	17	39780437	17	41624185	66188	77085
6	NM_000422.2(KRT17):c.309T > C (p.Arg103=)	KRT17	Not provided	Not provided	17	39780453	17	41624201	66187	77084
7	NM_000422.2(KRT17):c.304G > A (p.Val102Met)	KRT17	PC 2	Pathogenic (Mar 1, 2002)	17	39780458	17	41624206	14599	29638
8	NM_000422.2(KRT17):c.296T > C (p.Leu99Pro)	KRT17	PC 2	Pathogenic (Jun 9, 2015)	17	39780466	17	41624214	14598	29637
9	NM_000422.2(KRT17):c.292T > G (p.Tyr98Asp)	KRT17	PC 2	Pathogenic (Feb 1, 1997)	17	39780470	17	41624218	14588	29627
10	NM_000422.2(KRT17):c.284T > C (p.Leu95Pro)	KRT17	PC 2	Pathogenic (May 14, 2015)	17	39780478	17	41624226	14596	29635
11	NM_000422.2(KRT17):c.284T > A (p.Leu95Gln)	KRT17	PC 2	Pathogenic (May 1, 2001)	17	39780478	17	41624226	14595	29634
12	NM_000422.2(KRT17):c.281G > C (p.Arg94Pro)	KRT17	PC 2	Pathogenic (May 1, 2001)	17	39780481	17	41624229	14594	29633
13	NM_000422.2(KRT17):c.281G > A (p.Arg94His)	KRT17	PC 2| SM	Pathogenic (Dec 1, 2001)	17	39780481	17	41624229	14590	29629
14	NM_000422.2(KRT17):c.280C > T (p.Arg94Cys)	KRT17	PC 2|	Pathogenic(Aug 15, 2016)	17	39780482	17	41624230	14591	29630
15	NM_000422.2(KRT17):c.275A > G (p.Asn92Ser)	KRT17	PC 2	Pathogenic (Jul 26, 2016)	17	39780487	17	41624235	14587	29626
16	NM_000422.2(KRT17):c.274A > C (p.Asn92His)	KRT17	SM	Pathogenic (Feb 1, 1997)	17	39780488	17	41624236	14589	29628
17	NM_000422.2(KRT17):c.274A > G (p.Asn92Asp)	KRT17	PC 2	Pathogenic (Nov 3, 2016)	17	39780488	17	41624236	14586	29625
18	NM_000422.2(KRT17):c.263T > A (p.Met88Lys)	KRT17	Not provided	Not provided	17	39780499	17	41624247	66182	77079
19	NM_000422.2(KRT17):c.263T > C (p.Met88Thr)	KRT17	PC 2	Pathogenic (Nov 1, 1999)	17	39780499	17	41624247	14592	29631
20	NM_000422.2(KRT17):c.-6G > C	KRT17	Not specified	Benign (Apr 28, 2016)	17	39780767	17	41624515	380281	375886

PC pachyonychia congenita, *SM* steatocystoma multiplex

K16 and K17 in mild psoriasis (Fig. 2). Also, in moderate psoriasis, a similar mutation pattern was shown (Figs. 3 and 4) using Mutation Surveyor software. The mutation's pathogenicity was predicted by using Alamut Visual software; we found about 34 and 15% of K14 and K10 mutated sequences in mild psoriasis that were predicted to be tolerated, and the remaining sequences were predicted to have damaging effect. Based on Mutation Assessor, all mutated sequences in mild psoriasis have medium effect on the alteration of these protein functions (Table 5; Additional file 1: Fig. S1) where, as in moderate psoriasis, all mutated sequences are predicted to have a damaging role with high effect on the alteration of protein functions (Table 6; Additional file 1: Fig. S2). Totally, we identified 44 mutations among which 16 mutations were found in both mild and moderate psoriasis, whereas 28 mutations were found only in moderate psoriasis.

Comparison of mutated keratins with ExAC databases

When we compared K14, K10, K16, and K17 missense mutated variants in ExAC database with their respective K14, K10, K16, and K17 mutated variants observed in our psoriasis patients, we perceived that one K14 c1237G > A variant with MAF 0.01 and one K17 c986C > T variant with MAF < 0.001 existed in the ExAC database; additionally, none of the K10 and K16 variants were found to occur in the ExAC database. Based on the analysis, our result showed that 99% of K14 and K17 and 100% of K10 and K16 missense mutations in our psoriasis patients were considered to be as novel missense mutation which did not exist in the ExAC database. These novel mutations might be one of the reasons causing severe damage in psoriasis patients (Additional file 2: Table S1).

Identification of deleterious mutations

Keratin 14, 10, 16, and 17 CDS region of amino acid sequence in Fasta format and 44 missense mutations, which were obtained from Mutation Surveyor and Visual Alamut, were loaded to PredictSNP1.0, and all available integrated tools were selected for prediction. PredictSNP1.0 provided predictions for each integrated tool and a consensus prediction as percentages (expected accuracies) and the effect of mutation on protein function as "neutral" and "deleterious" by PredictSNP and all the integrated tools, except for nsSNPAnalyzer, which did not give any prediction for any mutations. In mild psoriasis, about 70% of mutated sequences in both K14 and K10 were found to be deleterious, whereas in moderate psoriasis, all K14 and K10; one K16 and six K17 mutated sequences were found to be deleterious. Out of 44 mutations, 33 mutations were predicted to be as deleterious by PredictSNP and all the integrated tools, except for nsSNPAnalyzer, which did not give any prediction for any mutations (Tables 7 and 8).

Location of the deleterious mutations on the secondary structure and 3D structure of keratin protein

Position of these deleterious mutations in the keratin secondary and 3D structure is important because amino acid sequences of keratin are mainly involved in the assembly of keratin filaments and also binding of keratins and keratin filaments to cell adhesion complexes or signaling molecules. The secondary structure of these keratin proteins has three sub-domains, namely, head domain, central α-helical rod domain, and tail domain. The rod domain is mainly composed of sub-domain coils 1A, 1B, 2A, and 2B connected by linkers L1, L12, and L2 (Fig. 5a). We detected that these 33 mutations were located in the rod domain of these keratin proteins. The deleterious mutations in the rod domain were

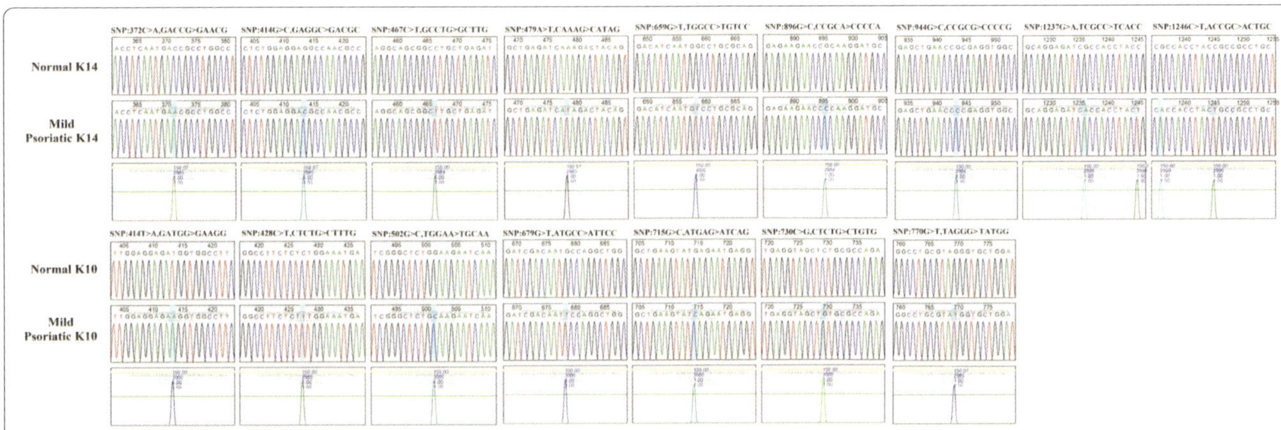

Fig. 2 Sanger sequencing of mutated K14 and K10 in mild psoriasis analyzed by Mutation Surveyor. Sanger sequencing of K14 and K10 CDS region of mild psoriatic samples in scf format and reference sequence of NCBI CDS region of all keratins in Gb file format were analyzed by using Mutation Surveyor; the positions are annotated according to the genetic code

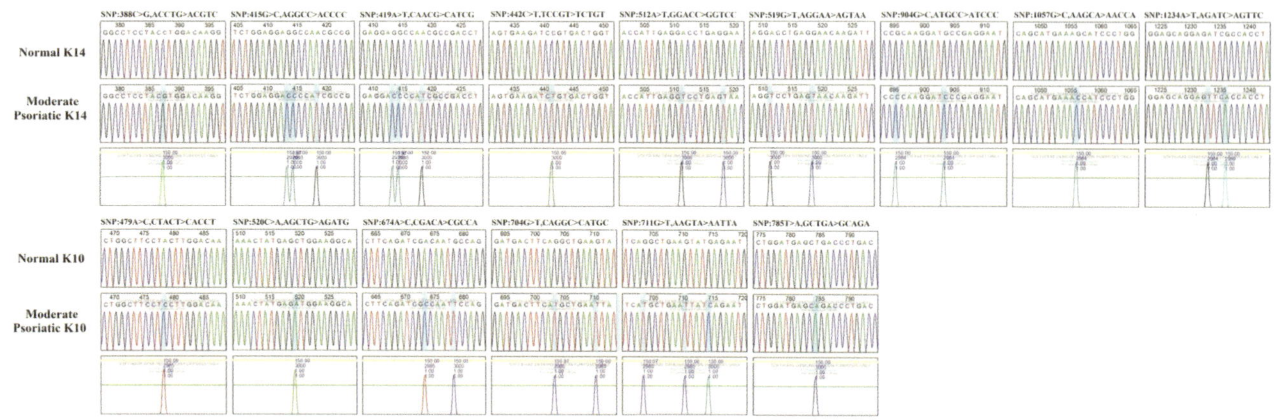

Fig. 3 Sanger sequencing of mutated K14 and K10 in moderate psoriasis analyzed by Mutation Surveyor. Sanger sequencing of K14 and K10 CDS region of moderate psoriatic samples in scf format and reference sequence of NCBI CDS region of all keratins in Gb file format were analyzed by using Mutation Surveyor; the positions are annotated according to the genetic code

mainly noticed in coil 1 and 2 regions, which are critical for the protein activity and structure of these keratins.

Pathogenic K14 mutated sequences are mainly located in exon 1 and exon 6. In keratin 14, exon 1 (1–586 nucleotide) mainly forms the head and rod (coil 1A, L1, and 1B) region and exon 6 (1115–1335 nucleotide) forms the coil 2 of the rod domain. In K14, coil 1A region has five mutated amino acids, L1 region has one mutated amino acid, coil 1B has three mutated amino acids, and coil 2 region has six mutated amino acids. All appeared in close proximity in the folded protein (Fig. 5b).

Exons 1 and 2 are the major regions affected by the mutation in K10; they mainly form the head and rod domain region of 1A and 1B. We found three mutations in coil 1A region and eight mutations in coil 1B region of the rod domain. In K16, one mutation in coil 1B region was found to be deleterious. However, in K17, one mutation in coil 1B region of peptide epitope S2, two mutations in 1B region of peptide epitope S3, and three mutations in coil 2 region of peptide epitope S4 of the rod domain were found (Fig. 5b) The deleterious mutations in the rod domain of all these keratins were mainly noticed in coil 1 and 2 regions, which are critical for the protein activity and structure of these keratins.

Our results showed that the predicted deleterious mutations highly located in the α-helical rod domain, which forms a coiled structure to these keratins, are important to maintain the structural integrity of the skin.

Effect of deleterious mutation on keratin protein stability

After predicting the deleterious effect and position of these mutated sequences in protein, it is imperative to analyze the stability of this protein. Therefore, we have

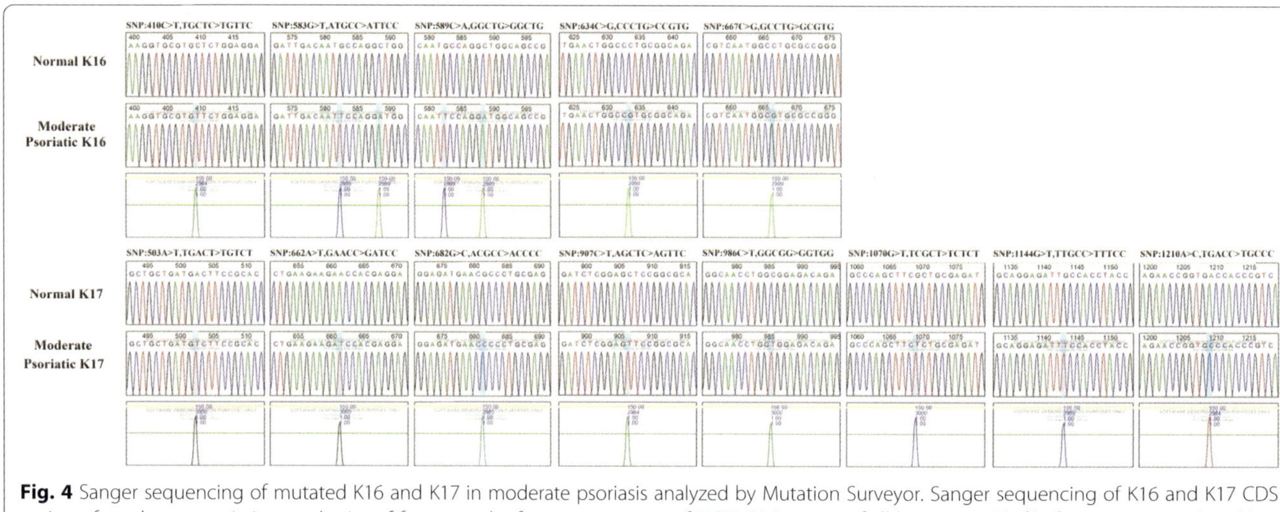

Fig. 4 Sanger sequencing of mutated K16 and K17 in moderate psoriasis analyzed by Mutation Surveyor. Sanger sequencing of K16 and K17 CDS region of moderate psoriatic samples in scf format and reference sequence of NCBI CDS region of all keratins in Gb file format were analyzed by using Mutation Surveyor; the positions are annotated according to the genetic code

Table 5 Prediction of epidermal keratin mutation's pathogenicity in mild psoriasis using Alamut Visual software

S. no.	MT position	Exon	seq.MT	Type of MT	AA change	Variant in protein domain	SIFT			Mutation taster			Mutation assessor		
							Prediction	Score	Range score	Prediction	Range score	*P* value	Prediction	Score	Range score
	K14														
1	372	1	C > A	Missense	p.(Asp124Glu)	IF	Damaging	0.017	0.5119	DC	0.4153	0.992	Medium	2.875	0.8364
2	414	1	G > C	Missense	p.(Glu138Asp)	IF	Tolerated	0.057	0.3792	DC	0.4441	0.998	Medium	2.0099	0.5492
3	467	1	C > T	Missense	p.(Pro156Leu)	IF	Damaging	0.006	0.6138	DC	0.8103	1	Medium	3.335	0.9109
4	479	1	A > T	Missense	p.(Lys160Ile)	IF	Damaging	0.019	0.5008	Polymorphism	0.08979	1	Medium	3.125	0.8823
5	659	2	G > T	Missense	p.(Gly220Val)	IF protein, keratin type I	Damaging	0	0.9122	DC	0.8103	1	Medium	2.565	0.7524
6	896	4	G > C	Missense	p.(Arg299Pro)	IF protein, prefoldin	Damaging	0.008	0.5857	DC	0.4637	0.999	Medium	3.1099	0.8799
7	944	4	G > C	Missense	p.(Arg315Pro)	IF protein, prefoldin	Damaging	0.006	0.6138	DC	0.3752	0.946	Medium	2.3399	0.6737
8	1237	6	G > A	Missense	p.(Ala413Thr)	IF protein (conserved site), IF	Tolerated	0.099	0.3061	Polymorphism	0.4614	0.001	Medium	2.2999	0.6591
9	1246	6	C > T	Missense	p.(Arg416Cys)	IF protein (conserved site), IF	Tolerated	0.132	0.2648	DC	0.8103	1	Medium	2.9349	0.8489
	K10														
10	414	1	T > A	Missense	p.(Asp138Glu)		Tolerated	0.828	0.02894	DC, polymorphism	0.8103	0.992	Medium	2.1549	0.6042
11	428	1	C > T	Missense	p.(Ser143Phe)		Damaging	0.016	0.518	DC	0.8103	0.55	Medium	2.14	0.6007
12	502	1	G > C	Missense	p.(Glu168Gln)	IF protein	Damaging	0.005	0.6317	DC	0.8103	1	Medium	3.4849	0.9277
13	679	2	G > T	Missense	p.(Ala227Ser)	IF protein, keratin type I	Damaging	0.023	0.4813	DC	0.8103	1	Medium	2.6349	0.7736
14	715	2	G > C	Missense	p.(Glu239Gln)	IF protein, keratin type I	Damaging	0.001	0.7842	DC	0.8103	1	Medium	2.7799	0.8138
15	730	2	C > G	Missense	p.(Leu244Val)	IF protein	Damaging	0.005	0.6317	DC	0.8103	0.97	Medium	2.8199	0.8237
16	770	3	G > T	Missense	p.(Arg257Met)	IF protein, keratin type I	Damaging	0	0.9122	DC	0.8103	0.916	Medium	3.25	0.9002

DC disease causing, *IF* intermediate filament, *MT* mutation, *AA* amino acid

Table 6 Prediction of epidermal and hyperproliferative keratin mutation's pathogenicity in moderate psoriasis using Alamut Visual software

S. no.	MT position	Exon	seq.MT	Type of MT	AA change	Variant in protein domain	SIFT			Mutation taster			Mutation assessor		
							Prediction	Score	Range score	Prediction	Range score	*P* value	Prediction	Score	Range score
	K14														
1	388	1	C > G	Missense	p.(Leu130Val)	IF protein	Damaging	0.001	0.7842	DC	0.537	1	High	3.8199	0.9566
2	415	1	G > C	Missense	p.(Ala139Pro)	IF protein	Damaging	0.006	0.6138	DC	0.8103	1	High	4.3049	0.9832
3	419	1	A > T	Missense	p.(Asn140Ile)	IF protein	Damaging	0	0.9122	DC	0.5881	1	High	4.425	0.9876
4	442	1	C > T	Missense	p.(Arg148Cys)	IF protein	Damaging	0	0.9122	DC	0.5881	1	High	3.75	0.9513
5	512	1	A > T	Missense	p.(Asp171Val)	IF protein	Damaging	0	0.9122	DC	0.8103	1	High	3.835	0.9576
6	519	1	G > T	Missense	p.(Arg173Ser)	IF protein	Damaging	0.001	0.7842	DC	0.4122	0.991	High	4.025	0.9697
7	904	4	G > C	Missense	p.(Ala302Pro)	IF protein, prefoldin	Damaging	0.001	0.7842	Polymorphism	0.2979	0.735	High	4.085	0.9729
8	1057	6	G > C	Missense	p.(Ala353Pro)	IF protein, keratin type I	Tolerated	0.189	0.2119	DC	0.4816	0.999	High	3.875	0.9604
9	1234	6	A > T	Missense	p.(Ile412Phe)	IF protein (conserved site), IF	Damaging	0	0.9122	DC	0.8103	1	High	4.65	0.9939
	K10														
10	479	1	A > C	Missense	p.(Tyr160Ser)	IF protein	Damaging	0	0.9122	DC	0.8103	1	High	4.5549	0.9916
11	520	1	C > A	Missense	p.(Leu174Met)	IF protein	Damaging	0.001	0.7842	DC	0.8103	0.991	High	3.5099	0.9302
12	674	2	A > C	Missense	p.(Asp225Ala)	IF protein	Damaging	0	0.9122	DC	0.8103	1	High	3.9549	0.9656
13	704	2	G > T	Missense	p.(Arg235Met)	IF protein, keratin type I	Damaging	0	0.9122	DC	0.8103	0.84	High	4.2849	0.9824
14	711	2	G > T	Missense	p.(Lys237Asn)	IF protein, keratin type I	Damaging	0	0.9122	DC	0.8103	0.983	High	3.66	0.944
15	785	3	T > A	Missense	p.(Leu262Gln)	IF protein, prefoldin, keratin I	Damaging	0	0.9122	DC	0.8103	0.834	High	4.2399	0.9805
	K16														
16	410	1	C > T	Missense	p.(Ala137Val)	IF	Damaging	0.002	0.7209	Polymorphism	0.3052	0.65	Medium	3.39	0.9174
17	583	1	G > T	Missense	p.(Ala195Ser)	IF protein, keratin type I	Damaging	0.029	0.457	DC	0.4734	1	Medium	2.805	0.8202
18	589	1	C > A	Missense	p.(Leu197Met)	IF protein, keratin type I	Damaging	0.028	0.4608	DC	0.4467	0.998	Medium	2.88	0.8371
19	634	1	C > G	Missense	p.(Leu212Val)	IF	Damaging	0.009	0.5743	DC	0.4067	0.988	Medium	2.9849	0.8585
20	667	1	C > G	Missense	p.(Leu223Val)	IF protein, keratin type I	Damaging	0.001	0.7842	DC	0.4434	1	Medium	3.3	0.9406
	K17														
21	503	1	A > T	Missense	p.(Asp168Val)	IF protein, keratin type I	Damaging	0	0.9122	DC	0.8103	1	Medium	3.3	0.9473
22	662	2	A > T	Missense	p.(Asn221Ile)	IF protein, prefoldin	Damaging	0.01	0	Polymorphism	0.4721	0.999	Medium	2.605	0.7645
23	682	3	G > C	Missense	p.(Ala228Pro)	IF protein, prefoldin	Damaging	0.016	0.518	Polymorphism	0.1948	1	Medium	3.25	0.9409
24	907	4	C > T	Missense	p.(Leu303Phe)	IF protein, prefoldin	Damaging	0.03	0, 0.001	Polymorphism	0.5164	1	Medium	3.4749	0.9267
26	986	5	C > T	Missense	p.(Ala329Val)	IF protein	Damaging	0.51	0.017	Polymorphism	0.4593	0.999	Medium	3.17	0.8891
26	1070	5	G > T	Missense	p.(Arg357Leu)	IF protein, keratin type I	Damaging	0	0.9122	DC	0.8103	1	Medium	3.17	0.9796
27	1144	6	G > T	Missense	p.(Ala382Ser)	IF protein (conserved site), IF	Tolerated	0	0.122	Polymorphism	0.4437	0.998	Medium	2.265	0.6465
28	1210	6	A > C	Missense	p.(Thr404Pro)	IF protein (conserved site), IF	Tolerated	0	0.075	Polymorphism	0.5199	1	Medium	2.6099	0.7658

DC disease causing, *IF* intermediate filament, *MT* mutation, *AA* amino acid

Table 7 The expected accuracy results of the missense mutations of epidermal keratins in mild psoriasis predicted as deleterious in PredictSNP and integrated tool

Gene	CDS mutation	AA mutation	Predict SNP		MAPP		PhD-SNP		PolyPhen-1		PolyPhen-2		SIFT		SNAP		PANTHER	
			Prediction	Accuracy	Prediction	Accuracy	Prediction	Accuracy	Prediction	Accuracy	Prediction	Accuracy	Prediction	Accuracy	Prediction	Accuracy	Prediction	Accuracy
K14	c.372C > A	p.D124E	DEL	0.55	DEL	0.59	DEL	0.68	NEU	0.67	DEL	0.59	DEL	0.53	NEU	0.67	DEL	0.69
	c.414G > C	p.E138D	NEU	0.65	NEU	0.64	DEL	0.59	NEU	0.67	NEU	0.72	DEL	0.43	NEU	0.71	DEL	0.66
	c.467C > T	p.P156L	NEU	0.60	DEL	0.48	NEU	0.66	NEU	0.67	DEL	0.40	DEL	0.53	NEU	0.58	DEL	0.67
	c.479A > T	p.K160I	DEL	0.55	DEL	0.41	NEU	0.66	DEL	0.74	NEU	0.61	DEL	0.45	DEL	0.62	DEL	0.57
	c.659G > T	p.G220V	DEL	0.51	NEU	0.73	NEU	0.45	DEL	0.74	DEL	0.65	DEL	0.79	NEU	0.55	DEL	0.74
	c.896G > C	p.R299P	DEL	0.87	DEL	0.75	DEL	0.88	DEL	0.59	DEL	0.50	DEL	0.53	DEL	0.72	DEL	0.74
	c.944G > C	p.R315P	DEL	0.76	DEL	0.62	DEL	0.82	DEL	0.59	DEL	0.50	DEL	0.79	NEU	0.50	DEL	0.70
	c.1237G > A	p.A413T	NEU	0.65	DEL	0.62	NEU	0.51	NEU	0.67	DEL	0.40	NEU	0.67	NEU	0.71	NEU	0.47
	c.1246C > T	p.R416C	DEL	0.61	DEL	0.57	DEL	0.88	DEL	0.59	DEL	0.50	NEU	0.71	NEU	0.55	DEL	0.78
K10	c.414T > A	p.D138E	NEU	0.83	NEU	0.77	NEU	0.66	0	0	0	0	NEU	0.81	NEU	0.83	NEU	0.67
	c.428C > T	p.S143F	NEU	0.60	NEU	0.75	DEL	0.61	0	0	0	0	DEL	0.53	NEU	0.55	DEL	0.74
	c.502G > C	p.E168Q	DEL	0.76	DEL	0.59	DEL	0.86	DEL	0.59	DEL	0.63	DEL	0.53	NEU	0.50	DEL	0.74
	c.679G > T	p.A227S	DEL	0.52	DEL	0.41	DEL	0.77	NEU	0.67	DEL	0.50	DEL	0.46	NEU	0.71	DEL	0.57
	c.715G > C	p.E239Q	DEL	0.76	DEL	0.48	DEL	0.68	DEL	0.59	DEL	0.63	DEL	0.79	NEU	0.55	DEL	0.74
	c.730C > G	p.L244V	DEL	0.55	DEL	0.59	DEL	0.68	NEU	0.67	DEL	0.50	DEL	0.53	NEU	0.71	DEL	0.66
	c.770G > T	p.R257M	DEL	0.76	DEL	0.51	DEL	0.73	DEL	0.74	DEL	0.54	DEL	0.79	NEU	0.58	DEL	0.74

DEL deleterious, *NEU* neutral

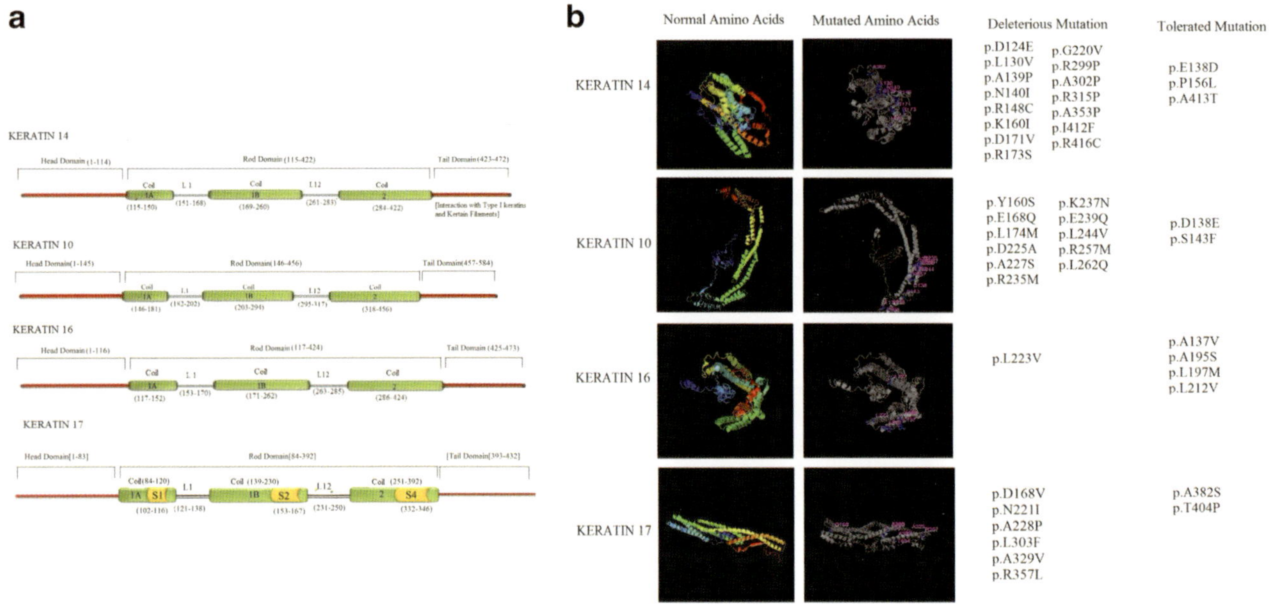

Fig. 5 Protein structure of epidermal and hyperproliferative keratins. **a** Schematic representation of secondary structure of all four keratins with their domain and sub-domain, whereas, S = peptide epitope and L = linker. **b** Specific regions of 33 deleterious mutation localizations. The figures in the left side are the 3D structure of all four keratin CDS regions. The figures in the right side are the 3D structures of domains with mutated residues. The mutated residues are numbered according to their position on the regions. The position of mutated amino acids (aa) on all four keratins and on CDS regions are provided

analyzed the protein stability of these 33 deleterious mutated sequences on MUpro server and I-Mutant 2.0. Our results showed that in mild psoriasis, about two third of K14 and K10 mutation decrease the protein stability. However, in moderate stage, 90% of all mutated K14, K10, K16, and K17 sequences showed decreased protein stability (Table 9).

Immunofluorescence analysis of K14, K10, K16, and K17 antibodies

Our immunofluorescence analysis of normal epidermis shows nuclei stained blue with DAPI throughout all the epidermal layers, whereas K14-positive cells are found only in the basal epidermal cell. Merging discloses co-expression of K14 and DAPI nuclear stain in most of the basal epidermal cells in control samples. In lesional samples, no staining of K14 was seen in the basal layer, whereas DAPI staining was seen throughout the elongated rete ridges, and merged results show there is no staining of K14 in the basal layer (Fig. 6).

DAPI stain was seen throughout all the epidermal layers, and K10 antibodies were stained in the spinosum of the epidermal layer in normal epidermis. K10-positive cells were seen marginally in the elongated rete ridges of the suprabasal epidermal layer. Merging of two stains shows marginal expression of K10 and strong DAPI staining in the nuclei of cells of the suprabasal epidermal layer (Fig. 6).

To confirm the expression of abnormal proteins K16 and K17 on the protein level, we performed immunofluorescence analyses in the corresponding control and lesional psoriatic skin samples. These analyses clearly reflected that there is no K16 expression, and blue DAPI stain stained the nuclei present in the normal epidermal layer. Psoriasis samples showed a strong expression of K16 throughout the suprabasal with nuclei stained with DAPI (Fig. 6). In addition, we analyzed there is no K17 protein in the normal epidermal layer, but nuclei were stained with DAPI and merging showed the blue nuclei staining throughout the epidermis, whereas in psoriasis, the K17 protein was seen in the stratum corneum along with DAPI staining (Fig. 6).

Expression of keratins and their correlation with PASI in both mild and moderate psoriases

In mild psoriatic samples, the mRNA expression of K14 and K10 was significantly elevated to 2.5- and 4.4-folds compared to nonlesional, respectively, whereas in moderate case, these expressions were decreased significantly. In contrast to K14 and K10 expression, decrease in K16 and K17 expression was found in mild psoriasis; as the disease progresses in moderate psoriasis, the expression of K16 and K17 significantly elevated at 4.9- and 4.4-folds compared to nonlesional, respectively (Fig. 7a). Further, these results were confirmed by the Western blot analysis (Fig. 7b). We strongly believed that the changes in keratin

Table 9 Protein stability change prediction results of MUpro and I-Mutant2.0 for the 33 deleterious missense mutations of epidermal and hyperproliferative keratins in mild and moderate psoriasis patients

Stages of psoriasis	Gene	CDS mutation	AA mutation	MUpro				I-Mutant 2.0	
				SVM	SVMCS	NN	NNCS	Stability	DDG
Mild	K14	c.372C > A	p.D124E	Increase	0.05	Increase	0.71	Decrease	− 0.52
		c.479A > T	p.K160I	Decrease	− 0.54	Decrease	− 0.89	Decrease	0.61
		c.659G > T	p.G220V	Increase	0.41	Increase	0.65	Decrease	− 0.46
		c.896G > C	p.R299P	Decrease	− 0.57	Decrease	− 0.75	Decrease	− 2.22
		c.944G > C	p.R315P	Decrease	− 0.53	Decrease	− 0.86	Decrease	− 1.26
		c.1246C > T	p.R416C	Decrease	− 0.16	Decrease	− 0.58	Decrease	− 0.3
	K10	c.502G > C	p.E168Q	Increase	0.39	Increase	0.70	Decrease	− 0.01
		c.679G > T	p.A227S	Decrease	− 1	Decrease	− 0.71	Decrease	− 0.19
		c.715G > C	p.E239Q	Decrease	− 0.12	Decrease	− 0.64	Decrease	− 0.28
		c.730C > G	p.L244V	Decrease	− 1	Decrease	− 0.94	Decrease	− 2.03
		c.770G > T	p.R257M	Increase	0.53	Increase	0.81	Decrease	− 0.47
Moderate	K14	c.388C > G	p.L130V	Decrease	− 1	Decrease	− 1	Decrease	− 1.67
		c.415G > C	p.A139P	Decrease	− 0.63	Decrease	− 0.88	Decrease	− 1.89
		c.419A > T	p.N140I	Decrease	− 0.23	Decrease	− 0.67	Increase	1.57
		c.442C > T	p.R148C	Decrease	− 1	Decrease	− 1	Decrease	− 0.28
		c.512A > T	p.D171V	Decrease	− 0.37	Decrease	− 1	Decrease	− 0.36
		c.519G > T	p.R173S	Decrease	− 1	Decrease	− 1	Decrease	− 2.37
		c.904G > C	p.A302P	Increase	0.63	Increase	0.73	Decrease	− 3.34
		c.1057G > C	p.A353P	Decrease	− 0.58	Decrease	− 0.65	Increase	− 0.65
		c.1234A > T	P.I412F	Decrease	− 1	Decrease	− 0.69	Decrease	− 0.95
	K10	c.479A > C	p.Y160S	Decrease	− 0.47	Decrease	− 0.64	Decrease	− 1.16
		c.520C > A	p.L174M	Decrease	− 1	Decrease	− 1	Decrease	0.12
		c.674A > C	p.D225A	Decrease	− 0.39	Decrease	− 0.78	Decrease	− 0.76
		c.704G > T	p.R235M	Decrease	− 0.45	Decrease	− 0.89	Decrease	− 0.59
		c.711G > T	p.K237N	Decrease	− 0.60	Decrease	− 1	Increase	0.26
		c.785T > A	p.L262Q	Decrease	− 1	Decrease	− 1	Decrease	− 1.82
	K16	c.667C > G	p.L223V	Decrease	− 1	Decrease	− 1	Decrease	− 1.39
	K17	c.503A > T	p.D168V	Decrease	− 0.30	Decrease	− 0.60	Decrease	− 0.73
		c.662A > T	p.N221I	Decrease	− 0.70	Increase	0.62	Increase	1.64
		c.682G > C	p.A228P	Decrease	− 0.04	Increase	0.61	Decrease	− 2.48
		c.907C > T	p.L303F	Decrease	− 1	Decrease	− 1	Decrease	0.95
		c.986C > T	p.A329V	Decrease	− 0.34	Decrease	− 0.88	Decrease	0.12
		c.1070G > T	p.R357L	Increase	0.15	Increase	0.68	Increase	0.66

CDS coding sequences, *AA* amino acid, *SVM* support vector machine, *SVMCS* SVM confidence score, *NN* neural network, *NNCS* neural network confidence score, *DDG* free energy change value

expression in the psoriatic epidermis might be due to some pathogenic variants in these keratin genes.

Correlation analysis of keratins and PASI in two stages of psoriasis is shown in Fig. 8. There was a significant inverse correlation between normal epidermal keratins K14 and K10 and PASI score ($r = -0.998$; $r = -0.996$; $P < 0.001$), respectively, in mild psoriasis, whereas the abnormal hyperproliferative keratins K16 and K17 showed a positive correlation with PASI score ($r = 0.999$; $r = 0.997$; $P < 0.001$) in mild psoriasis. In moderate case, Spearman's coefficient correlation analysis showed a negative correlation between K14 and K10 and PASI score ($r = -0.993$; $r = -0.997$; $P < 0.001$), respectively, and showed a strong positive correlation between K16 and K17 with PASI score, which was statistically significant ($r = 0.998$; $r = 0.998$; $P < 0.001$), respectively. We report that the

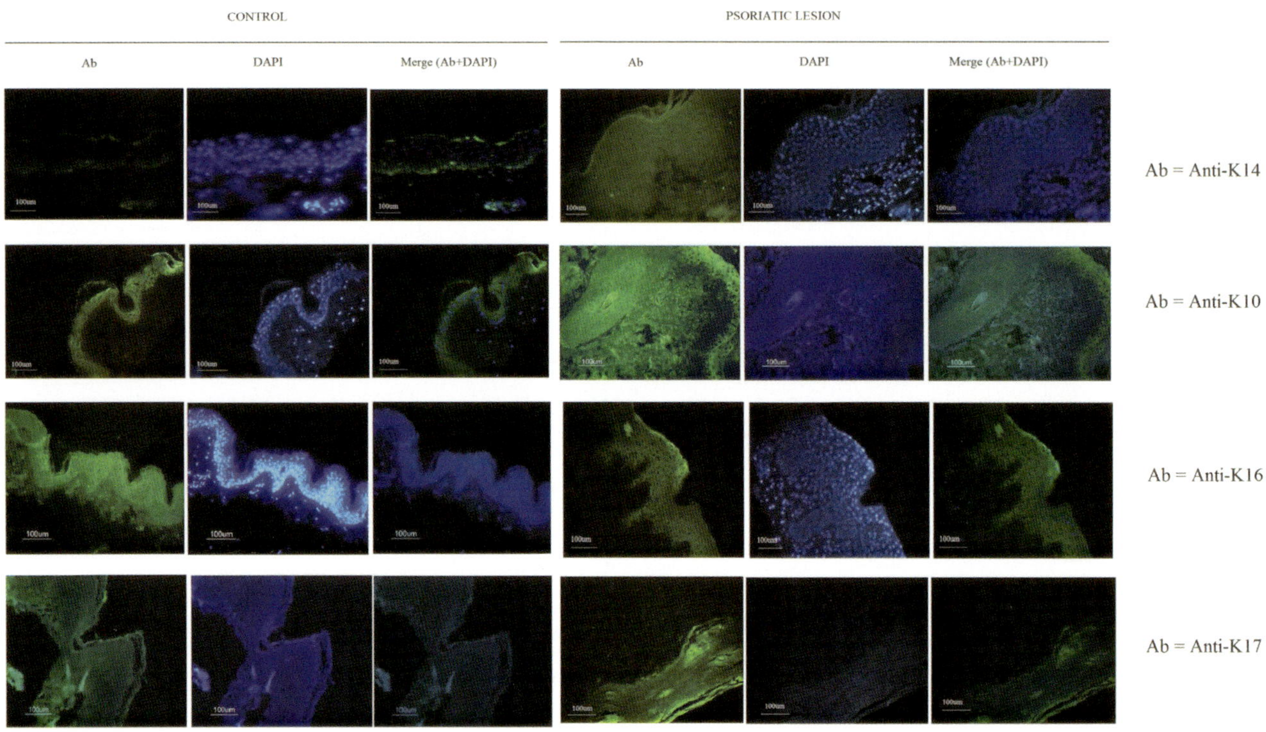

Fig. 6 Immunofluorescence analysis of keratins in nonlesional and lesional psoriatic skin. Immunofluorescence analysis of epidermal and hyperproliferative type I keratins in frozen skin sections from patients with psoriasis in nonlesional and lesional skin (× 20 magnification, respectively), and nuclei were visualized with 4′-6-diamidino-2-phenylindole (DAPI). Bar = 100 μm; Ab antibody

degree of severity of the clinical phenotype has been directly linked to the position of the pathogenic mutation along the keratin polypeptide backbone.

Discussion

The epidermal barrier is formed by keratinocytes contributing tight junctions and the cornified envelope [1]. Barrier dysfunction and cutaneous sensitization can give rise to chronic inflammatory disorders like atopic eczema and psoriasis. Keratin plays an important role in maintaining epidermal barrier as well as in the formation of tight junction and cornified envelope in skin [40]. However, mutations of keratins in psoriasis have not been fully investigated. In this present study, we have identified 18 mutations in the CDS region of K14 out of which nine mutations are slightly pathogenic variants in the psoriatic samples. Numerous mutations in K5 and K14 identified in EBS are dominant pathogenic mutations. There are a few cases of recessive mutations which nearly all lead to loss of function or a natural knockout in K14 [41–45]. Related to our result, studies showed that in EBS, the pathogenic mutations of K14 usually occur within two segments (1A and 2B) of the rod domain [46]. Cells expressing mutated K14 are more prone to stress damage and resistance to apoptosis [47, 48]. Thus, we propose that the mutation of K14 in psoriatic skin might lead to "unnatural" keratin pair; this will drastically alter the assembly of network filament as well as mechanical support in epidermal skin and also increase the degradation of keratin filaments by various stressors, all these leading to acanthosis in psoriasis.

Moreover, we have also identified 13 mutated sequences in keratin 10 protein. Of these, six sequences are considered as highly pathogenic, and the remaining seven sequences are considered as slightly pathogenic. Similar to our study, in epidermal hyperkeratosis, most of the pathogenic missense mutations of K10 usually occur within highly conserved regions of the α-helical rod domains and the non-helical HI domain [49, 50]. Reichelt et al. [51] reported that defects in keratin 10 gene may lead to hyperproliferation of basal cells, induction of c-Myc, cyclin D1, 14-3-3σ, K6, and K16. K10 is essential to control cell proliferation and also for the expression of filaggrin and cornified envelope proteins [52]. In epidermolytic ichthyosis (EI) patients, mutation of K10 proteins showed increased proliferation of suprabasal keratinocytes which leads to ichthyosiform lesions, suprabasal cytolysis, blister formation, and hyperkeratosis [53, 54]. Thus, the mutation in K10 might cause irregularly shaped pathognomonic keratin intermediate filament (KIF) clumps in suprabasal keratinocytes which disrupt the structural stability in the suprabasal

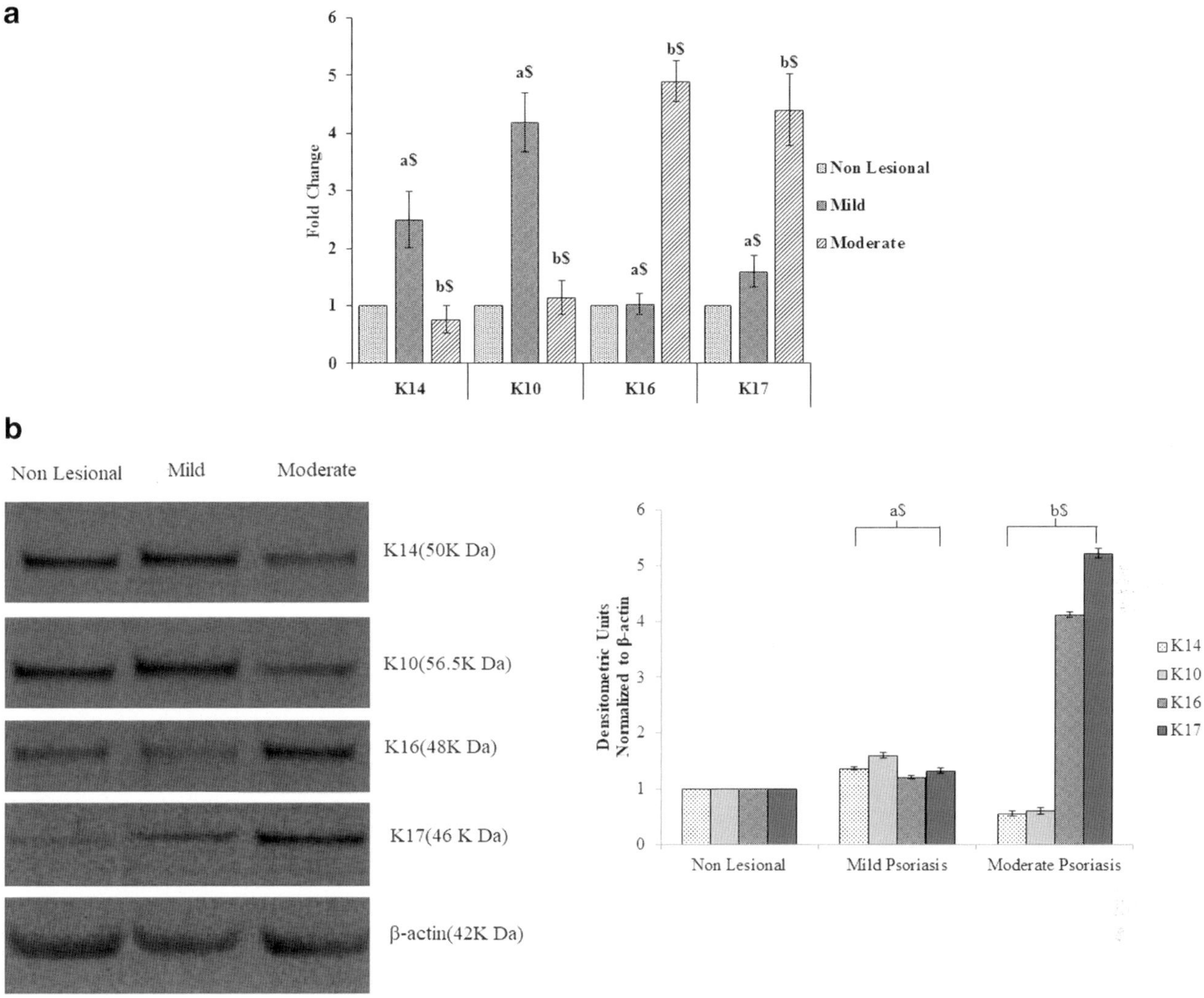

Fig. 7 mRNA and protein expression of epidermal and hyperproliferative type I keratins in mild and moderate psoriasis. **a** Quantification of keratin 14, 10, 16, and 17 mRNA by real-time PCR using the comparative C_T method. The C_T values were normalized on the basis of GADPH and analyzed relative to that of the normal control. Gene expressions were given as fold change. **b** Western blot and densitometric analysis of keratins in mild and moderate psoriasis. All values were expressed as mean ± SD, where the dollar sign denotes $P < 0.001$, "a" denotes comparison of non-lesional with mild psoriatic lesional skin biopsy, and "b": denotes comparison of mild and moderate psoriatic lesional skin biopsy

keratinocytes and also increase cyclin D, cyclin E, and phosho-Akt levels, all of which drive to hyperproliferation of keratinocytes in psoriasis.

Rapid psoriasis recurrence or new morphologies have been reported after discontinuation of traditional therapy or biological [55–58]. Interestingly, psoriatic lesions preferentially appeared at sites of wound healing (Koebner phenomenon). These relapse and Koebner phenomenon in psoriasis might be due to the variants in hyperproliferative keratin genes. In order to reveal this, we studied K16 and K17 psoriatic sequences for mutational analysis. In this, we did not find any mutation and expression of these keratins in mild psoriasis. As disease progresses, we found a pathogenic variant of K16 and K17 in moderate psoriasis. Early studies showed that an inherited dominant mutation in K16 and K17 is causative for pachyonychia congenita (PC) [59–63]. Lessard et al. [64] showed that in PC, loss of K16 function in mice causes the development of prominent calluses on the plantar side of the front and hind paws, which significantly compromise mobility and eventually lead to overt loss of barrier properties and also deletion of K16-produced spontaneously arising palmoplantar keratoderma-like lesions in mice. However, some studies have reported that in the context of epidermal wound healing, K16 mainly promotes a reorganization of the cytoplasmic array of keratin filaments, an event that precedes the onset of keratinocyte migration into the wound site [65], and also, K17-associated

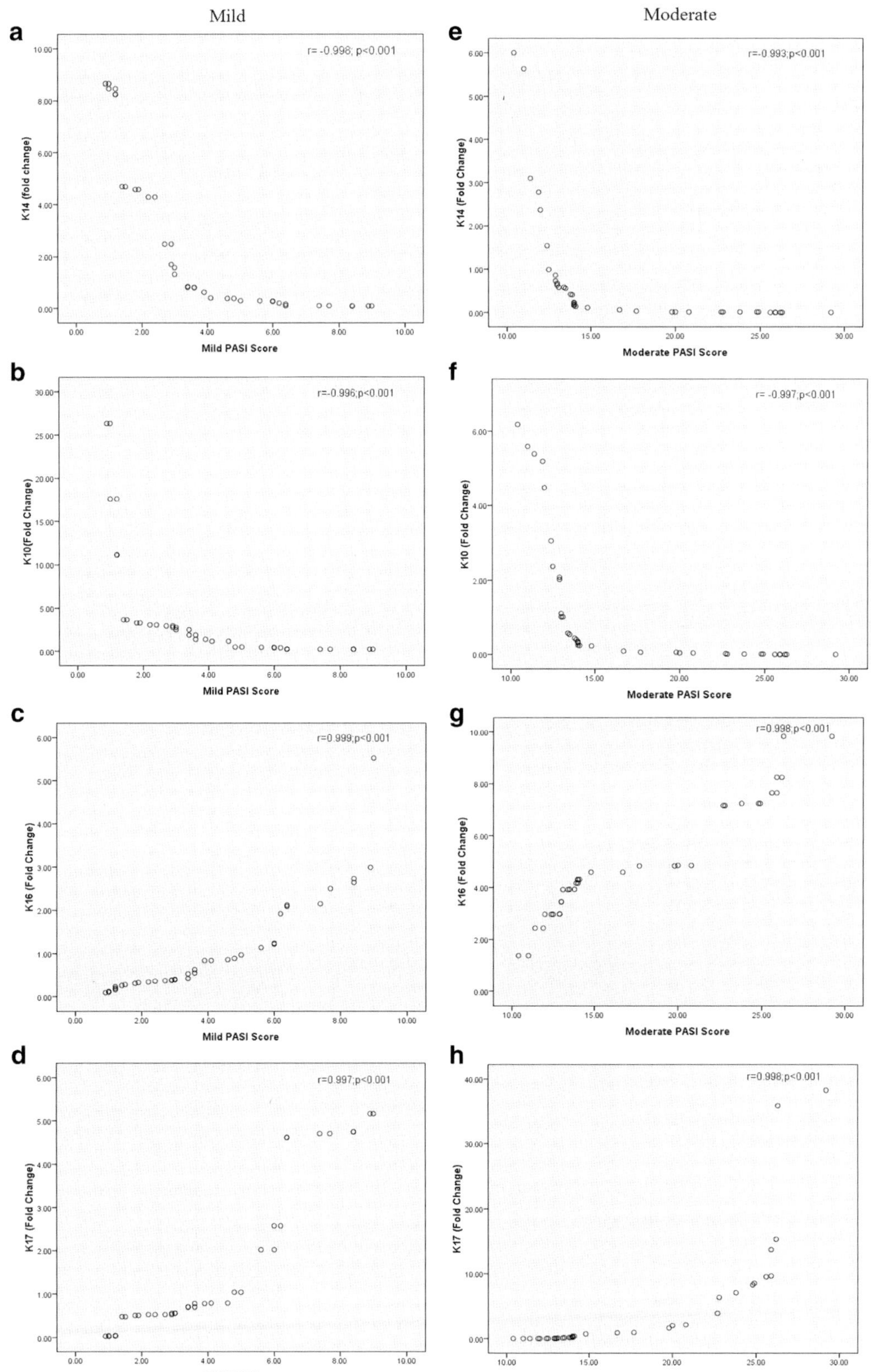

Fig. 8 Correlation between keratins with PASI score. **a** Keratin 14 vs. mild PASI score. **b** Keratin 10 vs. mild PASI score. **c** Keratin 16 vs. mild PASI score. **d** Keratin 17 vs. mild PASI score. **e** Keratin 14 vs. moderate PASI score. **f** Keratin 10 vs. moderate PASI score. **g** Keratin 16 vs. moderate PASI score. **h** Keratin 17 vs. moderate PASI score. The correlation coefficient (*r*) and significant value (*P*) are given in this figure

activation process is believed to be essential in reepithelization of the injured area [66]. In contrast to wound healing, K17 and K16 expression in psoriasis failed to resolve the deregulated inflammatory response which leads to the persistent activation of keratinocytes; these responses might be due to the mutation in these genes. Thus, mutation in K16 and K17 in psoriasis might be one of the factors for disease severity and Koebner phenomenon, accompanied with early relapse even with therapy.

In this study, we showed increased K14 and K10 expression at protein and mRNA levels in mild psoriatic skin biopsies compared to nonlesional skin biopsies; in contrast to this, moderate lesional biopsy showed decreased expression of K14 and K10. Similar to our results, other studies also showed that in lesional biopsy, the level of K14 was considerably higher with downregulation of K10 compared with normal epidermis [11, 13, 67]. Also, we found that the hyperproliferative keratin K16 and K17 expressions were low in mild psoriasis; as diseases progress, these expressions were increased in moderate psoriasis compared to nonlesional. Consistent with our results, many authors also showed an upregulation of K6 and K16 [68, 69] in psoriatic epidermis. Similarly, a study by de Jong et al. [69] also showed the overexpression of K17 in psoriatic epidermis. Earlier reports said that the K17 is considered as a therapeutic target and marker of antipsoriatic therapies used for the treatment of psoriasis [70, 71]. These finding suggests that the changes in keratin expressions might trigger and exacerbate psoriasis.

Finally, we also found a negative correlation between epidermal keratins and PASI score and positive correlation between hyperproliferative keratins and PASI score; these further added that alteration in these keratins in skin might cause severity of psoriasis. Previous studies have reported that the degree of severity of the clinical phenotype has been directly linked to the position of the pathogenic mutation along the keratin polypeptide backbone, although more recent reports provide some exceptions to this, whereby also milder disease phenotypes are caused by pathogenic mutations in the conserved hot spot region of the keratin genes [72, 73]. We demonstrate that the novel mutation of keratins found in psoriasis patients after comparison with ExAC database will be considered as efficient filtering of candidate psoriasis-causing variants and are useful for the discovery of human "knockout" psoriasis variants in protein-coding genes. Overall, we strongly believed that these novel keratin mutations in the psoriatic epidermis might be one of the main causative factors for psoriasis.

Conclusion

Even though there are many highly psoriasis-risk genes identified, in 2009, GWAS have found the importance of keratin pattern in psoriasis. Also, studies have found that keratin plays a critical role in the pathogenesis of psoriasis. Based on all these aspects, we focused on this first and foremost study in which we have identified mutation in K14, K10, K16, and K17 genes in the two stages of psoriasis. Our findings suggest that this mutation leads to decreased expression of highly regulated keratins which in turn causes defective barrier accompanied with acanthosis, hyperplasia, and infiltration of inflammatory mediators in psoriatic epidermis. These findings will offer a clue to better understanding the pathogenesis of psoriasis.

Additional files

Additional file 1: Figure S1. Comparison of the identified K14 and K10 nucleotide sequences of mild psoriasis obtained in this study with those of respective NCBI CDS sequences using BioEdit software (version 7.2). The mutated sequences are indicated by red arrows. **Figure S2.** Comparison of the identified K14, K10, K16, and K17 nucleotide sequences of moderate psoriasis obtained in this study with those of respective NCBI CDS sequences using BioEdit software (version 7.2). The

Additional file 2: Table S1. K14, K10, K16, and K17 missense mutated variants retrieved from ExAC database. The mutated sequences identical both in our study and ExAC database are indicated by boldfaced words.

Abbreviations

CDS: Coding sequences; EBS: Epidermolysis bullosa simplex; EI: Epidermolytic ichthyosis; GWAS: Genome-wide association studies; IF: Intermediate filament; K10: Keratin 10; K14: Keratin 14; K16: Keratin 16; K17: Keratin 17; KIF: Keratin intermediate filament; PC: Pachyonychia congenita; SNP: Single nucleotide polymorphism

Acknowledgements

We thank all patients who have assisted with this study.

Funding

The study was supported by the postdoctoral funding grant given by Anhui Medical University, National Natural Science Foundation of China (81602397), and the Natural Science Foundation of Shanghai (15ZR1405700).

Authors' contributions

TE performed the experiments and data analysis, interpreted the results, and drafted the manuscript. JS and CZ participated in the sample collection and performed the experiments and data analysis. FZ and YZ contributed to the sequence analysis. LS and SY contributed to the patients' recruitment. XJZ provided guidance on the experimental design and received funding. All authors read and approved the final manuscript.

Competing interests

The authors declare that they have no competing interests.

Author details
[1]Institute and Department of Dermatology, The First Affiliated Hospital, Anhui Medical University, Hefei, China. [2]Key Laboratory of Dermatology, Ministry of Education, Anhui Medical University, Hefei, China. [3]Collaborative Innovation Center for Complex and Severe Dermatosis, Anhui Medical University, Hefei, China. [4]Institute of Dermatology, Huashan Hospital, Fudan University, Shanghai, China. [5]Anhui Medical University, 81 Meishan Road, Hefei, Anhui Province, China.

References

1. Simpson CL, Patel DM, Green KJ. Deconstructing the skin: cytoarchitectural determinants of epidermal morphogenesis. Nat Rev Mol Cell Biol. 2011;12: 565–80.
2. Kim S, Coulombe PA. Intermediate filament scaffolds fulfill mechanical, organizational, and signaling functions in the cytoplasm. Genes Dev. 2007; 21:1581–97.
3. Magin TM, Vijayaraj P, Leube RE. Structural and regulatory functions of keratins. Exp Cell Res. 2007;313:2021–32.
4. Lane EB, McLean WH. Keratins and skin disorders. J Pathol. 2004;204(4): 355–66.
5. Omary MB, Ku NO, Strnad P, Hanada S. Toward unraveling the complexity of simple epithelial keratins in human disease. J Clin Invest. 2009;119:1794–805.
6. Oriolo AS, Wald FA, Ramsauer VP, Salas PJ. Intermediate filaments: a role in epithelial polarity. Exp Cell Res. 2007;313:2255–64.
7. Fuchs E, Cleveland DW. A structural scaffolding of intermediate filaments in health and disease. Science. 1998;279:514–9.
8. Osborn M. Intermediate filaments as histologic markers: an overview. J Invest Dermatol. 1983;81:104s–9s.
9. Nestle FO, Kaplan DH, Barker J. Psoriasis. N Engl J Med. 2009;61:496–509.
10. Fuchs E, Green H. Changes in keratin gene expression during terminal differentiation of the keratinocyte. Cell. 1980;19:1033–42.
11. Thewes M, Stadler R, Korge B, Mischke D. Normal psoriatic epidermis expression of hyperproliferation-associated keratins. Arch Dermatol Res. 1991;283(7):465–71.
12. Korver JE, van Duijnhoven MW, Pasch MC, et al. Assessment of epidermal subpopulations and proliferation in healthy skin, symptomless and lesional skin of spreading psoriasis. Br J Dermatol. 2006;155(4):688–94.
13. Elango T, Thirupathi A, Subramanian S, et al. Methotrexate normalized keratinocyte activation cycle by overturning abnormal keratins as well as deregulated inflammatory mediators in psoriatic patients. Clin Chim Act. 2015;451(Pt B):329–37.
14. Arnold I, Watt FM. c-Myc activation in transgenic mouse epidermis results in mobilization of stem cells and differentiation of their progeny. Curr Biol. 2001;11:558–68.
15. Waikel RL, Kawachi Y, Waikel PA, Wang XJ, Roop DR. Deregulated expression of c-Myc depletes epidermal stem cells. Nat Genet. 2001;28:165–8.
16. Schweizer J, Bowden PE, Coulombe PA, et al. New consensus nomenclature for mammalian keratins. J Cell Biol. 2006;174:169–74.
17. Schweizer J, Langbein L, Rogers MA, Winter H. Hair follicle-specific keratins and their diseases. Exp Cell Res. 2007;313:2010–20.
18. Uitto J, Richard G, McGrath JA. Diseases of epidermal keratins and their linker proteins. Exp Cell Res. 2007;313:1995–2009.
19. de Cid R, Riveira-Munoz E, Zeeuwen PL, et al. Deletion of the late cornified envelope LCE3B and LCE3C genes as a susceptibility factor for psoriasis. Nat Genet. 2009;41(2):211–5.
20. Zhang XJ, Huang W, Yang S, et al. Psoriasis genome-wide association study identifies susceptibility variants within LCE gene cluster at 1q21. Nat Genet. 2009;41(2):205–10.
21. Mrowietz U, Kragballe K, Reich K, et al. Definition of treatment goals for moderate to severe psoriasis: a European consensus. Arch Dermatol Res. 2011 Jan;303(1):1–10.
22. Livak KJ, Schmittgen TD. Analysis of relative gene expression data using real-time quantitative PCR and the 2(-delta deltaC(T)) method. Methods. 2001;25:402–8.
23. Dong C, Yu B. Mutation surveyor: an in silico tool for sequencing analysis. Methods Mol Biol. 2011;760:223–37.
24. Kumar P, Henikoff S, Ng PC. Predicting the effects of coding non-synonymous variants on protein function using the SIFT algorithm. Nat Protoc. 2009;4:1073–81.
25. Alamut®: gene mutation interpretation software: http://www.interactive-biosoftware.com. Accessed 8 Dec 2014.
26. Karbassi I, Maston GA, Love A, et al. A standardized DNA variant scoring system for pathogenicity assessments in Mendelian disorders. Hum Mutat. 2016;37(1):127–34.
27. Lek M, Karczewski KJ, Minikel EV, et al. Analysis of protein-coding genetic variation in 60,706 humans. Nature. 2016;536(7616):285–91.
28. Bendl J, Stourac J, Salanda O, et al. Predict SNP: robust and accurate consensus classifier for prediction of disease related mutations. PLoS Comput Biol. 2014;10(1):e1003440.
29. Sucularli C, Arslantas M. Computational prediction and analysis of deleterious cancer associated missense mutations in DYNC1H1. Mol Cell Probes. 2017;34:21–9.
30. Cheng J, Randall A, Baldi P. Prediction of protein stability changes for single-site mutations using support vector machines. Proteins. 2006;62(4):1125–32.
31. Capriotti E, Fariselli P, Casadio R. I-Mutant2.0: predicting stability changes upon mutation from the protein sequence or structure. Nucleic Acids Res. 2005;33(Web Server issue):W306–10.
32. Quan L, Lv Q, Zhang Y. STRUM: structure-based prediction of protein stability changes upon single-point mutation. Bioinformatics. 2016;32(19): 2936–46.
33. Johansen C, Funding AT, Otkjaer K, et al. Protein expression of TNF-alpha in psoriatic skin is regulated at a post transcriptional level by MAPK-activated protein kinase 2. J Immunol. 2006;176:1431–8.
34. Raul U, Sawant S, Dange P, et al. Implications of cytokeratin 8/18 filament formation in stratified epithelial cells: induction of transformed phenotype. Int J Cancer. 2004;111:662–8.
35. Meng L, Du J, Li W, et al. Study of a family with epidermolysis bullosa simplex resulting from a novel mutation of KRT14 gene. Zhonghua Yi Xue Yi Chuan Xue Za Zhi. 2017;34(4):504–8.
36. Wang WH, Zhang L, Li LF, et al. Ichthyosis hystrix Lambert type and Curth-Macklin type are a single entity with affected (KRT1 mutation) or unaffected (KRT10 mutation) palms and soles? Eur J Dermatol. 2016;26(5):493–5.
37. Chen PJ, Li CX, Wen J, et al. S159P mutation of keratin 10 gene causes severe form of epidermolytic hyperkeratosis. J Eur Acad Dermatol Venereol. 2016;30(10):e102–4.
38. Dai L, Wu J, Guo H, et al. Mutation p.Leu128Pro in the 1A domain of K16 causes pachyonychia congenita with focal palmoplantar keratoderma in a Chinese family. Eur J Pediatr. 2014;173(6):737–41.
39. Jiang M, Sun Z, Dang E, et al. TGFß/SMAD/microRNA-486-3p signaling axis mediates keratin 17 expression and keratinocyte hyperproliferation in psoriasis. J Invest Dermatol. 2017;137(10):2177–86.
40. Segre JA. Epidermal barrier formation and recovery in skin disorders. J Clin Invest. 2006;116(5):1150–8.
41. Rugg EL, McLean WH, Lane EB, Pitera R, McMillan JR, Dopping-Hepenstal PJ, et al. A functional "knockout" of human keratin 14. Genes Dev. 1994;8(21): 2563–73.
42. Chan Y, Anton-Lamprecht I, Yu QC, Jäckel A, Zabel B, Ernst JP, et al. A human keratin 14 "knockout": the absence of K14 leads to severe epidermolysis bullosa simplex and a function for an intermediate filament protein. Genes Dev. 1994;8(21):2574–87.
43. Jonkman MF, Heeres K, Pas HH, van Luyn MJ, Elema JD, Corden LD, et al. Effects of keratin 14 ablation on the clinical and cellular phenotype in a kindred with recessive epidermolysis bullosa simplex. J Invest Dermatol. 1996;107(5):764–9.
44. Schuilenga-Hut PH, Vlies PV, Jonkman MF, Waanders E, Buys CH, Scheffer H. Mutation analysis of the entire keratin 5 and 14 genes in patients with epidermolysis bullosa simplex and identification of novel mutations. Hum Mutat. 2003;21(4):447.
45. Homberg M, Ramms L, Schwarz N, Dreissen G, Leube RE, Merkel R, et al. Distinct impact of two keratin mutations causing epidermolysisbullosa simplex on keratinocyte adhesion and stiffness. J Invest Dermatol. 2015; 135(10):2437–45.
46. Szeverenyi I, Cassidy AJ, Chung CW, et al. The Human Intermediate Filament Database: comprehensive information on a gene family involved in many human diseases. Hum Mutat. 2008;29:351–60.

47. D'Alessandro M, Russell D, Morley SM, et al. Keratin mutations of epidermolysis bullosa simplex alter the kinetics of stress response to osmotic shock. J Cell Sci. 2002;115:4341–51.
48. Russell D, Ross H, Lane EB. ERK involvement in resistance to apoptosis in keratinocytes with mutant keratin. J Invest Dermatol. 2010;130:671–81.
49. Syder AJ, Yu QC, Paller AS, et al. Genetic mutations in the K1 and K10 genes of patients with epidermolytic hyperkeratosis. Correlation between location and disease severity. J Clin Invest. 1994;93:1533–42.
50. McLean WH, Morley SM, Higgins C, et al. Novel and recurrent mutations in keratin 10 causing bullous congenital ichthyosiformerthroderma. Exp Dermatol. 1999;8:120–3.
51. Reichelt J, Magin TM. Hyperproliferation, induction of c-Myc and 14-3-3σ, but no cell fragility in keratin-10-null mice. J Cell Sci. 2002;115:2639–50.
52. Reichelt J, Furstenberger G, Magin TM. Loss of keratin 10 leads to mitogen-activated protein kinase (MAPK) activation, increased keratinocyte turnover, and decreased tumor formation in mice. J Invest Dermatol. 2004;123(5):973–81.
53. Ishidayamamoto A, Iizuka H, Manabe M, et al. Altered distribution of keratinization markers in epidermolytic hyperkeratosis. Arch Dermatol Res. 1995;287:705–11.
54. Porter RM, Lane EB. Phenotypes, genotypes and their contribution to understanding keratin function. Trends Genet. 2003;19:278–85.
55. Cacoub P, Artru L, Canesi M, Koeger AC, Camus JP. Lifethreatening psoriasis relapse on withdrawal of cyclosporin. Lancet. 1988;2:219–20.
56. Georgala S, Koumantaki E, Rallis E, Papadavid E. Generalized pustular psoriasis developing during withdrawal of short-term cyclosporin therapy. Br J Dermatol. 2000;142:1057–8.
57. Fabiano A, De Simone C, Gisondi P, Piaserico S, Lasagni C, Pellacani G, et al. Management of patients with psoriasis treated with biological drugs needing a surgical treatment. Drug Dev Res. 2014;75(Suppl 1):S24–6.s.
58. Masson Regnault M, Konstantinou MP, Khemis A, Poulin Y, Bourcier M, Amelot F, et al. Early relapse of psoriasis after stopping brodalumab: a retrospective cohort study in 77 patients. J Eur Acad Dermatol Venereol. 2017;6 [Epub ahead of print]
59. McLean WH, Rugg EL, Lunny DP, et al. Keratin 16 and keratin 17 mutations cause pachyonychia congenita. Nat Genet. 1995;9:273–8.
60. Connors JB, Rahil AK, Smith FJ, et al. Delayed-onset pachyonychia congenita associated with a novel mutation in the central 2B domain of keratin 16. Br J Dermatol. 2001;144:1058–62.
61. Smith FJ, Corden LD, Rugg EL, et al. Missense mutations in keratin 17 cause either pachyonychia congenita type 2 or a phenotype resembling steatocystoma multiplex. J Invest Dermatol. 1997;108:220–3.
62. Smith FJ, Fisher MP, Healy E, et al. Novel keratin 16 mutations and protein expression studies in pachyonychia congenita type and focal palmoplantar keratoderma. Exp Dermatol. 2000;9:170–7.
63. Smith FJ. Nail that mutation-keratin 17 defect in late-onset pachyonychia. J Invest Dermatol. 2004;122:x–xi.
64. Lessard JC, Coulombe PA. Keratin 16-null mice develop palmoplantar keratoderma, a hallmark feature of pachyonychia congenita and related disorders. J Invest Dermatol. 2012;132(5):1384–91.
65. Paladini RD, Takahashi K, Bravo NS, Coulombe PA. Onset of re-epithelialization after skin injury correlates with a reorganization of keratin filaments in wound edge keratinocytes: defining a potential role for keratin 16. J Cell Biol. 1996;132(3):381–97.
66. Kim S, Wong P, Coulombe PA. A keratin cytoskeletal protein regulates protein synthesis and epithelial cell growth. Nature. 2006;441:362–5.
67. Castelijns FA, Gerritsen MJ, van Vlijmen-Willems IM, et al. Proliferation is the main epidermal target in the treatment of psoriatic plaques with once daily application of tacalcitol ointment. Acta Derm Venereol. 1999; 79(2):111–4.
68. van de Kerkhof PCM, JornBovenschen H, et al. In vivo effects of topical anti-psoriatic treatments on cutaneous inflammation, epidermal proliferation and keratinisation. Current Drug Therapy. 2007;2:21–6.
69. de Jong EMG, Ferrier CM, de Zwart A, et al. Effects of topical treatment with budesonide on parameters for epidermal proliferation, keratinization and inflammation in psoriasis. J Dermatol Sci. 1995;9:185–94.
70. de Jong EM, van Vlijmen IM, van Erp PE, Ramaekers FC, Troyanovski SM, van de Kerkhof PC. Keratin 17: a useful marker in anti-psoriatic therapies. Arch Dermatol Res. 1991;283(7):480–2.
71. Fu M, Wang G. Keratin 17 as a therapeutic target for the treatment of psoriasis. J DermatolSci. 2012;67(3):161–5.
72. Bowden PE, Knight AG, Liovic M. A novel mutation (p.Thrl98Ser) in the 1A helix of keratin 5 causes the localized variant of epidermolysis bullosa simplex. ExpDermatol. 2009;18(7):650–2.
73. Glasz-Bona A, Medvecz M, Sajo R, Lepesi-Benko R, Tulassay Z, Katona M, et al. Easy method for keratin 14 gene amplification to exclude pseudogene sequences: new keratin 5 and 14 mutations in epidermolysis bullosa simplex. J Invest Dermatol. 2009;129:229–31.

Permissions

All chapters in this book were first published in HG, by BioMed Central; hereby published with permission under the Creative Commons Attribution License or equivalent. Every chapter published in this book has been scrutinized by our experts. Their significance has been extensively debated. The topics covered herein carry significant findings which will fuel the growth of the discipline. They may even be implemented as practical applications or may be referred to as a beginning point for another development.

The contributors of this book come from diverse backgrounds, making this book a truly international effort. This book will bring forth new frontiers with its revolutionizing research information and detailed analysis of the nascent developments around the world.

We would like to thank all the contributing authors for lending their expertise to make the book truly unique. They have played a crucial role in the development of this book. Without their invaluable contributions this book wouldn't have been possible. They have made vital efforts to compile up to date information on the varied aspects of this subject to make this book a valuable addition to the collection of many professionals and students.

This book was conceptualized with the vision of imparting up-to-date information and advanced data in this field. To ensure the same, a matchless editorial board was set up. Every individual on the board went through rigorous rounds of assessment to prove their worth. After which they invested a large part of their time researching and compiling the most relevant data for our readers.

The editorial board has been involved in producing this book since its inception. They have spent rigorous hours researching and exploring the diverse topics which have resulted in the successful publishing of this book. They have passed on their knowledge of decades through this book. To expedite this challenging task, the publisher supported the team at every step. A small team of assistant editors was also appointed to further simplify the editing procedure and attain best results for the readers.

Apart from the editorial board, the designing team has also invested a significant amount of their time in understanding the subject and creating the most relevant covers. They scrutinized every image to scout for the most suitable representation of the subject and create an appropriate cover for the book.

The publishing team has been an ardent support to the editorial, designing and production team. Their endless efforts to recruit the best for this project, has resulted in the accomplishment of this book. They are a veteran in the field of academics and their pool of knowledge is as vast as their experience in printing. Their expertise and guidance has proved useful at every step. Their uncompromising quality standards have made this book an exceptional effort. Their encouragement from time to time has been an inspiration for everyone.

The publisher and the editorial board hope that this book will prove to be a valuable piece of knowledge for researchers, students, practitioners and scholars across the globe.

List of Contributors

Luluah Alhusain and Alaaeldin M. Hafez
College of Computer and Information Sciences, King Saud University, Riyadh, Saudi Arabia

Abdulaziz Alsemari
Department of Neurosciences, King Faisal Specialist Hospital and Research Centre, Riyadh, Saudi Arabia
Saudi Human Genome Project, King Abdulaziz City for Science and Technology, Riyadh, Saudi Arabia

Banan Al-Younes, Ewa Goljan, Dyala Jaroudi, Faisal BinHumaid, Brian F. Meyer and Dorota Monies
Department of Genetics, King Faisal Specialist Hospital and Research Centre, MBC 03, Riyadh 11211, Saudi Arabia
Saudi Human Genome Project, King Abdulaziz City for Science and Technology, Riyadh, Saudi Arabia

Stefan T. Arold
King Abdullah University of Science and Technology (KAUST), Computational Bioscience Research Center (CBRC), Division of Biological and Environmental Sciences and Engineering (BESE), Thuwal 23955-6900, Saudi Arabia

Rita M. C. de Almeida
Biocomplexity Institute and Department of Physics, Indiana University, Bloomington, IN 47405, USA
Instituto de Física and Instituto Nacional de Ciência e Tecnologia, Universidade Federal do Rio Grande do Sul, 91501-970 Porto Alegre, RS, Brazil

Sherry G. Clendenon and James A. Glazier
Biocomplexity Institute and Department of Intelligent Systems Engineering, Indiana University, Bloomington, IN 47405, USA

William G. Richards, Michael Boedigheimer and Michael Damore
AMGEN Inc., One Amgen Center Drive, Thousand Oaks, CA 91320-1799, USA

Sandro Rossetti and Peter C. Harris
Division of Nephrology, Mayo Clinic, 200 First Street SW, Rochester, MN 55905, USA

Britney-Shea Herbert
Department of Medical and Molecular Genetics, Indiana University School of Medicine, Indianapolis, IN 46202, USA

Wei Min Xu and Robert L. Bacallao
Division of Nephrology, Department of Medicine, Richard Roudebush VAMC and Indiana University School of Medicine, Indianapolis, IN 46202, USA

Angela Wandinger-Ness
Department of Pathology MSC08-4640 and Cancer Research and Treatment Center, University of New Mexico Health Sciences Center, Albuquerque, NM 87131, USA

Heather H. Ward
Division of Nephrology, Department of Medicine, University of New Mexico Health Sciences Center, Albuquerque, NM 87131, USA

Simon Crawford Harvey
Biomolecular Research Group, School of Human and Life Science, Canterbury Christ Church University, Canterbury CT1 1QU, UK

Yiru Anning Wang
Biomolecular Research Group, School of Human and Life Science, Canterbury Christ Church University, Canterbury CT1 1QU, UK
Laboratory of Nematology, Wageningen University, 6708 PB Wageningen, The Netherlands

Jan Edward Kammenga
Laboratory of Nematology, Wageningen University, 6708 PB Wageningen, The Netherlands

Lidiia Zhytnik
Department of Traumatology and Orthopedics, University of Tartu, Puusepa 8, 51014 Tartu, Estonia

Katre Maasalu and Aare Märtson
Department of Traumatology and Orthopedics, University of Tartu, Puusepa 8, 51014 Tartu, Estonia
Clinic of Traumatology and Orthopedics, Tartu University Hospital, Puusepa 8, 51014 Tartu, Estonia

Ene Reimann and Sulev Kõks
Centre of Translational Medicine, University of Tartu, Ravila 14a, 50411 Tartu, Estonia
Department of Pathophysiology, University of Tartu, Ravila 19, 50411 Tartu, Estonia

Ele Prans
Department of Pathophysiology, University of Tartu, Ravila 19, 50411 Tartu, Estonia

Eric S. Ho
Department of Biology, Lafayette College, Easton, PA 18042, USA
Department of Computer Science, Lafayette College, Easton, PA 18042, USA

Christopher Q. Zhang
Department of Biology, Lafayette College, Easton, PA 18042, USA
Weis Research Center, Geisinger Medical Center, Danville, PA 17822, USA

Heinric Williams and Thomas L. Prince
Urology Department, Geisinger Medical Center, Danville, PA 17822, USA
Weis Research Center, Geisinger Medical Center, Danville, PA 17822, USA

Ana Lígia Buzolin, Caroline Mônaco Moreira, Patricia Rossi Sacramento, Andre Yuji Oku, Alexandre Ricardo dos Santos Fornari, David Santos Marco Antonio, Caio Robledo D Angioli Costa Quaio, Wagner Rosa Baratela and Miguel Mitne-Neto
Research and Development, Fleury Group, Av. General Valdomiro de Lima, 508, São Paulo/SP 04344-070, Brazil

Ye Wang, Songqing Deng, Yanmin Luo and Qun Fang
Fetal Medicine Centre, Department of Obstetrics and Gynaecology, The First Affiliated Hospital of Sun Yat-Sen University, Guangzhou, China

Xueli Wu
Department of Dermatology, Guangzhou Institute of Dermatology, Guangzhou, China

Liu Du, Ju Zheng and Hongning Xie
Department of Ultrasonic Medicine, The First Affiliated Hospital of Sun Yat-Sen University, Guangzhou, China

Xin Bi
Guangzhou KingMed Center for Clinical Laboratory, Guangzhou, China

Qiuyan Chen
Dongguan Women and Children's Hospital, Dongguan, China

Claude Férec
UMR1078 "Génétique, Génomique Fonctionnelle et Biotechnologies", INSERM, EFS - Bretagne, Université de Brest, CHRU Brest, Brest, France

Jian-Min Chen
UMR1078 "Génétique, Génomique Fonctionnelle et Biotechnologies", INSERM, EFS - Bretagne, Université de Brest, CHRU Brest, Brest, France
INSERM UMR1078, EFS, UBO, 22 avenue Camille Desmoulins, 29238 Brest, France

David N. Cooper
Institute of Medical Genetics, School of Medicine, Cardiff University, Cardiff, UK

Danielle Carpenter, Laura M. Mitchell and John A. L. Armour
School of Life Sciences, University of Nottingham, Nottingham NG7 2UH, UK

Yung-Chang Chen
Kidney Research Center, Department of Nephrology, Chang Gung Memorial Hospital, Linkou Medical Center, Taoyuan, Taiwan

Pei-Chun Fan
Kidney Research Center, Department of Nephrology, Chang Gung Memorial Hospital, Linkou Medical Center, Taoyuan, Taiwan
Graduate Institute of Clinical Medical Sciences, Chang Gung University, Taoyuan, Taiwan

Chia-Chun Chen and Yu-Sun Chang
Molecular Medicine Research Center, Chang Gung University, Taoyuan, Taiwan

Pao-Hsien Chu
Division of Cardiology, Department of Internal Medicine, Chang Gung Memorial Hospital, College of Medicine, Chang Gung University, Taipei, Taiwan
Healthcare Center, Chang Gung Memorial Hospital, College of Medicine, Chang Gung University, Taipei, Taiwan
Heart Failure Center, Chang Gung Memorial Hospital, College of Medicine, Chang Gung University, Taipei, Taiwan
Department of Cardiology, Chang Gung Memorial Hospital, College of Medicine, Chang Gung University, 199 Tung Hwa North Road, Taipei 105, Taiwan

Ahmad H. Mufti, Anas Dannoun, Hassan Kordi and Mohammed T. Tayeb
Department of Medical Genetics, Medicine College, Umm Al-Qura University, Mecca 21955, Saudi Arabia

Nasser A. Elhawary
Department of Medical Genetics, Medicine College, Umm Al-Qura University, Mecca 21955, Saudi Arabia
Department of Molecular Genetics, Faculty of Medicine, Ain Shams University, Cairo 11566, Egypt

Essam H. Jiffri and Osama H. Jiffri
Department of Medical Laboratory Technology, Faculty of Applied Medical Sciences, King Abdul-Aziz University, Jeddah, Saudi Arabia

Samira Jambi
Department of Pediatrics, Al Hada Military Hospital, Al Hada, Saudi Arabia

Asim Khogeer
Department of Plan and Research, General Directorate of Health Affairs, Mecca Region, Ministry of Health, Mecca, Saudi Arabia

Abdelrahman N. Elhawary
Department of Pediatrics, Faculty of Medicine, Cairo University, Giza, Egypt

Kuo Wang, Mingyue Yang and Xiaosong Wang
Institute of Translational Medicine, the First Hospital of Jilin University, Changchun 130061, China

Genhong Cheng
Institute of Translational Medicine, the First Hospital of Jilin University, Changchun 130061, China
Department of Microbiology, Immunology and Molecular Genetics, University of California Los Angeles, Los Angeles, CA 90095, USA

Man Gao, Fanzheng Meng, Deli Li, Ruihua Lu, Yan Wang and Huadong Zhuang
Department of Pediatrics, the First Hospital of Jilin University, Changchun 130021, China

Mengyao Li
Bethune Medical School of Jilin University, Changchun 130021, China

Ana R. Cardoso, Manuela Oliveira, Antonio Amorim and Luisa Azevedo
Instituto de Investigação e Inovação em Saúde, Universidade do Porto, Rua Alfredo Allen 208, 4200-135 Porto, Portugal
IPATIMUP-Institute of Molecular Pathology and Immunology, University of Porto, Rua Júlio Amaral de Carvalho 45, 4200-135 Porto, Portugal
Department of Biology, Faculty of Sciences, University of Porto, Rua do Campo Alegre S/N, 4169-007 Porto, Portugal

Vasiliki Chondrou, Vlasia Kastrinou and Theodora Katsila
Department of Pharmacy, School of Health Sciences, University of Patras, University Campus, Rion, GR-265 04 Patras, Greece

George P. Patrinos
Department of Pharmacy, School of Health Sciences, University of Patras, University Campus, Rion, GR-265 04 Patras, Greece
Department of Pathology, College of Medicine & Health Sciences, United Arab Emirates University, Al-Ain, United Arab Emirates
Zayed Bin Sultan Center for Health Sciences, United Arab Emirates University, Al-Ain, United Arab Emirates

Alexia Pavlidaki
Department of Pharmacy, School of Health Sciences, University of Patras, University Campus, Rion, GR-265 04 Patras, Greece
Institut de Génétique et de Biologie Moléculaire et Cellulaire IGBMC/CNRS/INSERM/UDS, 67404 ILLKIRCH, BP 10142 CU de Strasbourg, France

Petros Kolovos
Biotech Research and Innovation Centre (BRIC), University of Copenhagen, Copenhagen, Denmark

Argyro Sgourou
Hellenic Open University, Patras, Greece

Alexandra Kourakli and Argiris Symeonidis
Hematology Division, Department of Internal Medicine, Faculty of Medicine, University of Patras, Patras, Greece

Anne John
Department of Pathology, College of Medicine & Health Sciences, United Arab Emirates University, Al-Ain, United Arab Emirates

Bassam R. Ali
Department of Pathology, College of Medicine & Health Sciences, United Arab Emirates University, Al-Ain, United Arab Emirates
Zayed Bin Sultan Center for Health Sciences, United Arab Emirates University, Al-Ain, United Arab Emirates

Adamantia Papachatzopoulou
Laboratory of General Biology, Faculty of Medicine, University of Patras, Patras, Greece

Angeliki Balasopoulou, Angeliki Panagiotara, Effrosyni Mendrinou, Apostolos Stratopoulos, Aigli Ioanna Legaki, Vasiliki Stathakopoulou, Aristoniki Tsolia, Nikolaos Govaris, Sofia Govari, Zoi Zagoriti, Konstantinos Poulas and Theodora Katsila
Department of Pharmacy, School of Health Sciences, University of Patras, University Campus, Rion, 265 04 Patras, Greece

George P. Patrinos
Department of Pharmacy, School of Health Sciences, University of Patras, University Campus, Rion, 265 04 Patras, Greece
Department of Pathology, College of Medicine and Health Sciences, United Arab Emirates University, Al Ain, United Arab Emirates

Biljana Stanković, Gordana Nikčevic, Sonja Pavlovic and Branka Zukic
Institute of Molecular Genetics and Genetic Engineering, University of Belgrade, Belgrade, Serbia

Brock A. Peters and Radoje Drmanac
Complete Genomics Inc., Mountain View, CA, USA
BGI Shenzhen, Shenzhen 51803, People's Republic of China

Anne John and Bassam R. Ali
Department of Pathology, College of Medicine and Health Sciences, United Arab Emirates University, Al Ain, United Arab Emirates

Maria Kanariou, Nikki Constantinidou and Kleopatra Spanou
Department of Immunology and Histocompatibility, "Aghia Sophia" Children's Hospital, Athens, Greece

Eleftheria Roma, Maro Krini and George Chrousos
First Department of Pediatrics, National and Kapodistrian University of Athens Medical School, Athens, Greece

Nedeljko Radlovic
Department of Gastroenterology and Nutrition, University Children's Hospital, Medical Faculty, University of Belgrade, Belgrade, Serbia

Joseph Borg
Department of Applied Biomedical Science, Faculty of Health Sciences, University of Malta, Msida, Malta

Cameron J. McDonald and Lesa Ostini
QIMR Berghofer Medical Research Institute, Brisbane, Australia

Daniel F. Wallace, Gautam Rishi, Eriza S. Secondes and V. Nathan Subramaniam
Institute of Health and Biomedical Innovation and School of Biomedical Sciences, Queensland University of Technology (QUT), 60 Musk Avenue, Kelvin Grove, Brisbane, Queensland 4059, Australia

Darrell H. G. Crawford
Faculty of Medicine and Biomedical Sciences, The University of Queensland, Brisbane, Australia

Hanlon Sia
ICON Cancer Care, Southport, Australia

Paul Clark
Princess Alexandra and Mater Hospitals, Brisbane, Australia

Weiwei Duan, Ruyang Zhang, Yang Zhao, Sipeng Shen, Yongyue Wei and Feng Chen
Department of Biostatistics, School of Public Health, Nanjing Medical University, 101 Longmian Avenue, Nanjing 211166, Jiangsu, China
China International Cooperation Center for Environment and Human Health, Nanjing Medical University, 101 Longmian Avenue, Nanjing 211166, Jiangsu, China
Joint Laboratory of Health and Environmental Risk Assessment (HERA), Nanjing Medical University School of Public Health / Harvard School of Public Health, 101 Longmian Avenue, Nanjing 211166, Jiangsu, China
Key Laboratory of Biomedical Big Data of Nanjing Medical University, 101 Longmian Avenue, Nanjing 211166, Jiangsu, China

Jingying Sun, Caihong Zhu and Fusheng Zhou
Institute and Department of Dermatology, The First Affiliated Hospital, Anhui Medical University, Hefei, China

Index